Laura Hillerman
941-456 0475
IF Misplaced
Thanks

of Chinese Medicine

Scent of Samadhi.

Essentials of Chinese Medicine

Internal Medicine

Anshen Shi

Bridge Publishing Group

Editors:

Shih-Shun Lin
Leigh Caldwell

NOTICE

The contents of this publication are for educational purpose only. It is not intended to replace the diagnosis, treatments, prescriptions, and services of a trained practitioner or physician. The publisher and writers of this book have made every effort to confirm the accuracy of the information presented in accordance with current recommendations, regulations and standard practice at the time of publication. However, the authors, editors and publisher are not responsible for errors of omission or for any consequence from application of the information in this book and make no warranty, express or implied, with respect to the contents of the publication. Readers are advised to check the contents constantly for new and updated researches, clinical experiences, and government regulations might influence the practice of Chinese medicine and/or herbal therapy.

Printed in Hong Kong by Imago

Library of Congress Cataloging-in-Publication Data

Essentials of Chinese medicine : internal medicine/ Anshen Shi ;
p. ; cm.
Includes bibliographical references and index.
ISBN 0-9728439-5-7 (hard cover)
1. Medicine, Chinese. I. Title
[DNLM: 1. Medicine, Chinese Traditional. WZ 80.5.06 S555e 2003]
R601.S528 2003
610'.951--dc22

2003020988

Bridge
Publishing Group
P. O. Box 1673
Walnut, California 91788-1673
U.S.A.
http://www.schisandrae.com

Foreword

Essentials of Chinese Medicine is a unified series consisting of multiple volumes. The first six volumes are Fundamental Theories, Diagnosis, Materia Medica, Formulas, Acupuncture and Moxibustion, and Internal Medicine. It is our intention to use concise, accurate and simple language to devote the essential knowledge of traditional Chinese medicine to our readers.

Consideration was taken into account to depict the characteristics of "essentials" when designing this series. "Essentials" signifies that each volume must clearly introduce to our readers the essence of the selected subject. In addition, the text is structured to be user-friendly for our readers to comprehend the contents. For that reason, this series was provided to the academy of Chinese medicine as a study tool for instructors and students.

This series is a collective achievement from a dedicated team of scholars. The principal author for each volume has extensive academic background and knowledge in the corresponding subject, and has been teaching in this field for decades. This qualification assures the scientific integrity and theoretical accuracy of the contents, as well as meets the practical needs of instructors and students from the oriental medical schools in the United States.

When organizing this series as a unity base on the systematic integrity of Chinese medical theories, we also emphasize the continuity among the subjects. We intend to minimize unnecessary repetitions or discontinuations in the contents among volumes. It is in our best interest to assure the consistency and accuracy in the interpretation and explanation of the Chinese medical terminology. We hope that *Essentials of Chinese Medicine* will form the framework, and that by expanding and building upon it, a comprehensive set of textbooks on Chinese medicine will be completed.

As you read these books, we wish you find them helpful and stimulating.

Bridge
Publishing Group

Preface

I would like to dedicate this book to my two instructors who prepared me with a substantial theoretical and clinical foundation in internal medicine and Integration of Traditional Chinese and Western Medicine. After graduating from Beijing University of TCM, I had the privilege to be Master Yingqiu Ren's assistant instructor and researcher in TCM theories and classics research. During my pursuit of graduate studies in Integration of Traditional Chinese and Western Medicine, my advisor, the famous professor Dr. Dianbang Shi, the President of China Academy of TCM, exposed me to the connections between theory and clinical practice, and between Traditional Chinese and Western medicine. For the last two decades, I have benefited from these experiences in my internal medicine career, including clinical practice, teaching and research.

Internal medicine is a fundamental subject of all the clinical sciences of TCM. It actualizes the integration of TCM theories with clinical practice. To a great extent, the development of internal medicine reflects the academic growth of TCM. The lack of an ideal textbook of internal medicine containing the original TCM theories and integrating current clinical practice has been a barrier during my ten-year teaching career in the United States. This difficulty motivates me to put my experience in internal medicine into writing. It is my wish that this book will meet the current academic and clinical demands of internal medicine in the United States and benefit my students and healthcare providers.

The body of this book is divided into two parts. Part I consists of 47 common internal medical conditions (including addendums) presented according to the traditional medical practice of differentiation and treatment. Derived from the analysis of etiology, pathogenesis, diagnosis and differential diagnosis, patterns for the selected condition are differentiated and identified, and guidelines for treatment are provided. Part II presents 37 Western medical conditions for which TCM treatment has proven effective. The approach in Part II integrates Western medical diagnosis and TCM differentiation of the condition. Based on the analysis of the primary symptoms, the characteristics and progressions of the patterns are elaborated, and appropriate TCM treatment measures are suggested. Current TCM studies for each condition are also introduced in Part II. It is not by omission, but to prevent dissemination of misleading information, that those Western medical conditions with few or no proven TCM therapies are excluded from Part II. Some medical conditions for which both Western medicine and TCM share common concepts are referred to the corresponding chapters in Part I for a comprehensive discussion of the TCM perspective. The contents of Part II are designed to meet the great demand for Chinese medicine from a large population suffering from Western medical diseases, and to create a new path for academia while providing an opportunity for internal medicine in clinical actualization.

I have received great support from my family, teachers, colleagues, and especially the team of Bridge Publishing Group. I would like to extend my appreciation to them here.

I am truly grateful for those who contribute to this book.

Anshen Shi
Los Angeles
July 4, 2003

Format Guide

Part I:

A. Chapter Title: The exact English name for the medical condition (such as Common Cold for *Gan Mao*), the closest English literal translation (Wasting and Thirsting Disorder vs. *Xiao Ke*), and the best English interpretation of the original meaning (Painful Urinary Syndrome vs. *Lin Zheng*) are adopted as the chapter titles, supplemented by traditional Chinese pinyin titles. We wish to establish a standardized naming system for the diseases of internal medicine.

B. Introduction.

C. Relevant Diseases: A list of Western diseases that can be referred to the selected condition for TCM differentiation and treatment.

D. Etiology and Pathogenesis.

E. Diagnosis.

F. Differentiation and Treatment: Presented as follows:

1···· Cold invading the stomach

Sudden onset of severe colic epigastric pain alleviated by application of warmth or drinking warm beverages; aggravated by cold and pressure. ······················2

3···· **S:** No thirst and/or desire for warm beverages.

4···· **T:** Thin and white coating. **P:** Wiry and tight. ································5

6···· • Disperse cold, warm the stomach and alleviate pain.

• *Liang Fu Wan*
- *Gao Liang Jiang* warms the stomach and disperses cold. ························7
- *Xiang Fu* facilitates the qi flow and alleviates pain.

8···· • Excessive cold. + *Wu Zhu Yu, Sheng Jiang*

1. Pattern
2. Primary symptoms
3. **S:** Secondary symptoms
4. **T:** Tongue
5. **P:** Pulse
6. Treatment principle for the selected pattern
7. Suggested formula: Following the suggested formula is the analysis of the primary ingredients. Refer to page 521 for the complete ingredients of the formula.

8. Modification of the formula based on clinical findings

The Chinese pinyin names for formulas and herbs have been adopted. The pinyin and Latin names of the individual herbs are standardized according to the Pharmacopoeia (2000 ed.) published by The People's Republic of China. A cross reference of pinyin and Latin names for individual herbs is listed in page 515.

G. Acupuncture Treatment: The names of the points, including pinyin and abbreviated channel naming and numbering, are recommended by the World Health Organization.

H. Practical Hints.

Part II:

A. Introduction: An overview of the disease from the Western medical perspective, according to current research and standard source texts.

B. Cross Reference for TCM Perspective: For those conditions where both Western medicine and TCM share a common concept, refer to the corresponding chapters in Part I as indicated.

C. Analysis of Symptom: This section gives primary symptoms of the diagnosed Western medical disease with a thorough analysis from the TCM perspective. Following a holistic approach, the affected organs and channels, pathogenesis, and progression of patterns are identified. Via analysis of the symptoms, patterns are differentiated, providing a guideline for TCM treatment. Therefore, the Western medicine and TCM perspectives and comprehension of the disease are incorporated, thus integrating disease diagnosis and pattern differentiation.

D. Pattern and Suggested Measure: Suggested measures refer to effective treatments for the corresponding TCM pattern and may not be exclusively proven effective for treating the Western medical disease component. This point is made clear to avoid controversy.

The ingredients and dosages of suggested formulas are provided.

E. Other Modality: This section provides common and proven clinical TCM modalities, including acupuncture and experiential herbs or formulas, among others, for the selected condition.

Table of Contents

Part I - TCM Internal Medicine

Part II- TCM Differentiation and Treatment for Western Medical Diseases

PART I

TCM Internal Medicine

CHAPTER 1

Common Cold

感冒 *Gan Mao*

Common cold is a frequently recurring disorder caused by attacks of exterior pathogenic wind. The underlying pathologies are failure of lung qi to disperse and inability of protective qi to consolidate the surface of the body. Common cold manifests with nasal congestion, runny nose and sneezing, coughing, headache, aversion to cold, fever and general discomfort. Common cold is not season specific; however, it is more common in winter and spring. Common cold, including mild and severe cold, has a short course and rapid recovery. In contrast, epidemic cold and cold in those with weak constitutions, such as the elderly and infants, tend to develop complications that make recovery difficult. To a certain degree, common cold is contagious in that it may spread from one person to another.

Relevant Diseases

- Flu
- Influenza
- Stomach flu
- Upper respiratory infection

Etiology and Pathogenesis

There are two perspectives to consider with occurrence of common cold, the presence of exterior factors and the insufficiency of righteous qi. If the righteous qi is intact, exterior pathogens will not be able to penetrate through the protective qi. Therefore, people with low resistance to exterior pathogens are more susceptible to catching cold than those with strong resistance.

Exterior pathogenic influences: Common cold may be caused by any of the six exterior pathogenic factors with wind being the primary factor. Wind is present throughout the year and combines with the changing seasonal pathogenic factors to invade the body. The most frequently occurring pathogenic combinations are wind-cold, wind-heat and summer heat-dampness.

Interior pathogenic influences: The insufficient righteous qi manifests as deficient lung qi failing to disperse; therefore, protective qi fails to consolidate the surface. Susceptibility to invasion by exterior pathogenic factors results.

In the case of pre-existing phlegm-fire or accumulation of phlegm-dampness in the lung, the lung is not able to regulate the protective qi and therefore a combination of interior and exterior pathogens occurs.

Persons with yang deficiency are susceptible to wind-cold; persons with yin deficiency tend to catch wind-heat or dry-heat; those with excessive phlegm-dampness are susceptible to invasion by dampness.

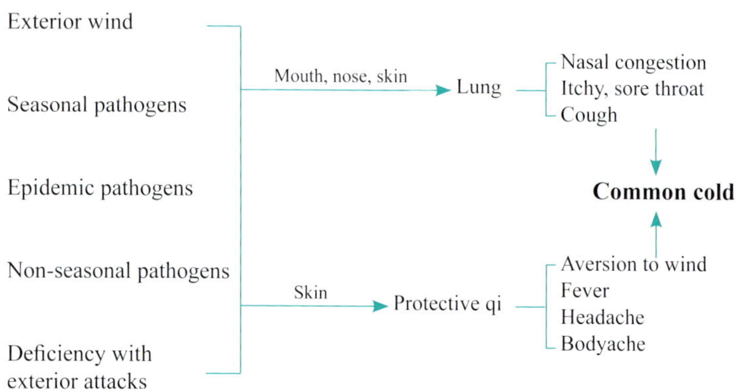

Diagnosis

A. Identification of mild, severe and epidemic cold:

	Pathogens	Season	Severity	Progress
Common Cold	Exterior pathogenic factors, primarily wind.	Winter-spring; sporadic occurrence.	Mild and no significant systemic symptoms.	Mild and superficial with mild or no internal invasion.
Epidemic Cold	Epidemic contagious pathogens.	Non-seasonal; pandemic occurrence in local population.	Severe systemic involvement.	Fast invasion into the interior with primary or secondary complications.

Both mild and severe cold are known as common cold.

Mild cold is caused by common pathogens pertaining to the corresponding seasons, such as wind-cold in winter and spring.

Severe cold is caused by invasion of pathogens at times other than their normal seasons, such as wind-cold in summer and summer heat in winter.

Epidemic cold is caused by epidemic pathogenic factors that are highly contagious; it resembles influenza in modern medicine.

B. Differential diagnosis of common cold and wind-warm febrile disease:
Both common cold and wind-warm febrile disease have signs and symptoms, such as aversion to wind and fever, pertaining to exterior syndromes at the initial stage.

Common cold: High fever is not common; sometimes, there is no fever at all. Common cold responds to herbs that release the exterior. After diaphoresis, fever is reduced and systemic symptoms are also relieved.

Wind-warm febrile disease: Usually manifests with high fever or with fever that is not reduced by sweating. After treatment with herbs that release the exterior, the fever may be temporarily lowered; however, the pulse remains rapid, fever recurs, and the progress of the disease persists as pathogens invade further into the body. Cough, chest pain and severe headache, even severe symptoms of convulsion, delirium and loss of consciousness, may be present as the disease progresses.

Basic Patterns

- Exterior wind-cold
- Exterior wind-heat
- Exterior summer heat-dampness
- Pre-existing qi deficiency with invasion of exterior pathogens
- Pre-existing yin deficiency with invasion of exterior pathogens

Differentiation and Treatment

Treatment principle:
Follow the principle that states, "For those pathogenic factors that stay in the superficial layer, induce sweating to release them". The primary treatment principle for common cold is to release the exterior by inducing sweating. On the other hand, epidemic cold is much severe, highly contagious and rapidly progressive; it also has many severe complications. Considering the critical features of epidemic cold, in addition to inducing sweating and releasing the exterior, it is very essential to greatly clear heat and relieve toxicity. Such method prevents it from progressing into severe conditions and from developing complications.

Wind-cold: Use acrid and warm herbs to induce sweating.

Wind-heat: Use acrid and cool herbs to clear and release the exterior.

Summer heat-dampness: Clear summer heat, eliminate dampness and release the exterior.

Exterior conditions with pre-existing deficiency: Support the righteous qi to release the exterior.

Exterior wind-cold

Aversion to cold, fever, no sweating, headache and general body ache.
S: Nasal congestion with clear discharge, itchy throat, cough with thin white sputum, and no thirst.
T: Thin white coating. **P:** Floating or floating and tight.

- Use acrid and warm herbs to release the exterior.
- *Jing Fang Bai Du San*
  - *Jing Jie*, *Fang Feng* and *Sheng Jiang* release the exterior and disperse cold.
  - *Qiang Huo* and *Du Huo*, acrid and warm, disperse wind-cold-dampness affecting the entire body.
  - *Chai Hu* and *Bo He* release the exterior pathogens and reduce fever.
  - *Chuan Xiong* invigorates the blood and expels wind to alleviate pain.
  - *Qian Hu*, *Jie Geng* and *Zhi Qiao* transform phlegm and facilitate the qi flow to stop coughing.
- For significant condition of aversion to cold, strengthen the acrid and warm effects to disperse cold. + *Ma Huang*, *Gui Zhi*
  Copious sputum. + *Chen Pi*, *Ban Xia*
  Significant qi stagnation. + *Xiang Fu*, *Su Geng*
  Cold at the exterior and heat in the interior, use *Ma Xing Shi Gan Tang*.

Exterior wind-heat

Fever, slight aversion to wind, obstructed and sluggish sweating, and distending headache.
S: Nasal congestion with yellow discharge, swollen sore throat, cough with sticky yellow sputum, and thirst.
T: Red tip or edge of the tongue with thin white or slightly yellow coating.
P: Floating and rapid.

- Use acrid and cool herbs to release the exterior.
- *Yin Qiao San*
  - *Jin Yin Hua* and *Lian Qiao*, acrid and cool, vent heat from the surface of the body.
  - *Bo He* and *Niu Bang Zi*, acrid and cool, disperse heat and relieve toxicity.
  - *Jing Jie* and *Dan Dou Chi*, acrid and warm, when used together with the acrid

and cool herbs above, strengthen the venting and dispersing effects to release the exterior.

- *Jie Geng* disperses lung qi and benefits the throat.
- *Zhu Ye* and *Lu Gen* clear heat and generate the fluid.

- Severe distending headache. + *Sang Ye, Ju Hua*
  Cough with excessive sputum. + *Bei Mu, Qian Hu, Xing Ren*
  Yellow viscous sputum. + *Huang Qin, Zhi Mu, Gua Lou Pi*
  Swollen sore throat. + *Xuan Shen*
  Wind-heat turning into dryness and injuring the fluid with scanty sputum, dry mouth, throat, lips and nose. + *Sha Shen, Tian Hua Fen*

Exterior summer heat-dampness

Fever, slight aversion to wind, slight sweating, heaviness and soreness of the body, headache with a heavy, distended and cloudy sensation.
S: Cough with sticky sputum, nasal congestion with turbid discharge, irritability, thirst with or without desire to drink, congested chest, nausea and scanty urination.
T: Thin yellow greasy coating. **P:** Soft and rapid.

- Clear summer heat, dispel dampness and release the exterior.

- *Xin Jia Xiang Ru Yin*
  - *Xiang Ru*, acrid, warm and aromatic, eliminates summer heat, transforms dampness and releases the exterior.
  - *Jin Yin Hua* and *Lian Qiao*, acrid, cool and aromatic, clear and eliminate summer heat.
  - *Hou Po*, bitter and warm, facilitates the qi flow and transforms dampness.
  - *Bai Bian Dou* transforms dampness and harmonizes the middle burner.

- Extreme summer heat. + *Huang Lian, Qing Hao, He Ye, Lu Gen*
  Excessive exterior dampness. + *Huo Xiang, Pei Lan*
  Dampness lingering in the middle burner with thick greasy tongue coating. + *Cang Zhu, Bai Dou Kou, Ban Xia*
  Dark scanty urine. + *Hua Shi, Gan Cao, Chi Fu Ling*

Pre-existing qi deficiency with invasion of exterior pathogens

Aversion to cold, fever, headache, nasal congestion, cough with white sputum, recurrent cold or propensity to catch cold.
S: Spontaneous sweating, pale complexion, lassitude and fatigue, shortness of breath and reluctance to speak.
T: Pale tongue with thin white coating. **P:** Floating and forceless.

- Augment the qi and release the exterior.
- *Shen Su Yin*
  - *Zi Su Ye*, *Ge Gen* and *Qian Hu* disperse wind and release the exterior.
  - *Ren Shen* and *Fu Ling* support the righteous qi to release the exterior.
  - *Zhi Qiao*, *Jie Geng* and *Ban Xia* disperse and open up lung qi, dry dampness, transform phlegm and stop coughing.
  - *Chen Pi* and *Mu Xiang* regulate the qi flow and transform phlegm.
  - *Gan Cao* augments the qi, harmonizes the middle burner, and moderates the formula.
- Severe qi deficiency. + *Huang Qi*
  Constitutional qi deficiency with spontaneous sweating and recurrent cold, use *Yu Ping Feng San*.

Pre-existing yin deficiency with invasion of exterior pathogens

Slight aversion to wind, fever, headache, no sweating, slight sweating or night sweating, and dry cough with scanty sputum.

S: Thirst, dry throat, irritability and dizziness or five-centers heat and insomnia.

T: Red tongue with dry scanty coating or no coating. **P:** Thready and rapid.

- Nourish the yin and release the exterior.
- *Jia Jian Wei Rui Tang*
  - *Yu Zhu* generates the fluid to replenish the source of sweat.
  - *Cong Bai*, *Dan Dou Chi* and *Bo He* disperse the exterior pathogenic factors.
  - *Jie Geng* disperses lung qi and releases the exterior.
  - *Bai Wei* clears heat and nourishes the yin.
- Excessive exterior pathogen. + *Jing Jie*, *Fang Feng*
  Dry throat, and cough with sticky sputum that is difficult to expectorate. + *Niu Bang Zi*, *Gua Lou Pi*
  Yin deficient heat with irritability and thirst. + *Zhu Ye*, *Tian Hua Fen*

Acupuncture Treatment

Exterior wind-cold:

- **Manipulation:** Reducing method; even method or add moxibustion for deficient constitution.
- **Prescription:** GV16 Fengfu, BL12 Fengmen, GB20 Fengchi, LU7 Lieque, LI4 Hegu

Exterior wind-heat:

- **Manipulation:** Reducing method.
- **Prescription:** GV14 Dazhui LI11 Quchi TE5 Waiguan LI4 Hegu LU10 Yuji LU11 Shaoshang

Exterior summer heat-dampness:

- **Manipulation:** Reducing method.
- **Prescription:** LU6 Kongzui LI4 Hegu ST36 Zusanli CV12 Zhongwan TE6 Zhigou

Pre-existing qi deficiency with invasion of exterior pathogens:

- **Manipulation:** In addition to the method and point prescription for wind-cold, add:
- **Prescription:** ST36 Zusanli BL13 Feishu

Pre-existing yin deficiency with invasion of exterior pathogens:

- **Manipulation:** In addition to the method and point prescription for wind-heat, add:
- **Prescription:** KI7 Fuliu BL43 Gaohuangshu

Prophylactic measures:

- **Manipulation:** Moxibustion.
- **Prescription:** BL12 Fengmen ST36 Zusanli

Practical Hints

• **Differentiating wind-cold and wind-heat is important in guiding the treatment**. When acrid and cool herbs are inappropriately used for wind-cold conditions, not only will the exterior not be released but also sweating will not occur. Consequently, the disease process is prolonged and the condition is exacerbated. Similarly, if acrid and warm herbs are wrongly prescribed for wind-heat conditions, heat builds up and the blood is disturbed. The result may be complications, such as epistaxis or lung heat with congestive chest pain and yellow sputum, due to internal invasion of the disease. If the nature of the disease is not particularly hot or cold, gentle formulas with acrid and neutral herbs should be used.

• **Avoid excessive diaphoresis.** In order to prevent further consumption of righteous qi by imposing sweating, acrid and dispersing herbs must not be overused in the cases with pre-existing deficiency; supporting the righteous qi to expel the pathogens should be adopted as the treatment principle. Add different types of tonic herbs to the formulas that disperse and release the exterior, according to the type of deficiency present.

• **Constitutional deficiency is associated with susceptibility to certain exterior pathogens.** A person with constitutional qi or yang deficiency has a propensity to be attacked by wind-cold, and a person with constitutional blood or yin deficiency is more susceptible to wind-heat. The treatment strategy of "supporting the righteous qi to expel the pathogenic influences" should be adopted in these cases.

• **Prophylactic method for complications.** The most common patterns in epidemic cold are wind-heat and fire-toxicity due to their severity and highly contagious natures. Treatment should emphasize clearing heat and relieving toxicity. Adding large doses of *Guan Zhong*, *Jin Yin Hua*, *Ban Lan Gen*, *Lian Qiao* and *Gan Cao* to the formula may effectively reduce fire toxicity, prevent complications, such as pneumonia, lung abscess, acute glomerulonephritis, rheumatic myocarditis or rheumatic fever, and inhibit the spread of disease.

CHAPTER 2

Cough

咳嗽 *Ke Sou*

Cough is one of the most commonly seen symptoms in respiratory disorders, occurring when the function of lung qi fails to disperse and descend. Cough may be silent or audible, productive of sputum or dry.

The two characters of its Chinese name, *ke sou*, originally referred to two different types of cough. *Ke* denotes coughing with sound but without production of sputum, while *sou* denotes productive cough with sputum but without sound. *Ke sou,* combination of the two characters, includes coughs that are audible and productive. In the clinical setting, sound and sputum occur together and are difficult to separate; therefore, TCM calls this disorder *ke sou* (cough).

Relevant Diseases

- Trachitis and bronchitis
- Bronchiolectasis
- Pneumonia
- COPD
- Tuberculosis
- Pleurisy
- Bronchial carcinoma
- Heart failure

Etiology and Pathogenesis

Exterior pathogenic influences attacking the lung: "All six pathogenic factors can cause cough, especially wind-cold." When the lung's defensive function is weakened, the six pathogenic factors can enter the body through the skin or nose, which is controlled by the lung. The pathogenic factors inhibit the dispersing and descending functions of lung qi and therefore, induce coughing.

Disharmony among interior organs affecting the lung: Dysfunctions of the internal organs can induce coughing. There may be dysfunctions of other organs that affect the lung or of the lung itself. The lung can be affected by the liver and spleen. Liver qi stagnation or liver fire, caused by emotional stress, may attack the lung and inhibit the descent of lung qi. Impaired spleen function of transforming and transporting, caused by improper diet, generates phlegm-dampness and disturbs the lung. Pathology of the lung includes chronic pulmonary illness that exhausts lung qi and injures lung yin, impairing the lung's ability to disperse and descend, and thereby inducing coughing.

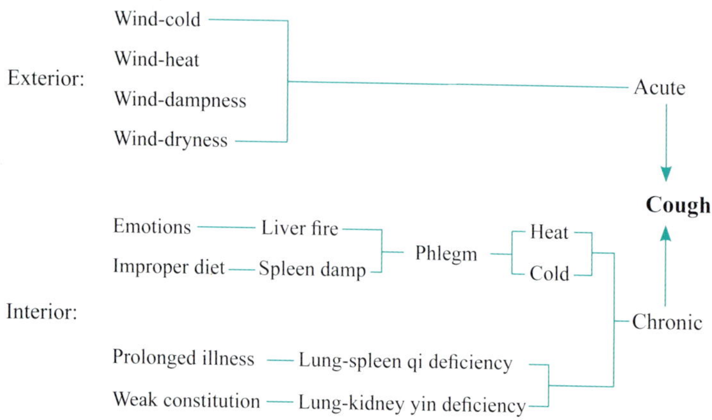

Diagnosis

A. Identification of exterior and interior:

An exterior condition is an early-stage illness with acute onset, a short course, and the presence of exterior excess pathogenic factors. An interior condition is a chronic, intermittently symptomatic illness, with a long course and the presence of excess pathogenic factors and/or deficient righteous qi.

B. Identification of patterns of cold, heat, deficiency and excess:

Identify patterns of cold, heat, deficiency and excess based on time of attack and the sound of cough, and characteristics of sputum.

- Time:

  - Cough occurs mostly during the daytime, severe cough, loud sound, and itchy or sore throat – Exterior wind-cold or wind-heat.
  - Cough is worse in the afternoon and evening or at night – Lung dryness or lung yin deficiency.
  - Cough is worse after eating greasy, raw and cold food – Phlegm-dampness.
  - Cough is accompanied or aggravated by emotional excitement, depression, and anger – Liver qi stagnation, possibly transforming into liver fire.
  - Cough is aggravated by exterior factors, including cold weather and cold food, and catching cold – Cold phlegm or deficient cold.

- Sound:

  - Hoarseness with acute onset – Exterior wind-cold or wind-heat.

- Hoarseness with chronic onset and long course – Yin or qi deficiency.
- Low and weak – Deficiency.
- Loud and strong – Excess.

- Characteristics of sputum:
  - Scanty sputum – Dry heat or yin deficiency.
  - Copious sputum – Phlegm-dampness or deficient cold.
  - Thin white sputum – Wind or cold.
  - Thick yellow sputum – Heat.
  - Blood-tinged sputum – Lung heat or lung yin deficiency.
  - Sputum with purulent blood – Phlegm-heat or lung abscess.

Basic Patterns

Cough due to exterior pathogenic factors:

- Wind-cold attacking the lung
- Wind-heat attacking the lung
- Wind-dryness attacking the lung

Cough due to interior injuries:

- Phlegm-dampness accumulation in the lung
- Phlegm-heat accumulation in the lung
- Liver fire insulting the lung
- Lung yin deficiency

Differentiation and Treatment

Treatment principle:

Exterior cough: Expel the pathogenic factors and restore the descending function of lung qi.

Interior cough: Eliminate the pathogenic factors, stop cough, support the righteous qi and tonify the deficiency; treat both root and branch of the condition.

Cough due to exterior pathogenic factors:

Wind-cold attacking the lung

Acute cough that is loud and constant, thin clear or white sputum that is easily expectorated, and itchy throat.

S: Aversion to cold, no sweating, headache, general body ache, stuffy nose and watery nasal discharge.

T: Thin white coating. **P:** Floating or floating tight.

- Release the exterior, expel wind-cold, disperse lung qi and stop coughing.
- *San Ao Tang*
  - *Ma Huang* disperses lung qi, dispels cold and releases the exterior.
  - *Xing Ren* descends lung qi and transforms phlegm. When used with *Ma Huang*, one disperses and the other descends, mutually assisting each other to restore the function of lung qi.
- To strengthen the effects of stopping coughing and transforming phlegm. *+ Zi Wan, Bai Qian, Bai Bu*

  To enhance the effects of dispersing and descending lung qi. *+ Jie Geng*

  Phlegm-dampness with sticky sputum, chest congestion and greasy tongue coating. *+ Ban Xia, Hou Po, Fu Ling*

  Accompanied by interior heat with tachypnea, sticky sputum, thirst and irritability. *+ Shi Gao, Sang Bai Pi, Huang Qin*

Wind-heat attacking the lung

Acute cough that is loud, sticky yellow sputum that is difficult to expectorate, dry and sore throat, and thirst.

S: Aversion to wind, fever, sweating, headache and yellow nasal discharge.

T: Thin yellow coating. **P:** Rapid floating or floating slippery.

- Release the exterior, expel wind-heat, disperse lung qi and stop coughing.
- *Sang Ju Yin*
  - *Sang Ye*, *Ju Hua*, *Bo He* and *Lian Qiao* dispel wind and disperse heat.
  - *Jie Geng* and *Xing Ren* disperse and descend lung qi to stop coughing.
  - *Lu Gen* clears lung heat and generates the fluid.
  - *Gan Cao* clears heat and relieves toxicity to benefit the throat.
- Excessive lung heat. *+ Huang Qin, Zhi Mu*

  Dry mouth and throat. *+ Sha Shen, Tian Hua Fen*

  Sore throat with hoarse voice. *+ Chan Tui, Niu Bang Zi, She Gan*

Wind-dryness attacking the lung

Warm-dryness (dryness combined with wind-heat): Dry cough, or cough with scanty or blood-tinged sputum, dry nose, dry lips, and dry sore throat.

S: Slight aversion to cold, fever and nasal congestion.

T: Red tongue with dry thin yellow coating. **P:** Floating and rapid.

Cool-dryness (dryness combined with wind-cold): Dry cough with white scanty sputum or no sputum, dry nose and throat.

S: Aversion to cold, headache and no sweating.

T: Dry thin white coating. **P:** Floating and tight.

- Release the exterior, moisten dryness and stop coughing.
- *Sang Xing Tang* for warm-dryness.
  - *Sang Ye* and *Dan Dou Chi* disperse wind and release the exterior.
  - *Xing Ren* and *Bei Mu* transform phlegm, moisten lung dryness, and stop coughing.
  - *Sha Shen* and *Li Pi* moisten the lung and generate the fluid.
  - *Zhi Zi* clears heat.
- Severe fluid injury with intense thirst. + *Mai Men Dong, Yu Zhu*
  Significant heat signs. + *Shi Gao, Zhi Mu*
  Blood-tinged sputum. + *Bai Mao Gen, Ou Jie*
- *Xing Su San* for cool-dryness.
  - *Zi Su Ye* and *Qian Hu* release the exterior and disperse pathogens.
  - *Xing Ren* and *Jie Geng* disperse and descend lung qi.
  - *Ban Xia* and *Fu Ling* transform phlegm and eliminate dampness.
  - *Chen Pi* and *Zhi Qiao* facilitate the qi flow and transform phlegm.
- To strengthen the moistening effect on the lung to stop coughing. + *Zi Wan, Kuan Dong Hua, Bai Bu*
  Aversion to cold, no sweating. + *Jing Jie, Fang Feng*

Cough due to interior injuries:

Phlegm-dampness accumulation in the lung

Recurrent cough with a rattling sound, copious thin watery or white sticky sputum that is easily expectorated, cough that is worse in the morning or after eating sweet and greasy food.
S: Chest congestion, focal distention in the epigastrium, bloating, nausea and poor appetite, and fatigue.
T: White greasy coating. **P:** Slippery.

- Strengthen the spleen and dry dampness, transform phlegm and stop coughing.
- *Er Chen Tang* and *San Zi Yang Qin Tang*
  - *Ban Xia* and *Fu Ling* dry dampness and transform phlegm.
  - *Chen Pi* facilitates the qi flow, transforms phlegm and stops coughing.
  - *Gan Cao* augments the qi and harmonizes the middle burner.
  - *San Zi Yang Qin Tang* transforms phlegm, descends lung qi and arrests coughing.
- Dampness accumulation in the middle burner with abdominal distention and thick greasy tongue coating. + *Cang Zhu, Hou Po*
  Significant spleen deficiency. + *Dang Shen, Bai Zhu*

Phlegm-heat accumulation in the lung

Cough with rapid respiration, thick sticky yellow sputum that is difficult to expectorate, possibly bloody sputum.
S: Stifling sensation in the chest and hypochondriac region, chest pain when coughing, and thirst.
T: Red tongue with thin yellow greasy coating. **P:** Rapid and slippery.

- Clear heat, transform phlegm, direct lung qi downwards and stop coughing.
- *Qing Jin Hua Tan Tang*
  - *Sang Bai Pi* and *Huang Qin* clear lung heat to stop coughing.
  - *Zhi Zi* and *Zhi Mu* clear heat, drain fire and generate the fluid.
  - *Bei Mu* and *Gua Lou* clear phlegm-heat and arrest coughing.
  - *Jie Geng* transforms phelgm and stops coughing.
  - *Ju Hong* and *Fu Ling* facilitate the qi flow, expel dampness and transform phlegm.
  - *Mai Men Dong* and *Gan Cao* augment the qi and generate the fluid.
- Yellow sputum or purulent sputum with foul smell. + *Yu Xing Cao, Yi Yi Ren, Dong Gua Ren*

  Chest congestion, copious sputum and constipation. + *Ting Li Zi, Mang Xiao*
  Phlegm-heat injuring the fluid. + *Tian Hua Fen, Sha Shen*

Liver fire insulting the lung

Paroxysmal coughing spells often elicited by emotional stress, dry throat, scanty sputum, and chest and hypochondriac pain when coughing.
S: Red face, dry throat, bitter taste in the mouth, irritability, dry stool and dark urine.
T: Thin yellow coating. **P:** Rapid and wiry.

- Drain liver fire, clear lung heat, direct lung qi downwards and stop coughing.
- *Xie Bai San* and *Dai Ge San*
  - *Sang Bai Pi* and *Di Gu Pi* clear and drain lung heat.
  - *Gan Cao* and *Jing Mi* harmonize the middle burner and augment lung qi.
  - *Qing Dai* and *Hai Ge Ke* clear and drain liver heat, and transform phlegm.
- To strengthen the effects of clearing heat and draining fire. + *Zhi Zi, Huang Qin, Mu Dan Pi*

  To enhance the effects to transform phlegm and descend lung qi. + *Su Zi, Zhu Ru, Pi Pa Ye*

  Sticky sputum that is difficult to expectorate. + *Fu Hai Shi, Bei Mu*
  Chronic cough with dry throat and mouth. + *Sha Shen, Mai Men Dong*

Lung yin deficiency

Chronic dry cough in short bursts, scanty or blood tinged sputum and hoarse voice.

S: Dry throat and mouth, tidal fever with red cheeks, five-centers heat, night sweating, irritability and insomnia.

T: Red tongue with scanty coating. **P:** Thready and rapid.

- Nourish and moisten lung yin, transform phlegm and stop coughing.
- *Sha Shen Mai Dong Tang*
  - *Sha Shen*, *Mai Men Dong*, *Yu Zhu*, *Tian Hua Fen* and *Bai He* nourish lung yin, generate the fluid and stop coughing.
  - *Sang Ye* disperses lung heat.
  - *Bian Dou* and *Gan Cao* augment the qi and harmonize the middle burner.
- To strengthen the effects of moistening the lung and transforming phlegm.
  + Chuan Bei Mu, Xing Ren
  To enhance the effect to clear lung heat. *+ Sang Bai Pi, Di Gu Pi*
  Restrain lung qi. *+ Wu Wei Zi, Wu Mei*
  Blood-tinged sputum. *+ Mu Dan Pi, Zhi Zi, Ou Jie*
  Significant yin deficiency with tidal fever and night sweating. *+ Yin Chai Hu, Qing Hao, Bie Jia, Fu Xiao Mai*

Acupuncture Treatment

Cough due to exterior pathogenic factors

Wind-cold attacking the lung:

- **Manipulation:** Reducing method, combine needling and moxibustion.
- **Prescription:** LU7 Lieque, LI4 Hegu, BL13 Feishu, TE5 Waiguan

Wind-heat attacking the lung:

- **Manipulation:** Reducing method.
- **Prescription:** LU5 Chize, BL13 Feishu, LI11 Quchi, GV14 Dazhui

Wind-dryness attacking the lung:

- **Manipulation:** Reducing method.
- **Prescription:** BL12 Fengmen, BL13 Feishu, LI1 Shangyang, KI7 Fuliu, KI6 Zhaohai

Cough due to interior injuries

Phlegm-dampness accumulation in the lung:

- **Manipulation:** Combination of reinforcing and reducing methods, moxibustion is applicable.
- **Prescription:** BL13 Feishu, BL20 Pishu, ST36 Zusanli, ST40 Fenglong, LU5 Chize, CV12 Zhongwan

Liver fire insulting the lung:

- **Manipulation:** Reducing method.
- **Prescription:** BL13 Feishu, BL18 Ganshu, LU8 Jingqu, LR3 Taichong

Lung yin deficiency:

- **Manipulation:** Even method.
- **Prescription:** BL13 Feishu, LU1 Zhongfu, LU7 Lieque, KI6 Zhaohai

Practical Hints

• **Adopt a holistic treatment plan to address the lung and the other organs involved.** Cough is the chief complaint for various respiratory diseases. It can be classified into two categories according to causes and pathogenesis. In addition to restoring the dispersing and descending functions of lung qi in order to stop coughing, adopt a holistic treatment plan, such as spreading liver qi, draining liver fire, strengthening the spleen, and tonifying the kidney. The holistic approach treats the lung as well as the other organs involved in the occurrence of coughing.

• **Use antitussives with caution.** Cough is a pathological phenomenon as well as a physiological defensive mechanism. It is essential to treat the root pattern when treating cough. Symptom management to stop coughing is not appropriate for all cases. It is not advisable to use astringent and binding herbs or formulas in the treatment of cough due to exterior pathogens, because they may retain the pathogenic factors and extend the course of the disease. Dispersing and ventilating the lung is the preferred treatment in this pattern.

CHAPTER 3

Wheezing

哮 證 *Xiao Zheng*

Wheezing, or *xiao*, is a paroxysmal episode of difficult breathing that produces whistling sounds. The symptoms during an acute episode include the sound of rattling sputum in the throat, rapid and shallow breathing, tachypnea, dyspnea, and the need to sit upright to breathe.

One of the major predisposing factor to wheezing, in TCM, is exterior wind, which is analogous to the western concept of allergens. The triggers of wheezing, including fecal matter from the house dust mites, pollen, animal dender or chemicals in the air, are carried by exterior wind to invade the lung system.

Relevant Diseases

- Allergic asthma
- Bronchial asthma
- Asthmatic bronchitis
- Cardiac asthma
- Eosinophilia

Etiology and Pathogenesis

Wheezing is caused by exterior pathogenic influences stirring latent phlegm that hides in the lung. When phlegm and the congested lung qi fuse, they obstruct the airway, making it difficult to breathe. The wheezing sound is produced when air passes through the congested phlegm in the respiratory tract during respirations.

Exterior pathogenic influences attacking the lung: Delayed treatment for exterior wind-heat or wind-cold allows the pathogens to linger in the lung, obstructing lung qi and producing phlegm. Also, extrinsic factors, such as pollen, smoke, dust and polluted air, affect the dispersion and descent of lung qi, inducing wheezing.

Improper diet: Excessive consumption of cold, raw, sour, salty, sweet or greasy food can interrupt the spleen's function of transformation and transportation and generate phlegm that is stored in the lung.

Deficiency or status post-illness: These two etiologies involve both the lung and the kidney. When there is a constitutional weakness due to deficiency of the kidney, or weakness following an illness that exhausts the lung, water metabolism will be impaired. Deficient qi therefore fails to transform fluids and phlegm is generated.

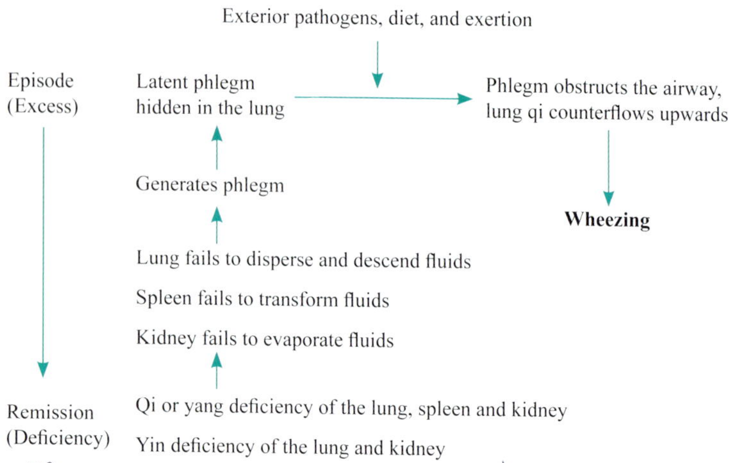

wind type wheezy → Yin Deficiency Qi stagnation Blood stasis — internal obstruction

Diagnosis

A. Identification of excess and deficiency:

Excess patterns include acute episodes with high-pitched, forceful, heavy breathing accompanied by a strong pulse.

Deficient patterns follow a prolonged course with low-pitched, weak, shallow breathing and a deep thready pulse. Inhalation is relatively more difficult than exhalation.

B. Identification of the stages of wheezing:

Wheezing is recurrent and paroxysmal, with an episode being as brief as a few minutes or hours or lasting as long as several days. Usually the episode is relatively short and the recovery is fast.

Aura: Symptoms of the aura stage that precedes an acute episode include sudden onset, itchiness in the nose and throat, sneezing, clear watery nasal discharge, tightness in the chest and anxiety.

Acute phase: Symptoms during an acute episode of wheezing include a sensation of congestion in the throat and chest, choking cough, dyspnea, prolonged exhalation, wheezing sound in the throat, and scanty sputum that is difficult to expectorate. In severe cases the manifestations include breathing through an open mouth, raised shoulders, sitting upright to breathe, panic, pale complexion with cyanotic lips and nails, extended jugular veins and profuse cold sweating.

Remission phase: If the obstructive sputum is expectorated, the suffocation and dyspnea will gradually be alleviated. As the airway clears, the wheezing breath will diminish and a normal breathing pattern will resume.

C. Differential diagnosis of wheezing and breathlessness:

Dyspnea is a common symptom in both wheezing and breathlessness.

Wheezing: Denotes difficult breathing with a whistling sound. As a recurrent paroxysmal disorder, wheezing is always accompanied by breathlessness. When the disorder lingers and becomes chronic, wheezing will turn into a phlegm-type of breathlessness.

Breathlessness: Characterized by shallow, rapid and labored breathing. It can be a symptom of various diseases. Breathlessness is not necessarily accompanied by wheezing. Unlike wheezing, breathlessness is relatively constant.

Basic Patterns

Acute phase:

- Cold pattern
- Heat pattern

Remission phase:

- Lung deficiency
- Spleen deficiency
- Kidney deficiency

Differentiation and Treatment

Treatment principle:

Treat the branch during an acute episode and treat the root during remission.

During the acute phase, expel phlegm and unblock the obstructed airway.

During the remission phase, support the righteous qi by warming the yang and nourishing the yin to reduce the frequency and severity of acute episodes.

Acute phase:

Cold pattern

Rapid breathing with a wheezing sound in the throat, stifling sensation in the chest and diaphragm, scanty sputum that is difficult to expectorate, and wheezing aggravated by cold weather.

S: Dull complexion, no thirst, aversion to cold and cold limbs.

T: White and moist coating. **P:** Wiry tight or floating tight.

- Warm the lung, disperse cold, transform phlegm and calm wheezing.

- *She Gan Ma Huang Tang*
  - *She Gan* and *Ma Huang* disperse lung qi, expel phlegm, calm wheezing and benefit the throat.
  - *Gan Jiang* and *Xi Xin* warm the lung and transform congested fluids.
  - *Ban Xia* dries dampness and transforms phlegm.
  - *Zi Wan* and *Kuan Dong Hua* transform phlegm and stop coughing.
  - *Wu Wei Zi* restrains lung qi.

- Excessive sputum, sitting upright to breathe. + *Ting Li Zi*
  In the case of exterior cold and interior congested fluids with preponderance of cold signs, use *Xiao Qing Long Tang*.
  Chronic frequent episodes with low-pitched wheezing, shortness of breath, clear sputum, pale complexion, spontaneous sweating, cold limbs, pale tongue with a white coating and a deep thready pulse, use *Su Zi Jiang Qi Tang*.

Heat pattern

Heavy breathing sound with high-pitched wheezing, choking cough, and thick sticky yellow sputum that is difficult to expectorate.
S: Anxiety, sweating, red face, thirst with desire to drink, headache, fever and aversion to wind.
T: Red tongue with yellow greasy coating. **P:** Slippery rapid or slippery wiry.

- Clear heat, disperse lung qi, transform phlegm, and direct lung qi downwards.

- *Ding Chuan Tang*
  - *Ma Huang* disperses lung qi and calms wheezing.
  - *Huang Qin* and *Sang Bai Pi* clear and drain lung heat.
  - *Xing Ren*, *Ban Xia*, *Kuan Dong Hua* and *Su Zi* transform phlegm and descend rebellious qi.
  - *Bai Guo* restrains lung qi.

- Exterior cold with excess lung heat. + *Sheng Shi Gao*
  Lung heat with the sound of rattling phlegm and sitting upright to breathe. + *Ting Li Zi*, *Di Long*
  Thick sticky yellow sputum that is difficult to expectorate. + *Zhi Mu*, *Hai Ge Ke*, *Yu Xing Cao*, *Zhu Li*

Remission phase:

During remission, wheezing is not evident. However, the underlying deficiency of the lung, spleen and kidney should be addressed because the deficiency generates phlegm, which remains latent until exterior pathogens or other factors trigger another acute episode.

Lung deficiency

Spontaneous sweating, aversion to wind, and slight wheezing sound in the throat, induced by changes in the weather. In the aura stage there will be sneezing and nasal congestion with a clear, watery discharge.
S: Shortness of breath, low voice, pale complexion and clear white sputum.
T: Pale tongue with thin white coating. **P:** Weak and thready.

- Tonify the lung and consolidate the protective qi.
- *Yu Ping Feng San*
  - *Huang Qi* tonifies the qi and consolidates the surface.
  - *Bai Zhu* strengthens the spleen and augments the qi, assists Huang Qi to consolidate the surface.
  - *Fang Feng* disperses exterior wind; when used with Huang Qi, the combination will disperse and tonify.
- Significant aversion to wind. + *Gui Zhi, Bai Shao, Sheng Jiang*
  Deficiency of both qi and yin with dry cough and scanty sticky sputum, dry mouth and throat, use *Sheng Mai San*.

Spleen deficiency

Poor appetite, epigastric and abdominal distention, loose stool, and wheezing elicited by excessive consumption of cold, raw, sweet and greasy food.
S: Shortness of breath, low weak voice and fatigue.
T: Thin greasy or white moist coating. **P:** Thready weak and soft.

- Strengthen the Spleen and transform phlegm.
- *Liu Jun Zi Tang*
  - *Dang Shen*, *Bai Zhu*, *Fu Ling* and *Gan Cao* tonify spleen qi.
  - *Ban Xia*, bitter and warm, dries dampness and transforms phlegm.
  - *Chen Pi* facilitates the qi flow and transforms dampness.
- Accompanied by spleen yang deficiency. + *Gan Jiang*

Kidney deficiency

Shortness of breath, shallow rapid breathing aggravated by exertion, more difficulty inhaling than exhaling, wheezing triggered by exertion and fatigue, and soreness and weakness of the lower back and knees.
S: Kidney yang deficiency- cold intolerance, cold limbs, pale complexion and spontaneous sweating. **T:** Swollen tongue with white coating. **P:** Deep thready.
S: Kidney yin deficiency- red cheeks, irritability, sensation of heat and night sweating. **T:** Red tongue with scanty coating. **P:** Thready rapid.

- Tonify the Kidney to grasp the qi.
- *Jin Gui Shen Qi Wan* for kidney yang deficiency
  - *Jin Gui Shen Qi Wan* warms the kidney and assists the yang.
- *Qi Wei Du Qi Wan* for kidney yin deficiency
  - *Qi Wei Du Qi Wan* assists the kidney to grasp the qi.
- To strengthen the effect of tonifying the kidney to grasp the qi. + *Hu Tao Rou*

Acupuncture Treatment

Acute phase:

- **Manipulation:** Reducing method; moxibustion for cold patterns.
- **Prescription:** CV22 Tiantu PC6 Neiguan Extra14 Dingchuan
- **Supplementary points:**
  - Cold wheezing. + LU7 Lieque; LI4 Hegu
  - Heat wheezing. + LU5 Chize; ST40 Fenglong; LU6 Kongzui

Remission phase:

- **Manipulation:** Reinforcing method; moxibustion is applicable.
- **Prescription:** BL13 Feishu LU9 Taiyuan ST36 Zusanli
- **Supplementary points:**
  - Spleen deficiency. + BL20 Pishu; CV12 Zhongwan
  - Kidney deficiency. + BL23 Shenshu; CV4 Guanyuan

Practical Hints

• **Constitution is relevant to therapeutic effect.** This disorder tends to be stubborn and recurrent. The elderly, those with deficiencies due to chronic illness, and patients with kidney deficiency may respond poorly to therapy. Children, adolescents and young adults are more likely to respond well to herbal therapy because their kidney qi is waxing full and their righteous qi is growing stronger as they mature.

• **Be alert that wheezing could develop into yang collapse.** In severe heart and kidney yang deficiency with imminent yang collapse, there will be signs of distress including breathing through an opened mouth, raised shoulders, irritability and panic, cyanotic complexion and lips, clammy cold skin, and a large but rootless or knotted pulse. The patient may be comatose. The prognosis in this case is poor.

CHAPTER 4

Breathlessness

喘證 *Chuan Zheng*

Breathlessness is a respiratory condition characterized by audible labored breathing that is rapid and shallow. There will be difficult inhalation accompanied by open-mouthed breathing, lifted shoulders and dilated nostrils. The symptoms are aggravated by physical exertion. In severe cases, persistent breathlessness results in orthopnea (difficulty breathing while lying down) and prostration. Breathlessness may occur during the course of many acute and chronic diseases.

Relevant Diseases

- Asthma
- Bronchitis
- Pneumonia
- COPD
- Bronchial carcinoma
- Pulmonary embolism
- Cardiac asthma
- Left ventricular failure
- Cor pulmonale
- Hysterical dyspnea
- Silicosis
- Anemia

Etiology and Pathogenesis

The underlying pathogenesis of breathlessness is failure of lung qi to descend, which can be elicited by two different etiologies. Excess pathogenic influences, including exterior wind-cold, and interior stagnant phlegm, qi or heat, obstruct lung qi. Deficiency of the lung and kidney contribute to failure of lung qi to descend.

Exterior pathogens: Wind-cold obstructs lung qi and contracts the superficial region, inhibiting the dispersion of lung qi. Wind-heat obstructs lung qi and forms phlegm to block the descent of lung qi.

Improper diet injures the middle burner and the spleen fails to transform and transport food essence, resulting in the accumulation of phlegm-dampness, which blocks the descent of lung qi.

Emotional stress: Worry causes lung qi stagnation; anger causes liver qi to rebel; both contribute to the dysfunction of lung qi in dispersing and descending.

Chronic illness consumes lung qi and yin, eventually damaging kidney essence. Breathlessness occurs when lung's function is weakened and the deficient kidney is not able to receive the qi.

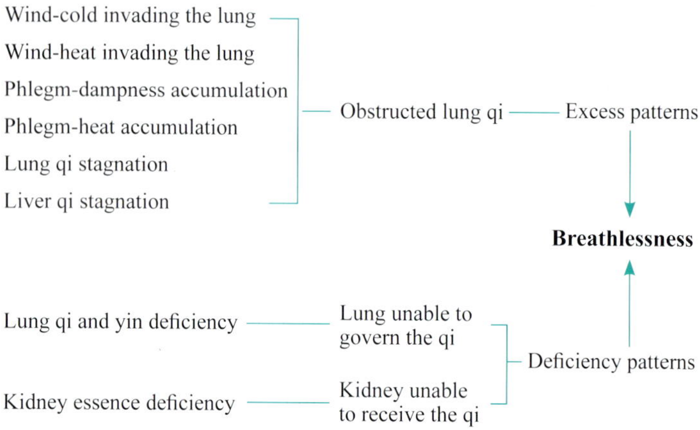

Diagnosis

A. Identification of excess and deficiency:

Excess patterns usually arise from lung pathology (external pathogens, phlegm turbidity and stagnant qi inhibiting the dispersion and descent of lung qi).

Deficient patterns derive from the lung and kidney (qi, yin and essence deficiency lead to impaired respiratory function).

The heart may be involved during the critical phase of breathlessness. Manifestations include a cyanotic complexion with cyanotic lips, tongue and nails and profuse perspiration, which can cause qi collapse and depletion of yang or yin.

- The heart vessels fill the lung and lung qi moves the blood. When there is lung qi deficiency, failure of heart qi to circulate the blood results.
- Kidney yang is the foundation of heart yang. When kidney yang is deficient, the *ming-men* fire fails to warm the heart. Fluids are not transformed and they accumulate in the lung and heart. This pattern is identified as "kidney yang deficiency with water overflowing towards the lung and heart."

B. Identification of cold and heat:

Cold patterns can be identified by thin watery or white frothy sputum, bluish-gray complexion, no thirst, preference for warm beverages, white tongue coating, and floating tight or slow wiry pulse.

Heat patterns can be identified by yellow viscous or white sticky sputum that is difficult to expectorate, red face, thirst with desire to drink, red tongue with yellow greasy or dry yellow coating, and rapid slippery pulse.

C. Differential diagnosis of breathlessness and shortness of breath:

Breathlessness is characterized by audible sighing dyspnea, open-mouthed breathing, lifted shoulders and needing to sit upright to breathe.

Shortness of breath is characterized by shallow breathing, fatigue, low voice, reluctance to speak and a weak pulse. It is primarily caused by qi deficiency. In its most severe stage, it may be accompanied by deficient breathlessness.

Basic Patterns

Excess patterns:

- Wind cold invading the lung
- Exterior cold with lung heat
- Turbid phlegm accumulation in the lung
- Phlegm-heat accumulation in the lung
- Stagnant qi obstructing the lung

Deficient patterns:

- Lung deficiency
- Kidney deficiency

Differentiation and Treatment

Treatment principle:

Excess: Focus the treatment on the lung by expelling pathogenic factors and restoring the function of lung qi, using methods such as warming and dispersing, clearing and descending, and transforming phlegm.

Deficiency: Treat both the lung and kidney, primarily the kidney. Depending on the pathogenesis and organ involvement, the methods should be tonifying the lung, assisting the kidney to grasp the qi, augmenting the qi and nourishing the yin.

Deficiency-excess complex or deficiency below with excess above: It is important to differentiate the root and branch and provide the proper treatment.

Excess patterns:

Wind-cold invading the lung

Audible sighing dyspnea with coughing and gasping, rapid breathing, stifling sensation in the chest, and abundant thin white sputum.

S: Aversion to cold, fever, headache, absence of sweating and no thirst.

T: Thin white slippery coating. **P:** Floating and tight.

- Expel wind-cold; restore the dispersing and descending function of lung qi.
- *Ma Huang Tang*
  - *Ma Huang* and *Gui Zhi* disperse lung qi, expel cold and release the exterior.
  - *Xing Ren* descends lung qi. When used with *Ma Huang*, one disperses and the other descends, mutually assisting each other to restore the function of lung qi to resolve breathlessness.
  - *Gan Cao* moderates the aggressive actions of *Ma Huang* and *Gui Zhi*, as well as harmonizes the formula.
- Cold-phlegm in the lung. + *Ban Xia, Ju Hong, Su Zi, Bai Qian*
  Breathlessness with sweating, use *Gui Zhi Jia Hou Po Xing Zi Tang*.
  Exterior wind-cold with pre-existing cold congested fluids in the lung, use *Xiao Qing Long Tang*.

Exterior cold with lung heat

Audible sighing dyspnea, rapid breathing, chest distention or pain, dilated nostrils, and sticky yellow sputum that is difficult to expectorate.
S: Slight aversion to cold, fever with or without sweating, thirst, irritability and headache.
T: Thin white or yellow coating. **P:** Floating or slippery and rapid.

- Disperse lung qi and drain internal heat.
- *Ma Xing Shi Gan Tang*
  - *Shi Gao* is acrid and extremely cold to clear and drain lung heat.
  - *Ma Huang* disperses lung qi, expels pathogens and calms wheezing.
  - *Xing Ren* descends lung qi and transforms phlegm.
  - *Gan Cao* harmonizes and moderates the formula.
- In the case of high fever with profuse sweating and dyspnea, increase the dosage of *Shi Gao*; if chest congestion with sputum is difficult to expextorate, sluggish perspiration and dyspnea, increase the dose of *Ma Huang*. In general, dosage of *Shi Gao* has to be greater than that of *Ma Huang*.
  To strengthen the effects of clearing and transforming phlegm-heat. + *Huang Qin, Sang Bai Pi, Gua Lou*
  Abundant sputum. + *Ting Li Zi, She Gan*

Turbid phlegm accumulation in the lung

Audible sighing dyspnea, stifling sensation in the chest, cough, and copious sticky white sputum that is difficult to expectorate.
S: Poor appetite, sticky sensation in the mouth, no thirst, nausea and vomiting.
T: Thick white greasy coating. **P:** Slippery.

- Resolve phlegm and restore the descending function of lung qi.
- *Er Chen Tang* and *San Zi Yang Qin Tang*
  - *Ban Xia*, bitter and warm, dries dampness and transforms phlegm.
  - *Chen Pi* facilitates the qi flow, transforms phlegm and expels dampness.
  - *Fu Ling* strengthens the spleen and augments the qi to transform dampness.
  - *Su Zi*, *Bai Jie Zi* and *Lai Fu Zi* transform phlegm, descend rebellious qi and resolve breathlessness.
- To strengthen the effects of drying dampness and regulating the qi. + *Cang Zhu, Hou Po*

Phlegm-heat accumulation in the lung

Audible sighing dyspnea, heat sensation in the chest with distention and pain, and coughing up copious thick yellow sputum that might be blood-tinged.
S: Thirst with desire to drink cold beverages, irritability, red face, dry throat, dark urine and constipation.
T: Yellow greasy coating. **P:** Slippery and rapid.

- Clear lung heat and transform phlegm.
- *Sang Bai Pi Tang*
  - *Sang Bai Pi*, *Huang Qin*, *Huang Lian* and *Zhi Zi* clear and drain lung heat.
  - *Bei Mu* and *Xing Ren* moisten the lung and transform phlegm.
  - *Su Zi* and *Ban Xia* descend rebellious qi and transform phlegm.
- Fever. + *Shi Gao, Zhi Mu*
  Thirst and dry throat. + *Tian Hua Fen, Xuan Shen*
  Thick and sticky sputum. + *Hai Ge Ke*
  Severe case with orthopnea, profuse sputum and constipation. + *Ting Li Zi, Da Huang, Mang Xiao*
  Coughing up sputum with a foul smell. + *Yu Xing Cao, Yi Yi Ren, Dong Gua Ren*

Stagnant qi obstructing the lung

Sudden attacks of breathlessness elicited by emotional stress, rapid short breathing with a suffocating sensation or constriction in the throat, and chest oppression and pain.
S: Insomnia, palpitations, stuffiness and pain in the hypochondriac and chest regions.
T: Thin white coating. **P:** Wiry.

- Soothe the liver, activate the qi flow and direct lung qi downwards.
- *Wu Mo Yin Zi*
  - *Wu Yao* soothes the liver and releases constrained qi.

- *Chen Xiang*, *Zhi Qiao*, *Mu Xiang* and *Bing Lang* descend rebellious qi and resolve breathlessness.

- Palpitations and insomnia. + *Bai He, He Huan Hua, Suan Zao Ren*
  Qi stagnation progressing to heat or fire, use *Dan Zhi Xiao Yao San*.

Deficient patterns:

Lung deficiency

Audible sighing dyspnea with shortness of breath; possible low and weak voice, cough with a low sound and thin white sputum; or possible scanty and sticky sputum, dry throat and mouth.
S: Spontaneous sweating and aversion to wind, pale complexion and lassitude.
T: Pale or red tongue. **P:** Thready weak or rapid.

- Tonify the lung, augment the qi and nourish the yin.

- *Sheng Mai San*
  - *Ren Shen* is sweet, and it benefits the lung and greatly tonifies the basal qi.
  - *Mai Men Dong*, sweet and cold, generates the body fluid. When used with *Wu Wei Zi*, the combination of sour and sweet properties will generate the yin.
  - *Wu Wei Zi* is sour to restrain lung qi.

- Significant lung qi deficiency. + *Huang Qi*
  Significant lung yin deficiency. + *Sha Shen, Yu Zhu, Bai He*
  To enhance the effect of transforming phlegm. + *Zi Wan, Sang Bai Pi*
  Accompanied by spleen qi deficiency with poor appetite, abdominal distention and loose stool, use *Bu Zhong Yi Qi Tang*.

Kidney deficiency

Longstanding audible sighing dyspnea with difficult inhalation that is aggravated by exertion.
S: Cold intolerance, clammy skin and cold limbs, soreness and weakness of the lower back and knees, fatigue, lassitude, ankle edema, and cyanotic complexion or lips.
T: Pale tongue. **P:** Deep and thready.

- Warm the yang and tonify the kidney to receive the qi.

- *Jin Gui Shen Qi Wan* and *Shen Ge San*
  - *Jin Gui Shen Qi Wan* warms and fortifies kidney yang.
  - *Ren Shen* and *Ge Jie* assist the kidney to receive the qi.

- To strengthen the effects of tonifying the kidney and grasping the qi. + *Wu Wei Zi, Hu Tao Rou*

Kidney qi deficiency with breathlessness, coughing, shortness of breath and copious sputum, use *Su Zi Jiang Qi Tang*.

Kidney yang deficiency with cold water overflowing towards the heart and lung, manifesting as breathlessness, coughing, palpitations, edema and scanty urination, use *Zhen Wu Tang*.

Acupuncture Treatment

Excess patterns

Wind-cold:

- **Manipulation:** Reducing method; moxibustion is applicable.
- **Prescription:** BL13 Feishu, GV14 Dazhui, LU7 Lieque, BL12 Fengmen, LI4 Hegu

Phlegm-heat:

- **Manipulation:** Reducing method.
- **Prescription:** BL13 Feishu, CV22 Tiantu, Extra14 Dingchuan, LU5 Chize, ST40 Fenglong

Deficient patterns

Lung deficiency:

- **Manipulation:** Reinforcing method; moxibustion is applicable.
- **Prescription:** BL13 Feishu, LU9 Taiyuan, ST36 Zusanli, SP3 Taibai

Kidney deficiency:

- **Manipulation:** Reinforcing method; moxibustion is applicable.
- **Prescription:** KI3 Taixi, BL23 Shenshu, BL13 Feishu, CV17 Tanzhong, CV6 Qihai, GV12 Shenzhu, BL43 Gaohuang

Practical Hints

• **Two possible patterns of excess above with deficiency below relate to altered breathing.** The first pattern is breathlessness caused by deficient kidney qi and phlegm-turbidity obstruction in the lung. The treatment principle for this pattern is to transform phlegm, descend lung qi, and warm the kidney to receive the qi. The second pattern of excess above with deficiency below pertains to a pathological pattern of edema in which kidney yang is deficient and water overflows towards the heart and lung. This pattern can worsen and develop into heart yang deficiency and heart blood stasis. The manifestations include systemic edema, palpitations, coughing, breathlessness, wheezing and oliguria. As the disorder progresses, cyanotic complexion, lips, nails and tongue, and stabbing chest pain will appear. The treatment principles are to warm and activate the yang, promote metabolism of water, and transform stasis.

• **Prognosis.** Excess patterns usually respond well to treatment as soon as the pathogenic factors are resolved. Deficiency patterns are caused by chronic dysfunction of the lung and kidney in governing and receiving the qi; therefore, tonifying methods may not produce an immediate therapeutic effect. Due to chronic deficiencies, the patient is susceptible to invasion by exterior pathogens, which complicate the pattern and cause recurrent episodes of breathlessness.

CHAPTER 5

Lung Abscess

肺 癰 *Fei Yong*

As one of the internal abscesses, lung abscess is referred to suppurated sores and boils in the lung. It is characterized by chest pain, fever, coughing up foul smelling opaque sputum. At its severe stage, sputum mixed with pus and blood is present. Lung abscess is mainly caused by wind-heat and fire toxicity. When these pathogens accumulate in the lung, the circulation of blood is interrupted. The combination of heat, stagnant qi, blood stasis and fire toxicity will decompose the local tissues and form boils. Therefore, the major treatment principle is to clear heat and relieve toxicity, transform stasis and promote purulent discharge.

Relevant Diseases

- Pulmonary abscess
- Suppurative pneumonia
- Infectious bronchiectasis

Etiology and Pathogenesis

Wind-heat attacking the lung: Through the nose, mouth and skin, wind-heat may enter and attack the lung. Also, unresolved wind-cold may transform into heat and stagnate in the lung. Steamed and smoked by these types of heat pathogens, lung qi fails to descend and disperse, further leading to toxic heat accumulation and blood stasis. Decomposed by these types of stagnant pathogens, the lung forms boils at the affected area.

Phlegm-heat hidden in the lung: The formation of damp-heat is closely related to overindulgence of alcohol or a greasy, spicy and rich diet. When heat consumes the fluid, the pre-formed dampness secondary to improper diet becomes concentrated, resulting in phlegm-heat. When phlegm-heat stagnates in the lung, it will steam and smoke the tissue and cause boils.

Exterior pathogenic influences, especially wind-heat, can easily trigger the formation of lung abscess in those patients who have pre-existing phlegm-heat in the lung. When righteous qi is deficient and a person's resistance to exterior pathogens is weak, the propensity to catch wind-heat will be increased. The deficient righteous qi can be a result of chronic illness or constitutional insufficiency.

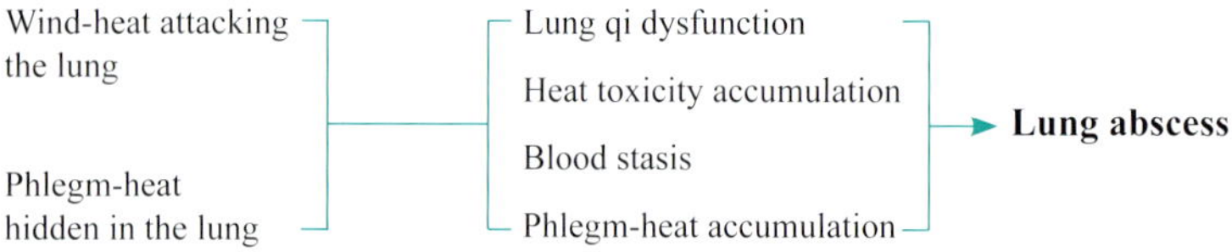

Diagnosis

A. Identification of the progressive stages:

Exterior stage: At this stage, the lung is attacked by exterior wind-heat. Both protective layer and lung organ are affected. Symptoms of exterior condition are manifested as aversion to wind, fever, cough and possible sweating.

Suppurative stage: At this stage the accumulated heat consumes lung fluid and forms phlegm-heat. Heat toxicity also consumes fluid in the blood; blood becomes concentrated and forms blood stasis. Phlegm-heat and blood stasis, when obstructed in the lung, start to decompose the tissues. Dead tissues and these pathogens fuse and form boils. Clinical manifestations during this stage include high fever, chills, cough, tachypnea and chest pain.

Perforating stage: As the phlegm-heat, blood stasis, heat toxicity and dead tissues continue to damage the lung and lung vessels, boils burst and copious discharge of purulent bloody sputum are expectorated.

Recovery stage: At this stage, the accumulated pathogens are discharged along with the sputum. Systemic symptoms are decreased as fever is reduced, cough is relieved and sputum is cleared, indicating that the righteous qi is recovering and the lung tissue is healing. However, if righteous qi was exhausted during the course, pathogenic factors would retain internally when deficient qi failed to expel them out. Chronic recurrent lung abscess will result. Manifestations include low grade fever, constant expectoration of purulent bloody sputum and general weakness.

B. Differential diagnosis of lung abscess and warm-febrile disease:

Lung abscess: It is manifested by chills and fever in the early stage and coughing with opaque and turbid sputum that is foul smelling. Due to the nature of the formation of abscess in the lung, this disease usually progresses with the stages as explained above.

Initial stage of warm-febrile disease: It is characterized by acute onset with fever, cough, irritability and thirst, possible tachypnea and chest pain. Having similar symptoms of lung abscess, early stage of warm-febrile disease can be easily misdiagnosed as lung abscess. Prompt treatment can stop the course of warm-febrile disease at the qi level. However, if the fever is not reduced after a week of treatment or if the fever reoccurs during treatment, consider the possibility of lung abscess.

Basic Patterns

- Exterior stage
- Suppurative stage
- Perforating stage
- Recovery stage

Differentiation and Treatment

Treatment principle:

Clear heat, relieve toxicity, transform stasis and expel purulent discharge.

Exterior stage: Clear the lung and disperse the pathogens.

Suppurative stage: Clear heat and relieve toxicity, and transform stasis and reduce abscess.

Perforating stage: Promote purulent discharge and relieve toxicity.

Recovery stage: Nourish the yin and tonify the qi in yin injury and qi exhaustion, or support the righteous qi to expel pathogens in chronic conditions with lingering pathogen.

Exterior stage

Aversion to cold, fever, and productive cough with white sticky sputum.

S: Painful sensation in the chest aggravated by coughing, dyspnea, and dry mouth and nose.

T: Thin white or thin yellow coating. **P:** Floating, rapid and slippery.

- Clear the pathogen from the lung and release the exterior.
- *Yin Qiao San*
  - *Jin Yin Hua* and *Lian Qiao* are acrid and cool; they vent heat from the surface of the body and relieve toxicity.
  - *Bo He*, acrid and cool, vents and disperses heat.
  - *Niu Bang Zi* clears heat and relieves toxicity.
  - *Jing Jie* and *Dan Dou Chi*, acid and warm in nature, when used together with acrid and cool herbs above, strengthen the venting and dispersing effects to release the exterior.
  - *Jie Geng* disperses lung qi, benefits the throat and transforms phlegm.
  - *Zhu Ye* and *Lu Gen* clear heat and generate the fluid.

- To strengthen the effect of clearing lung heat. + *Shi Gao, Huang Qin*
  Productive cough with copious sputum. + *Xing Ren, Chuan Bei Mu, Sang Bai Pi, Dong Gua Ren, Pi Pa Ye*
  Painful sensation in the chest with dyspnea. + *Gua Lou Pi, Yu Jin*

Suppurative stage

High fever following chills, sweating, irritability, cough, tachypnea, and opaque sputum or yellowish-green sputum, stifling and painful sensation in the chest, pain aggravated by changing position or deep breathing.
S: Subjective foul smell in the throat, and dry mouth and throat.
T: Yellow greasy coating. **P:** Slippery and rapid.

- Clear the lung, transform stasis and reduce abscess.
- *Qian Jin Wei Jing Tang*
  - *Dong Gua Ren*, *Yi Yi Ren* and *Tao Ren* transform phlegm-turbidity, resolve stasis and dissipate clumps.
  - *Lu Gen* clears lung heat, relieves toxicity and reduces abscess.
- To strengthen the effects of clearing heat and reducing abscess. + *Zhi Zi, Huang Qin, Jie Geng*
  To reinforce the effects of clearing heat and relieving toxicity. + *Jin Yin Hua, Hong Teng, Yu Xing Cao*
  Productive cough with yellow sticky sputum. + *Sang Bai Pi, She Gan*
  Phlegm obstructing in the lung with coughing and wheezing, and opaque sputum. + *Ting Li Zi*

Perforating stage

Productive cough with copious purulent bloody sputum which is foul smelling, possible hemoptysis, and stifling and painful sensation in the chest.
S: Irritability, dyspnea and orthopnea, fever, red face, thirst and desire to drink.
T: Red tongue with yellow greasy coating. **P:** Slippery and rapid.

- Promote purulent discharge and relieve toxicity.
- *Jia Wei Jie Geng Tang*
  - *Jie Geng* is the imperial herb for promoting purulent discharge and reducing abscess; large dose is recommended.
  - *Yi Yi Ren*, *Bei Mu* and *Ju Hong* transform phlegm and dissipate clump.
  - *Jin Yin Hua* and *Gan Cao* clear heat and relieve toxicity.
  - *Bai Ji* astringes the blood and stops bleeding.
- To reinforce the effects of clearing heat, relieving toxicity and promoting purulent discharge. + *Yu Xing Cao, Bai Jiang Cao, Huang Qin*

Hymoptysis. + *Mu Dan Pi, Zhi Zi, Ou Jie, Bai Mao Gen*
Intense thirst. + *Tian Hua Fen, Zhi Mu*
Insufficient fluid with dry mouth. + *Sha Shen, Mai Men Dong*
Qi deficiency failing to discharge pus. + *Huang Qi*

Recovery stage

The condition is improving with the confirmation by a reduction of fever, cough, purulent bloody discharge and foul odor, as well as clear sputum, increasing energy, and improving appetite. Secondary symptoms may still exist and would include dull pain in the hypochondria and chest, shortness of breath, spontaneous sweating or night sweating, low grade fever, tidal fever in the afternoon, irritability, dry mouth and throat, emaciation and lassitude.
On the contrary, if the condition turns chronic due to the pathogen lingering, there will be unremitting constant or recurrent fever and cough with purulent bloody discharge.
T: Red or slightly red tongue with thin coating. **P:** Thready or thready rapid and forceless.

- Nourish the yin and tonify the lung.
- *Sha Shen Qing Fei Tang*
  - *Sha Shen*, *Huang Qi* and *Tai Zi Shen* nourish the yin and augment the qi.
  - *Dong Gua Ren* and *Yi Yi Ren* transform phlegm and reduce abscesses.
  - *Jie Geng* disperses and opens up lung qi, and transforms phlegm.
  - *Bai Ji* astringes the blood, stops bleeding and generates the tissue.
  - *Sheng Gan Cao* augments the qi and harmonizes the formula.
- To strengthen the effects of nourishing the yin and moistening the lung. + *Mai Men Dong, Bai He*
  To reinforce the effects of nourishing the yin and stopping hemorrhage. + *E Jiao*
  Persistent low grade fever. + *Qing Hao, Bai Wei, Di Gu Pi*
  Lack of appetite and loose stool. + *Bai Zhu, Shan Yao, Fu Ling*
  Unremitting coughing up purulent bloody sputum. + *Bai Lian*

Acupuncture Treatment

Exterior stage:

- **Manipulation:** Reducing method.
- **Prescription:** GV14 Dazhui, LI11 Quchi, TE5 Waiguan, LI4 Hegu, LU7 Lieque, BL13 Feishu

Suppurative and perforating stages:

- **Manipulation:** Reducing method.
- **Prescription:**

CV22 Tiantu	LU5 Chize	ST40 Fenglong
LU7 Lieque	LI11 Shaoshang	BL13 Feishu

- **Supplementary points:**

  - Blood-tinged sputum or hemoptysis. + LU6 Kongzui; BL17 Geshu

Recovery stage:

- **Manipulation:** Combination of reinforcing and reducing methods.
- **Prescription:**

BL13 Feishu	LU1 Zhongfu	LU7 Lieque
KI6 Zhaohai	LU9 Taiyuan	SP3 Taibai

Practical Hints

• **Perforating stage is a critical phase for determining the prognosis.** If fever reduces, chest pain decreases, appetite improves and the speech is clear with strong tone; the prognosis is more likely optimistic. On the contrary, poor prognosis is suggested if the speech is slurred, hoarse and weak, discharge has a foul odor, fever is unremitting, chest pain is present with tachypnea, poor appetite, malar flush, cyanotic nails and lips, and short choppy or wiry pulse. These symptoms indicate a retrogressing condition and the lung is deteriorating. Therefore, perforating stage is the critical phase. The focus is on treating the branch. It is highly recommended to clear heat, relieve toxicity and promote purulent discharge. Using large dose of herbs that relieve toxicity and promote purulent discharge can greatly expel pathogens and prevent them from lingering.

• **Hospitalization may be required if abundant hemoptysis occurs.** Choking and suffocation might be a result from blood clots obstructing the airway. Referrals to an acute medical facility may be necessary.

CHAPTER 6

Palpitations

心悸 *Xin Ji*

Palpitations are typically a subjective sensation of a rapidly or irregularly beating heart. An involuntary, rapid heartbeat may be accompanied by feeling of anxiety or panic. Palpitations include changes in heart rate and rhythm. They are most often paroxysmal, elicited by emotional stress or exhaustion, but can also be a persistent symptom of organic heart disorders. Insomnia, forgetfulness, dizziness and tinnitus frequently occur in conjunction with palpitations.

Palpitations include two conditions, *jing ji* and *zheng chong*. *Jing ji* refers to intermittent palpitations due to panic attacks, fright and anger. *Zheng chong* refers to constant palpitations with restlessness and rapid heartbeat. Both conditions result from malnourishment of the heart from qi, blood, yin, and yang deficiency or from phlegm and blood stasis obstructing the heart channels.

Relevant Diseases

- Myocarditis
- Pericarditis
- Myocardial infarction
- Heart failure
- Menopause
- Arrhythmias
- Neurosis
- Hyperthyroidism
- Rheumatic fever

Etiology and Pathogenesis

Heart and gallbladder deficiency: Constitutional heart and gallbladder qi deficiency manifests with lack of self-confidence, timidity and indecisive behavior. The heart is malnourished and the spirit is easily disturbed by the shock of sudden frightening events.

Heart blood deficiency may be caused by severe loss of blood, or by pensiveness injuring the spleen, the source of blood. Deficient blood cannot nourish the heart and house the spirit.

Yin deficiency with empty fire: Excessive sexual activity injures kidney essence. If the essence is deficient, kidney yin (water) cannot nourish the heart (fire) and there will be loss of communication between the kidney and heart. Heart fire becomes overactive and causes palpitations.

Heart yang deficiency occurs when chronic or severe illness exhausts heart yang, which then fails to warm the heart vessels.

Cold congested fluids overflowing to the heart: Kidney yang fails to warm and steam water, thus fluids become congested. The fluids spill over and block the heart yang, giving rise to heart dysfunction and palpitations.

Blood stasis obstructing the channels can be caused by heart yang deficiency and inadequate circulation of the blood. Blood stasis may develop from *bi* syndromes in which wind, cold, and damp pathogens obstruct the channels in the early stages, then progress to the heart and block the heart vessels. Blood circulation is impaired, causing palpitations.

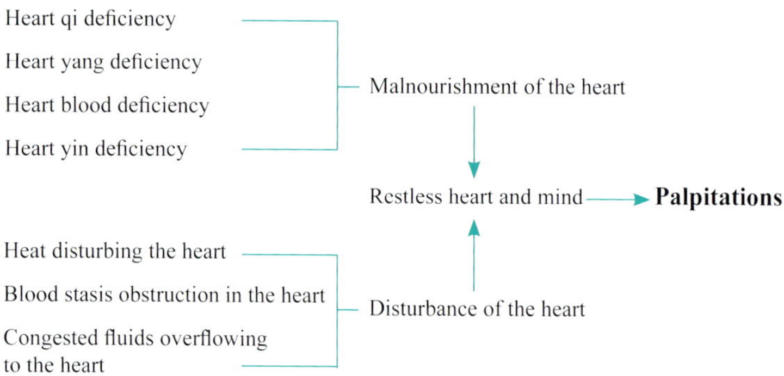

Diagnosis

A. Identification of *jing ji* and *zheng chong*:

	Jing Ji	*Zheng Chong*
Etiology	Triggered by emotional factors, e.g. fright, anger.	Occurs when there is dysfunction of the internal organs, elicited by exhaustion.
Condition	Mild, responds quickly to treatment, remits spontaneously.	Severe, poor prognosis, recurrent or persistent.
Chief Complaint	Palpitations.	Palpitations with systemic deficiency.
Character-istics	Excess, or mixed patterns of excess and deficiency; Functional disorder.	Primarily deficiency patterns; Organic disorder.

Clinically, *jing ji* and *zheng chong* both belong to one disorder. Long-standing *jing ji* can develop into *zheng chong*. If *zheng chong* is complicated by sudden exogenous stimulation, such as a sudden loud noise and unexpected tabbing on the back from someone, palpitations might be exacerbated.

B. Identification of excess and deficiency:

- Excess patterns are manifested as palpitations accompanied with:
  - Irritability, heat sensation in the chest, and insomnia or dream-disturbed sleep, nausea and lack of appetite – Phlegm-fire disturbing the heart.
  - Dizziness, stifling sensation in the chest, breathlessness or dyspnea, and edema – Congested fluids overflowing to the heart.
  - Agitation, stabbing chest pain, cyanotic lips, tongue with petechiae, and an irregular pulse – Heart blood stasis.
  - Rapid, slippery and forceful pulse – Phlegm-fire.
  - Slow pulse – Pathogenic cold.
- Deficient patterns are manifested as palpitations accompanied with:
  - An empty feeling in the heart, shortness of breath, fatigue, dizziness, and aggravated by exertion – Heart qi deficiency.
  - Weakness, irritability, and aggravated by mental strain – Heart blood or yin deficiency.
  - Thready, weak and rapid pulse – Yin deficiency with empty fire.
  - Deep and slow pulse – Yang deficiency with empty cold.

C. Identification of severity of the illness:

Mild case: These palpitations are triggered by emotional factors. Occurrences are paroxysmal and of short duration; remission is spontaneous.

Severe case: There are no emotional factors involved. Symptoms include persistent palpitations aggravated by exertion, breathlessness, dyspnea, edema, stabbing chest pain and cold extremities.

Critical situation: Collapse of heart yang is imminent when palpitations are accompanied by profuse sweating, frigid extremities, shallow breathing, cyanotic lips and tongue, faint pulse, and possibly loss of consciousness.

Basic Patterns

- Heart and gallbladder qi deficiency
- Heart blood deficiency
- Heart yin deficiency with empty fire
- Heart yang inactivity
- Cold congested fluids overflowing towards the heart
- Heart blood stasis

Differentiation and Treatment

Treatment principle:

Excess: Eliminate pathogenic factors by invigorating the blood and transforming stasis, clearing heat, and resolving phlegm and fluids.

Deficiency: Tonify deficiency by nourishing the blood and calming the spirit, warming heart yang and unblocking the vessels, and assisting the yang to resolve congested fluids.

Heart and gallbladder qi deficiency

Palpitations, easily frightened and agitated.
S: Restlessness, insomnia and excessive dreaming.
T: Thin white coating. **P:** Weak and rapid.

- Anchor and sedate the mind, nourish the heart to calm the spirit.
- *An Shen Ding Zhi Wan*
  - *Long Chi* sedates and tranquilizes the agitated heart.
  - *Fu Shen*, *Yuan Zhi* and *Shi Chang Pu* calm the spirit.
  - *Ren Shen* and *Fu Ling* augment the qi and tranquilize the mind.
- To enhance the effect of tonifying heart qi. + *Zhi Gan Cao*
  Complicated by heart yin deficiency. + *Bai Zhi Ren*, *Suan Zao Ren*
  Accompanied by irritability, nausea, loss of appetite and excessive sputum, yellow greasy tongue coating and slippery rapid pulse, use *Huang Lian Wen Dan Tang*.

Heart blood deficiency

Palpitations, dizziness and pale complexion.
S: Fatigue, insomnia and forgetfulness.
T: Pale tongue. **P:** Thready and weak.

- Augment the qi and blood, nourish the heart and calm the spirit.
- *Gui Pi Tang*
  - *Dang Gui* and *Long Yan Rou* tonify and nourish heart blood.
  - *Ren Shen*, *Huang Qi* and *Bai Zhu*, sweet and warm, strengthen the spleen and augment the qi to generate the blood.
  - *Suan Zao Ren*, *Yuan Zhi* and *Fu Shen* calm the spirit.
  - *Mu Xiang* regulates the qi flow.
  - *Gan Cao* harmonizes the middle burner and the formula.
- Palpitations with an irregular pulse, use *Zhi Gan Cao Tang*.
  Palpitations due to heart yin deficiency in the late stage of a warm-febrile disease, use *Sheng Mai San*.

Insomnia or dream-disturbed sleep. + *He Huan Pi, Ye Jiao Teng, Wu Wei Zi, Bai Zi Ren, Lian Zi Xin*

Heart yin deficiency with empty fire

Palpitations, irritability, restlessness, insomnia and five-centers heat.
S: Soreness of the lower back, tinnitus, dizziness and vertigo.
T: Red tongue with scanty or no coating. **P:** Thready and rapid.

- Tonify the yin, clear fire, nourish the heart and calm the spirit.
- *Tian Wang Bu Xin Dan*
  - *Sheng Di Huang*, *Xuan Shen*, *Mai Men Dong* and *Tian Men Dong* nourish the yin and clear heat.
  - *Dang Gui* and *Dan Shen* tonify the blood and nourish the heart.
  - *Ren Shen* and *Fu Ling* augment heart qi.
  - *Suan Zao Ren* and *Bai Zi Ren* nourish heart blood and calm the spirit.
  - *Wu Wei Zi* and *Yuan Zhi* astringe heart qi and calm the spirit.
- Significant heat signs with irritability, dry throat, and bitter taste in the mouth, use *Zhu Sha An Shen Wan*.
  Five-centers heat with nocturnal emission and soreness of the lower back, use *Zhi Bai Di Huang Wan*.
  Night sweating. + *Shan Zhu Yu, Wu Mei*

Heart yang inactivity

Palpitations with restlessness, stuffiness of the chest and shortness of breath.
S: Pale complexion, cold intolerance and cold extremities.
T: Pale tongue. **P:** Weak or deep and thready.

- Warm and activate heart yang, and calm the spirit.
- *Gui Zhi Gan Cao Long Gu Mu Li Tang*
  - *Gui Zhi* and *Zhi Gan Cao* warm and activate heart yang.
  - *Long Gu* and *Mu Li* sedate the agitated heart and calm the spirit.
- To enhance the effects of warming the yang and augmenting the qi. + *Ren Shen, Huang Qi*
  Severe systemic edema. + *Che Qian Zi, Ze Xie*
  Yang deficiency and blood stasis with stabbing pain in the chest, and cyanotic complexion. + *Dan Shen, Chi Shao, Hong Hua, Tao Ren*
  Unremitting profuse sweating. + *Ren Shen, Huang Qi, Shan Zhu Yu*
  Severe palpitations with perspiration, frigid extremities, cyanotic lips and tongue, and orthopnea. + *Shen Fu Tang*

Cold congested fluids overflowing towards the heart

Palpitations with dizziness, focal distention in the chest and epigastrium, scanty urination and edema.
S: Cold extremities, thirst with no desire to drink, nausea and vomiting clear fluids.
T: White slippery coating. **P:** Slippery and wiry.

- Warm and activate heart yang to transform cold congested fluids.
- *Ling Gui Zhu Gan Tang*
  - *Gui Zhi* and *Gan Cao* warm and unblock the flow of yang qi.
  - *Fu Ling* is bland to leach out and drain dampness.
  - *Bai Zhu* strengthens the spleen and dries dampness.
- Accompanied by nausea and vomiting. + *Ban Xia, Chen Pi, Sheng Jiang*
  Palpitations with coughing and wheezing, orthopnea, dysuria, and severe pitting edema, use *Zhen Wu Tang*.
  Oliguria and pitting edema. + *Da Fu Pi, Che Qian Zi, Ze Xie*
  Impaired dispersion of lung qi. + *Xing Ren, Qian Hu*
  Complicated by blood stasis. + *Ze Lan, Yi Mu Cao, Dang Gui*

Heart blood stasis

Palpitations with restlessness, chest stuffiness, and stabbing chest pain.
S: Cyanotic lips and nails.
T: Dark blue tongue with petechiae. **P:** Choppy, knotted or intermittent.

- Invigorate the blood, transform stasis and unblock the channels.
- *Xue Fu Zhu Yu Tang*
  - *Tao Ren* and *Hong Hua* invigorate the blood and dispel stasis.
  - *Dang Gui*, *Di Huang*, *Chuan Xiong* and *Chi Shao* nourish and invigorate the blood to expel stasis.
  - *Chai Hu* spreads the liver and regulates the qi.
  - *Zhi Qiao* facilitates the qi flow and expands the chest.
  - *Jie Geng* disperses lung qi and carries the formula upwards.
  - *Niu Xi* invigorates the blood and guides the movement of blood downwards.
- To strengthen the effect of warming yang qi. + *Gui Zhi, Zhi Gan Cao*
  Sedate the restless heart and calm the spirit. + *Long Gu, Mu Li*
  Accompanied by qi stagnation. + *Xiang Fu, Yu Jin, Yan Hu Suo, Chen Pi*
  Accompanied by qi deficiency. + *Huang Qi, Dang Shen*
  Significant palpitations. + *Long Gu, Mu Li, Ci Shi, Hu Po*

Acupuncture Treatment

- **Manipulation:** Reinforcing method for deficiency patterns, reducing or even method for excess patterns.
- **Prescription:** BL15 Xinshu CV14 Juque HT7 Shenmen PC6 Neiguan
- **Supplementary points:**

  - Qi deficiency. + HT5 Tongli; GB40 Qiuxu

  - Blood deficiency. + BL17 Geshu; BL20 Pishu; ST36 Zusanli

  - Empty fire. + BL14 Jueyinshu; KI3 Taixi; BL23 Shenshu

  - Phlegm-heat. + ST40 Fenglong; BL19 Danshu; LU5 Chize

  - Cold congested fluids. + CV9 Shuifen; CV4 Guanyuan; CV8 Shenque; SP9 Yinlingquan

  - Blood stasis. + PC3 Quze; HT3 Shaohai; CV6 Qihai; SP10 Xuehai

Practical Hints

• **Metal, shell and mineral substances tend to injure the spleen and stomach if use for long periods of time.** Since the main symptoms are palpitations and uneasiness related to heart dysfunction, herbs that anchor and sedate the heart spirit, or nourish the heart to calm the spirit, should be used accordingly to the excess or deficient nature of the pattern. However, herbs that anchor and sedate the heart spirit are not recommended for long-term use.

• **A comprehensive examination including both pulse and clinical manifestations is essential.** Palpitations are generally subjective. An irregular pulse might or might not be detected. Commonly occurring irregular pulses are hasty, knotted, and intermittent. These pulses can appear alone or in combination. Occasionally, an irregular pulse will be found in a patient with emotional trauma or extreme sadness; however, it only lasts for a short period of time. Palpitations accompanied by an irregular pulse usually indicate severe or critical depletion of heart qi or heart yang.

CHAPTER 7

Chest Painful Obstruction

胸痹 *Xiong Bi*

The Chinese definition of *bi* is closure, shutting down, or obstruction; therefore, chest *bi* refers to a group of symptoms caused by obstruction of qi and blood in the chest. Chest painful obstruction syndrome, or chest *bi*, is characterized by chest oppression and stabbing pain that radiates to the left upper back, shoulder and down to the arm. Accompanying respiratory symptoms are shortness of breath, dyspnea, and difficulty breathing when lying down. A stuffy sensation in the chest and difficulty breathing are present in mild cases, whereas a sharp crushing cardiac pain radiating through the thoracic cavity to the back is found in severe cases.

Relevant Diseases

- Angina pectoris
- Myocardial infarction
- Coronary artery disease
- Ischemic heart disease
- Rheumatic heart disease
- Bronchitis
- Pneumonia
- Pleurisy
- Pulmonary emphysema
- Carcinoma of the lung
- Intercostal neuralgia

Etiology and Pathogenesis

Invasion by external cold pathogenic factor: Exterior cold can directly invade the chest and obstruct the circulation of yang qi. Pre-existing yang deficiency, especially of the chest, creates susceptibility to exterior cold. When cold accumulates in the chest and yang qi is deficient, the conjunction leads to inadequate warming and circulation of qi and blood. The result is qi and blood stagnation, causing obstruction in the chest and, thus, chest pain.

Improper diet: Excessive consumption of greasy, raw and cold food hinders the function of the spleen and stomach. Water that is not transformed and transported into body fluid forms phlegm. Phlegm blocks the circulation of qi and blood in the channels and vessels and causes chest pain.

Emotional stress: The spleen is susceptible to worry and pensiveness. These two emotional factors weaken the spleen. Adequate amounts of the qi and blood cannot be generated when the spleen is weak. Insufficient qi fails to facilitate the circulation of blood, and the deficient blood fail to properly nourish the heart, leading to chest pain. In addition, anger and frustration can affect the liver and cause liver qi stagnation. Stagnant qi leads to blood stasis, resulting in chest pain.

Aging and deficient constitution: Deterioration of the kidney due to aging and constitutional deficiency may also be a factor causing chest pain. Kidney yang is the foundation of yang qi in the body; when kidney yang declines, heart yang becomes sluggish. Lack of warming by heart yang and poor circulation in the heart vessels can cause chest pain. Likewise, when kidney yin degenerates, heart yin and blood deficiency will follow. Consequently, circulation in the heart vessels becomes sluggish due to lack of nourishment from yin, causing pain.

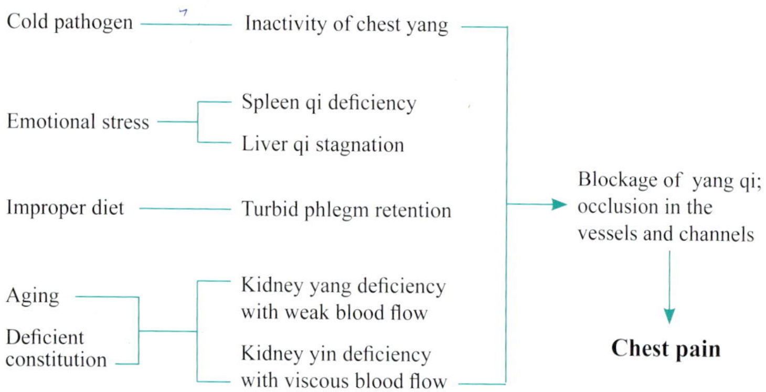

Diagnosis

A. Identification of excess and deficiency:

Chest *bi* is always a combination of deficiency and excess. The root is usually a deficiency of the spleen, heart, and kidney or a combined deficiency of these three organs. The branches are related to an excess of blood stasis, congealed cold, qi stagnation and/or phlegm accumulation.

B. Identification of the characteristics of pain:

- Oppressive pain, with
  - Altered severity depending on emotional status – Qi stagnation.
  - Distention and dull pain aggravated by exertion with shortness of breath, fatigue and spontaneous sweating – Heart qi deficiency.
  - Obesity, cough with excessive sputum and greasy tongue coating – Phlegm accumulation.

- Stabbing pain, with
  - Throbbing and crushing pain at a fixed location, and purple tongue with petechiae or dark purple sublingual veins – Blood stasis.
- Spasmodic pain, with
  - Sudden onset of excruciating pain accompanied by cold limbs, a sensation of suffocation, and symptoms aggravated by cold – Cold in the heart vessels.
  - Cold intolerance, lying in a fetal position and flabby pale tongue – Yang deficiency with empty cold.

C. Complications of chest painful obstruction syndrome:

Zhen xin tong (true cardiac pain): As the disorder progresses, paroxysmal chest *bi* can develop into true cardiac pain. This is characterized by sudden, severe and persistent chest pain due to complete occlusion of channels and vessels in the chest by blood stasis, turbid phlegm and excess cold.

Irregular pulse (arrhythmias): Paroxysmal chest *bi* may also give rise to an irregular pulse. This is caused by pathogenic influences obstructing the free flow of heart yang and blocking the blood circulation. Irregular pulse manifests as subjective palpitations or a palpable knotted, intermittent pulse.

Cold congested fluids overflowing towards the heart (heart failure): Extreme deficiency of heart and kidney yang causes cold water to spill over to the heart and deplete the heart yang. Clinical manifestations include cough, wheezing with copious watery sputum, palpitations and systemic pitting edema.

D. Differential diagnosis of similar disorders:

Chest *bi*: Pain is characteristically stabbing, with a sensation of oppression in the chest, and radiating to the left shoulder and arm. The pain is accompanied by palpitations, shortness of breath, cold limbs, perspiration and a knotted or intermittent pulse. It is frequently seen in middle-aged or elderly patients with a history of heart disease or hyperlipidemia. It is usually induced by overexertion, overeating or emotional stress. It occurs suddenly.

Zhen xin tong (true cardiac pain): As a severe complication progressing from chest *bi*, *zhen xin tong* is critical and fatal. This type of chest pain is constant, brutal and stabbing; it is usually accompanied by profuse sweating, clammy cold extremities, pale complexion and cyanotic tongue, lips, hands and feet. The pulse may be weak and deep, knotted or intermittent.

Epigastric pain: Atypical chest *bi* may present clinically as pain in the epigastrium, and can easily be confused with epigastric pain syndrome. True epigastric pain is a distending pain located in the epigastrium, and may radiate to the corresponding region in the back. Other symptoms include nausea, vomiting or acid regurgitation. The onset of epigastric pain is not age specific and is usually caused by improper diet.

Suspended fluids (*xuan yin*): Congested fluids accumulated in the chest and hypochondrium is known as suspended fluids. Manifestations include chest and hypochondriac pain aggravated by coughing, spitting, deep breathing and movement of the thorax.

Basic Patterns

- Heart blood stasis
- Congealed cold in the chest
- Qi and yin deficiency
- Turbid phlegm accumulation
- Heart and kidney yin deficiency
- Yang qi exhaustion

Differentiation and Treatment

Treatment principle:

Chest *bi* is rooted in deficiency and has an excess branch. It is a critical and fatal condition; therefore, the first priority is to treat the manifestation by expelling the pathogenic occlusion. Tonifying the righteous qi is a secondary concern once the patient's life is no longer threatened.

Methods of expelling pathogens include utilizing acrid and warm herbs to unblock the obstruction of yang qi, invigorate the blood and transform stasis, and dissolve turbid phlegm.

Methods of supporting the righteous qi include warming and tonifying yang qi, nourishing the yin and tonifying both qi and yin.

Heart blood stasis

Fixed stabbing chest pain, especially at night.

S: Palpitations, restlessness and cyanotic lips.

T: Dark purple tongue with petechiae or dark purple sublingual veins. **P:** Deep and choppy.

- Invigorate the blood, unblock the channels and alleviate pain.
- *Xue Fu Zhu Yu Tang*

  - *Tao Ren*, *Hong Hua*, *Chuan Xiong*, *Chi Shao* and *Dang Gui* invigorate the blood and expel stasis.

  - *Chai Hu* spreads constrained liver qi and *Zhi Qiao* promotes the movement of qi. In this combination, one ascends while the other descends to regulate the qi flow; therefore, qi moves and blood circulates.

- *Niu Xi* guides the movement of blood downwards.

- Strengthen the effect of invigorating the blood to alleviate pain. + *Yan Hu Suo*
  Expand the chest and regulate the qi. + *Gua Lou Pi, Qing Pi, Xuan Fu Hua*
  Mild chest *bi*, use *Dan Shen Yin*.

Turbid phlegm accumulation

Oppressive pain with a sensation of suffocation, possibly radiating through the left shoulder down the arm.
S: Obesity, sensation of heaviness, shortness of breath and copious sputum.
T: White greasy coating. **P:** Slippery.

- Unblock the obstruction of yang qi and resolve phlegm.
- *Gua Lou Xie Bai Ban Xia Tang*
  - *Gua Lou* expands the chest and transforms phlegm.
  - *Ban Xia* transforms phlegm and descends the rebellious qi.
  - *Xie Bai* unblocks the obstruction and dissipates clumps.
- Warm the yang and regulate the qi to resolve phlegm. + *Gan Jiang, Chen Pi*
  Complicated by blood stasis. + *Shi Xiao San*

Congealed cold in the chest

Acute onset of chest pain radiating to the back, aggravated or triggered by cold.
S: Oppressive pain with shortness of breath, palpitations, breathlessness, pale complexion and frigid extremities.
T: White coating. **P:** Deep and thready.

- Unblock the obstruction of yang qi and dispel cold.
- *Gua Lou Xie Bai Bai Jiu Tang*
  - *Xie Bai* and *Bai Jiu* are used to unblock the yang and dissipate clumps.
  - *Gua Lou* expands the chest and transforms phlegm.
- Strengthen the effect of warming the yang and dispelling cold. + *Gui Zhi*
  Strengthen the effect of invigorating the blood and regulating the qi. + *Zhi Shi, Tan Xiang, Dan Shen*
  For *zhen xin tong*, caused by severe congealed cold, use *Su He Xiang Wan*.

Heart and kidney yin deficiency

Intermittent chest oppression, dull and burning chest pain, and palpitations.
S: Night sweating, restlessness, insomnia, soreness and weakness of the lower back and knees, dizziness and tinnitus.
T: Red tongue with scanty coating or petechiae. **P:** Thready, rapid or choppy.

- Nourish kidney and heart yin, and calm the spirit.
- *Zuo Gui Yin*
  - *Shu Di Huang*, *Shan Zhu Yu* and *Gou Qi Zi* nourish the yin and benefit the kidney.
  - *Shan Yao*, *Fu Ling* and *Gan Cao* strengthen the spleen to support the generating source of qi and blood.
- Significant heart yin deficiency with irritability and insomnia. + *Mai Men Dong, Wu Wei Zi, Suan Zao Ren*
  Severe chest pain. + *Dang Gui, Dan Shen, Chuan Xiong, Yu Jin*
  Yin deficiency with yang rising. + *Gou Teng, Shi Jue Ming, Bie Jia*

Qi and yin deficiency

Intermittent dull and oppressive chest pain, shortness of breath, and palpitations aggravated by exertion.
S: Fatigue, reluctance to speak, dizziness and vertigo.
T: Slightly red tongue or with teeth marks. **P:** Knotted or intermittent, thready and weak.

- Tonify the qi and nourish the yin, invigorate the blood and unblock the obstruction in the channels.
- *Sheng Mai San* and *Ren Shen Yang Ying Tang*
  - *Ren Shen* greatly tonifies basal qi.
  - *Huang Qi*, *Fu Ling*, *Bai Zhu* and *Gan Cao* augment the qi and strengthen the spleen.
  - *Mai Men Dong*, *Bai Shao*, *Dang Gui* and *Di Huang* replenish the yin and nourish the blood.
  - *Yuan Zhi* and *Wu Wei Zi* nourish the heart and calm the spirit.
- Severe oppressive chest pain. + *Dan Shen, Yu Jin, Wu Ling Zhi*
  Deficiency of heart qi and blood with palpitations and an irregular pulse, use *Zhi Gan Cao Tang*.

Yang qi exhaustion

Chest oppression and shortness of breath, dull pain or colic pain, condition aggravated by cold, and chest pain radiating to the back in severe cases.
S: Palpitations, sweating, fatigue, cold intolerance, frigid extremities, pale complexion, and pale or cyanotic lips, nails and tongue.
T: Pale or dark purple tongue. **P:** Deep, thready or minute.

- Tonify yang qi, invigorate the blood and unblock the obstruction in the channels.

- *Shen Fu Tang* and *You Gui Yin*
  - *Ren Shen* greatly tonifies basal qi and rescues the collapsed qi.
  - *Fu Zi* and *Rou Gui* tonify the fire in the Gate of Vitality and assist the yang.
  - *Shu Di Huang*, *Shan Zhu Yu*, *Shan Yao*, *Gou Qi Zi* and *Du Zhong* tonify the kidney and augment the essence.
- Heart yang collapse with cyanotic complexion, lips and nails, profuse sweating, frigid extremities and minute pulse, increase the dosage of *Shen Fu Tang*, + *Long Gu*, *Mu Li*

  Kidney yang deficiency and cold congested fluids overflowing towards the heart with palpitations, breathlessness, orthopnea, oliguria and systemic edema, use *Zhen Wu Tang*.

Acupuncture Treatment

Heart blood stasis:

- **Manipulation:** Reducing method.
- **Prescription:**

CV17 Tanzhong	CV14 Juque	BL17 Geshu
HT6 Yinxi	BL15 Xinshu	

Turbid phlegm accumulation:

- **Manipulation:** Reducing method.
- **Prescription:**

CV17 Tanzhong	CV14 Juque	PC4 Ximen
LU9 Taiyuan	ST40 Fenglong	

Congealed cold in the chest:

- **Manipulation:** Reducing method and moxibustion.
- **Prescription:**

BL15 Xinshu	BL14 Jueyinshu	PC6 Neiguan
HT5 Tongli	CV4 Guanyuan	

Heart and kidney yin deficiency:

- **Manipulation:** Even method.
- **Prescription:**

BL15 Xinshu	BL23 Shenshu	HT6 Yinxi
KI3 Taixi	CV17 Tanzhong	BL17 Geshu

Qi and yin deficiency:

- **Manipulation:** Reinforcing method and moxibustion.
- **Prescription:**

BL15 Xinshu	PC6 Neiguan	CV17 Tanzhong
ST36 Zusanli	BL17 Geshu	

Yang qi exhaustion:

- **Manipulation:** Reinforcing method and moxibustion.
- **Prescription:** BL23 Shenshu, CV4 Guanyuan, CV17 Tanzhong, PC6 Neiguan, HT5 Tongli, BL15 Xinshu

Practical Hints

• **Use herbs that are acrid, warm and drying in nature with caution; avoid overuse of rich and cloying herbs.** Chest *bi* is a complicated disorder of excess and deficiency. Pure excess or deficiency patterns are rarely seen. Herbs with an acrid, warm and drying nature should be used to treat qi stagnation, blood stasis, cold pathogenic invasion or turbid phlegm retention in the excess patterns. Overuse of these herbs may injure the body fluid, disturb the blood and exacerbate the deficient condition. Herbs with a sweet, rich and cloying nature can be utilized to replenish the vital substances in treatments for heart qi deficiency, and heart and kidney yin or yang deficiency. Overuse of these herbs may contribute to qi stagnation, dampness accumulation or blood stasis.

• **Carefully differentiate excess and deficient cold.** Both excess and deficient cold share similar clinical presentations; however, they have different courses of progress and prognosis.

Excess cold is characterized by chest pain that radiates through the back, inability to lie flat, difficulty in breathing, cold limbs, deep and tight pulse. It can progress into *zhen xin tong* with constant severe chest pain. The progress of chest *bi* to *zhen xin tong* is similar to that of angina pectoris developing into myocardial infarction in modern medicine. Treatment is predominated by dispersing the cold pathogen.

Empty cold is characterized by chest pain that radiates to the back, profuse sweating, clammy cold extremities, and thready deep pulse. It can progress into heart yang collapse with profuse sweating, chest oppression, shortness of breath, cyanotic complexion, lips and nails, and minute pulse. The development of chest *bi* into heart yang collapse is similar to that of angina pectoris developing into cardiogenic shock or heart failure. Treatment is predominated by tonifying and rescuing the collapsed yang.

• **Manage diet appropriately.** It is essential to maintain a low-sodium and low-fat diet. Avoid dietary overindulgence. Preventing constipation is necessary because straining with bowel movements might elicit chest painful obstruction.

CHAPTER 8

Insomnia

失眠 *Shi Mian*

Insomnia is identified as the inability to experience normal sleep, and this is its major clinical manifestation. This disorder consists of various presentations, including difficulty falling asleep (difficulty sleeping), frequent waking during the night with inability to return to sleep (early awakening), a restless state between sleep and wakefulness, inability to enter a deep sleep or having nightmares (light sleep), dream-disturbed sleep, and inability to sleep the whole night through (sleeplessness). Headaches, dizziness, palpitations and forgetfulness commonly accompany insomnia.

Relevant Diseases

- Neurosis
- Hypertension
- Cerebral arteriosclerosis
- Anemia
- Mental disorders

Etiology and Pathogenesis

The amount and quality of sleep depend on the state of the mind, which is rooted in the heart and nourished by heart blood and heart yin. Insomnia is induced by pathogenic factors agitating the heart, or by malnourishment of the mind.

Emotional stress: Anger injures the liver, causing liver qi stagnation and blazing liver fire that disturbs the mind. Pensiveness injures the spleen, leading to deficient qi and blood, which fail to nurture the heart. Overexertion and excessive thinking exhaust heart blood, which fails to nourish the spirit.

Prolonged illness that weakens the constitution and exhausts kidney yin: Deficient kidney yin fails to nourish heart yin which also becomes deficient; heart yang becomes hyperactive and empty fire agitates the mind.

Qi deficiency of the heart and gallbladder: A constitutional weakness of both the heart and gallbladder may shape a personality that is timid, cowardly, fearful and indecisive. Sleep will be light with frequent awakenings during the night accompanied by panic, frightening dreams and palpitations.

Improper diet: Overeating or excessive consumption of greasy, spicy food can turn into food stagnation and phlegm-heat in the stomach. Stomach qi rebels upwards and phlegm-heat harasses the mind.

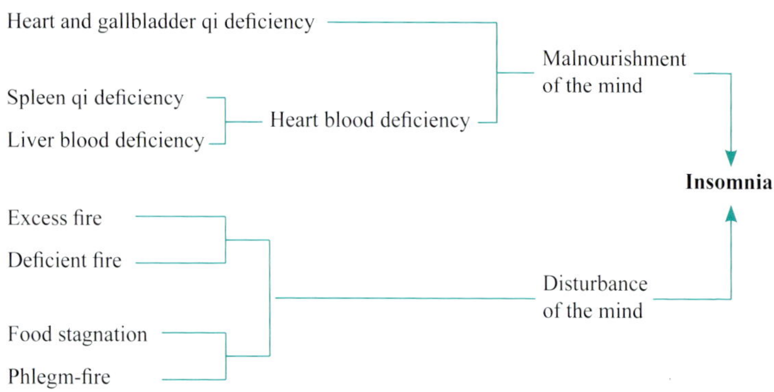

Diagnosis

A. Identification of excess and deficiency:

Excess: Insomnia is caused by excess pathogenic factors disturbing the mind. The pathogenic factors include fire (liver fire, heart fire, phlegm-heat and residual heat), food stagnation, phlegm accumulation, and disharmony of the stomach qi.

Deficiency: Insomnia is due to yin and blood deficiency which fails to nourish the heart and mind. Deficiency patterns involve the heart, spleen, liver and kidney.

B. Rule out temporary and secondary insomnia:

Primary insomnia is not caused by a sudden change in weather, drinking a lot of tea or coffee before bedtime, emotional distress or excitement, noise or stimulation by bright light. Do not diagnose insomnia when sleep is disturbed by other illnesses, such as asthma, cough, pain, or itching from a skin disorder.

Basic Patterns

Excess patterns:

- Liver qi stagnation turning into fire
- Phlegm-heat disturbance
- Disharmony of stomach qi

Deficiency patterns:

- Lack of communication between the heart and kidney
- Heart and spleen deficiency
- Heart and gallbladder qi deficiency

Differentiation and Treatment

Treatment principle:

Regulate the yin and yang, tonify deficiency and drain excess.

Excess: Clear fire, transform phlegm, and harmonize the middle burner to calm the mind.

Deficiency: Augment the qi, nourish the blood, and tonify the liver and kidney to nourish and calm the mind.

Excess patterns:

Liver qi stagnation turning into fire

Difficulty falling asleep, unpleasant dreams or nightmares, agitation and short temper.

S: Thirst, bitter taste in the mouth, red eyes, constipation and dark yellow urine.

T: Red tongue with yellow coating. **P:** Rapid and wiry.

- Soothe the liver, drain liver fire and calm the spirit.
- *Long Dan Xie Gan Tang*
  - *Long Dan Cao*, *Huang Qin* and *Zhi Zi* clear and drain liver fire.
  - *Ze Xie*, *Mu Tong* and *Che Qian Zi* clear and drain damp-heat.
  - *Dang Gui* and *Sheng Di Huang* nourish and cool the blood.
  - *Chai Hu* soothes the liver and regulates the qi.
- To strengthen the effect of tranquilizing the mind. + *Fu Shen, Long Gu, Mu Li, Zhen Zhu Mu*

  Accompanied by distention and pain in the hypochondriac region, relieved after sighing. + *Yu Jin, Xiang Fu, Chuan Lian Zi*

Phlegm-heat disturbance

Difficulty falling asleep, restless sleep, irritability, profuse sputum, chest stuffiness, and heaviness of the head.

S: Aversion to food, nausea, vomiting, sour regurgitation, bitter taste in the mouth and dizziness.

T: Yellow greasy coating. **P:** Rapid and slippery.

- Resolve phlegm, clear heat, harmonize the middle burner and calm the spirit.
- *Huang Lian Wen Dan Tang*
  - *Huang Lian* clears and drains fire from the heart.
  - *Ban Xia*, *Chen Pi* and *Fu Ling* dry dampness, resolve phlegm, descend rebellious qi and harmonize the stomach.
  - *Zhi Shi* descends rebellious qi and resolves phlegm.

- *Zhu Ru* clears heat, descends rebellious qi and transforms phlegm, as well as eliminates irritability and stops vomiting.

- Palpitations with terrors and mental restlessness. + *Zhen Zhu Mu, Long Chi*
  Phlegm and food stagnation. + *Shen Qu, Shan Zha, Lai Fu Zi*

Disharmony of stomach qi

Restless sleep, discomfort and distention in the epigastrium and abdomen.
S: Poor appetite, belching, sour and foul-smelling vomit containing undigested food, and irregular bowel movements.
T: Thick and greasy coating. **P:** Slippery.

- Reduce food retention and harmonize the stomach.

- *Bao He Wan*
  - *Shan Zha* is the chief herb; it reduces food stagnation of all kinds.
  - *Shen Qu* and *Lai Fu Zi* eliminate food retention and guide out stagnation.
  - *Ban Xia*, bitter and warm, dries dampness, transforms phlegm, descends rebellious qi and harmonizes the stomach.
  - *Chen Pi* regulates the qi and transforms phlegm.
  - *Fu Ling* strengthens the spleen and harmonizes the middle burner.
  - *Lian Qiao* clears and eliminates constrained heat.

- To enhance the effects of transforming phlegm and calming the spirit. + *Shi Chang Pu, Yuan Zhi*
  In severe cases of food stagnation. + *Mu Xiang, Zhi Shi, Bing Lang*
  Constipation. + *Tiao Wei Cheng Qi Tang*

Deficient patterns:

Lack of communication between the heart and kidney

Insomnia with irritability, palpitations, anxiety, dizziness, tinnitus and forgetfulness.
S: Soreness of the lower back, nocturnal emission, night sweating, five-centers heat and dry mouth.
T: Red tongue with scanty coating. **P:** Rapid and thready.

- Nourish the yin, drain fire, nourish the heart and calm the spirit.

- *Tian Wang Bu Xin Dan*
  - *Sheng Di Huang*, *Xuan Shen*, *Mai Men Dong* and *Tian Men Dong* nourish the yin and clear empty heat.
  - *Dan Shen* and *Dang Gui* nourish the blood.
  - *Ren Shen* and *Fu Ling* benefit the qi and quiet the heart.
  - *Suan Zao Ren* and *Bai Zi Ren* nourish the blood and calm the spirit.

- *Wu Wei Zi* astringes heart qi and calms the spirit.
- *Yuan Zhi* communicates the heart with the kidney.

- Yang hyperactivity with a slightly red face, dizziness and tinnitus. + *Mu Li, Gui Ban, Ci Shi*

  Yin deficiency with significant empty fire, manifested as five-centers heat, night sweating, and nocturnal emission, use *Huang Lian E Jiao Tang*.

Heart and spleen deficiency

Insomnia, excessive dreaming, easily awakened, palpitations and forgetfulness.
S: Dizziness and vertigo, fatigue, poor appetite and dull complexion.
T: Pale tongue with thin coating. **P:** Weak and thready.

- Tonify the heart and spleen to generate qi and blood.
- *Gui Pi Tang*
  - *Ren Shen*, *Huang Qi*, *Bai Zhu* and *Gan Cao* are sweet and warm herbs; they benefit the qi and strengthen the spleen.
  - *Dang Gui* and *Long Yan Rou* replenish the blood and nourish the heart.
  - *Suan Zao Ren*, *Fu Shen* and *Yuan Zhi* nourish the heart and calm the spirit.
  - *Mu Xiang* facilitates the qi flow, revives the spleen, and prevents stagnation from excessive tonification.
- Enhance the effects of sedating the restless heart spirit. + *Long Gu, Mu Li, Ye Jiao Teng*

  Liver blood deficiency with insomnia, irritability, palpitations and night sweating, use *Suan Zao Ren Tang*.

Heart and gallbladder qi deficiency

Light sleep, excessive dreaming, easily awakened with pavor, fearfulness and palpitations.
S: Timid, easily frightened or startled, shortness of breath, fatigue and clear abundant urine.
T: Pale tongue. **P:** Thready and wiry.

- Augment the qi, calm the spirit and settle the will.
- *An Shen Ding Zhi Wan*
  - *Ren Shen* and *Fu Ling* augment heart qi.
  - *Long Chi* sedates and tranquilizes the heart.
  - *Fu Shen*, *Yuan Zhi* and *Shi Chang Pu* calm the spirit.
- To strengthen the effects of nourishing the heart and calming the mind. + *Suan Zao Ren, Wu Wei Zi*

Acupuncture Treatment

- **Manipulation:** Reinforcing method in the deficient patterns, reducing method in the excess patterns. Use even method in the pattern of lack of communication between the heart and kidney.
- **Prescription:** HT7 Shenmen SP6 Sanyinjiao Extra13 Anmian
- **Supplementary points:**

  - Liver fire. + BL18 Ganshu; BL19 Danshu; GB12 Wangu

  - Phlegm-heat. + ST40 Fenglong; BL19 Danshu; LU5 Chize

  - Disharmony of stomach qi. +BL21 Weishu; ST45 Lidui; ST36 Zusanli

  - Lack of communication between the heart and kidney. + BL15 Xinshu; BL23 Shenshu; KI3 Taixi

  - Heart and spleen deficiency. + BL20 Pishu; BL15 Xinshu; SP1 Yinbai

  - Heart and gallbladder qi deficiency. + HT5 Tongli; GB40 Qiuxu

Practical Hints

• **When treating insomnia, treat the root causes first and foremost, then add herbs that anchor or nourish to calm the spirit according to the patterns of excess or deficiency.** To treat insomnia due to excess pathogenic factors that disturb the spirit, predominantly use herbs that anchor, settle and calm the mind, and add a small quantity of herbs that nourish the heart and calm the mind; vice versa for treating insomnia due to deficiency of qi, blood, yin and fluid.

• One of the traditional approaches to treating insomnia, known as "draining the south and tonifying the north", is appropriate for insomnia due to lack of communication between the heart and kidney. The herbal formulas *Tian Wang Bu Xin Dan*, *Huang Lian E Jiao Tang*, and *Jiao Tai Wan* all utilize this treatment method. The heart pertains to fire (south) while the kidney pertains to water (north). The heart and kidney must be in a state of balance as they represent the two fundamental poles of the yang and yin. In a harmonious state, they mutually support each other. In the case of kidney yin deficiency, water fails to nourish the heart and empty fire flares in the heart. Hyperactivity of heart fire leads to mental restlessness, insomnia, irritability and palpitations. **"Draining the south and tonifying the north" is draining heart fire and nourishing kidney water to restore communication between the heart and kidney, thus re-establishing their equilibrium.**

[Addendum]

Somnolence

多寐 *Duo Mei*

Somnolence is characterized by constant sleepiness, regardless of the time of day or night. A person with somnolence can be awakened, but falls back to sleep immediately.

Yang represents excitement, activity and a state of wakefulness. In insomnia, which is a state of imbalance between yin and yang, yang predominates.

Yin represents inhibition, inactivity and a state of sleepiness. In somnolence, also a state of imbalance between yin and yang, yin predominates.

Differentiation and Treatment

Excessive dampness

Most often seen during rainy seasons or in obesity condition; caused by excessive phlegm-dampness and deficiency of spleen yang. Manifestations include sleepiness, stifling sensation in the chest, poor appetite and a heavy sensation.
T: White greasy coating. **P:** Decelerating and soft.

- Dry dampness and strengthen the spleen.
- *Ping Wei San*
  - *Cang Zhu*, bitter and warm, dries dampness and strengthens the spleen.
  - *Hou Po* facilitates the qi flow, transforms dampness and reduces fullness.
  - *Chen Pi* facilitates the qi flow and strengthens the spleen.
  - *Gan Cao* augments the qi and harmonizes the middle burner.
- Increase the aromatic effect to dry dampness. + *Huo Xiang, Pei Lan*
  Excessive phlegm. + *Ban Xia, Shi Chang Pu*

Spleen qi deficiency

Deficient spleen qi is too weak to transform and transport efficiently. Manifestations include sleepiness aggravated after meals, sensation of heaviness and lassitude.
T: No significant change. **P:** No significant change.

- Augment the qi and strengthen the spleen.
- *Liu Jun Zi Tang*
  - *Si Jun Zi Tang* tonifies the qi and strengthens the spleen.
  - *Ban Xia* and *Chen Pi* dry dampness, transform phlegm, facilitate the qi flow and harmonize the middle burner.
- Complicated by food retention. + *Mai Ya, Shan Zha, Shen Qu*

Spleen yang deficiency

Usually occurs in prolonged illnesses or the elderly. Manifestations include sleepiness, lassitude, reluctance to speak, spontaneous sweating, cold intolerance and cold limbs.

T: Pale tongue. **P:** Weak.

- Warm the yang and augment the qi.
- *Li Zhong Wan*
  - *Gan Jiang* warms the middle burner and disperses cold.
  - *Ren Shen*, *Bai Zhu* and *Gan Cao* strengthen the spleen and augment the qi.
- Accompanied by kidney yang deficiency. + *Fu Zi*

CHAPTER 9

Epigastric Pain

胃脘痛 *Wei Wan Tong*

Epigastric pain refers to a painful sensation located between the lower margin of the sternum and the infracostal margins. Epigastric pain varies in severity and is accompanied by focal distention in the epigastrium, belching, acid regurgitation, lack of appetite, and hypochondriac and abdominal distention; the pain is often recurrent. Chronic epigastric pain that is accompanied by hematemesis, tarry stool, vomiting and dysphagia usually has a poor prognosis.

Relevant Diseases

- Acute or chronic gastritis
- Peptic ulcer
- Upper gastrointestinal bleeding
- Gastroptosis
- Prolapse of gastric mucosa
- Gastro-neurosis
- Duodenitis
- Pancreatitis
- Gastric cancer

Etiology and Pathogenesis

Exterior pathogens attacking the stomach, especially cold, will obstruct the flow of stomach qi by preventing it from descending. Various pathogens cause different types of pain; due to its congealing nature, a cold pathogen induces severe colic pain.

Improper diet injuring the stomach: Excessive indulgence in alcohol, tobacco and a greasy diet easily impairs the descending function of the stomach and leads to food retention, which results in stagnation of stomach qi.

Stagnated liver qi overacting on the stomach: Emotional stress impairs the function of the liver to ensure the smooth flow of qi. Liver qi stagnation can overact on the stomach and obstruct the movement of stomach qi.

Deficiency of the spleen and stomach: Improper diet, overexertion, chronic illness or an overdose of cold-natured medicinals may damage the spleen yang or stomach yin. Spleen yang deficiency generates internal cold which congeals the movement of qi and the circulation of blood, resulting in pain. Pain caused by stomach yin deficiency is due to malnourishment of the stomach.

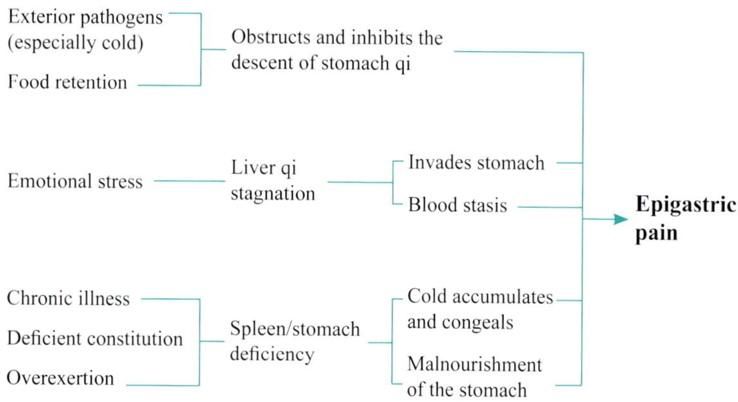

Diagnosis

A. Identification of cold and heat:

Cold patterns are characterized by absence of thirst and colic epigastric pain. The pain is triggered or aggravated by cold and raw foods and/or invasion by exterior cold; warm compresses or drinking warm beverages can alleviate this type of pain.

Heat patterns are characterized by thirst or a bitter taste in the mouth, bad breath and constipation. The pain is urgent and burning, and may be relieved by cold beverages or cold compresses.

B. Identification of excess and deficiency:

Excess patterns have an acute onset with constant intolerable pain which is aggravated by pressure, eating or taking tonics. Excess patterns are frequently seen in youths and adults. Deficiency patterns have a slow onset with dull pain that is relieved by pressure and eating. Overexertion or use of purgative herbs aggravates the pain. Deficiency patterns are often seen in elderly people or patients with chronic illness.

C. Identification of qi stagnation and blood stasis:

Qi stagnation: Patterns involving qi stagnation usually have a recent onset with distending and migrating pain. Pain is often accompanied by distention and fullness in the epigatrium and abdomen, and frequent belching.

Blood stasis: Patterns related to blood stasis have a chronic onset. The pain is stabbing with a fixed location or accompanied by hematemesis and tarry stool.

D. Identification of organ involvement:

Pain related to the liver is recurrent, migrating and distending, and is elicited by emotional stress. The pain radiates to the hypochondriac region.

Pain related to the spleen has a prolonged course. Dull pain is aggravated by hunger and alleviated after meals. Common manifestations include a sallow complexion, fatigue, loose stool and a decelerating pulse.

Pain related to the stomach has an acute onset and is usually caused by invasion of exterior pathogens or by improper diet. Constant pain with fullness and distention, frequent belching, irregular or incomplete bowel movements and a slippery pulse is a typical presentation.

E. Differential diagnosis of epigastric pain and true cardiac pain:

Epigastric pain: Is not usually age specific. A history of stomach disorders might be or might not be apparent. Frequent belching, acid regurgitation, poor appetite and irregular bowel movements are common in epigastric pain.

True cardiac pain (*zhen xin tong*): Usually occurs in middle-aged or elderly people with a history of heart disease. Left-sided chest pain is accompanied by chest congestion, palpitations, shortness of breath, profuse sweating, cold limbs, and cyanotic lips and nails. An intermittent or knotted pulse is evident. When encounter a patient who is at middle-aged or older complaining severe "epigastric pain", EKG and other laboratory tests are indicated to rule out possible cardiact conditions.

Basic Patterns

- Cold invading the stomach
- Retention of food
- Stagnant liver qi invading the stomach
- Congested liver fire invading the stomach
- Blood stasis in the stomach
- Stomach yin deficiency
- Yang deficiency of the spleen and stomach

Differentiation and Treatment

Treatment principle:

Regulate the qi, harmonize the stomach and descend rebellious qi.

When epigastric pain is related to the stomach, modify the methods of dispersing cold, eliminating food stagnation, clearing heat and transforming blood stasis according to the pattern differentiation. If the pain is related to the liver, soothe the liver qi, promote the movement of qi and blood, clear heat from the liver and expel stasis from the collaterals. To treat epigastric pain related to the spleen, strengthen the spleen and benefit the qi or warm spleen yang and raise sunken qi.

Cold invading the stomach

Sudden onset of severe colic epigastric pain alleviated by application of warmth or drinking warm beverages; aggravated by cold and pressure.
S: No thirst and/or desire for warm beverages.
T: Thin and white coating. **P:** Wiry and tight.

- Disperse cold, warm the stomach and alleviate pain.

- *Liang Fu Wan*
  - *Gao Liang Jiang* warms the stomach and disperses cold.
  - *Xiang Fu* facilitates the qi flow and alleviates pain.

- Excessive cold. + *Wu Zhu Yu, Sheng Jiang*
  Accompanied by a severe wind-cold exterior condition. + *Su Ye, Fang Feng*
  Accompanied by food stagnation. + *Zhi Qiao, Shen Qu, Ji Nei Jin, Ban Xia, Sheng Jiang*
  Mild cases, topical warm compression is appicable, or take decoction of *Sheng Jiang* with black sugar.

Retention of food

Dull epigastric pain with fullness and distention, belching, acid regurgitation and foul breath.
S: Nausea, vomiting undigested food, pain alleviated by belching, vomiting or passing flatus, and alternating loose stool and constipation.
T: Thick and greasy coating. **P:** Slippery.

- Eliminate food retention and promote digestion.

- *Bao He Wan*
  - *Shan Zha*, as the chief herb, reduces food stagnation of all kinds.
  - *Shen Qu* and *Lai Fu Zi* reduce food retention and guide out stagnation.
  - *Ban Xia* and *Chen Pi* dry dampness and facilitate the qi flow.
  - *Fu Ling* strengthens the spleen and harmonizes the middle burner.
  - *Lian Qiao* clears and disperses stagnant heat.

- To strengthen the effects of promoting the qi movement and reducing food retention. + *Zhi Shi, Bing Lang*
  Accompanied by constipation. + *Xiao Cheng Qi Tang*
  Accompanied by constipation, severe abdominal pain that resists pressure and a dry yellow tongue coating. + *Da Cheng Qi Tang*

Stagnant liver qi invading the stomach

Distending epigastric pain that radiates toward both hypochondriac regions, elicited or aggravated by emotional strain.
S: Poor appetite, belching, and long and deep sighing.
T: Thin and white coating. **P:** Deep and wiry.

- Soothe the liver and regulate the qi.
- *Chai Hu Shu Gan San*
  - *Chai Hu* spreads constrained liver qi and facilitates the qi flow.
  - *Xiang Fu*, *Chuan Xiong* and *Shao Yao* facilitate qi flow, invigorate the blood and transform stasis to alleviate pain.
  - *Chen Pi* and *Zhi Qiao* facilitate the qi flow, transform stagnation and harmonize the middle burner.
- Enhance the effects of regulating the qi and relieving stagnation to alleviate pain. + *Yu Jin, Yan Hu Suo, Qing Pi, Mu Xiang*
  Excessive belching. + *Chen Xiang, Xuan Fu Hua*
  Liver qi stagnation turning into liver fire. + *Zhi Zi, Mu Dan Pi*

Congested liver fire invading the stomach

Acute and sudden burning epigastric pain with acid regurgitation and gastric discomfort.
S: Irritability, short temper, dry mouth, and bitter taste in the mouth.
T: Red tongue with dry yellow coating. **P:** Wiry, slippery and rapid.

- Soothe liver qi, drain liver fire and harmonize the stomach.
- *Hua Gan Jian*
  - *Qing Pi* and *Chen Pi* spread constrained liver and regulate the qi flow to alleviate pain.
  - *Shao Yao* preserves the yin and softens the liver to alleviate pain.
  - *Mu Dan Pi* and *Zhi Zi* clear and drain liver fire.
- Acid regurgitation. + *Zuo Jin Wan*
  Significant stomach heat. + *Shi Gao, Zhi Mu*
  Co-existing stomach fire and yin deficiency, use *Yu Nu Jian*.

Blood stasis in the stomach

Stabbing epigastric pain with a fixed location, resistance to pressure, pain that worsens at night.
S: Recurrent or chronic attacks, possibly hematemesis with dark blood, or melena.
T: Dark purple tongue with petechiae. **P:** Choppy.

- Invigorate the blood and transform stasis.
- *Shi Xiao San* and *Dan Shen Yin*
  - *Shi Xiao San* invigorates the blood and dispels stasis to alleviate pain. This is an imperial formula for pain caused by blood stasis.
  - *Dan Shen* invigorates the blood and dispels stasis.
  - *Tan Xiang* and *Sha Ren* facilitate the qi flow and expand the middle burner to alleviate pain.
- Promote the movement of qi to circulate the blood. + *Xiang Fu, Zhi Qiao*
  Unblock the qi stagnation in the bowels to expel stasis via bowel movements. + *Da Huang, Gan Cao*
  Persistent hematemesis and melena. + *San Qi, Bai Ji*
  Spleen yang deficiency with hematemesis and melena, sallow complexion and cold limbs, use *Huang Tu Tang*.
  Blood stasis with blood deficiency. + *Si Wu Tang*
  Blood stasis with qi deficiency. + *Huang Qi, Dang Shen*

Stomach yin deficiency

Vague burning epigastric pain.
S: Hunger without desire to eat, dry mouth and throat, and dry stool.
T: Dry red tongue. **P:** Thready and rapid.

- Nourish stomach yin.
- *Yi Wei Tang* and *Shao Yao Gan Cao Tang*
  - *Sha Shen*, *Mai Men Dong*, *Sheng Di Huang* and *Yu Zhu* nourish stomach yin and generate the fluid.
  - *Shao Yao* and *Gan Cao* moderate spasm and alleviate pain.
- To reinforce the effects of regulating the qi and alleviating pain. + *Mei Gui Hua, Fo Shou*
  Dry stool. + *Yu Li Ren, Huo Ma Ren, Gua Lou Ren*
  Burning pain with stomach upset and acid regurgitation. + *Zuo Jin Wan*

Yang deficiency of the spleen and stomach

Vague dull epigastric pain, relieved by warmth, pressure and after meals, and aggravated by hunger.
S: Vomiting clear watery fluids, poor appetite, fatigue, cold limbs and loose stool.
T: Pale tongue with white coating. **P:** Weak slow and decelerating.

- Warm the middle burner and strengthen the spleen.
- *Huang Qi Jian Zhong Tang*

- *Huang Qi* augments the qi and tonifies the middle burner.
- *Xiao Jian Zhong Tang* warms the spleen, disperses cold and alleviates pain.

- Accompanied by acid regurgitation. + *Wu Zhu Yu, Wa Leng Zi*
  Excessively vomiting watery fluids. + *Gan Jiang, Chen Pi, Ban Xia*
  Severe cold pain with vomiting and cold limbs, use *Li Zhong Wan*.
  During the recovery stage, use *Xiang Sha Liu Jun Zi Tang*.

Acupuncture Treatment

- **Manipulation:** Reducing method for excess and reinforcing method for deficiency; moxibustion is applicable for cold patterns.
- **Prescription:** CV12 Zhongwan ST36 Zusanli PC6 Neiguan SP4 Gongsun
- **Supplementary points:**
  - Stomach cold. + CV6 Qihai; CV8 Shenque
  - Stomach heat. + ST44 Neiting
  - Stagnant liver qi invading the stomach. + LR14 Qimen; LR3 Taichong
  - Food retention. + Inner-Neiting (Extra)
  - Blood stasis. + BL17 Geshu; SP10 Xuehai

Practical Hints

Rule out gastric bleeding and gastric cancer. Herbal treatments, given parenterally, are usually very effective in treating epigastric pain. However, be alert for alterations in the rhythm or periodicity of the pain, especially if pain becomes protracted and is accompanied by epigastric distention and fullness, nausea, and dizziness. In this case, even though there is no hematemesis, a prompt referral should be made to rule out gastric bleeding. If a middle-aged patient complains of recurrent, irregular epigastric pain that responds poorly to herbal medicine, accompanied by emaciation, low grade fever and intermittent unexplained black stool, it is necessary to rule out gastric cancer.

[Addendum]

Acid Regurgitation

返 酸 *Fan Suan*

Acid regurgitation is the backward flow of acidic gastric fluid to the mouth from the stomach. In clinical situation, it is common that acid regurgitation occurs together with epigastric pain and stomach upset, especially when the stomch is empty, and it is alleviated by meal. Acid regurgitation involves both the liver and stomach.

Differentiation and Treatment

Heat pattern

Liver qi stagnation turning into liver fire which overacts on the stomach. Manifestations include acid regurgitation, bitter taste in the mouth, dry throat, distending pain in the hypochondria, and irritability.
T: Red tongue with yellow coating. **P:** Wiry and rapid.

- Clear heat from the liver and harmonize the stomach.
- *Zuo Jin Wan*
  - *Huang Lian*, bitter and cold, clears heat and drains fire.
  - *Wu Zhu Yu* enters the liver channel and descends rebellious qi.
- Control acidity. + *Wa Leng Zi*, *Hai Piao Xiao*
  Belching. + *Xuan Fu Hua*, *Dai Zhe Shi*
  Stomach upset. + *Bai He*, *Zhe Bei Mu*

Cold pattern

Spleen and stomach yang deficiency with empty cold which affects the normal transportation and transformation of food and drink. Manifestations include acid regurgitation with clear watery fluids, a stuffy sensation in the stomach, poor appetite, preference for warmth and pressure, cold limbs and loose stool.
T: Pale tongue with white and slippery coating. **P:** Wiry and thready.

- Warm the middle burner, strengthen the spleen and harmonize the stomach.
- *Xiang Sha Liu Jun Zi Tang*

- *Ren Shen*, *Bai Zhu*, *Fu Ling* and *Zhi Gan Cao* augment the qi, warm the middle burner and strengthen the spleen.
- *Ban Xia* descends rebellious qi and harmonizes the stomach.
- *Chen Pi*, *Xiang Fu* and *Sha Ren* facilitate the qi flow and harmonize the middle burner.

- To strengthen the effects of dispersing cold and descending rebellious qi. + *Wu Zhu Yu, Sheng Jiang*
Acid regurgitation occurring after meals. + *Shen Qu, Mai Ya, Gu Ya*
Dampness accumulated in the middle burner. + *Cang Zhu, Hou Po*
Epigastric dull pain. + *Chuan Jiao, Chen Xiang*
Gastric reflux. + *Ding Xiang, Mai Ya, Bai Dou Kou*

Stomach Upset

嘈 嘈 *Zao Za*

Stomach upset, or stomach discomfort, is characterized by an unexplainable sensation of non-specific pain or hunger. It may be accompanied by epigastric pain, acid regurgitation and belching.

Differentiation and Treatment

Stomach heat

Stomach upset with thirst, desire for cold beverages, irritability, and bad breath. **T:** Yellow coating. **P:** Rapid.

- Clear heat and harmonize the middle burner.

- *Huang Lian Wen Dan Tang*
- *Huang Lian* clears heat and drains fire.
- *Ban Xia*, *Chen Pi* and *Fu Ling* dry dampness, facilitate the qi flow and harmonize the stomach.
- *Zhu Ru* and *Zhi Shi* clear heat and descend the rebellious qi.

- Food stagnation turning into heat. + *Shan Zha, Gu Ya, Shen Qu*
Constipation. + *Da Huang*
Stomach pain radiating to hypochondriac region. + *Chai Hu, Chuan Lian Zi*

Stomach deficiency

Stomach upset with inability to taste, epigastric distention after meals, fatigue and lassitude.
T: Pale tongue with thin white coating. **P:** Thready and weak.

- Strengthen the spleen and harmonize the stomach.
- *Xiang Sha Liu Jun Zi Tang*

Blood deficiency

Stomach upset with pale complexion and lips, palpitations, dizziness, insomnia and dream-disturbed sleep.
T: Pale tongue. **P:** Thready.

- Tonify the qi and nourish the blood.
- *Gui Pi Tang*

CHAPTER **10**

Vomiting

嘔吐 *Ou Tu*

Vomiting is the ejection of the stomach's contents via the mouth due to a disharmony of the stomach and rebellion of the stomach qi. Ancient TCM practitioners distinguished heaving (*ou*) as vomiting with the ejection of emesis accompanied by sound, disgorgement (*tu*) as the ejection of emesis without any sound, and retching (*gan ou*) as the involuntary effort to vomit accompanied by the sound of vomiting without actual emesis. Despite these classical distinctions, given that sound and emesis are usually present simultaneously, vomiting (*ou tu*) is viewed and treated as one disorder.

Relevant Diseases

- Neurogenic vomiting
- Acute gastritis
- Acute hepatitis
- Acute pancreatitis
- Acute cholecystitis
- Acute appendicitis
- Prolapse of gastric mucosa
- Partial pyloric obstruction
- Meniere's disease
- End stage renal disease
- Morning sickness

Etiology and Pathogenesis

Exterior pathogens: Wind, cold, dampness and epidemic pathogens have a direct influence on the stomach. By hindering the descending function of stomach qi, these factors provoke rebellious qi and cause vomiting.

Improper diet: Excessive consumption of raw, cold, greasy food or contaminated food can injure the stomach and hinder the spleen; food stagnation ensues and prevents the stomach qi from descending.

Emotional stress: Anger and frustration have a direct impact on the liver, impairing its function to spread and ensure the free flow of qi. Stagnant liver qi overacts on the stomach and causes vomiting. Pensiveness and excessive worry impair the function of the spleen to digest food and drink ingested; the undigested stomach contents prevent stomach qi from descending.

Deficiency of the spleen and stomach: Constitutional deficiency, overexertion and chronic illness exhaust spleen yang and the spleen is unable to extract the essence from food and drink. Food and drink accumulate and stagnate in the stomach and turn into congested fluids, inducing vomiting. In the case of stomach yin deficiency and lack of stomach fluid to smooth the descending function may cause vomiting.

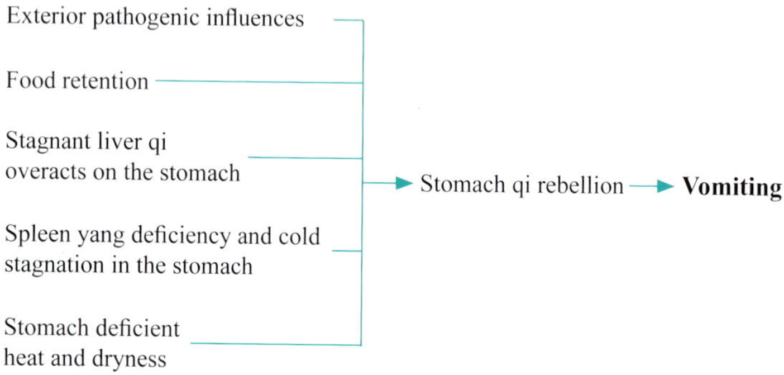

Diagnosis

A. Identification of excess and deficiency:

Excess patterns have an acute onset and short course. They are most often associated with exterior pathogenic influences, improper diet and the liver overacting on the stomach. Symptoms in excess patterns tend to be severe and constant.

Deficient patterns have a chronic onset and prolonged course. They are closely related to the declining function of the spleen and stomach to transform and transport. Symptoms in deficient patterns tend to be milder, intermittent and recurrent.

B. Differential diagnosis of similar disorders:

Vomiting, gastric reflux and hiccough are disorders of rebellious stomach qi.

Vomiting is characterized by sound and emesis. Vomiting is a forceful ejection of gastric contents due to rebellious stomach qi. Nausea is common.

Gastric reflux is characterized by a backflow of gastric contents into the mouth containing food consumed several hours previously. It is caused by impaired stomach qi failing to decompose and ripen the food. Nausea is not common.

Hiccough is a sequence of involuntary, spasmodic, frequent, short and sharp inhalations suddenly checked by closure of the glottis producing a characteristic sound. It is provoked by rebellious stomach qi that disturbs the qi flow in the diaphragm. Usually, nausea and vomiting are absent with hiccough.

Basic Patterns

Excess patterns:

- Exterior pathogens attacking the stomach
- Food retention
- Accumulation of congested fluids
- Stagnant liver qi overacting on the stomach

Deficient patterns:

- Deficient cold in the spleen and stomach
- Stomach yin deficiency

Differentiation and Treatment

Treatment principle:
The primary physiological function of the stomach as one of the six yang organs is to control descending of the qi. To treat stomach qi rebellion, consider restoring impaired stomach function. Descending the rebellious qi and harmonizing the stomach are the primary treatment principles.

Excess pattern: Expel pathogenic factors and transform turbidity, harmonize the stomach and descend rebellious qi.

Deficient pattern: Warm the middle burner and strengthen the stomach, or nourish and replenish stomach yin.

Excess patterns:

Exterior pathogens attacking the stomach

Sudden and urgent episodes of vomiting with a history of contracting an exterior illness.
S: Fever, aversion to cold, headache and general body ache, fullness and distention in the chest and epigastrium.
T: White greasy coating. **P:** Soft and decelerating.

- Release the exterior and utilize aromatic herbs to transform turbidity.
- *Huo Xiang Zheng Qi San*
  - *Huo Xiang*, *Zi Su Ye* and *Bai Zhi* are aromatic to disperse exterior pathogens and transform turbidity.
  - *Ban Xia* dries dampness, harmonizes the stomach and descends rebellion.
  - *Chen Pi*, *Hou Po* and *Da Fu Pi* facilitate the qi flow to transform dampness.

- *Bai Zhu* and *Fu Ling* strengthen the spleen and dry dampness.

- Significant focal distention in the epigastrium due to food retention. + *Shen Qu, Ji Nei Jin*
  Significant exterior wind-cold. + *Fang Feng, Jing Jie*
  Summer heat-dampness with thirst and irritability. + *Huang Lian, Pei Lan*

Food retention

Vomiting with sour and foul-smelling vomitus, aggravated by eating and relieved by vomiting.
S: Fullness and distention in the epigastrium and abdomen, belching, aversion to food, pasty stool with a strong odor or constipation.
T: Thick greasy coating. **P:** Slippery and forceful.

- Reduce food retention, harmonize the stomach and descend rebellious qi.

- *Bao He Wan*
  - *Shan Zha*, *Shen Qu* and *Lai Fu Zi* relieve food stagnation and accumulation.
  - *Ban Xia* harmonizes the stomach and descends rebellious qi.
  - *Chen Pi* and *Fu Ling* facilitate the qi flow and strengthen the spleen.
  - *Liang Qiao* clears constraint heat produced from food stagnation.

- Fullness and distention in the abdomen and constipation. + *Xiao Cheng Qi Tang*
  Stagnant food turning into heat with bad breath and instantaneous vomiting after eating. + *Huang Lian, Zhu Ru*

Accumulation of congested fluids

Nausea and vomiting clear liquids, and coughing up white or yellow sputum.
S: Dizziness, palpitations, fullness of the epigastrium, and poor appetite; often associated with obesity or a greasy, sweet and rich diet.
T: White greasy coating. **P:** Slippery.

- Warm and transform congested fluids, harmonize the stomach and descend rebellious qi.

- *Xiao Ban Xia Tang* and *Ling Gui Zhu Gan Tang*
  - *Ban Xia* and *Sheng Jiang* harmonize the stomach and descend rebellious qi.
  - *Fu Ling*, *Bai Zhu* and *Gui Zhi* strengthen the spleen, dry dampness, warm and transform cold congested fluids.

- Abundant clear watery emesis. + *Qian Niu Zi, Bai Jie Zi*
  Excessive sputum and significant focal distention in the chest and epigastrium. + *Chen Pi, Zhi Qiao*
  Congested fluids turning into heat with nausea, use *Wen Dan Tang*.

Stagnant liver qi overacting on the stomach

Vomiting of sour and bitter-taste vomitus, and frequent belching with a temporary sensation of relief after belching.
S: Fullness and pain in the chest and hypochondrium, focal distention in the epigastrium, and poor appetite.
T: Red tongue with thin greasy coating. **P:** Wiry and slippery.

- Spread and soothe liver qi, harmonize the stomach and descend rebellious qi.
- *Ban Xia Hou Po Tang* and *Zuo Jin Wan*
  - *Hou Po* and *Zi Su Ye* facilitate the qi flow.
  - *Ban Xia*, *Sheng Jiang* and *Fu Ling* descend rebellious qi, harmonize the stomach and stop vomiting.
  - *Huang Lian* and *Wu Zhu Yu*, acrid to disperse and bitter to descend, restore the function of the stomach to stop vomiting.
- Significant heat signs. + *Zhu Ru, Zhi Zi, Huang Qin*
  Bitter taste in the mouth, stomach upset and constipation. + *Da Huang*

Deficient patterns:

Deficient cold in the spleen and stomach

Recurrent vomiting with clear emesis induced by improper diet or fatigue.
S: Sallow complexion, fatigue, lack of strength, and loose stool; or pale complexion, cold limbs, and watery stool.
T: Pale tongue with thin white coating. **P:** Deep, thready and weak.

- Warm the middle burner, harmonize the stomach and descend rebellious qi.
- *Li Zhong Wan*
  - *Gan Jiang* warms the middle burner and disperses cold.
  - *Ren Shen*, *Bai Zhu* and *Gan Cao* benefit the qi and strengthen the spleen.
- To strengthen the effects of facilitating the qi and redirecting rebellious qi.
  + *Ban Xia, Sha Ren*
  Unremitting vomiting with watery emesis. + *Sheng Jiang, Wu Zhu Yu*
  Unremitting vomiting and frequent belching. + *Xuan Fu Hua, Dai Zhe Shi*

Stomach yin deficiency

Recurrent vomiting or dry heaves.
S: Hunger without desire to eat, dry mouth and throat, and dry stool.
T: Dry red tongue with scanty coating. **P:** Rapid and thready.

- Nourish and replenish stomach yin, descend rebellious qi and stop vomiting.
- *Mai Men Dong Tang*

- *Ren Shen*, *Mai Men Dong*, *Jing Mi* and *Gan Cao* nourish the stomach yin.
- *Ban Xia* descends rebellious qi and stops vomiting.

- Enhance the nourishing effect on the stomach. + *Tian Hua Fen*, *Sha Shen*
  Rebellion of both lung and stomach qi. + *Pi Pa Ye*, *Xuan Fu Hua*
  Yin injury with intestinal dryness. + *Huo Ma Ren*, *Gua Lou Ren*

Acupuncture Treatment

- **Manipulation:** Reducing method in excess patterns; reinforcing method in deficient patterns.
- **Prescription:** CV12 Zhongwan ST36 Zusanli PC6 Neiguan SP4 Gongsun
- **Supplementary points:**
  - Exterior pathogens attacking the stomach. + GB20 Fengchi; LI4 Hegu
  - Food retention. + CV10 Xiawan; CV21 Xuanji
  - Congested fluids. + CV17 Tanzhong; ST40 Fenglong
  - Liver overacting on the stomach. + LR3 Taichong; GB34 Yanglingquan
  - Deficiency of the spleen and stomach. + BL20 Pishu; LR13 Zhangmen

Practical Hints

• **Vomiting as a physiological defense mechanism.** Stomach qi rebelling upwards is the major pathogenesis of vomiting. In some cases, vomiting is a normal physiological defense mechanism by which pathogenic influences are expelled. Among the eight therapeutic strategies in TCM, the emetic method is used to expel pathogens from above the diaphragm and the stomach. Therefore, if vomiting is due to invasion of exterior pathogens or due to food retention, antiemetic treatment may not be appropriate. Instead, adopting methods to expel pathogens is recommended.

• **Dividing the daily dose of an herbal decoction into multiple doses of smaller quantity is advisable.** It may be difficult for a patient who is vomiting to take an herbal decoction. In this case, it is advisable to administer the decoction by dividing the daily dose into multiple doses of smaller quantity.

• **Referrals should be made as indicated.** Referral to an acute care medical facility is strongly recommended if dehydration due to severe vomiting is evident. Referral should also be made if there is projectile vomiting with blood in the vomitus, high fever, stubborn headache, irritability, lethargy or unconsciousness.

CHAPTER 11

Hiccough

呃逆 *E Ni*

Caused by stomach qi rebelling upwards to disturb the diaphragm, hiccough is characterized by an involuntary short, sharp and frequent inspiratory cough. Hiccough can be a mild discomfort that occurs alone in short duration and is relieved spontaneously. However, persistent and unremitting hiccough can also be a critical symptom in some acute or chronic diseases. Prolonged hiccough has serious consequences.

Relevant Diseases

- Indigestion
- Gastro-neurosis
- Hiatal hernia
- Status post gastric surgery
- Hysteria
- Phrenic nerve disturbance
- End stage of cirrhosis
- End stage renal disease
- Cerebral lesion

Etiology and Pathogenesis

The pathogenesis of hiccough involves two major organs and one tissue, the lung and the stomach, and the diaphragm. "The lung channel originates from the middle burner, and travels downwards to connect to the large intestine. As it travels upwards, it surrounds the stomach, passes through the diaphragm and infuses into the lung..." As connected by the lung channel, when stomach qi rebels upwards, it disturbs the diaphragm and attacks the lung.

Improper diet: Stagnation of cold in the stomach can be caused by intake of cold and raw food or cold herbs. Heat accumulating in the stomach can be the result from intake of hot, spicy or greasy food or herbs that are warm and hot in nature. When these pathogenic factors are obstructed in the stomach, they significantly disturb the proper movement of stomach qi. As stomach qi fails to descend it rebels up, disturbing the diaphragm and attacking the lung, leading to hiccough.

Emotional stress is the major cause of liver qi stagnation. Liver qi stagnation can further overact on the stomach leading to the backward flow of stomach qi; stagnant liver qi can also further insult the lung leading to rebellious lung qi. When stagnant qi fails to properly transport the body fluid, phlegm can accumulate and cause obstruction. Rebellious lung and stomach qi with phlegm can flow upwards to disturb the diaphragm, causing hiccough.

Insufficiency of righteous qi can be a result of chronic consumptive disorders, such as prolonged or critical illnesses, and from iatrogenic causes, such as misusage of purgatives or diuretics. Insufficient righteous qi have a direct impact on the stomach and kidney. When stomach qi and yin are insufficient, the stomach fails to descend smoothly, leading to hiccough. If the kidney is insufficient, it fails to receive the qi, causing qi rebelling. The qi failing to descend may join the rebellious stomach qi together to counterflow and disturb the diaphragm.

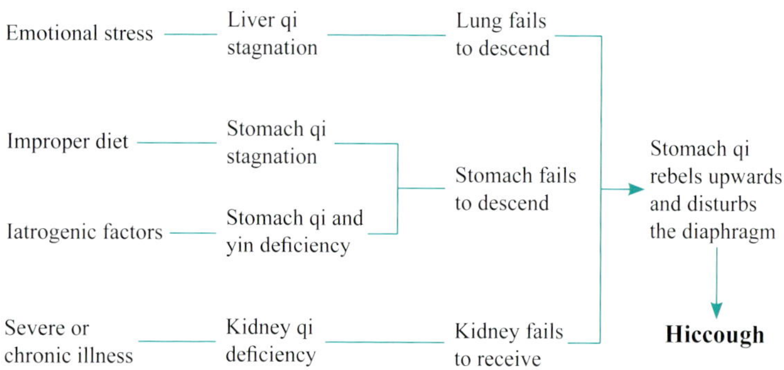

Diagnosis

A. Identification of cold, heat, deficiency and excess patterns:

- Excess patterns:
  - Loud and rigorous hiccough accompanied by belching, acid regurgitation and abdominal distention – Food stagnation.
  - Hiccough accompanied by stifling sensation in the chest, nausea, dizziness and greasy tongue coating – Phlegm accumulation.
  - Hiccough accompanied by fixed stabbing pain in the chest, and dark tongue or petechiae on the tongue – Blood stasis.
  - Hiccough elicited by emotional stress and accompanied by hypochondriac pain and wiry pulse – Liver qi stagnation.
  - Deep, slow and rigorous hiccough relieved by warmth and aggravated by cold and may accompanied by stomach cold pain – Stomach cold.
  - High pitch, loud and rigorous hiccough with bad breath, intense thirst and constipation – Stomach heat.

- Deficiency patterns:
  - Low pitch and weak hiccough accompanied by poor appetite, fatigue, lassitude, cold limbs, diarrhea, and sore weak lower back and knees – Spleen and kidney empty cold.
  - Short, frequent and abrupt hiccough accompanied by dry mouth, and red tongue with scanty coating – Stomach yin deficiency.

B. Identification of severity:

In most cases, hiccough is not a severe condition and it can be relieved without special treatments. However, hiccough can be a warning sign to a critical condition. When low-pitched and weak hiccough is accompanied by the inability to ingest, with a deep and hidden pulse, it may be a sign that the basal qi is devastated and the stomach qi is depleted. The prognosis is not optimistic.

C. Differential diagnosis of similar disorders:

Hiccough: A result from rebellious stomach qi and irregular qi flow in the diaphragm region, it is characterized by involuntary, sharp, short and frequent coughing sounds from the throat.

Retching: A relevant disorder caused by rebellious stomach qi, this involuntary and nonproductive attempt to vomit is characterized by the presence of vomiting sound without emesis.

Belching: A result from stomach gas rebelling upwards, it is manifested by escape of gas from the stomach and expelling through the esophagus and the mouth.

Basic Patterns

Excess patterns:

- Cold in the stomach
- Stomach fire blazing upwards
- Liver qi stagnation

Deficient patterns:

- Spleen and stomach yang deficiency
- Stomach yin deficiency

Differentiation and Treatment

Treatment principle:

The primary principle is to harmonize the stomach, descend rebellious qi, and calm hiccough. However, modifying the strategies according to the differentiations is recommended.

Excess patterns:

Cold in the stomach

Deep, slow and rigorous hiccough relieved by warmth and aggravated by cold.
S: Cold pain or discomfort in the epigastric and phrenic regions, and decreased appetite without thirst.
T: Moist white coating. **P:** Slow and decelerating.

- Warm the middle burner, expel cold and calm hiccough.
- *Ding Xiang San*
  - *Ding Xiang* and *Shi Di* descend rebellious qi and stop hiccough.
  - *Gao Liang Jiang* and *Zhi Gan Cao* warm the middle burner and expel cold.
- To strengthen the effects of warming the yang and expelling cold. + *Rou Gui, Wu Zhu Yu*

  Impaired digestive function of the stomach with epigastric distention and belching. + *Hou Po, Zhi Shi, Ban Xia, Chen Pi*

Stomach fire blazing upwards

Sudden projectile loud rigorous hiccough with bad breath and intense thirst.
S: Desire for cold beverages, dark scanty urine output and constipation.
T: Yellow coating. **P:** Slippery and rapid.

- Clear heat, descend rebellious qi and calm hiccough.
- *Xin Zhi Ju Pi Zhu Ru Tang*
  - *Zhu Ru* and *Shi Di* drain fire and descend rebellious qi.
  - *Sheng Jiang* and *Ju Pi* facilitate the qi flow, harmonize the stomach and descend rebellious qi.
- To reinforce the effects of clearing heat and draining fire. + *Shi Gao*

  Severe stomach fire with constipation, and fullness and distention of the abdomen. + *Xiao Cheng Qi Tang*

Liver qi stagnation

Persistent hiccough elicited or aggravated by emotional stress.
S: Stifling sensation in the chest, epigastric and hypochondriac regions, excessive borborygmus and passing flatus.
T: Thin white coating. **P:** Wiry.

- Pacify and descend rebellious qi.
- *Wu Mo Yin Zi*
  - *Wu Yao* and *Mu Xiang* promote the qi flow and spread constrained liver.
  - *Zhi Shi*, *Chen Xiang* and *Bing Lang* descend rebellious qi.

- To reinforce the effects of descending rebellious qi and calming hiccough. *+ Ding Xiang, Dai Zhe Shi.*
  To strengthen the effects of soothing the liver and relieving constraint. *+ Chuan Lian Zi, Yu Jin*
  Stagnant qi turning into fire with irritability, bitter taste in the mouth, and rapid wiry pulse. *+ Zhi Zi, Huang Lian*

Deficient patterns:

Spleen and stomach yang deficiency

Low pitch and weak hiccough, and shortness of breath.
S: Pale complexion, cold limbs and poor appetite.
T: Pale tongue with white coating. **P:** Deep, thready and forceless.

- Warm and tonify the spleen and stomach, harmonize the middle burner and descend rebellious qi.
- *Li Zhong Wan*
  - *Gan Jiang* warms the middle burner and disperses cold.
  - *Ren Shen*, *Bai Zhu* and *Gan Cao* augment the qi and strengthen the spleen.
- To strengthen the effects of descending rebellious qi and calming hiccough. *+ Wu Zhu Yu, Ding Xiang*
  Accompanied by kidney yang deficiency with cold intolerance, soreness and weakness of the lower back and knees, flabby tongue and deep slow pulse. *+ Fu Zi, Rou Gui*

Stomach yin deficiency

Abrupt intermittent hiccough, and dry mouth and throat.
S: Irritability, agitation, hunger without desire to eat, and dry stool.
T: Dry red tongue or cracked tongue. **P:** Thready and rapid.

- Generate the fluid, nourish the stomach and calm hiccough.
- *Mai Men Dong Tang*
  - *Mai Dong*, sweet and cold, generates the fluid and nourishes stomach yin.
  - *Ban Xia* descends rebellious qi and harmonizes the stomach.
  - *Ren Shen*, *Gan Cao* and *Jing Mi* tonify the qi and generate the fluid.
- To strengthen the effects of nourishing the yin and benefiting the stomach. *+ Shi Hu, Sha Shen, Yu Zhu*
  To reinforce the effects of descending rebellious qi and calming hiccough. *+ Shi Di, Pi Pa Ye*
  Severe stomach qi deficiency with lack of appetite. *+ Ju Pi Zhu Ru Tang*

Acupuncture Treatment

- **Manipulation:** Reducing method in excess patterns; reinforcing method in deficient patterns; puncture and moxibustion in pattern of yang deficiency.
- **Prescription:** CV12 Zhongwan PC6 Neiguan ST36 Zusanli BL17 Geshu
- **Supplementary points:**
  - Cold in the stomach. + ST21 Liangmen
  - Stomach fire. + ST43 Xiangu
  - Liver qi stagnation. + LR14 Qimen; LR3 Taichong
  - Spleen and stomach yang deficiency. + CV6 Qihai
  - Stomach yin deficiency. + KI3 Taixi

Practical Hints

Differentiate mild hiccough from critical pathology. Hiccoughs have various severities; they can be clinically insignificant or critical. Insignificant hiccough occurs occasionally and ceases spontaneously. As introduced by *Nei Jing*, stimulating the nasal cavity to induce sneezing can regulate the qi flow in the pathway from the stomach, diaphragm to the lung. As qi flows smoothly, hiccough will be relieved. However, if hiccough persists during the critical phase of any acute or chronic conditions, it indicates the retrogression of the course. This critical hiccough signifies devastated earth and depleted stomach qi, predicting a poor prognosis. According to TCM theory, stomach qi plays an extremely important role in the recovery phase from any disease. Recovery is optimal and predictable if stomach qi exists but unfavorable and may be life-threatening if stomach qi is depleted.

CHAPTER 12

Dysphagia and Gagging Syndrome

噎膈 *Ye Ge*

Ye, or dysphagia, is the inability to swallow or having difficulty swallowing. *Ge*, or gagging, implies the involuntary resistance to food and water after swallowing, as evidenced by immediate vomiting.

Dysphagia may occur alone; however, if persistent, it precipitates gagging syndrome. Pathophysiologically, dysphagia and gagging syndrome is an inexorable disorder in which two phases of rejecting oral intake follow from merely difficulty in swallowing to immediate vomiting right after food intake. Its pathology develops from a lack of moi-stening to a substantial obstruction in the passage into the stomach.

Relevant Diseases

- Dysphagia spastica
- Dysphagia paralytica
- Dysphagia lusoria
- Spasm of cardiac sphincter
- Hiatal hernia
- Esophagitis
- Esophageal diverticulosis
- Esophageal cancer

Etiology and Pathogenesis

Emotional stress: Worry and overthinking injure the spleen while anger and frustration injure the liver. Resulting from injury to the liver and spleen, qi becomes stagnant turning into blood stasis, and phlegm is generated and gets accumulated. Blood stasis, stagnant and rebellious qi, together with phlegm, obstructs the passage and entrance of the stomach, causing dysphagia and gagging.

Improper diet: Overindulgence of greasy, sweet and spicy food and alcohol can generate heat and phlegm. Phlegm may constrict or obstruct the passage and entrance of the stomach. Heat may injure the yin and deplete the blood and fluid. Lack of lubrication in the passage causes difficulty for food to pass through.

In order to prevent the occurrence of dysphagia and gagging, the stomach, spleen, liver and kidney organs have to remain in harmony. The spleen supplies the stomach with yin and fluid; the free flow of liver qi determines that the stomach qi is descending; kidney essence can reach the throat to nourish the passage into the stomach through the kidney channel. Proper accommodation and cooperation among these factors ensure the smooth flow of food and liquid into the stomach.

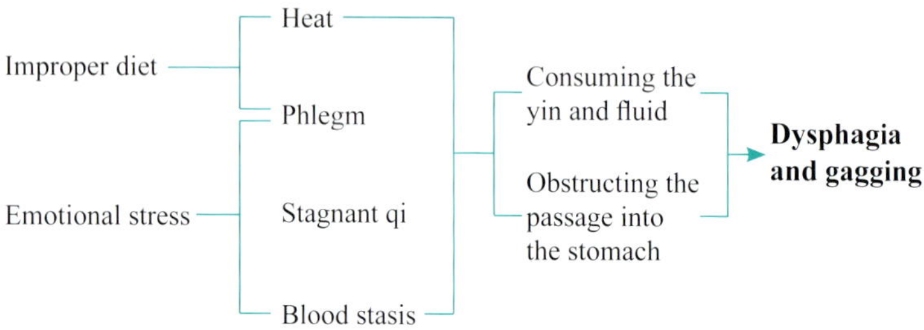

Diagnosis

A. Identification of deficiency and excess patterns:

In the early stage of disphagia and gagging syndrome, difficulty in swallowing is a major symptom, especially with solid food. As the condition progresses, immediate vomiting after indulgence will occur. There will be creamy dark red emesis with undigested food, retrosternal pain when swallowing, emaciation and lassitude.

- Excess pattern usually manifests in the early stage, in which qi stagnation, blood stasis and phlegm accumulation are combined and obstruct the passage into the stomach.
- Deficient pattern usually develops from chronic unremitting dysphagia and gagging syndrome. As the blood and fluid gradually depletes, dryness occurs and hinders the passage of food into the stomach.

B. Differential diagnosis of similar disorders:

Gastric reflux: Due to lack of stomach yang, the function of digesting food and water fails to perform. Food remaining in the stomach causes stomach qi to rebel. The classic manifestation is vomiting undigested food, resembling pyloric stenosis or spasm in western medicine. In contrary, dysphagia and gagging syndrome is characterized by inability to swallow, difficulty in swallowing or immediate vomiting after oral intake, analogous to esophageal and gastric pathologies.

Plum pit syndrome: Both dysphagia and gagging syndrome, and plum pit syndrome share the common subjective discomfort of an obstructive sensation in the throat. However, patient suffers from plum pit syndrome does not experience any difficulty in ingesting food whereas the patient of dysphagia and gagging syndrome has an obvious difficulty in swallowing.

Basic Patterns

- Constraint of phlegm and qi
- Fluid depletion and heat accumulation
- Internal accumulation of blood stasis
- Qi deficiency and yang devastation

Differentiation and Treatment

Treatment principle:

Excess: Choose herbs that facilitate the movement of qi, invigorate the blood and dispel stasis, and resolve phlegm, along with herbs that nourish the yin and moisten dryness.

Deficiency: Based upon the severity of depletion of blood and fluid or exhaustion of yang qi, modify the strategies to focus on replenishing the deficiency.

Constraint of phlegm and qi

Difficulty in swallowing, focal distention in the chest and phrenic region, condition is aggravated by emotional stress.
S: Dry mouth and throat and dry stool.
T: Red tongue with thin greasy coating. **P:** Wiry and slippery.

- Relieve the constraint, transform phlegm and moisten dryness.
- *Qi Ge San*
  - *Dan Shen*, *Yu Jin* and *Sha Ren* transform blood stasis and promote the movement of qi to unblock obstruction.
  - *Sha Shen*, *Chuan Bei Mu* and *Fu Ling* moisten dryness, transform phlegm and dissipate accumulation.
- To reinforce the effects of moving the qi and transforming phlegm. + *Gua Lou*, *Chen Pi*

  Constipation due to intestinal dryness. + *Zeng Ye Tang*

Fluid depletion and heat accumulation

Difficult and painful swallowing, unable to ingest solid food, and emaciation.
S: Dry mouth and throat, constipation and five-centers heat.
T: Dry red tongue with cracks. **P:** Wiry thready and rapid.

- Nourish the yin and generate the fluid.

- *Wu Zhi An Zhong Yin*
  - *Li Zhi*, *Ou Zhi* and *Niu Ru* nourish stomach yin and generate the fluid.
  - *Sheng Jiang Zhi* harmonizes the stomach and descends rebellious qi.
  - *Jiu Zhi* invigorates the blood and dissipates stasis.
- To enhance the effect to nourish the yin of kidney and stomach. + *Sha Shen, Shi Hu, Sheng Di Huang, Shu Di Huang*

  Constipation or fecal impaction due to severe intestinal dryness. + *Zeng Ye Cheng Qi Tang*

Internal accumulation of blood stasis

Stabbing pain in the center of the chest, inability to swallow food and drink, and immediate vomiting after ingestion, creamy dark red emesis with undigested food.
S: Dry and hard pebble-like stool, dusky complexion, severe emaciation, and dry and flaky skin.
T: Dry red or dark purple tongue. **P:** Thready and choppy.

- Nourish the yin and blood, break up stasis and invigorate the blood.
- *Tong You Tang*
  - *Sheng Di Huang* and *Shu Di Huang* nourish the yin and replenish the blood.
  - *Dang Gui* nourishes and invigorates the blood.
  - *Tao Ren* and *Hong Hua* break up and transform blood stasis.
- To enhance the effects of expelling stasis and invigorating the collaterals. + *San Qi, Ru Xiang, Mo Yao, Dan Shen, Wu Ling Zhi*

  To soften hardness. + *Hai Zao, Kun Bu, Bei Mu, Gua Lou*

Qi deficiency and yang devastation

Longstanding inability of ingestion, and vomiting clear liquid emesis.
S: Pale complexion, lassitude and listlessness, cold intolerance, facial and lower extremities edema, and abdominal distention.
T: Pale tongue with white coating. **P:** Thready and weak.

- Warm and tonify the spleen and kidney.
- *Liu Jun Zi Tang* and *You Gui Wan*
  - *Liu Jun Zi Tang* benefits the qi, harmonizes the stomach, dries dampness and descends rebellious qi.
  - *You Gui Wan* warms kidney yang and nourishes the essence and blood.
- To enhance the effect of descending the rebelling qi to stop vomiting. + *Xuan Fu Hua, Dai Zhe Shi*

Acupuncture Treatment

- **Manipulation:** Even method. Moxibustion is applicable in yang deficiency.
- **Prescription:** CV22 Tiantu CV17 Tanzhong
- **Supplementary points:**

  - Constraint of phlegm and qi. + CV14 Juque; PC6 Neiguan

  - Blood stasis. + BL17 Geshu; BL21Weishu

  - Qi deficiency and yang devastation. + BL20 Pishu; BL23 Shenshu; CV6 Qihai; CV4 Guanyuan

Practical Hints

• *Ye ge*, or dysphagia and gagging syndrome, is a pathology pertaining to the stomach and esophagus. The patterns are mostly a combination of excess branch and deficiency root. The deficiency is caused by depletion of the fluid and blood or by deficient yin leading to devastated yang. The excess is referred to the presence of pathological derivatives, such as qi stagnation, phlegm accumulation and blood stasis. Therefore, **the treatment usually addresses both the root and branch by replenishing the deficiency and expelling the excess accordingly.**

• Stomach is a yang organ that prefers moistness and dislikes dryness. Stomach yin is vulnerable to herbs that are warm and drying in the treatment for phlegm. Stomach yang is susceptible to herbs that are bitter and cold in the treatment for stomach heat. When using large doses of rich and cloying yin tonics to replenish stomach fluid, stomach qi can be stagnated. **Stomach qi determines the prognosis.** If stomach qi is rigorous, recovery is possible; if stomach qi is devastated, prognosis is not optimistic. Therefore, for stomach pathologies, the protection of stomach qi should be a vital part in the treatment of *ye ge*. Moist yet not cloying herbs that harmonize and descend the stomach qi are appropriate.

[Addendum]

Gastric Reflux

反 胃 *Fan Wei*

This disorder is characterized by vomiting of undigested food that has been ingested for hours. It is mainly caused by spleen and stomach deficient cold disrupting food digestion. Food retains in the stomach for hours and inhibits the descending of stomach qi, leading to gastric reflux. Chronic gastric reflux may induce kidney yang deficiency. "Secondary stomach yang deficiency caused by failure of fire in the lower burner fails to ripen the food and drink." Kidney yang deficiency predisposes exacerbation of the condition. This condition resembles pylori stenosis or spasm in western medicine.

Spleen and stomach yang deficiency

Distention and fullness after meals, vomiting undigested food that has been ingested hours ago; lassitude, fatigue and sallow complexion.
T: Pale tongue with thin coating. **P:** Decelerating, thready and forceless pulse.

- Warm the middle burner, strengthen the spleen, descend rebellious qi and harmonize the stomach.
- *Ding Chen Tou Ge San*
  - *Ren Shen* and *Bai Zhu* benefit the qi, warm the middle burner and strengthen the spleen.
  - *Mu Xiang* and *Sha Ren*, aromatic herbs, promote the movement of qi and harmonize the stomach.
  - *Shen Qu*, *Mai Ya*, *Ding Xiang* and *Chen Xiang* eliminate food retention and descend the qi.
- Severe vomiting. + *Xuan Fu Hua, Dai Zhe Shi*
  Kidney yang deficiency with pale complexion and frigid extremities, use *Fu Zi Li Zhong Wan*.
  Yin injury due to chronic gastric reflux, use *Mai Men Dong Tang*.

CHAPTER 13

Diarrhea

泄 瀉 *Xie Xie*

Diarrhea is characterized by changes in the frequency and quality of bowel movements. The disorder is defined by the frequent passage of unformed, loose or watery stool that may or may not contain undigested food. Diarrhea occurs in all seasons, but is more common during summer and autumn. Its pathophysiology involves excessive dampness, spleen and stomach dysfunction, impairment of the large intestine's transporting function, and failure to separate clear and turbid substances.

Related Diseases

- Stomach flu
- Acute gastritis
- Acute or chronic enteritis
- Acute or chronic colitis
- Intestinal tuberculosis
- Malabsorption syndrome
- IBS
- Food poisoning
- IBD
- Intestinal tumor
- Emotional diarrhea

Etiology and Pathogenesis

Exterior pathogenic factors: All six exterior pathogenic factors can induce diarrhea, especially cold, dampness, summer heat, and fire. The exterior influences can have a direct impact on the digestive system and may disturb the functions of the spleen and stomach. The spleen prefers a dry environment, dislikes dampness, and is particularly susceptible to exterior dampness.

Improper diet: Overeating that exceed the stomach's capability of receiving and ripenning can impair digestion and absorption. Additionally, consumption of cold raw food and contaminated food may directly injure the spleen and stomach and impair their ability to transform, transport, ascend and descend.

Emotional stress: Liver qi stagnation caused by excessive anger or longterm frustration may overact on the spleen, leading to secondary spleen qi deficiency and impaired function of transformation and transportation.

Deficiency of the spleen and stomach: Overexertion, irregular diet over a long period of time, and chronic illness can exhaust the spleen and stomach. The deficient stomach receives food but is unable to decompose it, and the deficient spleen is incapable of transforming and transporting food into essence. Consequently, the pure and turbid combine and drain out together as diarrhea.

Yang deficiency of the kidney: Deficient kidney yang, caused by chronic illness, degeneration in the elderly and constitutional weakness, will fail to warm spleen yang. This does not only impair the spleen's function to transform and transport food and water, but also hinder the kidney's function to control bowel movements, inducing diarrhea.

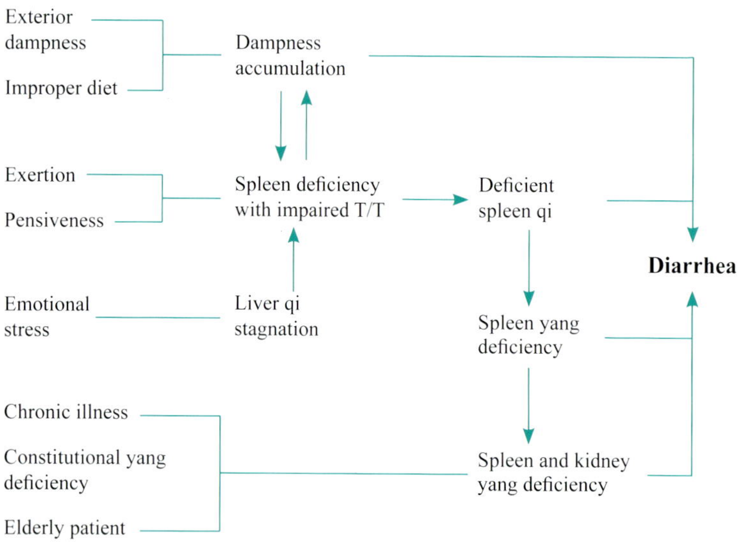

Diagnosis

A. Identification of excess and deficiency:

Excess patterns of diarrhea have an acute onset and short course; clinical manifestations include an increased frequency of bowel movements, abdominal pain aggravated by pressure and relieved by defecation.

Deficient patterns have a chronic onset and prolonged course; manifestations include intermittent episodes of diarrhea, abdominal pain relieved by pressure and aggravated by defecation.

B. Identification of cold and heat:

	Cold Pattern	Heat Pattern
Quality of the Stool	Loose or watery stool, containing undigested food.	Urgency, sticky yellow stool and burning sensation of the anus.
Abdominal Pain	Severe pain with loud borborygmus, relieved by warmth.	Burning pain with alteration of pain and diarrhea.
Thirst	No thirst or desire for warm beverages.	Intense thirst and preference for cold beverages.
Urination	Clear and abundant urine.	Dark and scanty urine.
Tongue	Moist white coating.	Red tongue with yellow coating.
Pulse	Deep and tight.	Slippery and rapid.

C. Identification of causes by stool characteristics:

- Yellow sticky or pasty stool with a strong foul odor, burning sensation of the anus – Damp-heat.
- Bluish-gray or bluish-black stool with a clear and thin or watery consistency without significant odor – Cold-dampness.
- Pasty stool containing undigested food with a foul odor like rotten eggs, and an uncomfortable sensation of incomplete defecation – Food stagnation.
- Paroxysmal loose stool triggered or aggravated by emotional stress – Liver overacting on the spleen.
- Unformed stool, loose bowel movements alternating with watery diarrhea, aggravated by fatigue or after meals – Spleen deficiency.
- Watery stool containing intact food particles that appear completely undigested, or abdominal pain with loose bowel movements occurring at dawn, also known as daybreak diarrhea – Kidney deficiency.

D. Differential diagnosis of diarrhea and dysentery disorder:

Diarrhea: The spleen or middle burner is affected. Diarrhea is caused by excessive dampness and spleen deficiency. Manifestations include abdominal pain, borborygmus and patent defecation without purulent or bloody stool. Pathological crisis is rarely seen with diarrhea.

Dysentery disorder: The intestines or lower burner are affected. Pathogenic factors accumulate internally; toxic heat rots the tissue, qi and blood, forming pus. Manifestations include purulent bloody stool, severe abdominal pain alternating with dysenteric bowel movements, and tenesmus caused by spasmodic contraction of the anal sphincter. Pathological crisis is common in dysentery disorder.

Basic Patterns

- Cold-dampness (wind-cold)
- Damp-heat (summer heat-dampness)
- Food retention
- Stagnant liver qi overacting on the spleen
- Spleen qi deficiency
- Kidney yang deficiency (daybreak diarrhea)

Differentiation and Treatment

Treatment principle:
Strengthening the spleen and draining dampness are the primary treatment principles.

Based on the various differentiations and patterns, there are ten treatment strategies for diarrhea. The ten strategies are: using bland medicinals to leach out dampness, raising and lifting sunken qi, clearing heat, pacifying the liver, unblocking obstruction, using sweet medicinals to moderate, using sour medicinals to astringe and bind, drying dampness from the spleen, warming the kidney, and restraining leakage and collapse.

Cold-dampness (wind-cold)

Acute onset, thin clear or loose watery stool with severe abdominal pain and borborygmus.
S: Aversion to cold, fever, headache, heaviness or soreness of the body, fullness and distention in the epigastrium, and poor appetite.
T: Thin white or white greasy coating. **P:** Decelerating and soft.

- Disperse cold to release the exterior and use aromatic medicinals to transform dampness.

- *Huo Xiang Zheng Qi San*
  - *Huo Xiang*, acting on the surface to disperse wind-cold, is also aromatic to transform dampness and harmonize the middle burner.
  - *Zi Su Ye* and *Bai Zhi* expel exterior wind-cold-dampness.
  - *Ban Xia*, *Chen Pi*, *Hou Po* and *Da Fu Pi* dry dampness and facilitate the movement of qi to stop diarrhea.

- *Bai Zhu* and *Fu Ling* strengthen the spleen, augment the qi and expel dampness to stop diarrhea.

- Significant symptoms of wind-cold attack. + *Jing Jie, Fang Feng*
  Dampness predominating with distention in the epigastrium and abdomen, oliguria, and white greasy tongue coating, use *Wei Ling Tang*.

Damp-heat (summer heat-dampness)

Urgent defecation with severe abdominal pain or an uncomfortable sensation of incomplete defecation, yellow-brown and sticky stool with an unpleasant odor.
S: Burning sensation of the anus, irritability, thirst and dark scanty urine.
T: Yellow greasy coating. **P:** Soft rapid or slippery rapid.

- Clear heat and eliminate dampness.

- *Ge Gen Qin Lian Tang*
  - *Huang Qin* and *Huang Lian*, bitter and cold, clear heat and dry dampness.
  - *Ge Gen* releases the pathogenic factors from the muscular layer and clears heat, as well as lifts the clear qi to stop diarrhea.

- Heat preponderance. + *Jin Yin Hua, Lian Qiao*
  Dampness preponderance. + *Che Qian Zi, Fu Ling, Mu Tong*
  During the summer. + *Huo Xiang, He Ye, Bian Dou*

Food retention

Frequent loose stool with a rotten smell and containing undigested food, and abdominal pain relieved by defecation.
S: Focal distention of the epigastrium and abdomen, belching with a foul smell or acid regurgitation, and lack of appetite.
T: Thick turbid greasy coating. **P:** Slippery.

- Reduce food retention and guide out stagnation.

- *Bao He Wan*
  - *Shan Zha*, *Shen Qu* and *Lai Fu Zi* reduce food retention.
  - *Ban Xia* and *Chen Pi* dry dampness, promote the qi flow, harmonize the stomach and descend rebellious qi.
  - *Fu Ling* augments the qi, strengthens the spleen and drains dampness.
  - *Lian Qiao* clears and disperses stagnant heat.

- Diarrhea due to overeating spicy, sweet or greasy food, with yellow tongue coating. + *Huang Qin, Huang Lian*
  Diarrhea due to overeating cold and raw food, with white tongue coating and decelerating pulse. + *Cang Zhu, Hou Po*

Severe food stagnation progressing to constrained heat with distention in the epigastrium and abdomen and an uncomfortable sensation of incomplete defecation, use *Zhi Shi Dao Zhi Wan*.

Stagnant liver qi overacting on the spleen

Recurrent painful diarrhea induced by emotional strain, abdominal pain temporarily relieved after bowel movements and recurring immediately, or a repetitive cycle of abdominal pain and diarrhea.
S: Distention and stifling sensation in the chest and hypochondriac regions, belching and poor appetite.
T: Slightly red tongue. **P:** Wiry.

- Pacify the liver, soothe the qi and strengthen the spleen.
- *Tong Xie Yao Fang*
  - *Bai Zhu* strengthens the spleen and dries dampness to stop diarrhea.
  - *Bai Shao* preserves the yin, and comforts and softens the liver.
  - *Fang Feng*, when used with *Bai Zhu*, augments the spleen and transforms dampness to stop diarrhea; when used with *Bai Shao*, spreads and soothes liver constraint.
  - *Chen Pi* regulates the movement of qi and harmonizes the middle burner.
- To strengthen the effects of spreading liver qi and comforting the liver. + *Wu Wei Zi, Mu Gua*

  To enhance the effects of strengthening the spleen and stopping diarrhea. + *Fu Ling, Bai Bian Dou, Shan Yao*

Spleen qi deficiency

Loose or watery stool that may contain undigested food, increased frequency of bowel movements with improper diet or exertion.
S: Sallow complexion, fatigue, poor appetite, fullness and distention in the epigastrium and abdomen.
T: Pale tongue with thin white coating. **P:** Weak and thready.

- Strengthen the spleen and benefit the stomach.
- *Shen Ling Bai Zhu San*
  - *Dang Shen, Bai Zhu, Fu Ling* and *Gan Cao* augment the qi and strengthen the spleen.
  - *Bian Dou* and *Yi Yi Ren* leach out dampness and stop diarrhea.
  - *Shan Yao* and *Lian Zi*, sweet and astringent, augment the qi as well as stop diarrhea.
  - *Sha Ren*, aromatic in nature, transforms dampness and facilitates the qi flow.

- Spleen yang deficiency with diarrhea, cold abdominal pain and cold limbs, use *Li Zhong Wan*.

  Unremitting chronic diarrhea, or qi sinking with prolapsed anus, use *Bu Zhong Yi Qi Tang*.

Kidney yang deficiency (daybreak diarrhea)

Cold abdominal pain accompanied by borborygmus and loose stool or diarrhea before dawn, pain relieved by defecation.

S: Cold intolerance and cold extremities; sore, cold and weak lower back and knees.

T: Pale tongue with white coating. **P:** Deep and thready.

- Warm the kidney, strengthen the spleen, bind the intestines and stop diarrhea.
- *Si Shen Wan*
  - *Bu Gu Zhi* warms and tonifies kidney yang.
  - *Rou Dou Kou* warms the spleen and kidney, and binds the intestines to stop diarrhea.
  - *Wu Zhu Yu* disperses cold and expels dampness.
  - *Wu Wei Zi* binds the intestines to stop diarrhea.
- Enhance the warming effect on the kidney and spleen. + *Fu Zi, Gan Jiang*

  Elderly patients with long-standing diarrhea developing into qi sinking.
  + *Huang Qi, Dang Shen, Bai Zhu, Sheng Ma*

Acupuncture Treatment

- **Manipulation:** Reducing method in the excess patterns; reinforcing method in the deficiency patterns; moxibustion is applicable in the cold patterns.
- **Prescription:** ST25 Tianshu ST36 Zusanli
- **Supplementary points:**
  - Cold-dampness. + CV12 Zhongwan; CV6 Qihai
  - Damp-heat. + ST44 Neiting; SP9 Yinglingquan
  - Food retention. + Inner Neiting (Extra)
  - Liver qi stagnation. + BL18 Ganshu; LR2 Xingjian
  - Spleen qi deficiency. + CV12 Zhongwan; BL20 Pishu; SP3 Taibai
  - Kidney deficiency. + CV4 Guanyuan; GV4 Mingmen; BL23 Shenshu; KI3 Taixi

Practical Hints

• **Excessive dampness and spleen deficiency are the two major causes of diarrhea.** With a mutual cause-effect relationship, these two etiologies influence each other. Accumulation of dampness may hinder the function of the spleen and cause diarrhea; bitter, warm and aromatic herbs should be used to dry dampness. The treatment principle emphasizes the action of expelling pathogenic factors. A deficient spleen may generate internal dampness and cause diarrhea; sweet and warm herbs should be used for strengthening the spleen to stop diarrhea. The treatment principle focuses on supporting the righteous qi.

• Since diarrhea is a common symptom present in various disorders, **symptomatic management by stopping diarrhea is not appropriate for all cases.** The underlying causes of diarrhea should be taken into consideration when forming the treatment plan. When treating the early stage of diarrhea, the binding and astringing method is not recommended because this strategy may retain pathogenic influences. In the case of chronic diarrhea, apply strategies of astringing and binding, and also consider integrating the method of raising yang qi.

• With proper treatment, most cases of diarrhea resolve in a few days; however, inappropriate treatment can prolong recovery and lead to chronic diarrhea. Pathological crisis related to diarrhea is rare. Clinically, **severe, excessive and unremitting diarrhea or incontinence of bowel movements will lead to great loss of the yin and body fluid, resulting in depletion of yin and devastation of yang.** Clinical manifestations include intense thirst with desire to drink, profuse sweating and cold extremities, pale complexion and minute pulse. Pathological crisis due to diarrhea is equivalent to fluid and electrolyte imbalance in modern medicine.

CHAPTER 14

Dysentery Disorder

痢疾 *Li Ji*

Dysentery disorder is characterized by abdominal pain, tenesmus, diarrhea with passage of blood, pus or mucous. It often occurs in the summer or fall season. Damp heat in the large intestine is the major predisposing factor to the occurrence of dysentery. Both sporadic and pandemic occurrences are possible. Dysentery disorder is considered one of the epidemic intestinal diseases.

Relevant Diseases

- Bacillary dysentery
- Amebic dysentery
- Viral dysentery
- Food poisoning
- Intoxication
- IBD

Etiology and Pathogenesis

Seasonal epidemic pathogens: Dysentery disorder is commonly seen in the summer or fall season. Summer heat-dampness as well as epidemic toxicity are two major contributors to dysentery disorder. These pathogens can attack the stomach and intestine, causing impaired qi flow and blood circulation. As these pathogens fuse together in the affected area and decompose the tissues, diarrhea with pus, blood or mucous is apparent.

Improper diet: Irregular diet habits or consuming contaminated food may generate damp-heat internally in those with pre-existing internal heat. Accumulated damp-heat can obstruct qi flow and blood circulation. In addition, a diet consisting of cold and raw food may also lead to cold-dampness accumulated internally in those with pre-existing internal cold. Cold-dampness can accumulate in the stomach or intestines to obstruct the qi flow and blood circulation. Stagnant qi, blood stasis and digested waste fuse together, transforming into pus and blood as tissue is being decomposed.

Although the intestines account for the primarily responsible organs, other organs play important roles in pathogenesis. In the case of chronic dysentery disorder that has severely injured stomach qi, patient will suffer from both severe diarrhea and anorexia. Unremitting dysentery disorder can also progress into an intermittent dysentery due to deficient righteous qi with residual pathogens. At advanced stage, constant diarrhea or fecal incontinence indicates kidney involvement.

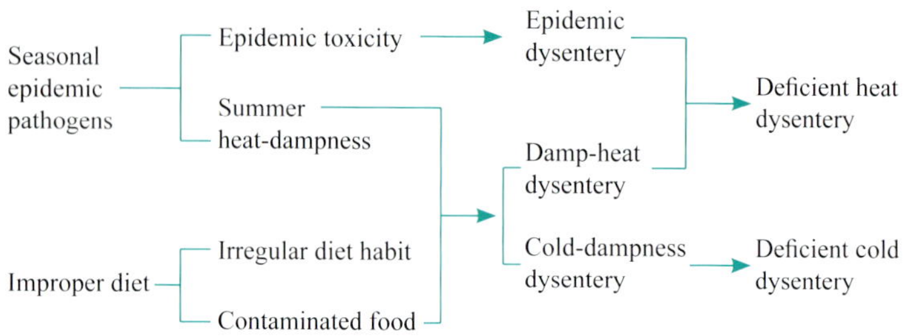

Diagnosis

Differential diagnosis of similar disorders:

Diarrhea: Both diarrhea and dysentery share some commonalities in their pathogenesis. They both have the tendency to occur during the summer and fall seasons; they both affect the stomach and intestines, and both are related to seasonal pathogens and improper diet. However, diarrhea is characterized by increasing frequencies of unformed bowel movements. Tenesmus is not evident in diarrhea. Abdominal pain may be present together with abdominal distention and borborygmus, and these symptoms are relieved after defecation. However, abdominal pain is severe and is accompanied by tenesmus in dysentery disorder. After defecation, abdominal pain and tenesmus remain problematic. Dysentery disorder is also characterized by the passage of pus, blood or mucous stool.

Bloody stool: Including hemotochezia and melena, it is a pattern from hemorrhagic disorder. Fresh bloody stool can be seen in dysentery disorder. However, tenesmus and abdominal pain are the primary symptoms for dysentery disorder.

Warm-febrile disease: Comatose with convulsions or contractions can be caused by acute heat toxicity consuming the yin and generating internal wind in epidemic dysentery, or caused by summer heat harassing the heart and mind in warm-febrile disease. To differentiate between these two disorders, other clinical manifestations obtained from history taking or physical examinations are necessary.

Basic Patterns

- Damp-heat dysentery
- Cold-dampness dysentery
- Deficient cold dysentery
- Epidemic dysentery
- Deficient heat dysentery
- Intermittent dysentery

Differentiation and Treatment

Treatment principle:

Clear febrile pathogens in heat patterns, warm the interior for cold patterns, unblock the obstructions during the early stage or in excess patterns, and tonify the insufficiency in chronic and deficient patterns.

Damp-heat dysentery

Abdominal pain, tenesmus, diarrhea with passage of blood and pus.
S: Burning pain at the perianal region and dark scanty urine output.
T: Yellow greasy coating. **P:** Slippery and rapid.

- Harmonize the qi and blood, clear heat and relieve toxicity.
- *Shao Yao Tang*
  - *Shao Yao* is the king herb; it harmonizes the nutritive qi and the blood when combining with *Dang Gui*; it moderates spasm and alleviates pain when used together with *Gan Cao*.
  - *Huang Qin*, *Huang Lian* and *Da Huang* are bitter and cold herbs; they clear heat and dry dampness to relieve toxicity.
  - *Mu Xiang* and *Bing Lang* promote the movement of qi.
- To strengthen the effects of clearing heat and relieving toxicity. + *Jin Yin Hua*
  Initial stage of dysentery, unresolved exterior with excessive internal heat manifested with fever, slight aversion to wind, sweating, and rapid abrupt pulse, use *Ge Gen Qin Lian Tang*.
  Resolved exterior condition and excessive internal damp-heat with unremitting dysentery. + *Xiang Lian Wan*
  Preponderance of dampness, use *Mu Xiang Bing Lang Wan*.
  Preponderance of heat, use *Zhi Shi Dao Zhi Wan*.

Epidemic dysentery

Acute onset, diarrhea with fresh blood and pus, excruciating pain in the abdomen and tenesmus.
S: High fever, thirst, headache, irritability, possible loss of consciousness or convulsions.
T: Dark red tongue with dry yellow coating. **P:** Slippery and rapid.

- Clear heat, cool the blood and relieve toxicity.
- *Bai Tou Weng Tang*
  - *Bai Tou Weng* cools the blood and relieves toxicity.
  - *Huang Lian*, *Huang Bai* and *Qin Pi* clear heat and dry dampness.

- To reinforce the effects of clearing heat, cooling the blood and relieving toxicity. + *Huang Qin, Jin Yin Hua, Chi Shao, Mu Dan Pi, Di Yu*

  Heat toxicity trapped in the heart, or the nutritive level with fever, loss of consciousness, delirium and convulsions. + *Shui Niu Jiao* (a substitute for *Xi Jiao*), *Ling Yang Jiao, Sheng Di Huang*

Cold-dampness dysentery

Diarrhea with passage of blood, pus and mucous, more pus and mucous than blood in the stool, abdominal pain and tenesmus.

S: Lack of appetite, abdominal and epigastric distention, and general heaviness.

T: Pale tongue with white greasy coating. **P:** Soft and decelerating. | Slow

- Warm and transform cold-dampness.
- *Wei Ling Tang*
  - *Cang Zhu* and *Hou Po* dry dampness and strengthen the spleen.
  - *Bai Zhu* and *Fu Ling* augment the qi and strengthen the spleen to dispel dampness.
  - *Gui Zhi* warms and transforms cold-dampness.
  - *Chen Pi* facilities the qi flow to alleviate distention.
- To reinforce the effects of dispelling cold and regulating the qi. + *Mu Xiang, Bing Lang, Pao Jiang*

  To invigorate the blood and harmonize nutritive qi. + *Bai Shao, Dang Gui*

Deficient heat dysentery

Diarrhea with passage of blood, pus and mucous, forceful efforts to defecate yet incomplete sensation after bowel movements, and burning pain in the abdomen.

S: Poor appetite, irritability and thirst.

T: Dark red tongue with scanty coating. **P:** Thready and rapid.

- Nourish the yin and clear the intestines.
- *Zhu Che Wan*
  - *Huang Lian*, bitter and cold, clears the intestines, dries dampness and stops dysentery.
  - *E Jiao* nourishes the blood and harmonizes the yin; it also astringes.
  - *Dang Gui* nourishes and invigorates the blood.
- To reinforce the effects of nourishing the yin, harmonizing the nutritive qi and alleviating abdominal pain. + *Bai Shao, Gan Cao*

  Significant thirst, scanty urine output and dry tongue. + *Sha Shen, Shi Hu*

  More blood than pus or mucous. + *Mu Dan Pi, Chi Shao, Han Lian Cao*

Deficient cold dysentery

Clear, watery diarrhea with mucous, dull pain in the abdomen, and fecal incontinence in severe cases.

S: Poor appetite, lassitude, cold limbs, and soreness and cold sensation in the lower back and knees.

T: Pale tongue with thin white coating. **P:** Deep, thready and weak.

- Warm and tonify the spleen and kidney, astringe and bind the essence.
- *Fu Zi Li Zhong Wan*
  - *Fu Zi* and *Gan Jiang* warm the yang and disperse cold.
  - *Ren Shen*, *Bai Zhu* and *Gan Cao* tonify the middle burner and benefit the qi.
- Chronic dysentery with rectal prolapse, use *Bu Zhong Yi Qi Tang*.
  Severe fecal incontinence, use *Tao Hua Tang*.

Intermittent dysentery

Recurrent, intermittent dysentery with abdominal pain, tenesmus, passage of blood and mucous.

S: Decreased appetite, fatigue, preference to lay down in fetal position and cold intolerance.

T: Pale tongue with greasy coating. **P:** Soft or deficient.

- Warm the middle burner, clear the intestines, and promote qi movement.
- *Lian Li Tang*
  - *Gan Jiang* warms the middle burner and disperses cold.
  - *Ren Shen*, *Bai Zhu* and *Gan Cao* augment the qi and strengthen the spleen.
  - *Huang Lian* clears and drains pathogens from the intestines.
- To promote the movement of qi and guide out the accumulation. + *Bing Lang, Mu Xiang, Zhi Shi*
  Stubborn dysentery manifested with combination of cold and heat pattern, use *Wu Mei Wan*.

Acupuncture Treatment

- **Manipulation:** Reducing method in heat patterns; moxibustion is applicable in cold patterns.
- **Prescription:** ST25 Tianshu ST37 Shangjuxu
- **Supplementary points:**
  - Damp-heat dysentery. + LI4 Hegu; LI11 Quchi

- Epidemic dysentery. + GV14 Dazhui; Extra24 Shixuan
- Cold-damp dysentery. + CV6 Qihai; SP9 Yinlingquan
- Deficient heat dysentery. + KI6 Zhaohai; SP10 Xuehai
- Deficient cold dysentery. + BL20 Pishu; BL23 Shenshu
- Intermittent dysentery. + CV4 Guanyuan; ST36 Zusanli

Practical Hints

• **"Regulate the qi to alleviate tenesmus; invigorate the blood to resolve pus."** Tenesmus is a subjective urgency and heavy sensation of the rectum. It is caused by qi stagnation and dampness accumulation. Therefore, by facilitating the qi flow, dampness can be resolved and tenesmus will be alleviated. Generation of pus is a result from decomposed tissues due to blood stasis and heat accumulation. By invigorating the blood to restore proper circulation, decomposition of the tissue can be prevented and tissues will have sufficient supply to recover.

• Modern medical application of antibiotics has greatly decreased the incidence and severity of dysentery disorders. However, long-term usage or misusage of antibiotics may induce an imbalance of normal bacteria flora in the intestines, complicating dysentery. Therefore, for chronic, stubborn, drug-resistant or complicated dysentery, herbal therapy has a considerable value.

CHAPTER 15

Abdominal Pain

腹痛 *Fu Tong*

Any subjective, unpleasant and painful sensation in the abdominal region is known as abdominal pain. Abdominal region is defined as the area from beneath the epigastrium to the suprapubic margin. Abdominal pain is the most common disorder that everyone may experience at least once in his/her lifetime. The abdomen covers a broad region in which many organs reside. The abdomen also is the merging area for the three hand and three foot yin channels, some hand and foot yang channels, and also the Penetrating, Reception and Girdle vessels. Abdominal pain signifies various disorders from the internal organs, as well as the channels and vessels.

In addition, surgical and gynecological disorders might contribute to abdominal pain. However, this chapter addresses only internal medical causes to abdominal pain.

Relevant Diseases

- Acute or chronic enteritis
- Intestinal tumor
- Intestinal tuberculosis
- Pancreatitis
- Cholecystitis
- Chronic non-perforated appendicitis
- Fecal impaction

Etiology and Pathogenesis

Invasion of seasonal exterior pathogens can instantly upset the organs in the abdomen. Cold invasion will slow down the movement of the qi and blood, leading to pain; cold transforming into heat or damp-heat invasion can inhibit the intestinal peristalsis and obstruct the qi flow in the intestines. Impairment of the spleen and stomach's function to transform and transport vital substances can therefore be caused by cold, summerheat and dampness invasion. Following stagnant pathogens in the middle burner, qi fails to flow smoothly and the end result is abdominal pain.

Improper diet: Consumption of food exceeding the spleen and stomach's capacity precipitates food stagnation. Indulgence of a greasy, sweet and rich diet contributes to the generation of damp-heat in the digestive system. Raw and cold food can injure the spleen yang and may inhibit normal functions of the spleen. Obstruction by food retention and damp-heat accumulation, and spleen deficiency lead to abdominal pain.

Emotional stress: Constrained liver qi secondary to emotional stress can progress into qi stagnation and blood stasis. Constrained liver qi can also overact on the spleen and stomach. Disharmony of the liver, spleen and stomach with stagnant qi and blood will then cause abdominal pain.

Constitutional yang deficiency: The result of yang qi deficiency is internal cold, which congeals and fails to warm the internal organs. Therefore, a deficient type of abdominal pain, which is a chronic type that has lingered for a long period of time, is now manifested.

Miscellaneous: Qi stagnation, blood stasis and obstruction in the channels and vessels resulting from surgeries and/or traumatic injuries are also causes for abdominal pain.

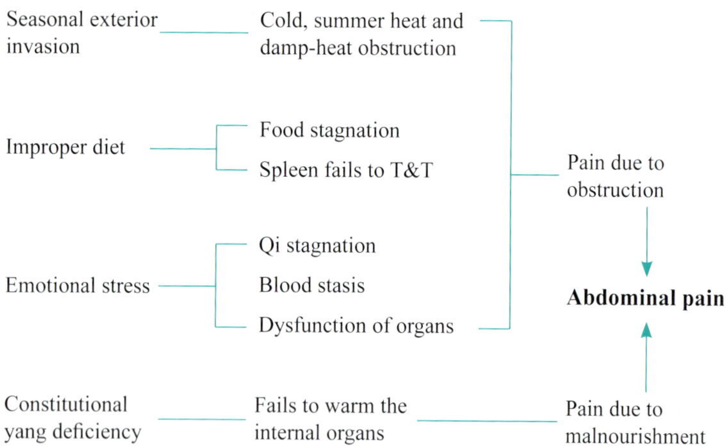

Diagnosis

A. Identification of cold, heat, excess and deficiency:

Based on the etiology, the affected area, and the characteristics of pain:

- Pain aggravated by pressure or after meals – Excess.
  Preference to pressure or pain aggravated by hunger – Deficiency.
- Pain alleviated by warmth – Cold.
  Pain alleviated by cold – Heat.

- Distending and migrating pain – Qi stagnation.
  Stabbing and fixed pain – Blood stasis.
- Pain localized at the lower flank radiating to the hypochondria – Involvement of the liver and gallbladder.
  Pain located at the suprapubic area and the periumbilical region – Involvement of the spleen, kidney and bladder.

B. Differential diagnosis of similar disorders:

Dysentery disorder, abdominal masses, intestinal abscess and hernia disorder may present with abdominal pain. However, they also possess various symptoms at different quadrants.

Dysentery disorder: It is manifested as abdominal pain with tenesmus, and severe diarrhea with purulent blood and mucous in the stool.

Abdominal masses: This disorder is characterized by visible or palpable abdominal masses, soft or hard to the touch, with abdominal pain.

Intestinal abscess: It is marked by pain localized at the right lower quadrant with rebound pain, muscle guard, tenderness and rigidity, and propensity to flexing the right lower extremity.

Hernia disorder: Lower abdominal cold pain radiating from the inguinal region to the scrotum, and protrusion of the abdominal wall is also evident.

Basic Patterns

- Cold invasion
- Damp-heat accumulation
- Food retention
- Qi stagnation and blood stasis
- Spleen and stomach yang deficiency

Differentiation and Treatment

Treatment principle:

Pain due to obstruction: Regulate the flow of qi, harmonize the blood, dispel cold, relieve food stagnation, and drain accumulation downwards to unblock the obstruction.

Pain due to malnourishment: Fortify yang qi to warm the internal organs.

Cold invasion

Sudden and urgent onset of severe abdominal pain, alleviated by warmth.

S: No thirst, clear and abundant urine output and loose stool.

T: White greasy coating. **P:** Deep and tight.

- Warm the middle burner and disperse cold.
- *Li Zhong Wan*
  - *Gan Jiang* warms and disperses cold.
  - *Dang Shen*, *Bai Zhu* and *Gan Cao* tonify the qi and warm the middle burner.
- To strengthen the effects of dispersing cold and facilitating the qi flow. + *Sheng Jiang, Wu Yao, Xiang Fu*

  Frigid limbs and minute pulse. + *Fu Zi, Cong Bai*

Damp-heat accumulation

Abdominal pain aggravated by pressure, stifling sensation in the chest, constipation or incomplete sense of evacuation after bowel movements.
S: Irritability, thirst, sweating and dark scanty urination.
T: Yellow greasy coating. **P:** Soft and rapid.

- Purge heat and unblock the bowel.
- *Da Cheng Qi Tang*
  - *Da Huang*, bitter and cold in nature, purges heat accumulation.
  - *Mang Xiao*, salty and cold in nature, softens hardness and moistens dryness.
  - *Zhi Shi* and *Hou Po* descend the qi and reduce clumps.
- Preponderance of damp-heat with significant sense of incomplete evacuation after bowel movements and mild constipation, take off *Mang Xiao* and + *Huang Qin, Zhi Zi*

  Abdominal pain radiating to the hypochondriac region. + *Chai Hu, Yu Jin*

Food retention

Abdominal distention, fullness and pain radiating to the epigastrium, aggravated by pressure, anorexia, and nausea after meals.
S: Belching, acid regurgitation, diarrhea with undigested food or constipation.
T: Greasy coating. **P:** Slippery.

- Relieve food stagnation and eliminate accumulation.
- *Bao He Wan*
  - *Shan Zha*, *Shen Qu* and *Lai Fu Zi* relieve food stagnation and eliminate accumulation to alleviate abdominal pain.
  - *Ban Xia* and *Chen Pi* dry dampness, expel phlegm and promote the qi flow.
  - *Fu Ling* strengthens the spleen and drains dampness.
  - *Lian Qiao* eliminates stagnant heat secondary to food retention.
- Severe cases of food stagnation accompanied by constipation, use *Zhi Shi Dao Zhi Wan*.

Qi stagnation and blood stasis

Distending and migrating abdominal pain, radiating to the lower flank if qi stagnation predominates; stabbing, sharp and fixed abdominal pain when blood stasis preponderates.
S: Pain aggravated by emotional stress and relieved by belching or passing gas.
T: Bluish purple tongue. **P:** Wiry or choppy.

- Spread liver constraint, invigorate the blood and transform stasis.
- *Chai Hu Shu Gan San* if qi stagnation is the principal cause
  - *Chai Hu*, *Xiang Fu*, *Chen Pi* and *Zhi Qiao* soothe liver qi and resolve constraint to alleviate pain.
  - *Chuan Xiong* facilitates the qi flow and invigorates the blood to alleviate pain.
  - *Shao Yao* and *Gan Cao* soften and comfort the liver to alleviate pain.
- *Shao Fu Zhu Yu Tang* if blood stasis is the principal cause
  - *Dang Gui*, *Chuan Xiong* and *Chi Shao* nourish and invigorate the blood.
  - *Pu Huang*, *Wu Ling Zhi* and *Yuan Hu* transform blood stasis to alleviate pain.
  - *Rou Gui*, *Gan Jiang* and *Xiao Hui Xiang* warm the meridians to alleviate pain.
- Abdominal pain secondary to surgical procedure. + *Ze Lan, Hong Hua*
  Abdominal pain related to traumatic injuries. + *Wang Bu Liu Xing, San Qi*

Spleen and stomach yang deficiency

Intermittent dull pain in the abdomen, preference for pressure and warmth, aggravated by hunger and exertion.
S: Loose stool, lassitude, shortness of breath and cold intolerance.
T: Pale tongue with white coating. **P:** Deep and thready.

- Warm the middle burner, moderate spasm and alleviate pain.
- *Xiao Jian Zhong Tang*
  - *Yi Tang*, sweet and warm, tonifies the middle burner.
  - *Gui Zhi*, acrid and warm in nature, unblocks yang qi.
  - *Bai Shao* benefits the yin and blood. Moderates spasm and alleviates pain when it is accompanied with *Gan Cao* and *Yi Tang*.
  - *Sheng Jiang* and *Da Zao* warm the middle burner, tonify the deficiency and disperse cold.
- To strengthen the effect of benefiting the middle burner. + *Huang Qi*
  Nausea, vomiting, cold limbs and minute pulse, use *Da Jian Zhong Tang*.
  Abdominal pain with severe diarrhea, cold limbs, and slow deep pulse, use *Fu Zi Li Zhong Wan*.

Acupuncture Treatment

Cold invasion:

- **Manipulation:** Reducing method and moxibustion.
- **Prescription:** CV12 Zhongwan CV8 Shenque ST36 Zusanli SP4 Gongsun

Damp-heat accumulation:

- **Manipulation:** Reducing method.
- **Prescription:** LI4 Hegu LI11 Quchi BL25 Dachangshu ST37 Shangjuxu ST25 Tianshu

Food retention:

- **Manipulation:** Reducing method.
- **Prescription:** CV12 Zhongwan ST25 Tianshu CV6 Qihai ST36 Zusanli

Qi stagnation:

- **Manipulation:** Reducing method.
- **Prescription:** CV17 Tanzhong LR3 Taichong PC6 Neiguan CV10 Xiawan GB34 Yanglingquan

Yang deficiency:

- **Manipulation:** Reinforcing method and moxibustion.
- **Prescription:** BL20 Pishu BL21 Weishu CV12 Zhongwan LR13 Zhangmen CV6 Qihai ST36 Zusanli

Practical Hints

Rule out all possible non-medical diagnoses before treatment. Abdominal pain can be a symptom of many disorders involving various organs. Gynecologic pathology, surgical conditions and traumatic injuries all can induce abdominal pain and mislead the medical diagnosis. Prompt diagnosis and identification of urgent and critical pathology are important to guide the treatments. Conservative medical measures are not adequate for gynecological, obstetrical or surgical conditions, such as ectopic pregnancy, bowel obstruction, perforated peptic ulcers, acute peritonitis, necrotic pancreatitis and acute appendicitis. Improper treatment due to misdiagnosis will mask symptoms. As a result, the patient will be placed at higher risk that might lead to possible death.

CHAPTER 16

Constipation

便秘 *Bian Bi*

Constipation refers to difficult and/or infrequent defecation with passage of unduly hard and dry stool, and also to sluggish bowel movements. Associated symptoms include abdominal pain, belching, focal distention in the epigastrium and abdomen, lack of appetite, dizziness and headache, all due to the blockage of qi circulation in the bowel and rebellious turbidity. Impairment of the large intestine's function to transport and guide turbidity downwards is an important factor in constipation; however, dysfunction of the spleen, stomach, lung and kidney can also promote constipation.

Relevant Diseases

- Habitual constipation
- Atonic constipation
- Spastic constipation
- Intestinal neurosis
- Bowel obstruction
- Intestinal tumor
- Perianal inflammation and infection (fissure or fistula)
- Hemorrhoids
- Overdose of antidiarrheal medication
- Adverse effect of medication

Etiology and Pathogenesis

Constitutional yang excess and accumulation of heat in the intestine and stomach: Overindulgence in alcohol, spicy and sweet foods when there is a pre-existing yang excess condition can exacerbate the accumulation of heat in the stomach and intestines. Residual heat following a warm-febrile disease consumes the body fluid and decreases lubrication in the intestines.

Qi stagnation: Worry, depression, stress or lack of physical activity can impair the transporting and descending function of the qi. If lung qi does not disperse and descend, it will affect the qi flow in the large intestine. Consequently, intestinal content accumulates and is not eliminated.

Qi and blood deficiency: When qi is deficient, the force for transporting the bowel contents is inadequate; when the blood, yin and essence are deficient, lack of lubrication in the intestines will lead to dryness of the bowel contents. Spleen qi deficiency due to improper diet, qi and blood deficiency due to chronic illness, post-partum status and aging are all factors contributing to constipation. Overuse of diaphoretics or purgatives injures the yin, while excessive bleeding, spermatorrhea and leukorrhea exhaust the essence, leading to constipation.

Yang deficiency with internal cold: Yang deficiency due to chronic illness, aging or overindulgence of food and herbs cold in nature produces internal cold, which accumulates in the intestines and stomach. Because cold congeals, the flow of yang qi and fluid in the intestine becomes sluggish and results in constipation.

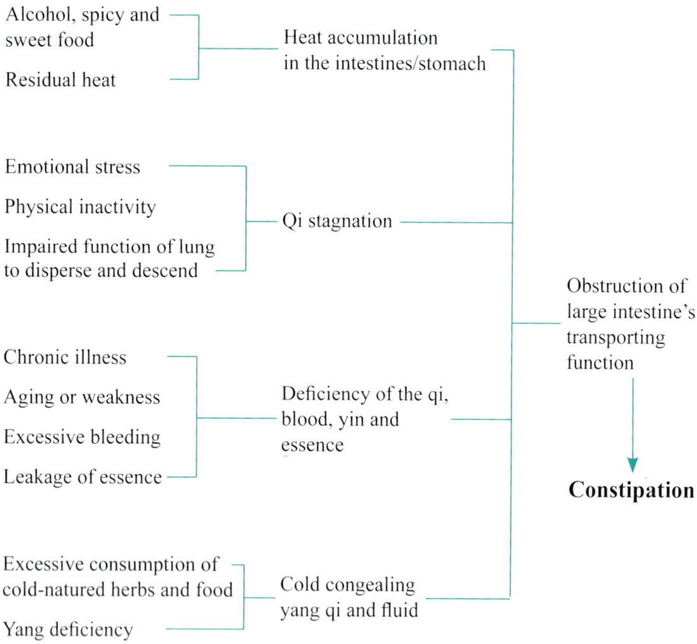

Diagnosis

A. Identification of excess and deficiency:

Excess pattern has a acute onset and a short course, and severe constipation; it responds well to treatment.

Deficient pattern has a chronic onset, a prolonged course, and mild to moderate constipation; it responds slowly to treatment and takes time for full recovery.

B. Identification of types of constipation:

- Dry impacted feces, infrequent and difficult defecation, accompanied by a red face, fever, bad breath, sores in the mouth, dark scanty urine, a dry yellow tongue coating, and forceful slippery pulse – Constipation due to heat.
- No significant alteration in the quality of stool, sense of incomplete defecation, sluggish defecation, frequent belching, focal distention in the chest and hypochondrium, distending abdominal pain, a thin greasy tongue coating and wiry pulse – Constipation due to qi stagnation.
- Normal desire for defecation, ineffective straining to force bowel movements, great effort and prolonged time required for defecation, a pale complexion, lassitude, spontaneous sweating and shortness of breath during defecation, a thin tongue coating and deficient pulse – Constipation due to qi deficiency.
- Normal frequency of bowel movements, dry pebble-like stool that is very difficult to evacuate, a sallow complexion, palpitations, dizziness, a pale tongue, and thready choppy pulse – Constipation due to blood deficiency.
- Normal stool similar to that of qi deficiency, difficult and sluggish defecation requiring great effort, cold limbs, abundant clear urine, preference for warmth and cold intolerance, a moist white tongue coating, and deep slow pulse – Constipation due to yang deficiency.

Basic Patterns

- Heat accumulation
- Qi stagnation
- Qi deficiency
- Blood deficiency
- Yang deficiency

Differentiation and Treatment

Treatment principle:

Unblocking obstruction of the bowel movement is the essential principle of treatment for constipation. Treatment methods are not limited to purging and draining. In clinical practice, depending on the pattern differentiation, other appropriate treatment methods include clearing heat to drain downwards, promoting qi flow to guide out accumulation, augmenting the qi and nourishing the blood, generating the body fluid to moisten dryness, and warming and unblocking cold obstruction.

Heat accumulation

Dry impacted feces, difficult and infrequent defecation, and dark scanty urine.
S: Fever, red face, bad breath, bitter taste in the mouth, sores in the mouth, irritability, short temper and abdominal distention.
T: Red tongue with dry yellow coating. **P:** Rapid and slippery.

- Drain heat, moisten the intestines and unblock the bowel obstruction.
- *Ma Zi Ren Wan*
  - *Huo Ma Ren* moistens the intestines and unblocks obstruction of the bowel movements.
  - *Da Huang* purges fire and unblocks obstruction of the bowel movements.
  - *Xing Ren* descends the qi and moistens the intestines.
  - *Bai Shao* and *Feng Mi* nourish the yin, generate the fluid and moisten intestinal dryness.
  - *Zhi Shi* and *Hou Po* promote the movement of qi and reduce distention.
- Excessive heat injuring the yin with dry mouth and intense thirst. + *Xuan Shen, Mai Men Dong, Sheng Di Huang*
  Perianal fissures and bleeding. + *Di Yu, Huai Hua*

Qi stagnation

Dry stool and sluggish bowel movements; aggravated by emotional stress.
S: Frequent belching, focal distention in the chest and hypochondrium, distending abdominal pain, and sighing; relieved after passing gas.
T: Thin greasy coating. **P:** Wiry.

- Promote the movement of qi and guide out accumulation.
- *Liu Mo Tang*
  - *Mu Xiang* and *Wu Yao* promote the movement of qi and dissipate clumps.
  - *Zhi Shi*, *Chen Xiang* and *Bing Lang* descend the qi and eliminate distention.
  - *Da Huang* purges fire and unblocks obstruction of the bowel movements.
- Qi stagnation turning into fire. + *Huang Qin, Zhi Zi*

Qi deficiency

Desire to defecate, normal quality of stool, ineffective straining to force bowel movements, great effort and prolonged time required for defecation.
S: Pale complexion, lassitude, spontaneous sweating and shortness of breath during defecation.
T: Pale tongue with thin white coating. **P:** Thready and weak.

- Strengthen the spleen and benefit the qi.

- *Huang Qi Tang*
  - *Huang Qi* and *Gan Cao* benefit the qi and strengthen the spleen. warm
  - *Huo Ma Ren* and *Bai Mi* moisten the intestines and unblock obstruction of the bowel movements.
  - *Chen Pi* regulates the qi.
- To enhance the effect of tonifying the qi. + *Dang Shen, Huang Jing*
  Deficient and sunken qi with heaviness of the anus. + *Sheng Ma, Chai Hu*

Blood deficiency

Dry pebble-like stool that is very difficult to evacuate.
S: Palpitations, dizziness, insomnia, dream-disturbed sleep, sallow complexion, pale lips and nails.
T: Pale tongue. **P:** Thready and choppy.

- Nourish the blood and moisten dryness.
- *Run Chang Wan*
  - *Dang Gui* and *Sheng Di Huang* nourish the yin and blood.
  - *Huo Ma Ren* and *Tao Ren* moisten dryness and unblock obstruction of the bowel movements.
  - *Zhi Qiao* facilities the flow of qi and dissipates accumulation.
- Five-centers heat, dry mouth and scanty tongue coating. + *Xuan Shen, Mai Men Dong, Sheng Shou Wu*
  Habitual constipation due to intestinal dryness, use *Wu Ren Wan*.

Yang deficiency

Dry or moist stool, difficult and sluggish defecation requiring great effort, and abundant clear urine.
S: Cold intolerance, cold limbs, abdominal cold pain, cold pain of the lower back and spine.
T: Pale and flabby tongue with moist white coating. **P:** Deep and slow.

- Warm the yang and open the bowels.
- *Ji Chuan Jian*
  - *Rou Cong Rong* warms the kidney, augments the essence and moistens the intestines.
  - *Dang Gui* nourishes the blood and moistens the intestines.
  - *Niu Xi* tonifies the liver and kidney and descends downwards.
  - *Zhi Qiao* regulates and descends the qi.
  - *Sheng Ma* and *Ze Xie* ascend the clear qi and descend turbidities.
- Warm and unblock the qi flow. + *Rou Gui, Wu Yao*

Acupuncture Treatment

- **Manipulation:** Reducing method in excess patterns; reinforcing method in deficiency patterns; add moxibustion in the cold patterns.
- **Prescription:** BL25 Dachangshu ST25 Tianshu TE6 Zhigou KI6 Zhaohai
- **Supplementary points:**
  - Heat accumulation. + LI11 Quchi; LI4 Hegu
  - Qi stagnation. + CV12 Zhongwan; LI3 Taichong
  - Qi and blood deficiency. + BL20 Pishu; BL21 Weishu; ST36 Zusanli
  - Cold. + CV8 Shenque; CV6 Qihai

Practical Hints

• Constipation itself is not a critical disorder; the **clinical significance is closely related to its complications.** Constipation is a cause of auto-intoxication via reabsorption of toxins that remain in the intestines. Auto-intoxication manifests with dizziness, headache, loss of appetite, irritability, insomnia, cracking and peeling skin and acne. Chronic constipation also contributes to stubborn perianal disorders that do not respond well to treatment, for example, hemorrhoids, perianal fissures and fistulas, and perianal abscesses. In addition, constipation can provoke a medical crisis; for example, cerebrovascular accident due to hemorrhage and myocardial infarction may be induced by forcing and straining during defecation.

• **Discontinue bitter and cold herbs that drain downwards once the therapeutic effect achieved.** The most common method for treating constipation is draining heat and unblocking the obstruction. This strategy incorporates herbs that are extremely bitter and cold and thus has the tendency to injure the stomach. Therefore, once the therapeutic effect is achieved, this strategy should be discontinued.

• **Support the righteous qi to restore normal bowel movements.** In the late stage of warm-febrile disease, constipation is a common symptom, caused by decreased food and water intake during the acute stage. Treatment to promote bowel movements might not be necessary. Instead, nourish stomach yin and tonify stomach qi. Once the righteous qi recovers and normal oral intake resumes, bowel movements will be restored.

CHAPTER **17**

Hypochondriac Pain

脅痛 *Xie Tong*

Hypochondriac pain refers to unilateral or bilateral pain in the infracostal regions. A subjective symptom, hypochondriac pain is usually associated with dysfunction of the liver and gallbladder. Clinically, the pain is accompanied by distention and pain in the epigastrium or by palpable masses in the infracostal regions.

Relevant Diseases

- Cholecystitis
- Cholelithiasis
- Gallbladder cancer
- Hepatitis
- Hepatosplenomegaly
- Liver cancer
- Acute pancreatitis
- Chronic pancreatitis
- Pleurisy

Etiology and Pathogenesis

The liver is located beneath the diaphragm and the liver channels are distributed bilaterally around the hypochondria. The gallbladder is attached to the liver and its channels travel through the same region. Pain in the hypochondria may indicate dysfunction of the liver and gallbladder.

Liver qi stagnation: Emotional stress, especially anger and frustration, is one of the major factors contributing to hypochondriac pain because it interferes with the liver's function to direct the free flow of qi.

Blood stasis in the liver channels: Prolonged qi stagnation or traumatic injury to the hypochondriac regions can develop into blood stasis obstructing the liver channels.

Liver and gallbladder damp-heat: Damp-heat derives from exterior dampness or from interior dampness caused by spleen injury due to improper diet. Accumulated dampness lingering for a long period of time can turn into heat and form a damp-heat complex. Damp-heat obstructs the free flow of liver qi.

Liver yin deficiency: Chronic illness or excessive sexual activity exhausts the essence and blood, which then fail to nourish the liver and its channels.

According to TCM theory, the causes of pain are two-fold. Obstructive pain is caused by stasis involving any pathogenic influence, e.g. liver or gallbladder qi stagnation, blood stasis in the liver channels, damp-heat accumulated in the liver and gallbladder, or congested fluids accumulated in the chest and hypochondria. Pain due to malnourishment is caused by lack of nourishment to the organs or tissues, e.g. liver yin or blood deficiency.

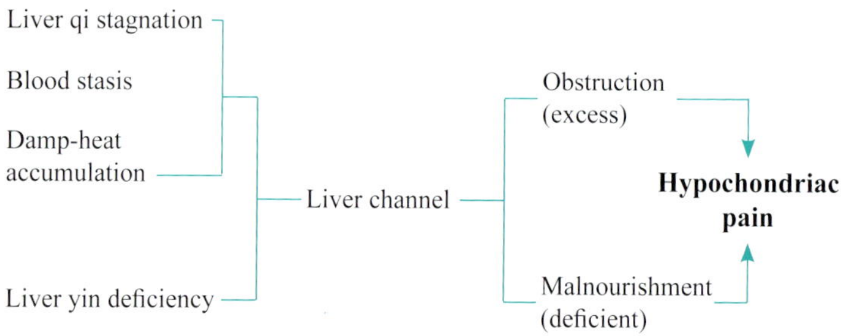

Diagnosis

A. Identification of exterior and interior patterns:

Exterior patterns are acute and usually related to damp-heat attacking the liver and gallbladder. Hypochondriac pain is accompanied by exterior symptoms, such as aversion to cold and fever, as well as nausea, vomiting and jaundice.

Interior patterns occur with gradual onset and without any presentation of exterior symptoms.

B. Identification of cold and heat patterns:

Cold patterns are usually seen in those with weak constitutions. Hypochondriac pain is accompanied by cold intolerance and absence of thirst. Pain is relieved by application of warmth and aggravated by exposure to cold. The pulse is slow, deep, choppy or wiry.

Heat patterns are usually associated with strong constitutions. Hypochondriac pain is accompanied by a red face, bitter taste in the mouth and thirst. Pain is relieved by application of cold and aggravated by warmth. The pulse is rapid, hasty, overflowing or wiry.

C. Identification of qi stagnation and blood stasis:

Qi stagnation: This pattern has an acute onset with distending and migrating hypochondriac pain.

Blood stasis: This pattern is related to prolonged illness. The pain is stabbing with a fixed location and becomes worse during the afternoon or at night. Petechiae on the lips and tongue may be observed. A history of traumatic injury may support the diagnosis.

D. Differential diagnosis of similar disorders:

	Hypochondriac Pain	Epigastric Pain	Chest Painful Obstruction
Location	Unilateral or bilateral infracostal regions.	Between the lower margin of the sternum and the infracostal margin.	Thoracic region.
Characteristics of Pain	Distending, stabbing, burning, dull or colic pain; patient has the desire to move and change position.	Distending, stabbing pain or focal distention.	Stabbing and congested pain; patient has the desire to remain still.
Accompanied Symptoms	Palpable hypochondriac masses or congested fluids.	Nausea, vomiting or acid regurgitation.	Shortness of breath, chest congestion, cold limbs and palpitations.
Etiology	Exterior pathogens or emotional stress.	Improper diet, emotional stress or cold invading the stomach.	Improper diet and emotional instability.
History	History of liver and gallbladder disease.	History of spleen and stomach disease.	History of heart or lung disease.
Pain Radiates to	Right shoulder and back.	Point on the back correponding to the stomach.	Left shoulder, upper back and arm.

Basic Patterns

- Liver qi stagnation
- Blood stasis in the liver channels
- Damp-heat in the liver and gallbladder
- Liver yin deficiency

Differentiation and Treatment

Treatment principle:

Based on the principle of "unblocking the obstruction to alleviate pain", select the methods of soothing liver qi, draining liver fire and drying dampness according to the pattern differentiation; nourish liver yin and blood if indicated.

Liver qi stagnation

Distending and migrating hypochondriac pain, which is aggravated by emotional stress.

S: Distending epigastric pain, chest stuffiness, and frequent belching.

T: Thin coating. **P:** Wiry.

- Soothe the liver and regulate the qi.
- *Chai Hu Shu Gan San*
  - *Chai Hu* soothes liver qi.
  - *Xiang Fu*, *Chen Pi* and *Zhi Qiao* regulate the qi and alleviate pain.
  - *Chuan Xiong* invigorates the blood, regulates the qi and alleviates pain.
  - *Shao Yao* and *Gan Cao* moderate spasm and alleviate pain.
- To enhance the effects of regulating the qi and alleviating pain. + *Qing Pi, Chuan Lian Zi, Yu Jin, Yan Hu Suo*

  Qi stagnation turning into fire with burning pain, irritability, bitter taste in the mouth and constipation. + *Mu Dan Pi, Zhi Zi, Huang Lian*

  Liver fire damaging the yin with vague pain that is worse on exertion, dizziness, irritability, and insomnia. + *Dan Shen, Mu Dan Pi, Dang Gui, Ju Hua*

  Liver qi invading the spleen with abdominal pain, borborygmus and diarrhea. + *Tong Xie Yao Fang*

  Rebellious stomach qi with nausea and vomiting. + *Xuan Fu Hua, Dai Zhe Shi, Ban Xia, Sheng Jiang*

Blood stasis in the liver channels

Stabbing hypochondriac pain with fixed location that becomes worse at night.

S: Palpable abdominal masses.

T: Dark red and purple tongue with petechiae. **P:** Deep and choppy.

- Dispel stasis and unblock obstruction in the channels.
- *Xuan Fu Hua Tang*
  - *Qian Cao* (substituting *Xin Jiang*) invigorates the blood, expels stasis and unblocks obstruction of the channels to alleviate pain.
  - *Xuan Fu Hua* regulates the qi and alleviates pain.

- To enhance the effects of regulating the qi and invigorating the blood. + *Yu Jin, Tao Ren, Dang Gui Wei, Yan Hu Suo*
  Pain related to traumatic injuries, use *Fu Yuan Huo Xue Tang*.
  Palpable abdominal masses. + *San Leng, E Zhu, Tu Bie Chong*

Damp-heat in the liver and gallbladder

Stuffy sensation and pain in the hypochondria, bitter taste in the mouth, focal distention of the chest and epigastrium, and poor appetite.
S: Nausea and vomiting; or yellow sclera, skin and urine.
T: Yellow greasy coating. **P:** Wiry, slippery and rapid.

- Clear heat and drain dampness.
- *Long Dan Xie Gan Tang*
  - *Long Dan Cao* clears and drains damp-heat from the liver and gallbladder.
  - *Zhi Zi, Huang Qin* and *Sheng Di Huang* clear heat and drain fire.
  - *Che Qian Zi, Mu Tong* and *Ze Xie* clear heat and drain dampness.
  - Chai Hu soothes liver qi.
- To strengthen the effects of soothing the liver, regulating the qi and alleviating pain. + *Chuan Lian Zi, Qing Pi, Yu Jin*
  Jaundice with fever. + *Yin Chen Hao, Huang Bai*
  Stones from accumulated damp-heat obstructing the gallbladder with radiating pain to the right shoulder and back. + *Jin Qian Cao, Hai Jin Sha, Yu Jin*

Liver yin deficiency

Persistent vague hypochondriac pain that is aggravated by exertion.
S: Dry mouth and throat, five-centers heat, tidal fever, night sweating, dizziness, and soreness of the lower back and knees.
T: Red tongue with scanty coating. **P:** Thready, wiry and rapid.

- Nourish the yin and soothe the liver.
- *Yi Guan Jian*
  - *Sheng Di Huang* and *Dang Gui* nourish the yin and blood, comfort and soften the liver to alleviate pain.
  - *Sha Shen* and *Mai Men Dong* nourish the yin and generate the fluid.
  - *Gou Qi Zi* tonifies the yin and blood, augments the liver and kidney.
  - *Chuan Lian Zi* soothes the liver, regulates the qi and alleviates pain.
- Irritability and heat sensation in the chest. + *Zhi Zi, Suan Zao Ren*
  Dizziness and blurred vision. + *Huang Jing, Nu Zhen Zi, Ju Hua*
  Restlessness and insomnia, use *Suan Zao Ren Tang*.

Acupuncture Treatment

Excess patterns:

- **Manipulation:** Reducing method.
- **Prescription:** LR14 Qimen TE6 Zhigou GB34 Yanglingquan
- **Supplementary points:**
  - Qi stagnation. + LR3 Taichong; GB40 Qiuxu
  - Blood stasis. + BL17 Geshu; BL18 Ganshu
  - Damp-heat. + GB24 Riyue; LR3 Taichong

Deficiency patterns:

- **Manipulation:** Reinforcing method.
- **Prescription:** LR14 Qimen BL18 Ganshu SP6 Sanyinjiao BL23 Shenshu

Practical Hints

• In general, qi stagnation, blood stasis and damp-heat accumulation are causative factors in excess patterns, whereas deficient liver yin or blood is the root of deficient patterns. **Patterns of excess and deficiency may mutually transform.** Chronic qi stagnation may lead to blood stasis; blood stasis or damp-heat accumulation can block the flow of qi; excess heat may injure the yin; slow metabolism due to functional deficiency may lead to qi stagnation. Clinically, patterns of hypochondriac pain are varied and complicated.

• **Acrid and neutral qi regulators are recommended to enhance the therapeutic effect.** Liver qi stagnation is the predominant pathogenesis for hypochondriac pain and can progress to the other patterns. Herbs that soothe the liver and regulate the qi are added to the selected formulas to enhance the therapeutic effect. Herbs that regulate the qi are acrid and drying in nature and may injure liver yin; therefore, long-term usage is not recommended. **Acrid and neutral qi regulators are recommended if indicated.**

CHAPTER 18

Jaundice

黃疸 *Huang Dan*

Jaundice is characterized by a yellowish discoloration of the sclera, skin and urine due to obstruction of bile and abnormal deposition of bile pigments into the body fluid and blood. Among all pigmentations, yellowish discoloration of the sclera is the marker of diagnosis of jaundice. It occurs when the liver and gallbladder are unable to direct the free flow and distribution of the qi, and drainage of bile is obstructed by damp-heat or cold-dampness.

Relevant Diseases

- Hemolytic jaundice
- Hepatitis or cirrhosis
- Liver cancer
- Acute or subacute yellow atrophy
- Cholecystitis or cholelithiasis
- Cholangioma
- Leptospirosis
- Pancreatic cancer

Su Wen had the first documentation of jaundice; treatments and herbal prescriptions for this disorder were discussed in *Shang Han Lun*. Later, based on the dominant pathology of damp-cold, damp-heat or heat-toxicity, jaundice was further subcategorized into yin, yang and heat-toxin jaundice, with higher prevalence of yang jaundice. Concept of jaundice in TCM is identical to that of the western medicine.

Etiology and Pathogenesis

Exterior pathogenic factors: Exterior damp-heat lingering in the middle burner interferes with the free flow of qi in the liver and gallbladder. Normal secretion of bile in the middle burner is interrupted and bile overflows into the blood and body fluid. Among all the exterior pathogens, epidemic contagious heat toxicity is the most common etiological factor because it has a strong effect to force the bile to detour from its physiological path. The resulting pathology is heat-toxin jaundice, or *ji huang*.

Improper diet generates damp-heat internally by hindering the functions of the spleen and stomach. Damp-heat can disturb liver and gallbladder function by obstructing the free flow of qi and the drainage of bile.

Spleen and stomach yang deficiency: Constitutional spleen yang deficiency following an illness produce internal cold, which can combine with either internal or external dampness and transform into cold-dampness. Cold-dampness will obstruct the middle burner and inhibit the secretion of bile.

Stones or parasites obstructing the bile ducts: According to TCM theory, stones are formed as the remainder when heat dries and condenses the body fluid. Damp-heat in the middle burner can easily lead to gallstones which obstruct the bile ducts. It is also possible for intestinal parasites to enter the bile ducts due to agitation from heat and cause obstruction.

Blood stasis obstructing the bile ducts: Chronic qi stagnation may progress to blood stasis in the bile ducts and cause obstruction. Consequently, there is abnormal secretion and drainage of bile resulting in jaundice.

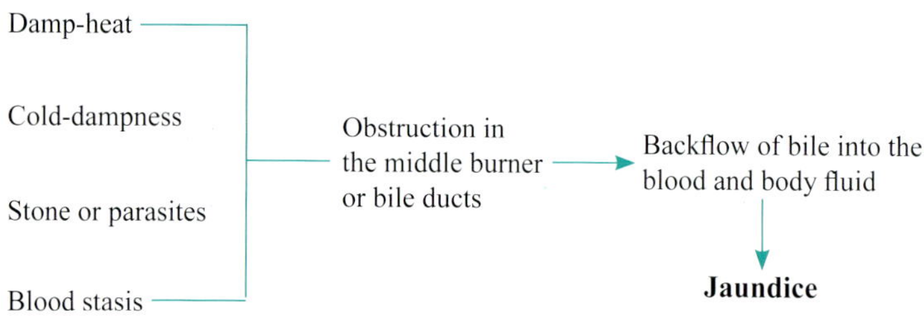

Diagnosis

A. Identification of yin jaundice and yang jaundice:

Patterns	**Yang Jaundice**	**Yin Jaundice**
Etiology and Pathogenesis	Damp-heat; mainly from exterior pathogens.	Cold-dampness; mainly from deficient spleen and stomach.
Characteristic Color	Bright lustrous yellow pigmentation like an orange peel.	Dusky and smoky yellow pigmentation.
Characteristic Symptoms	Excess heat pattern.	Deficient cold pattern or combination of excess and deficiency.
Course	Short.	Long.
Severity	Mild (excluding *ji huang*).	Severe.

B. Identification of heat toxin jaundice (*ji huang*):

Heat toxin jaundice, or *ji huang*, is categorized as yang jaundice. It is most often caused by excessive damp-heat or epidemic contagious heat toxicity, which flares up suddenly and exhausts the blood. It is marked by sudden onset, immediate golden-yellow discoloration of the sclera, skin and urine, high fever, and intense thirst. *Ji huang* can progress to coma, delirium, subcutaneous and mucosal hemorrhaging or hematuria.

C. Differential diagnosis of jaundice and sallow skin (*wei huang*):

Types	**Jaundice**	**Sallow Skin**
Pathogenesis	Dampness or blood stasis obstructing the middle burner and the bile ducts.	Inadequate supplies of qi and blood due to spleen and stomach deficiency, exhaustion of qi and blood due to severe bleeding, or chronic illness.
Symptoms	Yellowness of the sclera, skin and urine. Accompanied by symptoms of damp-heat, cold-dampness or blood stasis.	Yellowish skin that is dry and lusterless. Accompanied by dizziness, tinnitus, palpitations and insomnia.

Basic Patterns

Yang jaundice:

- Preponderance of heat
- Preponderance of dampness
- Heat toxin jaundice

Yin jaundice:

- Cold-dampness

Differentiation and Treatment

Treatment principle:

Drain dampness and promote urination.

Yang jaundice: In addition, utilize methods of clearing heat and draining downward to eliminate damp-heat.

Yin jaundice: In addition, incorporate methods of warming the middle burner and draining dampness to resolve cold-dampness.

Heat toxin jaundice *(ji huang)*: Clear heat, relieve toxicity, cool the blood and open the orifices.

Yang jaundice:

Preponderance of heat

Bright yellow sclera, skin and urine, with scanty urination.
S: Fever, intense thirst, irritability, fullness and distention of the abdomen, nausea, vomiting, bitter taste in the mouth and constipation.
T: Yellow greasy coating. **P:** Wiry and rapid.

- Clear heat, drain dampness and eliminate jaundice.
- *Yin Chen Hao Tang*
  - *Yin Chen Hao* drains damp-heat, and is the imperial herb for jaundice.
  - *Zhi Zi* unblocks the tripple burner and guides out damp-heat via urination.
  - *Da Huang* clears heat, purges fire and unblocks the bowel.
- Enhance the effect of draining dampness to expel damp-heat via urination.
  + Zhu Ling, Fu Ling, Che Qian Zi, Hua Shi
  Purge fire and descend rebellious qi to stop vomiting. *+ Huang Lian, Zhu Ru*
  Significant hypochondriac pain on the right side, possibly radiating to upper back and shoulder. *+ Chai Hu, Yu Jin, Chuan Lian Zi, Yan Hu Suo*
  Obstructed bile ducts by stones. *+ Jin Qian Cao, Hai Jin Sha, Ji Nei Jin*

Preponderance of dampness

Yellow sclera, skin and urine, but not as bright as in the previous pattern, with scanty urination.
S: Heavy sensation in the head and body, thirst with no desire to drink, focal distention in the chest and epigastrium, lack of appetite, nausea, vomiting and loose stool.
T: Slightly yellow, thick and greasy coating. **P:** Wiry and slippery.

- Drain dampness, eliminate turbidity and clear heat.
- *Yin Chen Wu Ling San* and *Gan Lu Xiao Du Dan*
  - *Yin Chen Hao* drains dampness, clears heat and eliminates jaundice.
  - *Wu Ling San* drains and leaches out dampness, warms the yang and assists qi transformation.
  - *Gan Lu Xiao Du Dan* transforms damp-turbidity and relieves toxicity.
- To enhance the effects of draining dampness and transforming turbidity.
  + Huang Qin, Mu Tong, Huo Xiang, Bai Dou Kou
  Initial stage of yang jaundice with exterior symptoms, use *Ma Huang Lian Qiao Chi Xiao Dou Tang*.

Heat toxin jaundice

Sudden onset, immediate golden-yellow discoloration of the sclera, skin and urine.
S: High fever, irritability, severe thirst, hypochondriac pain, abdominal fullness, delirium and loss of consciousness; or subcutaneous and mucosal hemorrhaging, blood in the stool and hematuria.
T: Dark red tongue with dry yellow coating. **P:** Wiry, slippery and rapid.

- Clear heat, relieve toxicity, cool the blood and open the orifices.
- *Xi Jiao San*
  - *Shui Niu Jiao* (substituted for *Xi Jiao*) clears heat and opens the orifices.
  - *Yin Chen Hao* clears heat and eliminates jaundice.
  - *Huang Lian*, *Zhi Zi* and *Sheng Ma* purge fire and relieve toxicity.
- To strengthen the effects of clearing heat and cooling the blood. + *Sheng Di Huang, Mu Dan Pi, Xuan Shen*
  Hemorrhaging. + *Di Yu Tan, Ce Bai Ye Tan*
  Delirium and unconsciousness. + *An Gong Niu Huang Wan* or *Zhi Bao Dan*

Yin jaundice:

Cold-dampness

Dusky, smoky yellow discoloration of the sclera, skin and urine.
S: Poor appetite, focal distention in the abdomen, loose stool, fatigue, cold intolerance and absence of thirst.
T: Pale tongue with white greasy coating. **P:** Soft and decelerating, or deep and slow.

- Strengthen the spleen, harmonize the stomach, warm and transform cold-dampness.
- *Yin Chen Zhu Fu Tang*
  - *Yin Chen Hao*, the imperial herb for eliminating jaundice, combines with *Fu Zi* to warm and transform cold-dampness to eliminate jaundice.
  - *Bai Zhu* and *Gan Cao* benefit the qi and strengthen the spleen.
  - *Gan Jiang* warms the middle burner to disperse cold-dampness.
- To strengthen the effect of promoting the movement of qi to drain dampness. + *Yu Jin, Hou Po, Ze Xie, Fu Ling*
  Chronic jaundice complicated by qi stagnation, blood stasis and dampness accumulation in the hypochondriac regions with hard palpable masses, use *Bie Jia Jian Wan* and *Xiao Yao San*.
  Significant spleen and stomach deficiency. + *Xiang Sha Liu Jun Zi Tang*

Acupuncture Treatment

- **Manipulation:** Reducing method for yang jaundice, even method and moxibustion for yin jaundice.
- **Prescription:** SP9 Yinlingquan ST36 Zusanli BL18 Ganshu BL19 Danshu GV9 Zhiyang
- **Supplementary points:**

  - Yang jaundice. + LR3 Taichong; GB34 Yanglingquan
  - Yin jaundice. + BL20 Pishu; BL48 Yanggang

Practical Hints

• **Continuing treatment can prevent lingering dampness from accumulating and progressing to *zheng jia ji ju*, or abdominal masses.** Yang jaundice has a shorter course and better response to treatment, whereas yin jaundice has a longer course and responds slowly. Jaundice involves accumulation of dampness, a yin pathogen that lingers within the body for a long time; therefore, after the yellowish discoloration fades, treatment to drain dampness and strengthen the spleen is still required.

• **Jaundice needs to be distinguished from yellowish skin discolorations associated with certain medicinal agents or food.** For instance, large doses of quinacrine, an antimalarial and an anthelmintic agent, may cause yellow discoloration of the sclera and the skin in sun-exposed areas. This side effect usually disappears spontaneously after a couple of months; thus, treatment may not be required. Ingesting fresh fruits and vegetables containing carotene, such as carrots, pumpkins, spinach, tomatoes, oranges or papayas, may also induce a yellowish discoloration. Taking a thorough history and physical examination are important when diagnosing jaundice.

CHAPTER 19

Painful Urinary Syndrome

淋 證 *Lin Zheng*

Painful urinary syndrome refers to a group of symptoms characterized by discomfort during urination, including various experiences of urgency, increased frequency, oliguria, and difficult, painful urination. Spasmodic pain and distention in the lower abdomen may radiate to the area of the costovertebral angle. Clinically, there are six common types of *lin* syndrome differentiated according to their pathogeneses: heat *lin*, qi *lin*, blood *lin*, stone *lin*, cloudy *lin* and exhaustion *lin*.

Relevant Diseases

- Urinary tract infection
- Urinary calculi
- Prostatitis
- Prostatic hypertrophy
- Chyluria
- Bladder tumor

Etiology and Pathogenesis

Damp-heat in the bladder can be caused by overindulging in damp-heat producing foods or by external damp-heat invasion. Damp-heat slows down the qi transformation function of the bladder and obstructs the water passages, leading to *lin* syndrome. Heat *lin,* caused by damp-heat, is characterized by burning pain during urination. Damp-heat can cause the excess pattern of blood *lin* when heat forces the blood to move recklessly; there will be burning, painful and bloody urination. If damp-heat disturbs the bladder's function to separate the clear from the turbid, the excess pattern of cloudy *lin* will occur. Chronic lingering damp-heat evaporates fluids and condenses dampness to form stones or sand, resulting in stone *lin*.

Spleen and kidney deficiency results from chronic *lin* syndrome, aging, weak constitution, overexertion and excessive sexual activity. Qi sinking due to severe spleen qi deficiency, and instability in the lower burner due to kidney deficiency, can lead to *lin* syndrome. *Lin* syndrome that occurs with or is aggravated by exertion is exhaustion *lin*; *lin* syndrome due to spleen qi deficiency or qi sinking is the deficient pattern of qi *lin*; cloudy urination due to instability and failure to secure essence in the lower burner is the deficient pattern of cloudy *lin*; *lin* syndrome with hematuria due to kidney yin deficiency and empty fire is the deficient pattern of blood *lin*.

Liver qi stagnation due to anger and frustration can transform into liver fire. Stagnant qi combining with fire disturbs the transformation function of the bladder qi and will cause pain in the lower abdomen, dysuria and frequent dribbling, all manifestations of the excess pattern of qi *lin*.

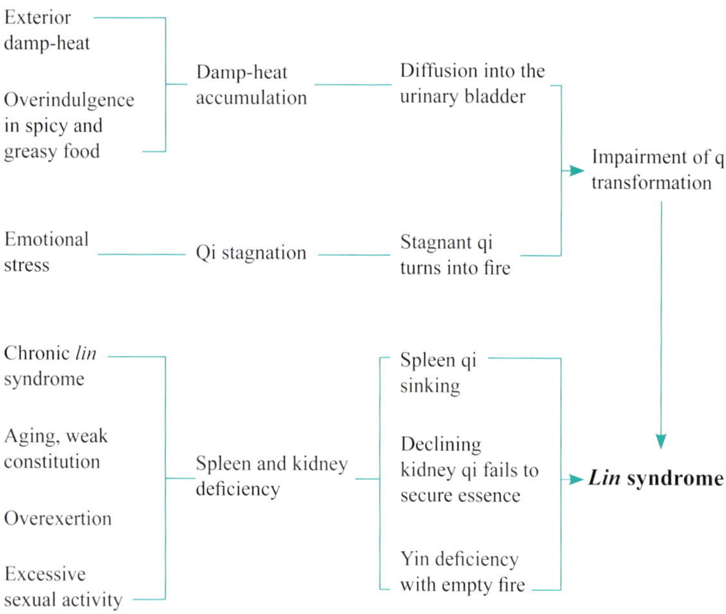

Diagnosis

A. Identification of excess and deficiency:

Excess: The initial stage or acute onset of *lin* syndrome due to damp-heat, qi stagnation or stone formation in the bladder is usually an excess pattern. Significant burning and pricking pain may be present when voiding. The color of the urine can be dark, turbid or red.

Deficiency: The later stage or chronic onset of *lin* syndrome due to spleen deficiency, kidney deficiency or qi and yin deficiency is usually a deficient pattern. In comparison to the excess pattern, there will only be a slight burning or pricking sensation when voiding. The color of the urine is light or clear.

Certain types of *lin* syndrome can be further differentiated into excess or deficient pattern. For instance, cloudy *lin* can be either the excess or deficient type depending on the etiology and pathogenesis. Damp-heat diffusing downward to the lower burner and disturbing qi transformation in the bladder will cause the excess pattern of cloudy *lin*, while kidney deficiency failing to secure the essence will lead to the deficient pattern of cloudy *lin*. Likewise, blood *lin* can be caused by damp-heat in the lower burner injuring the blood vessels (excess pattern of blood *lin*) or by yin deficiency with empty fire leading to reckless movement of the blood (deficient pattern of blood *lin*).

B. Identification of different patterns of *lin* syndrome:

The common symptoms of *lin* syndrome include urgency, increased frequency, oliguria, difficulty and pain during urination. Spasmodic pain and distention in the lower abdomen may radiate to the region around the costovertebral angle. In addition, the following features help differentiating patterns:

- Urine containing sand or stone – Stone *lin*.
- Turbid and cloudy urination with a milky or oily appearance – Cloudy *lin*.
- Hematuria or urine containing blood clots with sharp and burning pain during urination – Blood *lin*.
- Dysuria with frequent dribbling of urine, and distention and heavy sensation of the lower abdomen – Qi *lin*
- Burning and pricking pain during urination – Heat *lin*.
- Difficult urination and constant dribbling that are initiated or exacerbated by exertion – Exhaustion *lin*.

C. Differential diagnosis of similar disorders:

As its name indicates, painful urinary syndrome is characterized by painful and difficult urination that is accompanied by other symptoms, such as urgency, increased frequency, burning and prickling pain during voiding. It is important to rule out the following disorders, which can be easily confused with *lin* syndrome as they all present with similar symptoms.

Oliguria-anuria: Difficulty urinating characterized by decreased urine output with less than normal volume, or no urine output at all. Pain is absent with oliguria and anuria. In comparison, *lin* syndrome has significant pain when voiding and the daily volume of urine output is adequate.

Hematuria: Blood in the urine is a common symptom for both hematuria and blood *lin*; however, pain during urination is absent with hematuria and is always present with blood *lin*.

Turbid urination: Both turbid urination and cloudy *lin* manifest a milky or oily appearance of the urine. To differentiate, pain is a major symptom with cloudy *lin* but absent with turbid urination.

Blood Qi & Cloudy - Excess Def.

Basic Patterns

- Heat lin
- Excess pattern of qi lin
- Excess pattern of blood lin
- Excess pattern of cloudy lin
- Exhaustion lin
- Stone lin
- Deficient pattern of qi lin
- Deficient pattern of blood lin
- Deficient pattern of cloudy lin

Differentiation and Treatment

Treatment principle:

Excess pattern: Clear heat and drain dampness if there is damp-heat accumulation in the bladder. Cool the blood and stop bleeding if heat causes reckless movement of the blood. Unblock urinary obstruction and eliminate stones if there is sand or stone accumulation. Facilitate and improve the movement of qi when there is qi stagnation.

Deficiency pattern: Strengthen the spleen and benefit the qi. Tonify the kidney to secure the essence.

Heat lin

Frequent and scanty urination with burning pricking pain. Urine is dark yellow or red in color.

S: Spasmodic, distending pain in the lower abdomen that may radiate to the lower back; possibly with aversion to cold, fever, bitter taste in the mouth, nausea, vomiting or constipation.

T: Yellow greasy coating. **P:** Soft and rapid.

- Clear heat, drain dampness and unblock the obstruction in the urinary tract.
- *Ba Zheng San*
  - *Bian Xu*, *Qu Mai*, *Mu Tong*, *Che Qian Zi* and *Hua Shi* clear heat, drain dampness and unblock the obstruction in the urinary tract.
  - *Da Huang* and *Zhi Zi* clear heat and purge fire.
- For constipation or distending pain in the lower abdomen. + *Zhi Shi*

  Alternating chills and fever with a bitter taste in the mouth, and irritability. + *Xiao Chai Hu Tang*

  Damp-heat injuring the yin. + *Sheng Di Huang, Zhi Mu, Bai Mao Gen*

Stone lin

Difficult urination with sand or stones in the urine, urgent spasmodic pain in the urethra while urinating midstream, dark yellow urine or urine mixed with blood.
S: Spasmodic pain in the lower abdomen or at the flanks.
T: Red with thin yellow coating. **P:** Wiry and rapid.

- Clear heat, drain dampness, unblock the obstruction and eliminate the stones.
- *Shi Wei San*
  - *Shi Wei* unblocks the obstruction in the urinary tract and eliminates stones.
  - *Qu Mai*, *Dong Kui Zi*, *Hua Shi* and *Che Qian Zi* clear heat and unblock the obstruction in the urinary tract.
- Enhance the effect to unblock the obstruction in the urinary tract and eliminate stones. + *Jin Qian Cao, Ji Nei Jin, Hai Jin Sha*
  Colic pain in the lower back and abdomen. + *Chi Shao, Bai Shao, Gan Cao*
  Blood in the urine. + *Xiao Ji, Sheng Di Huang, Ou Jie, Bai Mao Gen*

Excess pattern of qi lin

Difficulty in urination and distention of the lower abdomen.
S: Fullness and discomfort in the chest and hypochondriac regions.
T: Thin white coating. **P:** Deep and wiry.

- Facilitate the movement of qi.
- *Chen Xiang San*
  - *Chen Xiang* and *Chen Pi* regulate the qi.
  - *Dang Gui* and *Bai Shao* nourish the yin and blood to soften the liver.
  - *Shi Wei*, *Hua Shi* and *Dong Kui Zi* promote urination and unblock the obstruction in the urinary tract.
- Severe fullness and discomfort of the chest and hypochondriac regions. + *Yan Hu Suo, Chuan Lian Zi, Qing Pi*
  Distending pain in the lower abdomen. + *Wu Yao, Mu Xiang, Xiang Fu*
  Stabbing pain in the chest, hypochondriac region and abdomen. + *Hong Hua, Chuan Niu Xi, Yi Mu Cao, Ze Lan*

Deficient pattern of qi lin

Difficult urination with frequent dribbling of clear urine, heavy sensation and pain in the lower abdomen.
S: Pale complexion, fatigue, lassitude and loose stool.
T: Pale tongue. **P:** Weak and thready.

- Tonify the spleen and raise yang qi.
- *Bu Zhong Yi Qi Tang*
  - This formula augments the qi, strengthens the spleen and raises the yang.
- Sallow complexion with dizziness and palpitations. + *Bai Shao, Di Huang*
  Soreness and weakness of the lower back and knees. + *Niu Xi, Du Zhong*

Excess pattern of blood lin

Urgent, frequent urination with burning, pricking pain. Urine is red or contains blood clots.
S: Fullness and distending pain in the lower abdomen with irritability and restlessness.
T: Red tongue with yellow coating. **P:** Rapid and slippery.

- Clear heat, unblock the obstruction, cool the blood and stop bleeding.
- *Xiao Ji Yin Zi*
  - *Xiao Ji*, the chief herb, cools the blood to stop bleeding.
  - *Pu Huang* and *Ou Jie* invigorate and cool the blood to stop bleeding.
  - *Hua Shi*, *Tong Cao*, *Zhu Ye* and *Zhi Zi* clear heat, drain dampness and unblock the obstruction in the urinary tract.
  - *Sheng Di Huang* nourishes the yin, clears heat and cools the blood.
- Severe bleeding and painful urination. + *Hu Po, San Qi*

Deficient pattern of blood lin

Urine that is slightly red, and mild pain during urination.
S: Soreness and weakness of the lower back and knees, fatigue and lassitude.
T: Red tongue with scanty coating. **P:** Thready and rapid.

- Nourish kidney yin, clear heat and stop bleeding.
- *Zhi Bai Di Huang Wan*
  - *Zhi Mu* and *Huang Bai* nourish the yin, clear heat and eliminate fire.
  - *Liu Wei Di Huang Wan* nourishes the liver and kidney.
- Enhance the effects to nourish yin and cool the blood. + *Han Lian Cao, Nu Zhen Zi, E Jiao*

Excess pattern of cloudy lin

Turbid, milky and oily urine, possibly with blood clots. Difficult urination accompanied by burning and pricking pain.
S: Abdominal distention and pain, thirst with no desire to drink.
T: Red tongue with yellow greasy coating. **P:** Slippery and rapid.

- Clear heat, drain dampness and separate the clear from the turbid.
- *Cheng Shi Bi Xie Fen Qing Yin*
  - *Bi Xie* and *Shi Chang Pu* clear and drain turbid dampness.
  - *Che Qian Zi* and *Huang Bai* clear heat and eliminate dampness.
  - *Bai Zhu* and *Fu Ling* strengthen the spleen and dry dampness.
  - *Lian Zi* and *Dan Shen* clear heat from the heart and invigorate the blood.
- Severe burning, pricking pain. + *Hua Shi, Mu Tong*
  Difficult urination with abdominal distention. + *Wu Yao, Qing Pi*
  Blood in the urine. + *Bai Mao Gen, Xiao Ji, Ou Jie*

Deficient pattern of cloudy lin

Chronic or recurrent *lin* syndrome with oily urine and insignificant pain.
S: Emaciation, soreness and weakness of the lower back and knees, dizziness and fatigue.
T: Pale tongue with greasy coating. **P:** Deep and weak.

- Tonify the kidney and restrain the leakage of essence.
- *Gao Lin Tang*
  - *Dang Shen* and *Shan Yao* tonify the spleen.
  - *Di Huang* and *Qian Shi* nourish the kidney.
  - *Long Gu*, *Mu Li* and *Bai Shao* restrain and bind the leakage of essence.
- Spleen and kidney deficiency with spleen qi sinking and kidney failing to stabilize the lower burner, use *Bu Zhong Yi Qi Tang* and *Qi Wei Du Qi Wan*.

Exhaustion lin

Difficult urination with continuous dribbling that occurs with or is exacerbated by exertion.
S: Fatigue, lassitude, and soreness and weakness of the lower back and knees.
T: Pale tongue. **P:** Weak.

- Strengthen the spleen and fortify the kidney.
- *Wu Bi Shan Yao Wan*
  - *Shan Yao*, *Shan Zhu Yu*, *Tu Si Zi* and *Wu Wei Zi* benefit the kidney and bind the essence.
  - *Fu Ling* and *Ze Xie* strengthen the spleen and drain dampness.
  - *Shu Di Huang*, *Du Zhong*, *Niu Xi* and *Rou Cong Rong* augment the kidney.
- Accompanied by sinking spleen qi. + *Bu Zhong Yi Qi Tang*
  Kidney yin deficiency with heat signs. + *Zhi Bai Di Huang Wan*
  Kidney yang deficiency with cold intolerance and cold limbs. + *You Gui Wan*

Acupuncture Treatment

- **Manipulation:** Reducing method or combination of reducing and reinforcing methods.
- **Prescription:** CV3 Zhongji SP9 Yinlingquan BL28 Pangguangshu
- **Supplementary points:**
  - Heat *lin*. + LI4 Hegu; TE5 Waiguan
  - Stone *lin*. + BL39 Weiyang; KI2 Rangu
  - Qi *lin*. + LR2 Xingjian
  - Blood *lin*. + SP10 Xuehai; SP6 Sanyinjiao
  - Cloudy *lin*. + BL23 Shenshu; KI6 Zhaohai
  - Exhaustion *lin*. + GV20 Baihui; CV6 Qihai; ST36 Zusanli

Practical Hints

• **Use diaphoretics and tonics provisionally.** In ancient TCM documents, diaphoresis and tonification are contraindicated as treatment methods for *lin* syndrome. In the initial stage of *lin* syndrome, aversion to cold, fever and general body ache may be present. Because frequent urination and excessive heat of *lin* syndrome can damage the yin, using acrid and warm herbs to induce sweating and release the exterior will further injure the yin and complicate the condition. However, if *lin* syndrome is caused by exterior wind-heat or exterior damp-heat with manifestations of aversion to wind, fever, cough and sore throat, acrid and cool herbs that induce sweating and release the exterior may be used. Tonification is contraindicated for excess *lin* syndrome. Tonification is appropriate and recommended for deficient l*in* syndrome, including spleen qi deficiency or qi sinking and kidney deficiency failing to secure the essence.

• According to TCM theory, **"Use the strategy of unblocking the obstruction to promote elimination in unremitting draining syndromes".** Unremitting draining syndromes include intractable diarrhea, frequent urination, and gushing and leaking syndrome caused by excess pathogenic influences. This treatment method is only applicable to excess patterns, including excess *lin* syndromes. By facilitating the movement of qi, clearing heat, draining dampness, invigorating the blood and dissolving stones, the treatment methods that unblock the obstruction and promote elimination will remove the excess pathogenic influences, unblock the obstruction in the urinary passages, and treat the root cause of the disorder.

CHAPTER 20

Oligurla-Anuria Syndrome

癃閉 *Long Bi*

Oliguria-anuria syndrome, or *long bi*, is characterized by a measurable decrease in the amount of urine output in relation to fluid intake. It occurs in primary or secondary failure of urine formation, or in retention of urine due to obstruction in the urinary passage. Gradual onset of scanty urination and dribbling is known as *long*, while acute onset of inability to urinate is called *bi*. *Long* and *bi* are not identical, but both involve some degrees of difficulty in urinating; therefore, they are known and treated as one disorder, *long bi* syndrome.

Relevant Diseases

- Renal calculi
- Atony of the bladder
- Urinary retention
- Prostatic hypertrophy
- Renal or bladder tumor
- Renal failure
- Spasm of the bladder sphincter
- Dehydration
- Excessive blood loss

Etiology and Pathogenesis

Normal formation and elimination of urine depend on proper function of the lung, spleen, kidney and triple burner. These organs are responsible for water metabolism in the upper, middle and lower burners. The lung disperses and descends to regulate the water passage; the spleen transforms and transports to distribute metabolized fluid to the entire body; the kidney dominates water, controls the two lower orifices, is internally-externally related to the bladder, and controls the bladder's function of excreting urine; the triple burner is the pathway for metabolized fluid.

Heat accumulated in the lung impairs the lung's descending function. As a result, fluid can not be metabolized and disseminated to the bladder.

Damp-heat accumulation in the middle burner infuses downwards to the bladder, interrupting the process of qi transformation and inducing oliguria-anuria.

Spleen qi failing to ascend: When clear yang from the spleen fails to ascend, turbid yin will not be able to descend. Turbid yin, including the metabolized fluid, cannot be eliminated via the lower burner.

Deficiency of the kidney: Kidney yang deficiency, or failure of the fire in the gate of vitality, leads to loss of control over the lower orifices. Primary or secondary kidney yin deficiency leads to failure to form urine.

Constrained liver qi disturbs the flow in the water passage or the triple burner.

Obstruction in the urinary passage: Substantial obstruction by blood stasis, masses and/or calculi is a direct cause of urinary retention.

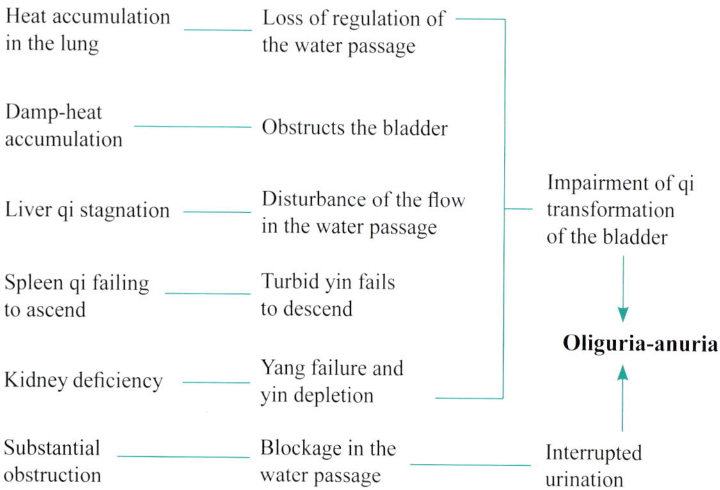

Diagnosis

A. Identification of urine formation:

The diagnosis and treatment plan is determined based on whether or not urine is being formed. Physical examination, especially inspection, palpation and percussion, is necessary to detect urine formation. Distention, discomfort on palpation, and solid resonance to percussion in the lower abdomen indicate formation of urine and a full bladder. The patient may express a desire to urinate but be unable to do so. Decreased urine output, lack of desire to urinate, hollow resonance and a flat lower abdomen indicate lack of urine formation in the bladder.

B. Identification of excess and deficiency:

Usually, detectable urine formation indicates excess while absent or scanty urine formation indicates deficiency.

- Excess patterns include damp-heat accumulation, lung heat accumulation, liver qi stagnation and substantial obstruction. The onset is acute, accompanied by distention and discomfort in the lower abdomen, dark scanty urine, a yellow greasy or thin yellow tongue coating, and a wiry, choppy or rapid pulse.

- Deficiency patterns include spleen qi sinking or kidney deficiency. The onset is slow, with lassitude, shortness of breath, weak voice, pale-sallow complexion, lack of strength to void, dribbling urine or anuria, pale tongue, and a weak, deep and thready pulse.

C. Identification of intoxication from urinary toxins:

When turbid yin, or metabolized waste, is not eliminated properly, internal accumulation of metabolic by-products interrupts normal physiological functions. Intoxication from metabolized waste leads to nausea, vomiting, a stifling sensation in the chest, dyspnea, systemic edema, constipation, irritability, spasms, delirium and loss of consciousness. This is a life-threatening complication.

D. Differential diagnosis of oliguria-anuria and painful urinary syndrome:

Decreased urine output and dysuria are common in both oliguria-anuria and painful urinary syndrome.

Oliguria-anuria: Urination is difficult and inadequate. Although discomfort may be present, pain is not significant. The total daily output of urine is less than normal. Anuresis, or no urine output, is possible.

Painful urinary syndrome: Increased frequency of urination and pricking pain during urination are characteristic. Although there is increased frequency of urination with a decreased amount each time, the total daily urine output is adequate.

Basic Patterns

- Lung heat accumulation
- Damp-heat accumulation in the bladder
- Liver qi stagnation
- Substantial obstruction in the urinary passage
- Spleen qi sinking
- Kidney yang deficiency

Differentiation and Treatment

Treatment principle:

Although the proper elimination of urine involves many organs, treatment of oliguria-anuria should focus on the bladder. Benefit the bladder, a yang organ, by maintaining its patent status.

Deficiency: Tonify the spleen and kidney and assist qi transformation.

Excess: Clear damp-heat, disperse stagnation and accumulation, facilitate the qi flow and unblock obstruction in the urinary passage.

Lung heat accumulation

Sluggish or dribbling urination, and scanty dark urine or anuria; rapid shallow respiration.
S: Cough, dry throat and intense thirst.
T: Thin yellow coating. **P:** Rapid.

- Clear heat from the lung and facilitate the flow in the water passage.
- *Qing Fei Yin*
  - *Huang Qin*, *Sang Bai Pi* and *Mai Men Dong* clear heat from the lung and nourish lung yin.
  - *Che Qian Zi*, *Mu Tong* and *Zhi Zi* clear heat through urination.
  - *Fu Ling* is bland and leaches out dampness.
- Complicated by excessive heart fire with irritability and red tongue tip. + *Huang Lian, Zhu Ye*
  Lung yin deficiency with dry red tongue. + *Sha Shen, Tian Hua Fen, Yu Zhu*
  Headache, nasal congestion and floating pulse. + *Bo He, Jie Geng*
  Constipation. + *Da Huang, Xing Ren*

Damp-heat accumulation in the bladder

Anuria or dark scanty urine, burning sensation during micturition, and distention in the lower abdomen.
S: Bitter taste and sticky sensation in the mouth, thirst without desire to drink, and a sense of incomplete defecation.
T: Red tongue with yellow greasy coating. **P:** Rapid.

- Clear heat and drain dampness, unblock obstruction and promote urination.
- *Ba Zheng San*
  - *Mu Tong*, *Che Qian Zi*, *Bian Xu*, *Qu Mai* and *Hua Shi* are herbs with effects to unblock the urinary passage; they drain damp-heat via urination.
  - *Zhi Zi* clears heat and drains dampness from all three burners.
  - *Da Huang* clears heat and drains fire.
- To strengthen the effects of clearing heat and drying dampness for yellow greasy tongue coating. + *Cang Zhu, Huang Bai*
  Irritability and sores in the mouth and on the tongue. + *Dao Chi San*
  Anuria with a dark, dusky complexion, stifling sensation in the chest, irritability, nausea and vomiting, breath smelling of ammonia, delirium and loss of consciousness. + *Huang Lian Wen Dan Tang*

Liver qi stagnation

Anuresis or difficult urination following emotional distress.
S: Distention and pain in the chest and hypochondriac regions, depression or irritability.
T: Red tongue with thin yellow coating. **P:** Wiry.

- Spread constrained liver qi, facilitate the qi flow and promote urination.
- *Chen Xiang San*
  - *Chen Xiang* and *Chen Pi* spread constrained liver qi and facilitate the qi flow.
  - *Dang Gui* and *Wang Bu Liu Xing* invigorate the blood.
  - *Hua Shi*, *Shi Wei* and *Dong Kui Zi* unblock urinary tract obstruction.
- To reinforce the effect to spread constrained liver qi and facilitate the qi flow. + *Xiang Fu, Yu Jin, Wu Yao*
  Qi stagnation transforming into fire with irritability, short temper and yellow tongue coating. + *Mu Dan Pi, Zhi Zi, Long Dan Cao*

Substantial obstruction in the urinary passage

Dribbling or weak urine stream, interrupted urination, or total urinary retention.
S: Distention and pain in the lower abdomen.
T: Dark purple tongue with petechiae. **P:** Choppy.

- Transform stasis, dissipate accumulation and unblock the obstruction.
- *Dai Di Dang Wan*
  - *Dang Gui Wei*, *Chuan Shan Jia* and *Tao Ren* invigorate the blood and transform stasis.
  - *Da Huang* and *Mang Xiao* expel stasis and soften hardness.
  - *Sheng Di Huang* nourishes the blood and tonifies the yin.
  - *Rou Gui* warms and unblocks the channels.
- To enhance the effects of invigorating the blood and dispelling stasis for severe abdominal stabbing pain and petechiae on the tongue. + *Hong Hua, Niu Xi*
  Hematuria. + *San Qi, Hu Po*
  Urinary calculi. + *Jin Qian Cao, Hai Jin Sha, Qu Mai, Bian Xu*

Spleen qi sinking

Distention and heaviness in the lower abdomen, urinary urgency with inability to urinate, or scanty urine output and hesitant urination.
S: Lassitude, weakness, shortness of breath, weak voice, poor appetite, chronic diarrhea and rectal prolapse or a sense of incomplete defecation.
T: Pale tongue with thin white coating. **P:** Weak.

- Raise clear yang and descend turbid yin, transform qi and promote urination.
- *Bu Zhong Yi Qi Tang* and *Wu Ling San*
  - *Bu Zhong Yi Qi Tang* augments the qi and strengthens the spleen; it is the imperial formula for spleen qi sinking.
  - *Wu Ling San* promotes urination, transforms dampness by warming the yang and transforming the qi.

Kidney yang deficiency

Anuria or dribbling and weak urine stream.
S: Soreness and weakness of the lower back and knees, cold intolerance, cold limbs and pale complexion.
T: Pale tongue with white coating. **P:** Deep, thready and weak at the posterior position.

- Warm the yang, augment the qi, tonify the kidney and promote urination.
- *Ji Sheng Shen Qi Wan*
  - *Rou Gui* and *Fu Zi* tonify the fire in the gate of vitality and assist the yang.
  - *Liu Wei Di Huang Wan* augments the kidney and replenishes the essence; it is the imperial formula for kidney essence deficiency. When combining with *Fu Zi* and *Rou Hui*, together they tonify the yang on the basis of yin nourishing.
  - *Niu Xi* tonifies the liver and kidney; it guides the water downwards.
  - *Che Qian Zi* promotes urination.
- Elderly patient with soreness and pain in the lower back and spine, listlessness or lethargy. + *Ren Shen, Lu Jiao Jiao, Yin Yang Huo, Xian Mao*

Acupuncture Treatment

Excess:

- **Manipulation:** Reducing method.
- **Prescription:** SP6 Sanyinjiao, SP9 Yinlingquan, CV3 Zhongji, BL28 Pangguangshu

Deficiency:

- **Manipulation:** Reinforcing method or moxibustion.
- **Prescription:** KI10 Yingu, BL23 Shenshu, BL20 Pishu, GV20 Baihui, CV4 Guanyuan, TE4 Yangchi

Practical Hints

Treat oliguria-anuria based on accurate differentiation. Oliguria-anuria is differentiated into two major types according to whether or not urine is being formed. In urinary retention, urine is formed and is retained in the bladder. This is a relatively manageable pattern. Use herbal therapy, acupuncture at ST36, CV3, SP6 and SP9, moxibustion at CV4 and CV6, and local heat compression or catheterization. In anuria, urine is not formed and the bladder is empty. This pattern is much more critical since metabolized waste accumulates inside the body, analogous to uremia or end stage renal disease in western medicine. Autointoxication can be a serious complication of this pattern. Elimination of the metabolic by-products is the most important treatment principle. Since waste is not eliminated via the urine, new avenues must be explored. Opening the bowels to eliminate by-products of metabolism has been a traditional treatment strategy in TCM for this specific pattern. Herbs including *Da Huang*, *Ban Xia* and harsh expellants are commonly used to expel the waste and reduce the harmful effects on the central nervous system. Herbs that break up stasis or invigorate the blood and promote urination, such as *Tao Ren*, *Shui Zhi*, *Meng Chong*, *Ze Lan* and *Yi Mu Cao*, can be used to unblock the obstruction in the water passage and promote the flow in the triple burner.

CHAPTER 21

Lower Back Pain

腰 痛 *Yao Tong*

Lower back pain is a subjective sensation of discomfort or pain and can be unilateral, bilateral or centered on the lumbar vertebrae. Lower back pain is strongly influenced by the kidney. According to TCM theory, "The lower back houses the kidney." Despite a localized manifestation, lower back pain can be complicated and the characteristics of the pain can vary depending on the pathogenic factors involved. Clinical complaints include cold pain, burning pain, soreness, heaviness, distending pain, stabbing pain, spasmodic pain, dull pain or pain with numbness. Pain is not necessarily limited to the lumbar region and may radiate to the upper back or down to the toes. Changes in weather or activities may elicit or aggravate lower back pain.

Relevant Diseases

- Rheumatoid spondylitis
- Herniated intervertebral disk
- Lumbar vertebral tuberculosis
- Sprain of the lumbar ligament
- Strain of the lumbar muscle
- Glomerulonephritis
- Pyelitis
- Prostatitis

Etiology and Pathogenesis

Kidney essence deficiency is the primary internal factor in the pathogenesis of lower back pain. Among all the exterior pathogens, dampness is the key contributor to lower back pain due to its heaviness, adhesive nature and tendency to infuse downwards. In addition, blood stasis frequently occurs in the lower back as a result of damage from falling, sprains, strains, heavy lifting, improper body mechanics or traumatic injuries.

Invasion by exterior pathogens: Exterior cold-dampness or damp-heat invading the channels can cause lower back pain. These factors inhibit the circulation of the qi and blood in the lower back.

Qi stagnation and blood stasis can be caused by traumatic injuries or prolonged and chronic illness. Obstructed qi flow may lead to blood stasis in the lower back and produce lower back ache.

Kidney essence deficiency: Constitutional weakness, advanced age, chronic illness or excessive sexual activity lead to kidney essence deficiency with failure to nourish the lower back, sinews and bones.

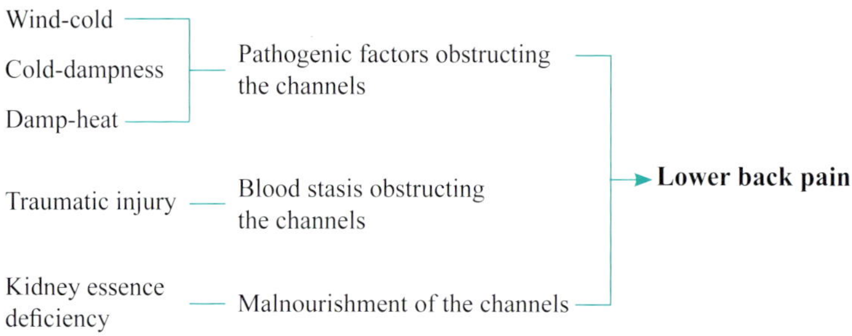

Diagnosis

A. Identification of excess and deficiency:

Excess patterns are usually associated with obstruction of exterior pathogenic factors or direct impact from trauma. They have an acute onset.

Deficiency patterns are commonly related to kidney essence deficiency and the onset is gradual.

A combination pattern of excess and deficiency is present when there is concurrent qi deficiency and blood stasis.

B. Differential diagnosis of similar disorders:

Lower back pain can be a symptom of both painful obstruction syndrome and painful urination syndrome. Before treating lower back pain, these two disorders should be ruled out.

Painful obstruction syndrome mainly affects the joints and muscles of the extremities, or it manifests as lower back pain with pain in the joints and extremities.

Painful urination syndrome: Severe lower back pain can accompany stone *lin*, heat *lin* and blood *lin*. In painful urination syndrome, lower back pain is accompanied by urgency, increased frequency and difficult urination.

Basic Patterns

- Cold-dampness invasion
- Damp-heat invasion
- Blood stasis
- Kidney essence deficiency

Differentiation and Treatment

Treatment principle:

Initial stage of an exterior condition: Expel pathogenic factors and unblock the obstruction in the channels.

Chronic and prolonged illness: Tonify kidney essence.

Combination of excess and deficiency: Treat both the root and branch simultaneously by augmenting the qi and invigorating the blood.

Cold-dampness invasion

Cold pain and heaviness in the lower back, with gradually diminishing range of motion and increasing pain.

S: Aggravated by cloudy, rainy or cold weather and relieved by warmth.

T: White greasy coating. **P:** Deep and slow.

- Expel cold-dampness, warm and unblock the channels.
- *Gan Jiang Ling Zhu Tang*
  - *Gan Jiang* and *Gan Cao* disperse cold and warm the middle burner.
  - *Fu Ling* and *Bai Zhu* strengthen the spleen and drain dampness.
- To strengthen the effects of eliminating dampness, warming and unblocking the obstruction in the channels. + *Gui Zhi, Xu Duan, Du Zhong, Niu Xi, Sang Ji Sheng*

  Cold predominating with cold pain and spasm. + *Fu Zi, Xi Xin*

  Dampness predominating with pronounced heaviness. + *Cang Zhu, Yi Yi Ren*

Damp-heat invasion

Burning pain and heaviness in the lower back, and red swollen joints.

S: Aggravated by rainy or hot weather and relieved by exercise, with dark scanty urination.

T: Yellow greasy coating. **P:** Soft and rapid.

- Clear heat and drain dampness, relax the sinews and alleviate pain.
- *Si Miao Wan*
  - *Cang Zhu*, bitter and warm, dries dampness.
  - *Huang Bai*, bitter and cold, clears heat and dries dampness.
  - *Yi Yi Ren* clears heat and drains dampness.
  - *Niu Xi* guides the formula downwards and tonifies the liver and kidney to strengthen the back and knees.
- Enhance the effects to relax the sinews, unblock the channels and alleviate pain. + *Mu Gua, Luo Shi Teng*

Heat predominating with thirst, irritability or scanty urination. + *Zhi Zi, Ze Xie, Mu Tong*

Damp-heat consuming kidney yin with soreness and weakness of the lower back and knees, five-centers heat and dry throat. + *Nu Zhen Zi, Han Lian Cao*

Blood stasis

Sharp, fixed lower back pain that becomes worse at night and limited range of motion at the lumbar joints aggravated by pressure.

S: Possibly a history of traumatic injury.

T: Dark purple tongue with petechiae. **P:** Choppy.

- Invigorate the blood, transform stasis, regulate the qi and alleviate pain.
- *Shen Tong Zhu Yu Tang*

  \- *Tao Ren*, *Hong Hua*, *Dang Gui* and *Chuan Xiong* invigorate the blood and transform blood stasis.

  \- *Mo Yao* and *Wu Ling Zhi* invigorate the blood, expel blood stasis, reduce swelling and alleviate pain.

  \- *Xiang Fu* facilitates the qi flow to activate the blood circulation.

  \- *Niu Xi* invigorates the blood and guides the movement of blood downwards; it tonifies the liver and kidney to strengthen the back and knees.

  \- *Di Long* unblocks the collaterals and expels stasis to alleviate pain.
- History of traumatic injury. + *Ru Xiang, Qing Pi, San Qi*

  Complicated by kidney deficiency. + *Du Zhong, Xu Duan, Shu Di Huang*

Kidney essence deficiency

Recurrent soreness and weakness of the lower back and knees, aggravated by exertion.

S: Predominantly yang deficiency: pale complexion, cold limbs, and cold pain in the lower abdomen. Predominantly yin deficiency: irritability, insomnia, dry throat, malar flush and five-centers heat.

T: Pale or red tongue with scanty coating. **P:** Deep and thready or thready and rapid.

- Tonify kidney essence.
- *You Gui Wan* or *Zuo Gui Wan*

  \- *You Gui Wan* warms the kidney yang and fortifies the fire.

  \- *Zuo Gui Wan* nourishes kidney yin and replenishes the essence.
- Kidney yin deficiency with heat signs. + *Da Bu Yin Wan*

  Kidney yang deficiency with shortness of breath, fatigue, poor appetite and loose stool. + *Huang Qi, Sheng Ma, Dang Shen*

Acupuncture Treatment

- **Manipulation:** Reducing method for lower back pain related to traumatic injuries. Reinforcing method or combination of needling and moxibustion for other patterns.
- **Prescription:** BL23 Shenshu BL40 Weizhong GV3 Yaoyangguan
- **Supplementary points:**
  - Cold-dampness. + BL25 Dachangshu; BL26 Guanyuanshu
  - Traumatic injuries. + GV26 Renzhong; Extra 29 Yaotongxue; Ahshi point
  - Kidney yang deficiency. + GV4 Mingmen; Extra21 Yaoyan
  - Kidney yin deficiency. + BL52 Zhishi; KI3 Taixi

Practical Hints

Lower back pain related to focal muscular pathology. Among the predisposing factors to lower back pain, muscular exertion and exhaustion is the most common. Unlike the differentiations discussed above, lower back pain related to muscular pathology can be confirmed by objective findings. During the physical examination, focal muscular tenderness, spasm, peripheral effusion, pain elicited by pressure, hematoma or ecchymosis, pain radiating to the upper back or lower extremities, and possibly numbness in the toes can be detected. The etiology and pathogenesis of lower back pain due to muscular pathology can be clarified with a detailed history intake. After ruling out exterior pathogenic factors and kidney deficiency, determine if the condition derives from a work related injury, automobile accident or physical exertion. To treat lower back pain related to muscle sprain and strain, employ internal and external therapeutic modalities. Herbal formulas can be administered orally to invigorate the blood and collaterals for a systemic effect. Physical therapy combined with acupuncture, cupping, acupressure, and hot or cold compresses can address localized pain. By promoting blood circulation and qi movement, the muscles will be nourished and relaxed. Symptoms caused by compressed nerves and inflammation will be relieved as well.

CHAPTER 22

Seminal Emission

遺 精 *Yi Jing*

Seminal emission is the spontaneous discharge of semen not induced by sexual activity. There are two types of seminal emission. The first type is nocturnal emission that occurs when there is ejaculation of semen during sleep and is commonly known as a wet dream. Spermatorrhea is the second type and involves frequent involuntary emission of semen while awake. Seminal emission may be considered physiologically normal if it occurs less than twice a month without any other significant symptoms. If seminal emission disturbs normal daily activities or is accompanied by dizziness, listlessness, insomnia, and soreness and weakness of the lower back and knees, evaluation and treatment may be medically necessary.

Relevant Diseases

- Neurosis
- Neurasthenia
- Prostatitis
- Prostatic hypertrophy
- Spermatocystitis
- Orchitis

Etiology and Pathogenesis

The primary pathogenesis for seminal emission is kidney qi failing to restrain the essence. The kidney qi must be firm in order to store essence and prevent leakage. The following are various predisposing factors to instability of kidney qi:

Lack of communication between the heart and kidney can induce nocturnal emission. Excessive mental exertion consumes heart yin and causes heart fire to become hyperactive. Hyperactive heart fire may harass the mind and lead to nocturnal emission accompanied by excessive dreaming. In addition, heart fire may injure kidney water. With hyperactive heart fire above and empty fire agitating the kidney below, the seminal vesicles are disturbed, leading to nocturnal emission.

Damp-heat infusing downwards: Damp-heat results when overindulgence in alcohol and a rich, greasy diet hinder the spleen. Damp-heat infuses downwards to harass the seminal vesicles and cause leakage of semen during the day and night.

Deficient qi failing to bind essence: Excessive physical or mental exertion can exhaust the qi of the heart and spleen. Deficient qi failing to constrain the essence will lead to spermatorrhea that is aggravated by exertion and exhaustion.

Kidney deficiency and seminal gate instability: When kidney yin is deficient, empty fire harasses the seminal vesicles, leading to nocturnal emission. Unremitting and chronic nocturnal emission will lead to deficiency of both the essence and qi. The deficiency is compounded, complicating the condition and causing spermatorrhea even when the person is awake.

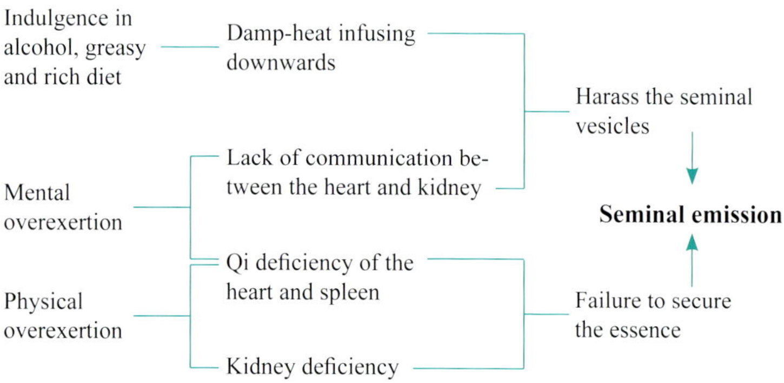

Diagnosis

A. Identification of organ involvement:

Nocturnal emission in its early stage is closely related to heart fire or damp-heat, patterns of relative excess. Unremitting and chronic nocturnal emission can progress to kidney deficiency and result in a deficiency pattern.

Spermatorrhea usually develops from nocturnal emission or is caused by constitutional deficiency. Kidney deficiency is usually responsible for spermatorrhea.

B. Differential diagnosis of seminal emission and premature ejaculation:

Seminal emission is subcategorized into nocturnal emission and spermatorrhea. The former occurs during sleep and is usually accompanied by erotic dreams. The latter refers to the involuntary discharge of semen while awake, possibly during bowel movements, urination or strenuous activities. As a disorder, seminal emission does not occur in the context of sexual activity.

Premature ejaculation occurs during preparation for sexual intercourse. It refers to the ejaculation of semen shortly after sexual arousal. The pathogenesis of premature ejaculation is similar to that of spermatorrhea. Both conditions result from a pathological failure to contain or secure the essence.

Basic Patterns

- Lack of communication between the heart and kidney
- Damp-heat infusing downwards
- Qi deficiency failing to bind the essence
- Kidney deficiency and seminal gate instability

Differentiation and Treatment

Treatment principle:

Because the kidney stores the essence and prevents it from leaking, treatment of seminal emission should tonify the kidney and secure the essence. However, as the other organs may also be involved in the pathogenesis, treatment should be modified based on the complete pattern differentiation.

Lack of communication between the heart and kidney

Nocturnal emission with erotic dreams, insomnia or dream-disturbed sleep, and irritability.

S: Dizziness, blurred vision, palpitations, dry mouth and dark scanty urine.

T: Red tongue with scanty coating. **P:** Thready and rapid.

- Clear heat from the heart, calm the spirit and nourish the yin.
- *Tian Wang Bu Xin Dan*
  - *Sheng Di Huang*, *Xuan Shen*, *Mai Men Dong* and *Tian Men Dong* nourish the yin and clear heat.
  - *Dan Shen* and *Dang Gui* nourish the blood.
  - *Suan Zao Ren*, *Bai Zi Ren*, *Wu Wei Zi* and *Yuan Zhi* nourish the heart, calm the spirit and restore communication between the heart and kidney
  - *Ren Shen* and *Fu Ling* augment the qi and quiet the heart.
- Chronic nocturnal emission injuring the kidney with yin deficiency and empty fire, use *Zhi Bai Di Huang Wan* or *Da Bu Yin Wan*.

Damp-heat infusing downwards

Frequent seminal emission, possibly spermaturia, dark turbid urine, and a burning sensation during urination.

S: Bitter taste in the mouth, pasty stool with foul odor, sensation of incomplete defecation, and possibly focal distention in the epigastrium and abdomen.

T: Yellow greasy coating. **P:** Soft and rapid.

- Clear heat and drain dampness.
- *Cheng Shi Bi Xie Fen Qing Yin*
  - *Bi Xie*, *Huang Bai*, *Fu Ling* and *Che Qian Zi* clear and drain damp-heat.
  - *Lian Zi*, *Dan Shen* and *Shi Chang Pu* clear the heart and calm the spirit.
  - *Bai Zhu* strengthens the spleen and dries dampness.

Qi deficiency failing to bind the essence

Seminal emission that occurs when fatigued, sallow complexion, and a heavy and fatigued sensation of the limbs.
S: Palpitations, insomnia, forgetfulness, poor appetite and loose stool.
T: Pale tongue with thin coating. **P:** Weak.

- Harmonize and tonify the heart and spleen, augment the qi and bind the essence.
- *Bu Zhong Yi Qi Tang*
  - *Bu Zhong Yi Qi Tang* is the imperial formula for augmenting the qi and raising the yang. Via lifting the collapse, it binds the essence.
- To enhance the effects of restraining and binding. *+ Shan Yao, Lian Zi, Qian Shi*

Kidney deficiency and seminal gate instability

Frequent nocturnal emission, possibly spermatorrhea, and soreness and weakness of the lower back and knees.
S: Dry throat, irritability, dizziness, forgetfulness, insomnia, low-grade fever, malar flush, emaciation, night sweating, hair loss and loose teeth.
T: Red tongue with scanty coating. **P:** Thready and rapid.

- Tonify and augment the kidney, bind the essence and prevent leakage.
- *Zuo Gui Yin*
  - *Zuo Gui Yin* nourishes kidney yin and replenishes kidney essence.
- Severe loss of essence with significant weakness and soreness of the lower back and knees, use *Zuo Gui Wan*.
  To strengthen the effects of binding and astringing in order to restrain seminal emission. *+ Jin Suo Gu Jing Wan*

Acupuncture Treatment

Nocturnal emission:

- **Manipulation:** Combination of reducing and reinforcing methods.
- **Prescription:** HT7 Shenmen, BL15 Xinshu, KI3 Taixi, BL52 Zhishi

Spermatorrhea:

- **Manipulation:** Reinforcing method and moxibustion.
- **Prescription:** BL23 Shenshu KI12 Dahe SP6 Sanyinjiao CV4 Guanyuan CV6 Qihai

Practical Hints

• Lack of communication between the heart and the kidney is the most common pattern of seminal emission. According to TCM theory, **"It is the heart fire that triggers the hyperactive empty fire of the kidney, which in turn forces the semen to leak out."** Therefore, clearing heart fire should be the primary treatment principle for seminal emission. Nourishing the yin and binding the essence could be utilized as auxiliary measures.

• **Lifting the clear qi to drain dampness.** Seminal emission is a disorder of leaking essence. In most cases, it requires herbs and formulas that stabilize and bind. However, utilizing the method of binding and astringing for the condition of damp-heat infusing downwards will result in the retention of pathogens, and thus this method is contraindicated, especially during the early stage of the disease. In addition, the formation of damp-heat is closely related to the dysfunction of the spleen and stomach. To properly treat the damp-heat pattern, one must also strengthen the spleen on the basis of clearing heat and draining dampness. By raising the clear qi, dampness will be transformed and turbidity will be drained.

[Addendum]

Impotence

陽痿 *Yang Wei*

Impotence is a male reproductive disorder manifesting with inability to achieve or maintain an erection. Impotence is one of the major reasons for sexual dissatisfaction. Clinically, impotence may present with seminal emission or premature ejaculation. Kidney yang deficiency or failure of the fire in the gate of vitality can result in impotence.

Differentiation and Treatment

Failure of the fire in the gate of vitality

Excessive sexual activity leading to kidney essence deficiency and failure of the fire in the gate of vitality.
Impotence, pale complexion, dizziness, listlessness, and soreness and weakness of the lower back and knees.
T: Pale tongue with a white coating. **P:** Deep and thready.

- Tonify the kidney and fortify the yang.
- *Wu Zi Yan Zong Wan*
  - *Gou Qi Zi*, *Tu Si Zi* and *Fu Pen Zi* warm the yang, augment the kidney and bind the essence.
  - *Wu Wei Zi* is sour to astringe the essence.
  - *Che Qian Zi* clears and drains turbid dampness; it provides a draining effect in this tonifying formula.

Deficiency of the heart and spleen

Excessive pensiveness and worry injure the heart and spleen, resulting in qi and blood deficiency.
Impotence, insomnia, lassitude and dull complexion.
T: Pale tongue. **P:** Thready.

- Tonify the heart and spleen.
- *Gui Pi Tang*
  - *Gui Pi Tang* is the primary formula for augmenting the qi and nourishing the blood; it strengthens the spleen to encourage the generation of qi and blood.

Shock and fear injuring the kidney

Fear and shock scatter the kidney essence, leading to kidney dysfunction.
Impotence, timidity, suspiciousness, palpitations and insomnia.
T: Slightly cyanotic tongue with thin greasy coating. **P:** Wiry and thready.

- Augment the kidney and quiet the mind.
- *Da Bu Yuan Jian*
  - *Shu Di Huang*, *Shan Yao* and *Shan Zhu Yu* tonify and augment the liver and kidney to bind the essence.
  - *Du Zhong* and *Gou Qi Zi* tonify the liver and kidney.
  - *Dang Gui*, *Ren Shen* and *Zhi Gan Cao* augment the qi and nourish the blood.
- To strengthen the tranquilizing effect. + *Suan Zao Ren*, *Yuan Zhi*

CHAPTER **23**

Manic-Depressive Psychosis

癲 狂 *Dian Kuang*

Manic-depressive psychosis is a bipolar affective disorder characterized by severe alterations in mood that are usually episodic and recurrent. Mood fluctuates between depression and mania. In TCM, depressive psychosis, or *dian*, is caused by qi stagnation complicated by phlegm misting the heart's orifice; it is characterized by depression, apathy, incoherent speech, dementia, subdued and non-violent behavior. In contrast, manic psychosis, or *kuang*, is induced by phlegm-fire disturbing the mind; it is characterized by mental hyperactivity and manic behavior, manifesting with shouting, hostility and violent behavior. Clinically, *dian* and *kuang* are not distinct disease entities; they are two aspects of one disorder and their clinical manifestations may be interchangeable.

Relevant Diseases

- Schizophrenic psychosis
- Bipolar disorder
- Psychiatric disorders
- Mania
- Major depression
- Senile dementia
- Alzheimer's disease
- Brain tumor
- Organic brain syndrome

Etiology and Pathogenesis

Lack of equilibrium between the yin and yang: "As the yin is even and the yang is firm, the physical and psychological equilibrium is preserved." If the equilibrium between the yin and yang is disturbed, mental disorders occur. Preponderance of the yin or yang determines the clinical presentations of mental disorders. Both absolute and relative excess of the yang can lead to manic psychosis, or *kuang*; whereas absolute or relative excess of the yin can lead to depressive psychosis, or *dian*.

Emotional factors (anger, joy, pensiveness, sadness, worry, fear and shock) can injure their corresponding internal organs and induce manic-depressive psychosis. Impaired spleen function results in inadequate production of the qi and blood, which leads to malnourishment of the heart and the mind. Deficient essence and blood due to injury to the liver and kidney lead to emptiness of the brain and marrow. Heart yin deficiency with hyperactivity of empty fire disturbs the spirit. Emotional change is closely related to mental and behavioral alterations, manifested by unusual behaviors, poor memory, and intellectual defects.

Turbid phlegm misting the heart's orifice hinders the heart's ability to govern the mind. The clarity of the mind is impaired and awareness of reality and the ability to form judgments are lost, leading to abnormal behavior and depressed demeanor. Turbid phlegm is the major pathogenic factor causing depressive psychosis. In the case of manic psychosis, turbid phlegm is further complicated by fire. The phlegm-fire complex obstructs the heart's orifice and also disturbs the mind, causing manic behavior.

Qi stagnation and blood stasis in the brain due to head injury obstruct the flow of qi and cause disassociation between the internal organs and the brain. The brain is one of the organs controlling thinking and mental activities. When it is inadequately supplied with qi, it cannot properly manage the mind. This condition can retrograde into manic-depressive psychosis.

Miscellaneous: Influences from other contributing factors, including heredity and a person's constitution, should not be underestimated. Individuals with weaker constitutions are susceptible to and unable to cope with emotional stress. Imbalance of the yin and yang is more likely to occur and equilibrium is more difficult to restore. Therefore, a weak constitution is associated with a higher risk of occurrence of manic-depressive psychosis. Family history is also relevant to the occurrence of mental disorders.

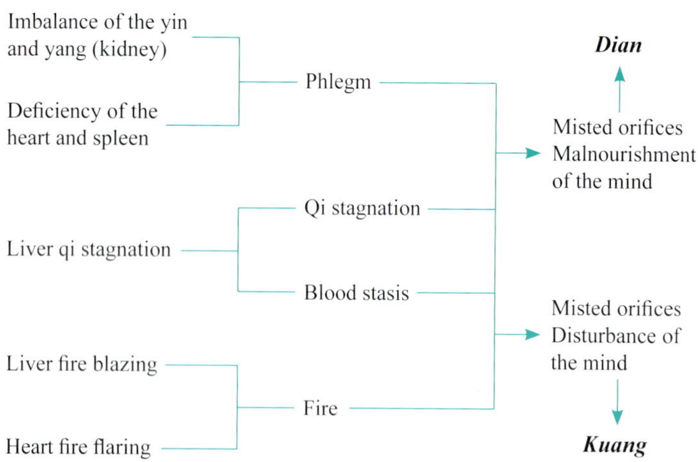

Diagnosis

A. Identification of depressive and manic psychosis:

Dian: With yin predominating, depressive psychosis presents clinically with depression, apathy, incoherent speech, dementia, quiet and non-violent behavior.

Kuang: With yang predominating, manic psychosis manifests with mental and behavioral hyperactivity; shouting, hostility and agitation, and violent behavior might also be apparent.

B. Differential diagnosis of manic-depressive psychosis and epilepsy:

Manic-depressive psychosis is categorized as a psychological disorder.

Epilepsy is a recurrent paroxysmal neurological disorder characterized by sudden, brief episodes of altered consciousness, motor activity or sensory perception. The symptoms of epilepsy are not evident during periods of remission.

Basic Patterns

Depressive psychosis (dian):

- Stagnated qi combining with phlegm
- Heart and spleen deficiency

Manic psychosis (kuang):

- Phlegm-fire disturbing the heart
- Excessive fire injuring the yin

Differentiation and Treatment

Treatment principle:

Manic psychosis: Sedate the heart, resolve phlegm, clear liver fire or nourish the yin and calm the spirit.

Depressive psychosis: Soothe liver qi, resolve phlegm, open the orifices or nourish the heart and calm the spirit.

Depressive psychosis (dian):

Stagnated qi combining with phlegm

Depression, apathetic expression, incoherent speech, subdued and non-violent behavior, suspicion, anxiety and mood swings.

S: Talking to oneself and no appetite.

T: Pale tongue with white greasy coating. **P:** Wiry and slippery.

- Regulate the qi, release constraint, resolve phlegm and open the orifices.
- *Xiao Yao San* and *Di Tan Tang*
  - *Chai Hu* soothes the liver and releases constrained qi.
  - *Dang Gui* and Bai Shao nourish the blood, preserve the yin, and comfort and soften the liver.
  - *Ban Xia* and *Ju Hong* dry dampness and transform phlegm.
  - *Dan Nan Xing*, *Zhu Ru* and *Zhi Shi* resolve phlegm and descend the qi.
  - *Shi Chang Pu* transforms phlegm and opens the orifice.
- Phlegm misting the heart's orifice with white greasy tongue coating, use *Su He Xiang Wan* first to open the orifices via its aromatic effect.

Heart and spleen deficiency

Protracted course with disturbed thoughts, incoherent speech, depression, crying spells, and panic attacks with palpitations.
S: Pale complexion, fatigue, lassitude, dream-disturbed sleep, loss of appetite and loose stool.
T: Pale, flabby tongue with teeth marks and thin white coating. **P:** Thready, weak and forceless.

- Strengthen the spleen, nourish the heart, benefit the qi and calm the spirit.
- *Yang Xin Tang*
  - *Ren Shen* greatly tonifies basal qi.
  - *Huang Qi*, *Fu Ling* and *Gan Cao* benefit the qi and strengthen the spleen.
  - *Dang Gui* and *Chuan Xiong* nourish and invigorate the blood.
  - *Suan Zao Ren* and *Bai Zi Ren* nourish heart blood to calm the spirit.
  - *Wu Wei Zi* and *Yuan Zhi* augment heart qi and quiet the heart to calm the spirit.
- To enhance the effects of nourishing the heart and calming the spirit. + *Gan Mai Da Zao Tang*

Manic psychosis (kuang):

Phlegm-fire disturbing the heart

Acute onset, rapid flushing of the face and eyes, manic and aggressive behavior, inability to sleep or eat.
S: Irritability, agitation, insomnia and distending headache before onset, dry mouth and throat, preference for cold drinks, and constipation.
T: Deep red with yellow greasy coating. **P:** Wiry, rapid and slippery.

- Purge fire, eliminate phlegm, sedate the irritated heart and tranquilize the mind.
- *Xie Xin Tang* and *Meng Shi Gun Tan Wan*

- *Huang Lian* and *Huang Qin*, bitter and cold, clear and drain fire from the heart and upper burner.
- *Da Huang* drains fire, clears heat and relieves toxicity.
- *Meng Shi Gun Tan Wan* strongly and aggressively eliminates phlegm and purges fire. It is the primary formula for phlegm-fire disturbing the heart.

- Heat trapped in the yang-brightness stage with constipation, dry yellow tongue coating, use *Da Cheng Qi Tang* first.

Excessive fire injuring the yin

Following excessive fire or protracted manic psychosis, with emotional instability, nervousness, impatience, insomnia, anxiety, and panic attacks with palpitations.
S: Five-centers heat, emaciation, and scanty and dark urination.
T: Red tongue with scanty or no coating. **P:** Thready and rapid; or wiry, thready and rapid.

- Nourish the yin, eliminate fire and calm the spirit.
- *Er Yin Jian* and *Ding Zhi Wan*
  - *Sheng Di Huang*, *Mai Men Dong* and *Xuan Shen* nourish the yin and generate the fluid to clear heat.
  - *Huang Lian*, *Mu Tong*, *Zhu Ye* and *Deng Xin Cao* clear and drain heat from the heart to calm the spirit.
  - *Fu Shen* and *Suan Zao Ren* benefit the heart and calm the spirit.
  - *Ding Zhi Wan* strengthens the spleen, nourishes the heart, calms the spirit and settles the will.
- Enhance the effect of eliminating empty heat. + *Bai Wei, Di Gu Pi*

Acupuncture Treatment

Depressive psychosis:

- **Manipulation:** Even method.
- **Prescription:** BL15 Xinshu, BL18 Ganshu, BL20 Pishu, HT7 Shenmen, ST40 Fenglong, PC7 Daling

Manic psychosis:

- **Manipulation:** Reducing method.
- **Prescription:** PC8 Laogong, GV26 Renzhong, GV14 Dazhui, GV16 Fengfu, PC6 Neiguan, ST40 Fenglong, KI4 Dazhong

Practical Hints

• "As the yin is even and the yang is firm, the physical and psychological equilibrium is preserved." A harmonious state between the yin and yang is the essential foundation for normal mental function. Therefore, **the ultimate aim of treatment is to readjust and restore equilibrium between the yin and yang.** When the yang predominates over the yin in manic psychosis, clinical manifestations that are yang in nature, such as excitement, aggressive behaviors and heat signs, are evident. When the yin predominates over the yang in depressive psychosis, clinical manifestations that are yin in nature, such as apathy, withdrawal, subdued demeanor and cold signs, are present.

• Phlegm is the most significant factor in the development of manic-depressive psychosis. Phlegm misting the heart's orifice is the primary pathogenesis in this disorder. During treatment, **in addition to transforming phlegm, it is equally important to break the cycle of phlegm production.** Improper diet can injure the spleen and generate phlegm internally; emotional stress may lead to constrained liver qi overacting on the spleen. Therefore, proper diet and emotional coping mechanisms should be taught and encouraged as prophylactic measures.

• **Family history and constitutional weakness are related to susceptibility.** Emotional factors may be triggers for manic-depressive psychosis. Temporary disharmony between the yin and yang can be induced by any emotional stressor; in most people, psychosis is unlikely to result. However, individuals with a significant family history, or who have a weak constitution, have relatively inadequate coping skills; therefore, they are more susceptible to developing manic-depressive psychosis once triggered, and they experience more difficulties in recovering from this disorder.

CHAPTER 24

Epilepsy

癇證 *Xian Zheng*

Epilepsy refers to a recurrent paroxysmal neurological disorder characterized by sudden, brief episodes of altered consciousness. During an epileptic seizure, the patient may emit a cry, fall, drool or froth at the mouth, fixate their eyes in an upward stare, and experience localized or general muscular contractions. These symptoms result from liver wind triggering turbid phlegm, whcih mists the clear orifices and obstructs the channels. However, during remission, these symptoms are abscent.

Relevant Diseases

- Seizure disorders
- Anxiety attack
- Gestational epilepsy

Etiology and Pathogenesis

Liver wind and phlegm are the two major factors in epileptic seizures. Pre-existing phlegm triggered by liver wind will travel to the heart and cover the orifice resulting in loss of consciousness; it also can travel and obstruct the channels, causing seizures.

Emotional stimulation: Extreme shock and fear, causing derangement of the qi and blood followed by deterioration of the organs, precede epilepsy. When deterioration of the organs results in liver and kidney yin deficiency, internal wind and heat are generated. Dampness and phlegm accumulate when there is spleen and stomach deficiency. Phlegm-dampness stirred by the movement of wind and heat will ascend and cover the heart's orifice, resulting in epilepsy.

Congenital exposure: Juvenile epilepsy is closely related to pre-natal exposure to shock and fear when a pregnant woman experiences these strong negative emotional stimuli. Strong emotional stimulation can cause derangement of the fetal qi and blood and can damage the fetal kidney essence.

Head trauma associated with a fall, head contusions, improper utilization of obstetric forceps or vacuum during delivery, and delayed or difficult labor can injure the brain, one of the organs responsible for cognitive activities. The resulting stagnation of the qi and blood manifests with altered consciousness and contraction of the extremities.

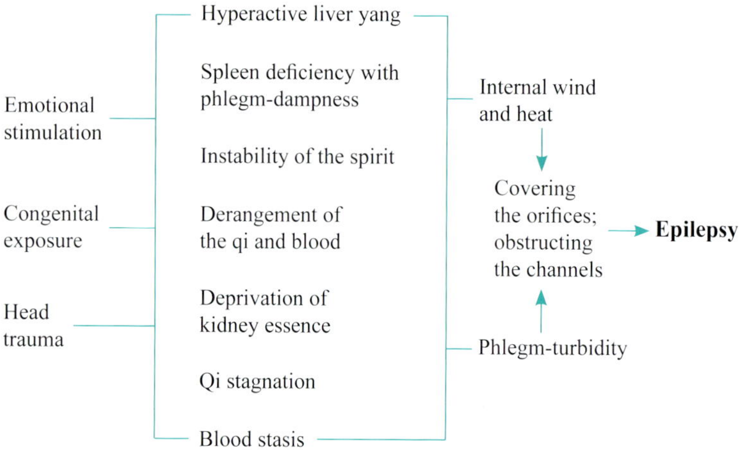

Diagnosis

A. Identification of yang and yin patterns during an epileptic episode:

Yang patterns pertain to excess heat and have an acute onset in persons with robust constitutions. They are characterized by sudden falling with a loud cry, contractions, drooling or frothing at the mouth, locked jaws, eyes rolled back in the head, and a wiry rapid or wiry slippery pulse.

Yin patterns pertain to deficient cold and have a recurrent onset in persons with weak constitutions. The manifestations include a pale complexion, trance, brief staring spells, apathy, lack of awareness of the surroundings, quiet and still demeanor, and a deep wiry or deep slippery pulse.

B. Identification of organ involvement during remission:

Good history taking during periods of remission is essential to identify patterns of organ involvement, such as spleen qi deficiency with excessive phlegm, and liver and kidney yin deficiency.

C. Differential diagnosis of similar disorders:

Epilepsy, wind stroke and hypertonicity disorders share the common symptom of loss of consciousness; they are distinguished by their secondary manifestations.

Epilepsy: During a seizure, the subject may fall down with a cry, drool or froth at the mouth, fix their eyes in an upward stare, and experience contractions of the four extremities. The subject will recover consciousness within seconds or minutes; sequelae are absent.

Wind stroke: Characterized by a sudden silent fall accompanied by facial paralysis, hemiplegia, and weakness or numbness of the affected side of the body followed by a slow recovery of consciousness. Various degrees of sequelae are present in most cases.

Hypertonicity disorder: Marked by tonic contractions of voluntary muscles or, in severe cases, opisthotonos with high fever, a prolonged period of unconsciousness and a difficult recovery.

Basic Patterns

Episode:

- Yang pattern
- Yin pattern

Remission:

- Spleen deficiency with excessive phlegm
- Liver and Kidney yin deficiency

Differentiation and Treatment

Treatment principle:

Considering the paroxysmal, recurrent and transient nature of epilepsy, a treatment strategy should be developed on the different phases of episode or remission and the different patterns of the illness. During or immediately following an epileptic seizure, treatment should focus on the branch by strongly expelling phlegm, extinguishing wind, opening the orifices, and arresting contractions. During remission, treatment should focus on the root by strengthening the spleen, resolving phlegm, tonifying the liver and kidney, and nourishing the heart and calming the spirit.

Episode:

Yang pattern

Aura with dizziness, headache and a stifling sensation in the chest; followed by a sudden fall with a cry, loss of consciousness, eyes staring upward, locked jaws, dark blue lips, contractions of the extremities, drooling or frothing at the mouth and/or a gurgling sound of sputum in the throat.

S: Possible fecal and urinary incontinence, feeling exhausted when consciousness returns.

T: White greasy or yellow greasy coating. **P:** Wiry slippery or wiry rapid.

- Clear and transform phlegm-heat, extinguish wind and arrest contractions.
- *Long Dan Xie Gan Tang* and *Di Tan Tang*
  - *Long Dan Cao*, *Zhi Zi* and *Huang Qin* clear and drain liver fire.
  - *Ban Xia*, *Dan Nan Xing*, *Ju Hong* and *Shi Chang Pu* transform phlegm and open the orifices.

Yin pattern

Pale, lusterless or sallow complexion, cold limbs, loss of consciousness with eyes remaining partially open, contraction of the entire body in a fetal position; or clonic contractions of the extremities, drooling and foaming at the mouth.
S: Absence of a cry or a weak cry, possibly absence of attention or loss of connection to reality, brief episodes of staring, trance, apathy, quiet and still demeanor, and a feeling of weakness and lack of strength when consciousness returns.
T: Pale tongue with white greasy coating. **P:** Deep thready or thready slippery.

- Resolve phlegm, open the orifices and extinguish wind.
- *Ding Xian Wan*
  - *Dan Nan Xing*, *Ban Xia* and *Bei Mu* resolve phlegm and open the orifices.
  - *Tian Ma* extinguishes wind and stops tremors.
- To enhance the effect of transforming phlegm. + *Zhu Ru, Shi Chang Pu*
  To enhance the effects of extinguishing wind and stopping tremors. + *Quan Xie, Bai Jiang Can*
  To enhance the effects of sedating the heart and calming the spirit. + *Long Gu, Hu Po, Fu Shen, Yuan Zhi*

Remission:

Spleen deficiency with excessive phlegm

Fatigue, lassitude, dizziness, sallow complexion, lack of appetite, abdominal distention and loose stool.
S: Nausea, vomiting, focal distention and fullness in the chest and epigastrium, and coughing up white sputum.
T: Pale tongue with white greasy coating. **P:** Soft slippery; or thready, wiry and slippery.

- Strengthen the spleen and resolve phlegm.
- *Liu Jun Zi Tang*
  - *Ren Shen*, *Bai Zhu*, *Fu Ling* and *Zhi Gan Cao* tonify the qi.
  - *Ban Xia* dries dampness and transforms phlegm.
  - *Chen Pi* promotes the movement of qi and transforms phlegm.

- Transform phlegm and calm the heart. + *Shi Chang Pu, Yuan Zhi*
  Copious and viscous yellow sputum, use *Wen Dan Tang*.

Liver and kidney yin deficiency

Declining memory, poor concentration, lusterless complexion, dizziness, vertigo and dry eyes.
S: Forgetfulness, insomnia, and soreness and weakness of the lower back and knees.
T: Red tongue with scanty coating. **P:** Thready and rapid.

- Tonify the liver and kidney, nourish the heart and calm the spirit.
- *Zuo Gui Wan*
  - *Shu Di Huang*, *Shan Yao* and *Shan Zhu Yu* nourish the liver and kidney to bind the essence.
  - *Tu Si Zi* and *Gou Qi Zi* tonify the yin and blood of the liver and kidney.
  - *Gui Ban Jiao* and *Lu Jiao Jiao* greatly tonify the essence and blood, and replenish the conception and governing vessels.
  - *Niu Xi* tonifies the liver and kidney, and strengthens the back and knees.
- To enhance the effects of nourishing the yin and subduing the yang. + *Mu Li, Long Gu, Bie Jia*
  Quiet the heart and calm the spirit. + *Bai Zi Ren, Ci Shi*
  To enhance the effect of transforming phlegm. + *Zhu Ru, Shi Chang Pu*

Acupuncture Treatment

Episode:

- **Manipulation:** Reducing method.
- **Prescription:** GV26 Renzhong, CV15 Jiuwei, PC5 Jianshi, LR3 Taichong, ST40 Fenglong
- **Supplementary points:**
  - Episode during the day. + BL62 Shenmai
  - Episode during the night. + KI6 Zhaohai

Remission:

- **Manipulation:** Even method.
- **Prescription:** BL15 Xinshu, Extra2 Yintang, HT7 Shenmen, SP6 Sanyinjiao, KI3 Taixi, Extra19 Yaoqi

Practical Hints

• During an epileptic seizure, **acupuncture may be effective as an emergency treatment to restore consciousness.** Herbal therapy is more appropriate during remission because it addresses the underlying causes of seizure by pacifying the liver and extinguishing wind, as well as by strengthening the spleen and transforming phlegm.

• **Preventing complications during a seizure** should not be overlooked. The airway should be kept clear; turn the head to one side to allow drainage of saliva; protect the head and body from possible trauma. Concurrent consultation and evaluation by western medical practitioners is advisable.

CHAPTER 25

Hypertonicity Disorder

痙 證 *Jing Zheng*

Hypertonicity disorder is characterized by rigidity and stiffness of the neck and upper back, contractions and tremors of the extremities, and, in extreme cases, opisthotonos. Disharmony between the yin and yang is the major predisposing factor for hypertonicity disorder. When there is insufficient yin to nourish the sinews, hyperactive yang manifests as rigidity and abnormal movement. Muscle regidity, stiffness and contractions can also be results of deep tissue trauma, injured by stepping over a rotten metal or a sharp. This disorder is known as tetanus, which is not subject to be covered in internal medicine.

Relevant Diseases

- Meningitis
- Encephalitis
- Febrile convulsions
- Parkinson's disease
- Opisthotonos

Etiology and Pathogenesis

Hypertonicity disorder involves pathology of the sinews. It is caused by exterior pathogenic factors invading and obstructing the sinews or by malnourishment of the sinews. Contractions and tremors occur when there are constrictions in the sinews connecting the muscle to the bone.

Pathogenic factors accumulating and obstructing the channels interrupt the blood circulation and the qi flow. When the sinews are deprived of the qi and blood they contract. According to Nei Jing, "All patterns of stiff neck and rigid back pertain to influences of dampness; ... all patterns of muscular hypertonicity are associated with wind; ... pathology of sinews presenting as severe contractions or opisthotonos are induced by cold."

Extreme heat: Extreme internal heat consumes the body fluid. Deficient yin and body fluid fail to nourish and moisten the sinews, resulting in hypertonicity disorder.

Deficiency of the yin and blood: Constitutional yin and blood deficiency, excessive loss of blood, and excessive diaphoresis and purgation all contribute to hypertonicity disorder by injuring the yin, which then fails to nourish the sinews.

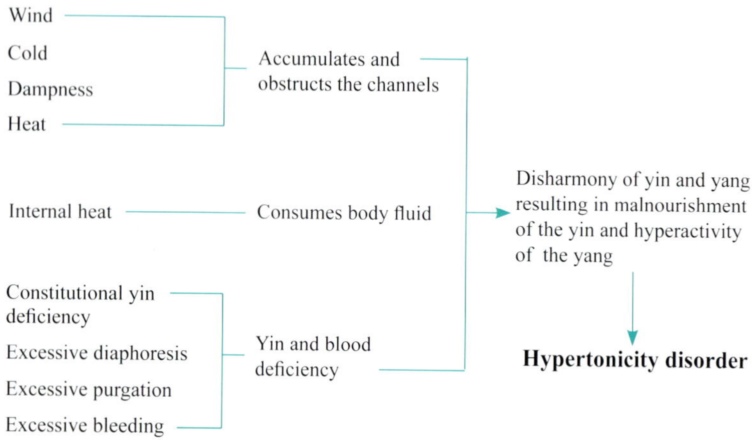

Diagnosis

Differential diagnosis of similar disorders:

Hypertonicity disorder, wind-stroke and epilepsy all share some common symptoms, such as loss of consciousness and contraction of the extremities.

Hypertonicity disorder: Primarily characterized by stiffness and rigidity of the neck and upper back accompanied by tremors, contractions or opisthotonos.

Wind-stroke: Contraction of the extremities may be accompanied by facial paralysis, hemiplegia, and stroke sequelae. Residual effects will become more apparent once consciousness has been recovered.

Epilepsy: Relatively short episodes of unconsciousness, with contractions of the extremities, drooling and foaming at the mouth, and utterance of a cry. Contractions are eased as soon as consciousness is recovered.

Basic Patterns

- Pathogenic factors accumulating and obstructing the channels
- Extreme heat inducing hypertonicity
- Yin and blood deficiency

Differentiation and Treatment

Treatment principle:

Excess patterns, usually related to exterior pathogens, should be treated by expelling the pathogenic influences, including dispelling wind, dispersing cold, eliminating dampness and clearing heat.

Deficient patterns, usually pertaining to impairment of the internal organs, should be treated by supporting the righteous qi via nourishing the yin and blood, extinguishing wind, relaxing the sinews and unblocking the collaterals.

Pathogenic factors accumulating and obstructing the channels

Headache, stiffness and rigidity of the neck and upper back.
S: Aversion to cold, fever, and soreness and heaviness of the extremities.
T: White greasy coating. **P:** Floating and tight.

- Dispel wind and disperse cold, dry dampness and harmonize nutritive qi.
- *Qiang Huo Sheng Shi Tang*
  - *Qiang Huo*, *Du Huo*, *Fang Feng* and *Gao Ben* dispel wind-dampness.
  - *Chuan Xiong* invigorates the blood and dispels wind to alleviate pain.
  - *Man Jing Zi* dispels wind and alleviates pain.
- Preponderance of cold with thin white tongue coating and floating tight pulse, use *Ge Gen Tang*.
  Preponderance of wind with aversion to wind, headache and sweating, use *Gui Zhi Tang* to harmonize the nutritive and protective qi; add *Tian Hua Fen* to generate the fluid and relax the sinews.
  Preponderance of damp-heat with focal distention and fullness in the chest and the epigastriac regions, thirst with no desire to drink, yellow greasy tongue coating and rapid slippery pulse, use *San Ren Tang*. + *Di Long, Qin Jiao, Si Gua Luo, Wei Ling Xian*

Extreme heat inducing hypertonicity

High fever, stifling sensation in the chest, locked jaw, stiffness and rigidity of the neck and upper back, contractions or, in extreme cases, opisthotonos.
S: Dry throat, thirst, abdominal distension, fecal impaction, irritability, impatience, or delirium and unconsciousness.
T: Yellow greasy coating. **P:** Wiry and rapid.

- Drain heat and nourish the yin to preserve the body fluid.
- *Zeng Ye Cheng Qi Tang*
  - *Da Huang* and *Mang Xiao* drain fire and relieve toxicity, soften hardness and

moisten dryness.

- *Xuan Shen*, *Mai Men Dong* and *Sheng Di Huang* nourish the yin and generate the fluid.

- Severe contractions. + *Di Long, Quan Xie, Ju Hua, Gou Teng*
  Severe irritability and agitation. + *Dan Zhu Ye, Zhi Zi*
  Excessive heat without fecal impaction, use *Bai Hu Jia Ren Shen Tang*.
  Extreme heat generating wind with unconsciousness, high fever, locked jaws and opisthotonos, use *Ling Jiao Gou Teng Tang*.

Yin and blood deficiency

Stiffness and rigidity of the neck and upper back with contractions and tremors of the four extremities, often seen following excessive blood loss or abundant sweating.

S: Dizziness, vertigo, lassitude and shortness of breath.

T: Pale-pink tongue. **P:** Wiry and thready.

- Replenish the yin and nourish the blood.
- *Si Wu Tang* and *Da Ding Feng Zhu*
  - *Si Wu Tang* nourishes and invigorates the blood; it is the basic formula for harmonizing the blood.
  - *Ji Zi Huang* and *E Jiao* greatly tonify the yin and fluid to extinguish wind.
  - *Gui Ban*, *Bie Jia* and *Bai Shao* nourish the yin to relax the sinews.
  - *Wu Wei Zi* and *Zhi Gan Cao*, a combination of sour and sweet properties transforming into the yin, soften and moderate spasms.
- Dizziness, irritability and insomnia. + *Zhi Zi, Zhu Ye, Ye Jiao Teng*
  Loose stool with a pale tongue and thready pulse. + *Dang Shen, Bai Zhu*

Acupuncture Treatment

Pathogenic factors accumulating and obstructing the channels:

- **Manipulation:** Reducing method.
- **Prescription:** LI4 Hegu, TE5 Waiguan, GV14 Dazhui, GV20 Fengchi, BL12 Fengmen

Extreme heat inducing hypertonicity:

- **Manipulation:** Reducing method.
- **Prescription:** GV14 Dazhui, LI11Quchi, LR3 Taichong, KI1 Yongquan, 12 Jing-well points

Yin and blood deficiency:

- **Manipulation:** Reinforcing method.
- **Prescription:** GV20 Baihui, SP6 Sanyinjiao, KI1 Yongquan, CV4 Guanyuan, ST36 Zusanli

Practical Hints

• Hypertonicity is a complex disease of internal wind and exterior pathogenic factors obstructing the channels. Due to a complicated pathogenesis involving excess and deficiency, exterior and interior, the qi and blood, and the yin and yang, prescribing herbs that heavily subdue the yang and extinguish wind are not adequate to address the root of the disease. Based on the differentiation and pathogenesis, **modify the treatment to support the righteous qi by nourishing the yin and blood,** because yin and blood deficiency are major predisposing factors for hypertonicity disorder.

• A crisis of hypertonicity may occur during the courses of other illnesses; **prevention and early treatment make a difference in the prognosis.** Take prompt measures to clear heat, replenish the yin and nourish the blood when there are excessive perspiration, heavy bleeding and severe diarrhea, or when there is extreme internal heat. Prompt treatment can prevent the occurrence of hypertonicity disorder.

CHAPTER 26

Syncope

厥證 *Jue Zheng*

The word *jue*, in TCM, refers to a subjective cold sensation or palpable coolness beginning in the fingertips and toes. Coldness can gradually progress from the distal ends of the extremities towards the medial part of the body. The worst scenario of *jue* occurs when the coldness reaches beyond the joints of the knees and elbows.

Jue also refers to a condition of fainting with cold limbs. Syncope, or *jue* syndrome, refers to a group of disorders in which sudden and transient loss of consciousness is accompanied by frigid extremities. Spontaneous recovery without any sequelae can be seen in mild cases, while delayed recovery may indicate a life-threatening condition. According to TCM theory, separation and disconnection between the yin and yang predisposes a person to syncope. If this separation and disconnection is temporary, consciousness will return spontaneously; however, unremitting separation of the yin and yang is life-threatening and death may occur.

Relevant Diseases

- Transient ischemic attack
- Hypoglycemia
- Hysterical syncope
- Cardiac syncope
- Hemorrhagic shock
- Heat stroke
- Defecation syncope
- Hypertensive encephalopathy
- Pulmonary encephalopathy
- Fainting spell during acupuncture

Etiology and Pathogenesis

The main pathogenesis of syncope is a sudden rebellion of qi causing an imbalance between qi movement and blood circulation. This disturbance triggers a temporary separation and disconnection between the yin and yang.

Qi syncope: There are excess and deficiency types of qi syncope. Extreme emotions often trigger an excess pattern. Qi syncope of the excess type is caused by qi rebelling upwards. Mental activities are blocked and there is sudden loss of consciousness with frigid extremities. The deficient pattern is caused by severe qi deficiency, in which clear yang fails to reach the head and the qi sinks. The mind, lacking qi support, cannot function properly, leading to sudden loss of consciousness with frigid extremities.

Blood syncope: The excess pattern of blood syncope commonly occurs when a sudden state of extreme anger exacerbates pre-existing hyperactivity of liver yang. Blood rebels upwards following the rebellious qi movement, sensory orifices are obstructed, and syncope occurs. The deficient pattern involves various types of hemorrhaging in which the qi is lost along with the blood. Malnourishment of the spirit due to blood deficiency also leads to syncope.

Phlegm syncope: Inability of the spleen to transform or transport water due to improper diet may result in phlegm formation. Phlegm obstructs the movement of qi and follows rebellious qi upwards to mist the sensory orifices, causing loss of consciousness.

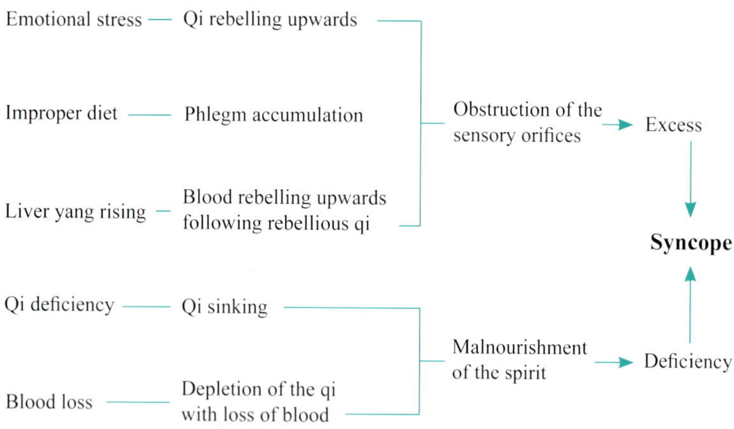

Diagnosis

A. Identification of precipitating factors:

It is important to obtain a detailed history to correctly diagnose the type of syncope. Determine if there is a preexisting condition, predisposing factor, or an aura preceding the event.

- Deficient constitution, severe exertion, lack of sleep or hunger prior to syncope – Deficient qi syncope.
- Excessive loss of blood prior to onset of syncope, including but not limited

to heavy menstrual flow, postpartum bleeding, and gastrointestinal bleeding – Deficient blood syncope.

- Middle-aged or older person, extreme emotional stress, dizziness, headache and/or vertigo prior to syncope – Excess qi or blood syncope.
- Elderly or obese person, history of overindulgence in greasy, sweet and rich foods, chronic coughing, wheezing and abundant sputum – Phlegm syncope.

B. Differential diagnosis of similar disorders:

Loss of consciousness is the common symptom in these three different disorders.

Syncope: Distinguished by the presence of frigid extremities.

Wind stroke: Characterized by hemiplegia, facial paralysis, dysphasia or aphasia; wind stroke has sequelae of muscular weakness and sensory-motor impairment following loss of consciousness.

Epilepsy: Seizures are marked by contractions, tremors, convulsions, drooling and upward-staring eyes, sequelae are absent during periods of remission.

Basic Patterns

- Excess qi syncope
- Excess blood syncope
- Phlegm syncope
- Deficient qi syncope
- Deficient blood syncope

Differentiation and Treatment

Treatment principle:

During the acute stage of syncope, treatment is based on the patterns of excess or deficiency.

Excess pattern: Open the orifices and awaken the consciousness.

Deficient pattern: Augment the qi, revive devastated yang and secure the yang from collapse.

During remission, the treatment principle should address the root of the disorder according to the pattern differentiation.

Excess qi syncope

Sudden loss of consciousness following strong emotional stimulation with rapid and heavy respiration.

S: Locked jaws, clenched fists and frigid extremities.

T: Thin white coating. **P:** Deep and wiry.

- Promote the movement of qi and spread constrained liver qi.
- *Wu Mo Yin Zi*
  - *Wu Yao* facilitates the qi movement and spreads liver constraint.
  - *Chen Xiang*, *Zhi Shi*, *Bing Lang* and *Mu Xiang* facilitate the qi flow and descend rebellious qi.
- To reinforce the effects of facilitating the movement of qi and expanding the chest. + *Tan Xiang, Bai Dou Kou, Ding Xiang*
  Liver yang rising with headache and dizziness. + *Gou Teng, Shi Jue Ming*
  Mood swings and insomnia during remission. + *Fu Shen, Yuan Zhi, Suan Zao Ren*
  Excessive phlegm and dyspnea. + *Dan Nan Xing, Bei Mu, Ju Hong*
  Prophylactic remedy for those susceptible to emotional stimulation, use *Xiao Yao San*.

Deficient qi syncope

Loss of consciousness following a feeling of dizziness and vertigo, accompanied by weak respiration.
S: Pale complexion and clammy cold skin.
T: Pale tongue. **P:** Deep and minute.

- Tonify the qi and restore the devastated yang.
- *Si Ni Jia Ren Shen Tang*
  - *Ren Shen* greatly tonifies basal qi.
  - *Fu Zi* and *Gan Jiang* restore the devastated yang to reverse the peripheral frigidity.
  - *Zhi Gan Cao* benefits the qi and warms the middle burner.
- Unremitting sweating. + *Long Gu, Mu Li*
  Palpitations and agitation. + *Suan Zao Ren, Yuan Zhi*
  Prophylactic remedy for those with a propensity to recurrent attacks, use *Xiang Sha Liu Jun Zi Tang* and *Gan Mai Da Zao Tang*.

Excess blood syncope

Sudden loss of consciousness following extreme emotional stimulation, red face and purple lips.
S: Locked jaws and frigid extremities.
T: Red tongue. **P:** Deep and wiry.

- Invigorate the blood and redirect the movement of qi.
- *Tong Yu Jian*
  - *Dang Gui Wei*, *Hong Hua* and *Shan Zha* invigorate the blood.

- *Qing Pi*, *Wu Yao*, *Mu Xiang* and *Xiang Fu* facilitate the qi flow and resolve constraint.
- *Ze Xie* descends and drains the turbidity.

- Impatience, short temper and dream-disturbed sleep. + *Gou Teng, Shi Jue Ming, Long Dan Cao, Mu Dan Pi, Yuan Zhi*
  Significant dizziness and headache. + *Ju Hua, Zhen Zhu Mu, Gou Qi Zi*

Deficient blood syncope

Sudden loss of consciousness, pale complexion, lusterless and pale lips.
S: Tremors, enophthalmos, opened mouth, clammy cold skin and weak respiration.
T: Pale tongue. **P:** Hollow; or rapid, thready and forceless.

- Nourish and tonify the blood and qi.
- *Du Shen Tang* for first aid purposes to restore consciousness, followed by the use of *Ren Shen Yang Ying Tang*
  - *Ren Shen* and *Huang Qi* augment the qi to prevent excessive blood loss.
  - *Dang Gui* and *Shu Di Huang* nourish the blood.
  - *Bai Shao* and *Wu Wei Zi* preserve and astringe the yin.
- Unremitting hemorrhage. + *Xian He Cao, Ou Jie, Ce Bai Ye*
  Clammy cold skin and weak respiration. + *Fu Zi, Gan Jiang*
  Palpitations and insomnia. + *Long Yan Rou, Yuan Zhi, Suan Zao Ren*
  Dry mouth and thrist. + *Mai Men Dong, Yu Zhu, Sha Shen*

Phlegm syncope

Sudden loss of consciousness and frigid extremities, accompanied by a rattling sound in the throat.
S: Rapid and heavy respiration, and vomiting white mucus.
T: White greasy coating. **P:** Deep and slippery.

- Promote the movement of qi and transform phlegm.
- *Dao Tan Tang*
  - *Ban Xia*, *Tian Nan Xing* and *Fu Ling* transform phlegm and dry dampness.
  - *Chen Pi* and *Zhi Shi* promote the qi movement and descend rebellious qi.
- To reinforce the effects of resolving phlegm and descending rebellious qi. + *Su Zi, Bai Jie Zi*
  Phlegm-dampness transforming into heat with thirst, constipation, yellow greasy tongue coating and rapid slippery pulse. + *Huang Qin, Zhi Zi, Zhu Ru, Gua Lou Ren*

Acupuncture Treatment

Excess:

- **Manipulation:** Reducing method.
- **Prescription:** GV26 Renzhong PC6 Neiguan
- **Supplementary points:**
  - Qi syncope. + LR3 Taichong
  - Blood syncope. + LR2 Xingjian; KI1 Yongquan
  - Phlegm syncope. + CV14 Juque; ST40 Fenglong

Deficiency:

- **Manipulation:** Reinforcing method; moxibustion is applicable.
- **Prescription:** GV20 Baihui CV6 Qihai
- **Supplementary points:**
  - Qi syncope. + ST36 Zusanli
  - Blood syncope. + CV4 Guanyuan

Practical Hints

Differentiate severe qi stagnation from yang qi deficiency. In most cases, frigidity of the extremities is induced by deficient yang qi that fails to reach the distal parts of the body. This pathogenesis is easily detected and can be treated by using very hot and acrid herbs including *Fu Zi*, *Gan Jiang* and *Rou Gui*, and the formula *Si Ni Tang*. The treatment principle is to restore the devastated yang and reverse peripheral frigidity. There is, however, another pathogenesis besides deficiency of yang qi. Severe qi stagnation that inhibits the qi flow from warming the digits is also a common predisposing factor to frigid extremities. This pathogenesis can be easily overlooked. The treatment for this type of peripheral frigidity should address the need to spread constraint and soothe the qi flow. Appropriate herbs are *Chai Hu*, *Xiang Fu*, *Zhi Qiao* and *Bai Shao*, and the formula of choice is *Si Ni San*.

CHAPTER 27

Wind Stroke

中風 *Zhong Feng*

Wind stroke refers to a disorder manifested by sudden loss of consciousness with unilateral weakness, numbness, paralysis and dysphasia, or to a disorder manifested by sudden onset of unilateral paralysis and facial paralysis without experiencing unconsciousness. Because of its sudden and acute onset, multiple symptoms and rapid alterations in manifestations, and the onset of sudden fall and contractions are similar to the natural characteristics of wind, which is moving, migrating and changing rapidly. Stroke, with the above characteristics, is therefore given the name wind stroke in TCM.

Relevant Diseases

- Hemorrhagic CVA
- Ischemic infarction CVA
- Transient ischemic attack
- Subarachnoid hemorrhage
- Brain tumor
- Cranial arteritis
- Bell's palsy
- Facial paralysis

Etiology and Pathogenesis

Unconsolidated channels with the invasion of exterior wind: Wind stroke involves exterior and interior causes. When protective qi is unconsolidated, it fails to defend the body from the exterior pathogenic invasion, causing stroke. In addition, exterior wind may also trigger the pre-existing phlegm hidden internally; together they obstruct the channels and lead to wind stroke. Without systemic symptom such as loss of consciousness, this type of wind stroke has clinical presentations of facial paralysis, and sensory or motor impairment.

Improper diet could impair the spleen's function to transform and transport; such impairment causes generation of phlegm, which can cover the heart's orifice or obstruct the flow in the channels. Corresponding manifestations include loss of consciousness or hemiplegia and aphasia.

Emotional stress: Excessive emotional stimulations affect both the heart and the liver. When disturbed by intense emotional stresses, heart fire explosively flares up whereas hyperactive liver yang would generate liver wind. Mutually aggravating each other, heart fire and liver wind will further cause qi and blood to ascend and rush upwards to the brain. Sudden loss of consciousness would result.

Prolonged exhaustion due to aging, chronic illness, excessive exertion and weak constitution can cause liver and kidney yin deficiency with liver yang rising. This is a complicated condition of deficiency below with excess above. In this condition, the qi and blood rebel upward following liver yang rising. Moreover, phlegm may also follow and ascend upwards to obstruct the flow in the channels or cover the clear orifices.

There are multiple pathogenesis to wind stroke. It involves *deficiency*, such as yin deficiency and qi deficiency; *fire*, which includes liver fire and heart fire; *wind*, such as liver wind and exterior wind; *phlegm*, or wind-phlegm and phlegm-dampness; and rebellious *qi* and *blood* stasis.

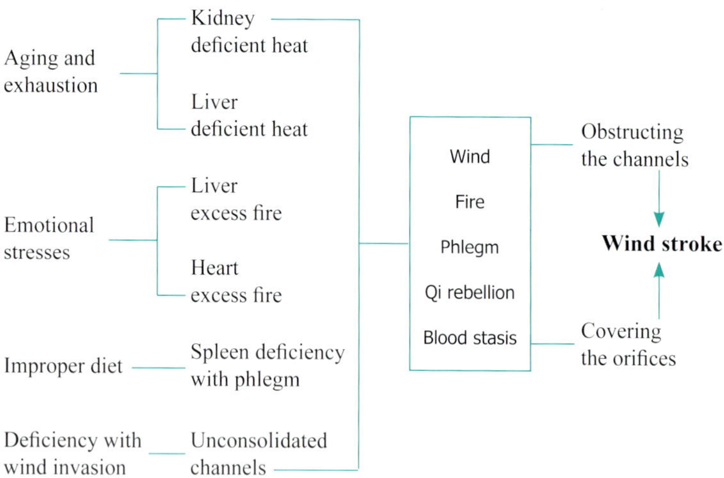

Diagnosis

A. Identification of channel and organ involvement:

Channel involvement: In patterns of wind stroke involving only the meridians and collaterals, the effects are limited to the peripheral areas and are considered non-systemic. It is relatively milder in severity and a person's consciousness and cognition remain intact. Clinical manifestations are numbness and weakness of the affected area, facial paralysis and alterations in speech.

Organ involvement: Once the organ is affected, there will be loss of consciousness and alterations in cognition. Clinically, this is a severe stage and its manifestations are considered systemic. Other clinical manifestations may include aphasia, difficulty in swallowing and hemiplegia.

B. Identification of closed disorder and abandon disorder:

Wind stroke in which there is organ involvement can be subcategorized as closed and abandon disorders, based on the pathogenesis of pathogenic factors trapped internally or that of yang qi devastation. Divergent therapeutic strategies are required for treatment of these two subtypes of wind stroke.

Closed disorder: Locked jaws, clenched fists, rigid limbs, fecal and urinary retention, and forceful pulse are manifested. Fire and turbid phlegm are the pathogens that are being trapped and are locked within.

Abandon disorder: In contrast to closed disorder, there is flaccidity of the muscles, fecal and urinary incontinence, profuse sweating and minute weak pulse due to collapse of yang qi.

C. Identification of prognosis:

The prognosis of wind stroke could be optimistic if the conditions of motor and sensory coordination remain following recovery of consciousness. If alterations of consciousness and cognition persist along with hiccough, contractions and frigidity of the four extremities, hematemesis and blood in the stool, this may indicate a poor prognosis.

D. Identification of true wind stroke and wind-like stroke:

True wind stroke refers to the actual presence of exterior wind invasion.

Wind-like stroke, or internal wind stroke, refers to the absence of exterior wind. The clinical presentations are caused by internal wind swirling.

E. Differential diagnosis of similar disorders:

There are four disorders with loss of consciousness being their common symptom. Identification and differentiation among these four disorders can help guide the treatment principle.

Wind stroke: In addition to being comatose, other manifestations include facial paralysis and hemiplegia due to loss of motor coordination, as well as various degrees of sequelae after consciousness has been resumed.

Epilepsy: Accompanied with loss of consciousness, there are tremors, muscle contractions and drooling of white froth. The sequelae are absent during remission.

Syncope: Clinical presentations, along with loss of consciousness, are pale complexion and frigid extremities. Neither paralysis nor contractions is noticed.

Hypertonicity disorder: With rigid posture of the neck and back as its primary symptoms, muscular spasm and tremors of the extremities may also be present. Opisthotonos occurs at its worst scenario.

Basic Patterns

Channel involvement:

- Exterior wind invading into the unconsolidated channels
- Wind-yang disturbing upwards with liver and kidney yin deficiency

Organ involvement:

- Heat-type of closed disorder
- Cold-type of closed disorder
- Abandon disorder

Sequelae:

- Hemiplegia associated with qi deficiency and blood stasis
- Hemiplegia associated with yin deficiency and yang rising
- Dysphasia associated with wind-phlegm obstructing the channels
- Dysphasia associated with kidney essence deficiency
- Facial paralysis

Differentiation and Treatment

Treatment principle:

During the acute phase, as the excess branch dominates, follow the guideline of treating the branch during the acute stage. Focus on expelling the pathogens. Open the orifices and awaken the spirit if there is loss of consciousness.

During the recovery phase, a combination of excess and deficiency manifests. As the pathogen is not completely expelled, there is also deficient righteous qi. Emphasize on supporting the righteous qi to expel the pathogens.

Channel involvement:

Exterior wind invading into the unconsolidated channels

Sudden weakness and numbness of the extremities, facial paralysis, slurred speech, drooling or hemiplegia.

S: Aversion to wind, fever, soreness and pain in the joints.

T: Thin white coating. **P:** Floating and rapid.

- Dispel wind, nourish the blood and unblock the channels.
- *Da Qin Jiao Tang*

- *Qin Jiao*, *Fang Feng*, *Bai Zhi*, *Xi Xin*, *Qiang Huo* and *Du Huo* dispel wind and unblock the obstruction in the channels.
- *Shu Di Huang*, *Dang Gui*, *Shao Yao* and *Chuan Xiong* nourish and invigorate the blood and relax the sinews.
- *Bai Zhu* and *Fu Ling* augment the qi and strengthen the spleen.

• Obstruction of phlegm-dampness or blood stasis with unresolved numbness of the extremities and facial paralysis. + *Dan Shen, Ji Xue Teng, Bai Jie Zi, Bai Fu Zi*
Accompanied with exterior wind-heat. + *Sang Ye, Ju Hua, Bo He*

Wind-yang disturbing upwards with liver and kidney yin deficiency

Sudden occurrence of facial paralysis, slurred speech or aphasia, numbness and heavy sensation of the extremities and hemiplegia.
S: Dizziness, headache, vertigo and tinnitus, dream disturbed sleep, soreness and weakness of the lower back and knees, dry throat, constipation and scanty dark urine output.
T: Red tongue with scanty or greasy coating. **P:** Wiry, thready and rapid, or wiry slippery.

• Nourish the yin, subdue the yang, extinguish wind and unblock the channels.

• *Zhen Gan Xi Feng Tang*
- *Gui Ban*, *Bai Shao*, *Xuan Shen* and *Tian Men Dong* nourish the yin, soften the liver and extinguish wind.
- *Long Gu*, *Mu Li* and *Dai Zhe Shi* are heavy substances that can subdue and anchor floating yang.
- *Niu Xi* guides the blood movement downwards as well as tonifies the liver and kidney.

• To reinforce the effects of pacifying the liver and extinguishing wind. + *Tian Ma, Gou Teng, Ju Hua*
Accompanied by phlegm-heat. + *Dan Nan Xing, Zhu Li, Chuan Bei Mu*
Severe headache. + *Ling Yang Jiao, Shi Jue Ming, Xia Ku Cao*

Organ involvement:

Heat-type of closed disorder

Sudden loss of consciousness with locked jaws, clenched fists, rigid limbs, and fecal and urinary retention as well as red face and fever.
S: Tachypnea, bad breath, excessive sputum or rattling sound in the throat, restlessness or agitation. Possible contractions and hiccoughs.
T: Red tongue with yellow greasy coating. **P:** Wiry slippery and forceful.

- Clear heat from the liver, extinguish wind and open the orifices.
- *Zhi Bao Dan* or *An Gong Niu Huang Wan* and *Ling Jiao Gou Teng Tang* (tube feeding)
  - *Ling Yang Jiao* and *Gou Teng* clear heat, cool the liver and extinguish wind.
  - *Sang Ye* and *Ju Hua* disperse wind and vent heat.
  - *Sheng Di Huang* and *Bai Shao* nourish the yin, soften the liver and relax the sinews.
  - *Bei Mu* and *Zhu Ru* clear heat and transform phlegm.
- To strengthen the effects of nourishing the yin and subduing the yang. + *Gui Ban, Shi Jue Ming*

  Excessive phlegm. + *Zhu Li, Dan Nan Xing*

  Contractions of the extremities. + *Quan Xie, Wu Gong, Jiang Can*

  Bad breath and constipation. + *Da Huang, Zhi Shi, Mang Xiao*

Cold-type of closed disorder

Sudden loss of consciousness with locked jaws, clenched fists, rigid limbs, and fecal and urinary retention as well as pale complexion and dark lips.

S: Quiet and still, cold extremities, distention and fullness in the abdomen, and excessive sputum.

T: White greasy coating. **P:** Deep, slippery and decelerating.

- Resolve phlegm, extinguish wind and open the orifices.
- *Su He Xiang Wan* and *Di Tan Tang* (tube feeding)
  - *Ban Xia*, *Ju Hong*, and *Fu Ling* dry dampness and transform phlegm.
  - *Zhu Ru* descends downwards and transforms phlegm.
  - *Shi Chang Pu* and *Dan Nan Xing* open the orifices and expel phlegm.
  - *Zhi Shi* descends the qi.
- To strengthen the effects of pacifying the liver and extinguishing wind. + *Tian Ma, Gou Teng*

Abandon disorder

Sudden loss of consciousness with flaccid extremities, closed eyes, opened mouth, fecal and urinary incontinence.

S: Shallow respirations, profuse sweating and clammy skin.

T: Flaccid tongue. **P:** Thready, weak or minute.

- Augment the qi, revive the yang and consolidate the collapse.
- *Shen Fu Tang* and *Sheng Mai San*
  - *Ren Shen* greatly tonifies the basal qi to consolidate the collapse.

- *Fu Zi* restores the devastated yang and reverses peripheral frigidity.
- *Mai Men Dong* nourishes the yin and generates the fluid.
- *Wu Wei Zi*, sour and astringent, when used with *Ren Shen* and *Mai Men Dong*, could greatly tonify the qi and yin.

• Unremitting profuse sweating. + *Huang Qi, Long Gu, Mu Li, Shan Zhu Yu*

Sequelae:

Hemiplegia associated with qi deficiency and blood stasis

Unilateral weakness, loss of sensory and motor coordination, fatigue and lassitude, numbness or edema of the extremities and facial paralysis.

S: Sallow complexion, poor appetite, loose stool and slurred speech.

T: Dark purple tongue with petechiae and white coating. **P:** Thready, choppy and weak.

• Augment the qi, invigorate the blood and unblock the channels.

• *Bu Yang Huan Wu Tang*
- *Huang Qi* in large dose greatly tonifies the qi to promote blood circulation.
- *Tao Ren*, *Hong Hua*, *Dang Gui Wei*, *Chuan Xiong* and *Chi Shao* invigorate the blood and transform stasis.
- *Di Long* unblocks the obstruction in the channels.

• To reinforce the effect of invigorating the collaterals. + *Quan Xie, Chuan Niu Xi, Wu Shao She, Sang Zhi*
Significant weakness of the lower extremities. + *Du Zhong, Sang Ji Sheng*
Significant weakness of the upper extremities. + *Gui Zhi*
Swelling of the affected extremities. + *Fu Ling, Ze Xie*

Hemiplegia associated with yin deficiency and yang rising

Unilateral contracture of the affected extremities, headache, and red flush on the face.

S: Agitation, dizziness, tinnitus, dysphasia and numbness of the extremities.

T: Red tongue with thin yellow coating. **P:** Wiry and forceful.

• Nourish the yin, subdue the yang and unblock the collaterals.

• *Tian Ma Gou Teng Yin*
- *Tian Ma*, *Gou Teng* and *Shi Jue Ming* pacify the liver and extinguish wind.
- *Zhi Zi* and *Huang Qin* clear heat and drain fire.
- *Yi Mu Cao* invigorates the blood and promotes urination.
- *Niu Xi* invigorates the blood and guides the movement of blood downwards.
- *Du Zhong* and *Sang Ji Sheng* tonify the liver and kidney.

- To reinforce the effects of clearing heat and nourishing the yin. + *Sheng Di Huang, Bai Shao, Mai Men Dong*
  To relax the sinews and unblock the collaterals. + *Mu Gua, Shen Jin Cao*

Dysphasia associated with wind-phlegm obstructing the channels

Rigid tongue and slurred speech, dysphagia, excessive sticky sputum that is difficult to expectorate.

S: Dizziness, headache and loss of motor coordination or numbness of the extremities.

T: Dark tongue with white greasy or yellow greasy coating. **P:** Wiry and slippery.

- Dispel wind-phlegm, disclose the orifices and unblock the channels.
- *Jie Yu Dan*
  - *Tian Ma*, *Quan Xie*, *Dan Nan Xing* and *Fu Zi* dispel phlegm, pacify the liver and extinguish wind.
  - *Yuan Zhi* and *Shi Chang Pu* transform phlegm and open the orifices.
  - *Qiang Huo* dispels wind.

Dysphasia associated with kidney essence deficiency

Weak and flaccid tongue with slurred speech, and soreness and weakness of the lower back and knees.

S: Palpitations, dizziness and blurred vision, or fecal and urinary incontinence.

T: Thin small tongue with scanty coating. **P:** Deep and thready.

- Nourish the yin, tonify the kidney and open the orifices.
- *Di Huang Yin Zi*
  - *Shu Di Huang* and *Shan Zhu Yu* nourish and tonify kidney yin.
  - *Rou Cong Rong* and *Ba Ji Tian* warm and tonify kidney yang.
  - *Mai Men Dong*, *Shi Hu* and *Wu Wei Zi* nourish the yin and generate the fluid.
  - *Shi Chang Pu*, *Yuan Zhi* and *Fu Ling* bring communication to the heart and kidney, open the orifices and transform phlegm.
- Due to the preponderance of yin deficiency, *Fu Zi* and *Rou Gui* are removed from the original formula.
  To improve speech and open the orifice. + *Xing Ren, Jie Geng*

Facial paralysis

Facial paralysis includes the loss of motor and sensory coordination of facial muscles, inability to properly open and close the affected eye, inability to control the movement of affected side of the mouth, and drooling.

- Dispel wind, resolve phlegm and unblock the channels.

- *Qian Zheng San*
  - *Bai Fu Zi* dispels wind, transforms phlegm and unblocks the collaterals.
  - *Jiang Can* and *Quan Xie* dispel wind, transform phlegm and alleviate spasm.
- To strengthen the effect of extinguishing wind. + *Tian Ma, Gou Teng, Shi Jue Ming*

  To strengthen the effects of relaxing the sinews and unblocking the channels. + *Bai Shao, Mu Gua*

Acupuncture Treatment

Channel involvement

- **Manipulation:** Even method on the healthy side first, then the affected side.
- **Prescription:** GV20 Baihui BL7 Tongtian GV16 Fengfu
- **Supplementary points:**

  - Paralysis of the upper limbs. + LI15 Jianyu; LI11 Quchi; TE5 Waiguan; LI4 Hegu

  - Paralysis of the lower limbs. + GB30 Huantiao; ST36 Zusanli; ST41 Jiexi; GB34 Yanglingquan

  - Facial paralysis. + ST4 Dicang; ST6 Jiache; LI4 Hegu; ST44 Neiting

Organ involvement

Closed disorder:

- **Manipulation:** Reducing method.
- **Prescription:** GV20 Baihui GV26 Renzhong ST40 Fenglong LR3 Taichong KI1 Yongquan 12 Jing-well points
- **Supplementary points:**

  - Locked jaws. + ST7 Xiaguan; ST6 Jiache; LI4 Hegu

  - Rigid tongue and aphasia. + GV15 Yamen; CV23 Lianquan; HT5 Tongli

Abandon disorder:

- **Manipulation:** Moxibustion.
- **Prescription:** CV8 Shenque CV6 Qihai CV4 Guanyuan

Practical Hints

• **Referral to an acute healthcare facility at the onset of wind stroke.** As a medical emergency, at the onset of a wind stroke, prompt treatment can make a difference between life and death. Referral to an acute medical facility is necessary.

• **Use TCM measurement for recovery and rehabilitation.** In spite of transient ischemic attack, the majority of patients who suffered from stroke will have various degrees of sequelae. Early recovery stage accounts for the best time to introduce TCM measurements such as acupuncture treatments and herbal therapies. Prompt intervention promotes the recovery and diminishes possible permanent impairments from wind stroke. The motor skills, such as speech, ambulation, and range of motion, as well as muscle tonicity, are the major focus during rehabilitation.

• **Early prophylactic measurements to prevent stroke.** Identifying warning signs of a stroke and implementing early interventions will help prevent a stroke from occurring. There may be an aura preceding the stroke that include dizziness, tinnitus and muscle twitching indicating hyperactive liver yang and liver wind swirling internally. Other signs are weakness, numbness or heaviness of the extremities, which indicates the obstruction of qi stagnation and blood stasis in the channels. These may be warning signs to the onset of wind stroke.

CHAPTER 28

Headache

頭痛 *Tou Tong*

Presenting as a diffuse pain in different areas of the head, headache is a subjective symptom commonly seen in clinical practice. It may occur independently or with other symptoms in the process of acute or chronic diseases. The entire head may be affected or pain may be localized to the frontal, temporal, occipital and/or vertex regions. Pain can radiate to the eyes, cheeks or teeth. The head is the merging area for the clear yang of the body as well as the location of the sea of marrow. Pain in the head results when the clear yang is obstructed or when nourishment to the head from the qi, blood and essence is inadequate. Characteristics of headaches vary according to different pathologies.

Relevant Diseases

- Meningitis
- Migraine headache
- Trigeminal neuralgia
- Sinusitis
- Glaucoma
- Hypertension
- Head injury

Etiology and Pathogenesis

Exterior pathogenic factors: Wind is the primary pathogenic factor. "When injured by wind, the upper part of the body will be affected first." Wind, yang in nature, has the ability to attack the merging point of all yang, which is the head. Wind, being the leader of all exterior pathogenic factors, carries other pathogens to invade the body. Wind-cold can congeal the qi and blood, obstructing the collaterals. Wind-heat can flare upwards, disturbing the clear orifices. Wind-dampness can injure yang qi and block the flow of qi, veiling the clear orifices and preventing clear yang from ascending.

Interior organ dysfunction: The brain relies on the essence and blood from the liver and kidney for nourishment. The brain also depends on the spleen and stomach to transform and transport water and food, and to distribute qi and blood upwards to the head. Therefore, dysfunction of the liver, kidney and spleen leads to malnourishment of the head. In addition, formation of phlegm secondary to dysfunction of the spleen can also inhibit clear yang to reach the head.

Miscellaneous: Trauma due to accidents that affect the head can disturb qi and blood flow and lead to obstruction and stasis in the blood vessels and meridians. The resulting headache will occur with a fixed location.

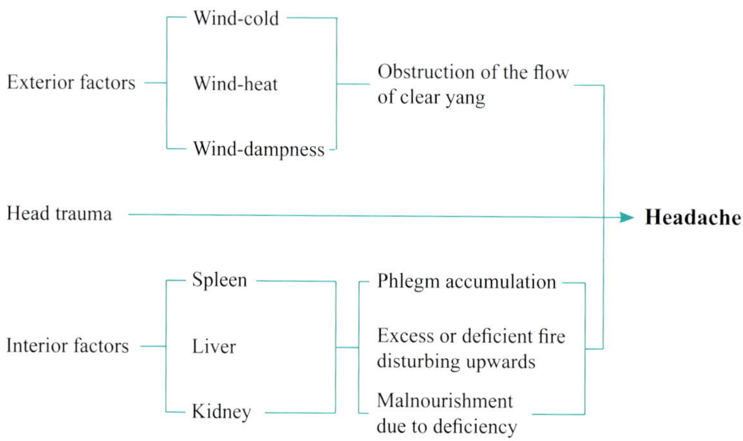

Diagnosis

A. Identification of exterior and interior conditions:

Type	**Exterior**	**Interior**
Onset	Sudden.	Gradual.
Severity	Severe.	Mild.
Characteristics of pain	Sharp, throbbing, burning, distending, heavy and constant.	Dull, empty, lingering, worsen on exertion, and intermittent.

B. Identification by channels:

- Headache starting from the back of the head, or occipital region, down to the neck – *Taiyang* headache.
- Forehead and eyebrow regions – *Yangming* headache.
- Bilateral temporal and/or auricular regions – *Shaoyang* headache.
- From the vertex and connecting to the eye system – *Jueyin* headache.
- Headache radiating to the cheeks and teeth – *Shaoyin* headache.

C. Identification of accompanying symptoms:

- Sharp and stabbing pain with fixed location, prolonged duration, and worse at night, presenting with a history of head trauma – Blood stasis headache.
- Accompanied by nausea and vomiting – Phlegm-turbidity headache.

Basic Patterns

Exterior:

- Wind-cold headache
- Wind-heat headache
- Wind-dampness headache

Interior:

- Liver yang headache
- Phlegm-turbidity headahce
- Blood stasis headache
- Blood deficiecy headache
- Kidney essence deficiency headache

Differentiation and Treatment

Treatment principle:

Exterior: Expel the exterior pathogenic factors.

Interior: Tonify the deficiency primarily. For complex patterns of excess and deficiency, determine the root and branch, and treat accordingly.

Exterior:

Wind-cold headache

Headache with radiating pain to the neck and back that is aggravated by windy weather.

S: Aversion to wind or cold, and no thirst.

T: Thin white coating. **P:** Floating and tight.

- Disperse and expel wind-cold.
- *Chuan Xiong Cha Tiao San*
  - *Chuan Xiong*, *Bai Zhi* and *Qiang Huo* dispel wind and alleviate headache.
  - *Jing Jie* and *Fang Feng* disperse cold and release the exterior.
  - *Xi Xin* disperses cold and alleviates pain.
  - *Bo He* disperses wind, clears and benefits the head and eyes.

- Exterior wind-cold with underlying yang deficiency presenting with headache in the occipital region, use *Ma Huang Fu Zi Xi Xin Tang*.
  Cold invading the *jueyin* channel with intense vertex headache, dry heaves or vomiting with clear watery emesis, cold extremities, white tongue coating and wiry pulse, use *Wu Zhu Yu Tang*.

Wind-heat headache

Headache with distention, possible with a sensation of "splitting".
S: Aversion to wind, fever, red face and eyes, thirst with desire to drink cold beverages, and swollen sore throat.
T: Dry red tongue with yellow coating. **P:** Floating and rapid.

- Disperse wind and clear heat.
- *Xiong Zhi Shi Gao Tang*
  - *Chuan Xiong* and *Bai Zhi* disperse wind, release the exterior and alleviate headache.
  - *Ju Hua* and *Shi Gao* clear heat.
- To strengthen the effects of dispersing and clearing heat. + *Bo He, Zhi Zi*
  Excessive heat injuring the yin with intense thirst. + *Zhi Mu, Xuan Shen, Tian Hua Fen*
  Constipation. + *Da Huang, Mang Xiao* .
  Severe sore throat. + *Jin Yin Hua, Ban Lan Gen, Pu Gong Ying*

Wind-dampness headache

Headache with sensation of heaviness, aggravated by cloudy or rainy weather.
S: Heaviness of the extremities, stuffy chest and epigastrium, poor appetite, dysuria and irregular bowel movements.
T: White greasy coating. **P:** Soft and decelerating.

- Expel wind and eliminate dampness
- *Qiang Huo Sheng Shi Tang*
  - *Qiang Huo* and *Du Huo* dispel wind-dampness to alleviate pain.
  - *Fang Feng* and *Gao Ben* dispel wind and disperse pathogens.
  - *Man Jing Zi*, ascending and dispersing, benefits the head and eyes.
  - *Chuan Xiong* invigorates the blood and promotes the movement of qi to alleviate headache.
- Accompanied by summer dampness. + *Huo Xiang, Pei Lan*
  Accompanied by accumulation of turbid dampness in the middle burner. + *Cang Zhu, Hou Po*
  Nausea and vomiting. + *Ban Xia, Sheng Jiang*

Interior:

Liver yang headache

Headache with throbbing or distending pain, dizziness, red eyes, unilateral or bilateral, and aggravated by emotional stress.
S: Distention and pain in the hypochondriac region, irritability, short temper, insomnia, red face, and bitter taste in the mouth.
T: Thin yellow coating. **P:** Wiry and forceful.

- Pacify the liver and subdue the yang.
- *Tian Ma Gou Teng Yin*
  - *Tian Ma*, *Gou Teng* and *Shi Jue Ming* pacify the liver and subdue the yang.
  - *Huang Qin* and *Zhi Zi* clear and drain liver fire.
  - *Du Zhong*, *Niu Xi* and *Sang Ji Sheng* tonify the liver and kidney.
  - *Ye Jiao Teng* and *Fu Shen* nourish the heart and calm the spirit.
- Enhance the effect to anchor and suppress the yang. + *Long Gu, Mu Li*
  Accompanied by liver and kidney yin deficiency. + *Sheng Di Huang, Bai Shao, He Shou Wu, Nu Zhen Zi, Han Lian Cao*

Phlegm-turbidity headache

Headache with dizziness and cloudiness of the head.
S: Full and stuffy sensation in the chest and epigastrium, nausea and vomiting of phlegm and saliva.
T: White greasy coating. **P:** Slippery, or wiry and slippery.

- Transform phlegm and descend rebellious qi.
- *Ban Xia Bai Zhu Tian Ma Tang*
  - *Ban Xia* and *Chen Pi* transform phlegm, descend rebellious qi, dry dampness and facilitate the qi flow.
  - *Bai Zhu* and *Fu Ling* strengthen the spleen and dry dampness.
  - *Tian Ma* pacifies the liver and extinguishes wind to alleviate headache.
  - *Man Jing Zi* clears and benefits the head and eyes.
- Phlegm turning into phlegm-heat with a bitter taste in the mouth, dry stool, a yellow greasy tongue coating and a rapid slippery pulse. + *Huang Qin, Zhu Ru, Zhi Shi*

Blood stasis headache

Prolonged lingering headache, fixed location and sharp stabbing pain.
S: Possibly with a history of head injury.
T: Purple tongue with thin white coating. **P:** Thready, or thready and choppy.

- Invigorate the blood and transform stasis.
- *Tong Qiao Huo Xue Tang*
  - *Tao Ren*, *Hong Hua*, *Chuan Xiong* and *Chi Shao* invigorate the blood and expel stasis.
  - *She Xiang* and *Cong Bai* unblock the flow of yang qi and open the orifices.
- Activate the qi and open the orifices. + *Yu Jin, Shi Chang Pu, Xi Xin*
  Severe headache. + *Quan Xie, Wu Gong*
  Chronic headache with qi and blood deficiency. + *Huang Qi, Dang Gui*

Blood deficiency headache

Headache and dizziness, palpitations, and restlessness.
S: Fatigue, lack of strength and pale complexion.
T: Pale tongue with thin white coating. **P:** Thready and weak.

- Nourish the blood.
- *Si Wu Tang* (Jia Wei Si Wu
  - *Shu Di Huang* and *Dang Gui* tonify the blood.
  - *Bai Shao* preserves the yin and nourishes the blood.
  - *Chuan Xiong* invigorates the blood, facilitates the qi flow, and nourishes the blood; it is the imperial herb for headache.
- Clear the head and eyes. + *Ju Hua, Man Jing Zi*
  Complicated by qi deficiency. + *Huang Qi, Dang Shen*
  Both liver blood and yin deficiency. + *He Shou Wu, Gou Qi Zi, Huang Jing*

Kidney essence deficiency headache

Headache with dizziness, and a sensation of emptiness in the head.
S: Soreness and weakness of the lower back and knees, lassitude, lack of strength, insomnia and tinnitus.
T: Red tongue with scanty or no coating. **P:** Thready and weak.

- Tonify the kidney, nourish the yin and replenish the essence.
- *Da Bu Yuan Jian*
  - *Shu Di Huang*, *Shan Yao*, *Shan Zhu Yu* and *Gou Qi Zi* nourish the liver and kidney, augment the yin and replenish the essence.
  - *Ren Shen* and *Dang Gui* tonify both the qi and blood.
  - *Du Zhong* tonifies the liver and kidney.
- During remission, use *Qi Ju Di Huang Wan*.
  Headache with cold intolerance, cold limbs, pale complexion, pale tongue, and deep thready and decelerating pulse, use *You Gui Wan*.

Acupuncture Treatment

Tx c̄ nourishing herbs

Exterior — Excess

Exopathic wind Dispel.

- **Manipulation:** Reducing method.
- **Prescription:** Point selection based on the location or channels affected.

Frontal headache:

ST8 Touwei, Extra2 Yintang, GV23 Shangxing, LI4 Hegu, ST44 Neiting

Vertex headache:

GV20 Baihui, SI3 Houxi, BL67 Zhiyin, LR3 Taichong

Occipital headache:

GB20 Fengchi, BL60 Kunlun, SI3 Houxi

Temporal headache:

Extra1 Taiyang, GB8 Shuaigu, TE5 Waiguan, GB41 Zulinqi

Interior — Deficiency. Reg. visceral Fx

Tx - Purging herbs

Liver yang headache:

- **Manipulation:** Reducing method.
- **Prescription:** GB20 Fengchi, GV20 Baihui, GB5 Xuanlu, GB43 Xiaxi, LR2 Xingjian

Phlegm-turbidity headache:

- **Manipulation:** Reducing method.
- **Prescription:** CV12 Zhongwan, ST40 Fenglong, GV20 Baihui, Extra2 Yintang

Blood stasis headache:

- **Manipulation:** Combination of reinforcing and reducing methods.
- **Prescription:** Ashi points, LI4 Hegu, SP6 Sanyinjiao

Blood and essence deficiency headache:

- **Manipulation:** Reinforcing method, moxibustion is applicable.
- **Prescription:** GV20 Baihui, CV6 Qihai, BL18 Ganshu, BL20 Pishu, BL23 Shenshu, ST36 Zusanli

Practical Hints

• When treating headache, follow the principle of differentiation and treatment to either expel pathogenic influences or adjust the functions of the *zang-fu* organs. In addition, **include guiding herbs in the formula according to the location of the headache and the channel involved.** This will greatly enhance the therapeutic effect.

The most commonly used guiding herbs are listed below: (Chuang Xiong)

Taiyang (headache at occipital, upper back and neck)	*Qiang Huo, Ge Gen*
Yangming (headache at forehead and supraorbital region)	*Man Jing Zi, Bai Zhi*
Shaoyang (headache at unilateral/bilateral temporal and auricular regions)	*Chai Hu, Huang Qin, Chuan Xiong*
Jueyin (headache at vertex and radiating to the eye system)	*Wu Zhu Yu, Gao Ben, Chuan Xiong*
Shaoyin (headache rediating to cheeks and teeth)	*Xi Xin*

• Unilateral headache is an uncommon type of headache. It is characterized by sudden onset of severe pain involving only one side of the head. Radiating pain to the eyes and teeth is apparent. It resembles trigeminal neuralgia in western medicine. The Chinese medical differentiation is wind-fire in the liver channel; therefore, the treatment principle is to pacify the liver, extinguish wind and clear heat. Commonly used herbs are *Ju Hua*, *Tian Ma*, *Chuan Xiong*, *Bai Zhi*, *Shi Gao*, *Gou Teng*, *Quan Xie* and *Di Long*.

• **To treat stubborn headache, incorporate herbs that invigorate the blood and unblock collaterals.** In chronic headache, the etiology involves a deep obstruction in the collaterals. The complication of obstructed circulation of blood and qi in these distal and extremely small collaterals causes a poor response to therapy and, therefore, a very stubborn headache. To enhance the therapeutic effect, add herbs that invigorate the blood and unblock the collaterals, such as *Tao Ren*, *Hong Hua*, *Chi Shao* and *Si Gua Luo*, or herbs that enter the collaterals to gather the pathogens, such as *Quan Xie*.

CHAPTER 29

Dizziness

眩 暈 *Xuan Yun*

Dizziness refers to subjective symptoms of blurred vision and a sensation of turning in space or of having objects moving about oneself. In Chinese medicine, it is known as *xuan yun*. *Xuan* refers to a sensation of blurred, dark or dull vision, while *yun* refers to a sudden spinning sensation or the perception that the surroundings are spinning. Dizziness may range from mild lightheadedness, sometimes only on changing posture, to severe vertigo with loss of balance and the sensation that everything around the person is spinning. Dizziness often occurs with blurred vision or sensory confusion, nausea and vomiting, perspiration or even fainting. Dizziness is believed to be closely related to deficiency, phlegm, and internal wind.

Relevant Diseases

- Hypertension
- Hypotension
- Hypoglycemia
- Anemia
- Labyrinthitis
- Meniere's disease
- Eighth cranial nerve injury
- Head injury

Etiology and Pathogenesis

Liver yang rising results from constitutional yang excess, liver yin deficiency and kdiney yin deficiency failing to nurture the liver. The rising yang ascending upwards to disturb the clear orifices will induce dizziness. "All manifestations of wind, such as dizziness, tremors and twitching, pertain to pathology of the liver."

Qi and blood deficiency can be secondary to chronic illness consuming the righteous qi, to status post excessive bleeding, and to spleen deficiency failing to generate the qi and blood. Qi deficiency leads to impaired distribution of yang qi to the brain; blood deficiency causes malnourishment to the brain. Both induce dizziness.

Kidney essence deficiency, whether congenital or acquired, presents to be lack of generation of the marrow and failure of fillment of the brain. "Insufficient sea of the marrow manifests as dizziness, vertigo, blurred vision, tinnitus..."

Phlegm-dampness accumulation is subsequent to improper diet, and deficient spleen and stomach. Turbid phlegm prevents clear yang from rising to the brain, or phlegm-fire creates an upwards disturbances and causes dizziness. "Dizziness will not occur if there is no phlegm."

The above stated eitologies influence and aggravate each others mutually. For instance, kidney essence deficiency may progress into deficiency of both yin and yang; it is not uncommon for accumulated phlegm tranform into phelgm-fire, further consuming the yin.

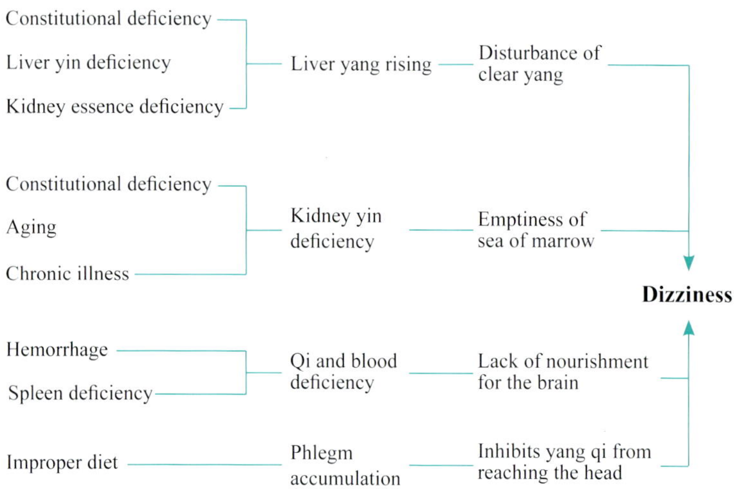

Diagnosis

A. Differential diagnosis of dizziness and headache:

Dizziness and headache can occur at the same time or separately.

	Headache	Dizziness
Etiology	Invasion by exterior pathogenic factors; interior disequilibriums.	Mostly interior disequilibriums.
Patterns	Mostly excess.	Mostly deficiency.

B. Differential diagnosis of dizziness and wind-stroke:

If dizziness occurs in a middle-aged or older adult due to liver yang rising, a high risk of wind stroke should be considered.

	Wind Stroke	Dizziness
Etiology	Interior or exterior influences.	Interior influences in most cases.
Manifestations	Usually accompanied by dizziness, with or without loss of consciousness, facial paralysis, hemiplegia and aphasia. Sequelae of varying severity.	No change in consciousness and no sequelae; vaying degrees of dizziness.

Basic Patterns

- Liver yang rising
- Qi and blood deficiency
- Phlegm-dampness obstruction
- Kidney essence deficiency

Differentiation and Treatment

Treatment principle:

Excess: Extinguish wind, subdue floating yang, clear fire and transform phlegm; focus on treating the manifestations.

Deficient: Tonify the qi and blood, nourish the kidney and liver, and strengthen the spleen; focus on treating the root.

Liver yang rising

Dizziness with distending headache, aggravated by anger, stress or exertion.

S: Tinnitus, flushed face, irritability, impetuosity, insomnia or dream-disturbed sleep, bitter taste in the mouth and nausea.

T: Red tongue with yellow coating. **P:** Rapid and wiry.

- Pacify the liver, subdue the yang and nourish the liver and kidney.
- *Tian Ma Gou Teng Yin*
  - *Tian Ma*, *Gou Teng* and *Shi Jue Ming* pacify the liver and extinguish wind.
  - *Zhi Zi* and *Huang Qin* clear heat and drain fire.
  - *Yi Mu Cao* and *Niu Xi* invigorate the blood and guide the movement of blood downwards.
  - *Du Zhong* and *Sang Ji Sheng* nourish and augment the liver and kidney.

- To strengthen the effect of clearing liver fire. + *Long Dan Cao, Mu Dan Pi*
  To strengthen the effects of pacifying the liver and extinguishing wind. + *Long Gu, Mu Li, Zhen Zhu Mu*
  Significant liver and kidney yin deficiency with soreness and weakness of the lower back and knees, and a rapid, wiry and thready pulse. + *Bie Jia, Gui Ban, E Jiao, Ji Zi Huang*

Phlegm-dampness obstruction

Dizziness with a sensation of heaviness and muzziness in the head, and difficulty in thinking and concentrating.
S: Obesity, stuffy chest, poor appetite, nausea and excessive sleepiness.
T: White greasy coating. **P:** Slippery.

- Dry dampness, resolve phlegm, augment the spleen and harmonize the stomach.

- *Ban Xia Bai Zhu Tian Ma Tang*
  - *Tian Ma* extinguishes wind and stops tremors to alleviate dizziness.
  - *Bai Zhu* and *Fu Ling* strengthen the spleen and augment the qi to break the cycle of phlegm formation.
  - *Ban Xia* and *Chen Pi* dry dampness, promote the movement of qi and transform phlegm.

- Frequent vomiting. + *Dai Zhe Shi, Zhu Ru, Sheng Jiang*
  Abdominal distention and loss of appetite. + *Sha Ren, Bai Dou Kou*
  Tinnitus and impaired hearing. + *Yu Jin, Shi Chang Pu*
  Congested phlegm transforming into fire with dizziness, distending pain of the head and eyes, irritability, short temper, bitter taste in the mouth and insomnia, use *Huang Lian Wen Dan Tang*.

Qi and blood deficiency

Dizziness aggravated by or recurring with exertion, sometimes occurring only on change of posture.
S: Pale complexion, dull-pale lips and nails, dry lusterless hair, palpitations, shortness of breath, insomnia, poor memory, fatigue and poor appetite.
T: Pale tongue. **P:** Thready and weak.

- Tonify the qi and nourish the blood.

- *Gui Pi Tang*
  - *Gui Pi Tang* augments the qi and strengthens the spleen; it assists the generating source of the qi and blood, as well as nourishes the blood and calms the spirit. This is the imperial formula for deficiency of the qi and blood.

- To tonify the qi and generate the blood for severe deficiency of the blood, increase the dosage of *Ren Shen* and *Huang Qi*. + *Shu Di Huang, E Jiao*.
  Qi sinking, or clear yang unable to ascend, with dizziness, diarrhea and organ prolapse, use *Bu Zhong Yi Qi Tang*.

Kidney essence deficiency

Persistent dizziness with a feeling of emptiness in the head, fatigue, tinnitus, insomnia, poor memory, and weakness and soreness of the lower back and knees.
S: More yang deficiency- cold intolerance, coldness and soreness of the lower back and knees, impotence or cold uterus. **T:** Pale. **P:** Deep and weak.
S: More yin deficiency- night sweating, five-centers heat, nocturnal emission, and irregular menstruation. **T:** Red tongue with scanty coating. **P:** Thready and rapid.

- Tonify the kidney and assist the yang or nourish the yin.
- *You Gui Wan* for kidney yang deficiency
  - *You Gui Wan* warms the yang, tonifies the kidney and replenishes the essence.
- *Zuo Gui Wan* for kidney yin deficiency
  - *Zuo Gui Wan* nourishes the yin, tonifies the kidney and replenishes the essence.
- To strengthen the effect of subduing floating yang. + *Long Gu, Mu Li*

Acupuncture Treatment

Liver yang rising:

- **Manipulation:** Combination of reinforcing and reducing methods.
- **Prescription:** GB20 Fengchi, BL18 Ganshu, BL23 Shenshu, KI3 Taixi, LR2 Xingjian

Phlegm-dampness obstruction:

- **Manipulation:** Even method.
- **Prescription:** ST8 Touwei, BL20 Pishu, CV12 Zhongwan, PC6 Neiguan, ST40 Fenglong

Qi and blood deficiency:

- **Manipulation:** Reinforcing method and moxibustion.
- **Prescription:** GV20 Baihui, BL20 Pishu, CV4 Guanyuan, ST36 Zusanli, SP6 Sanyinjiao

Kidney essence deficiency:

- **Manipulation:** Reinforcing method and moxibustion.
- **Prescription:** GV20 Baihui, BL17 Geshu, BL23 Shenshu, CV4 Guanyuan, KI6 Zhaohai

Practical Hints

• "Yin decreases tremendously when one passes age 40." After middle age, the risk of developing wind stroke increases. Dizziness caused by liver yang rising, especially liver yang stirring liver wind, will be very severe. Sudden loss of consciousness may follow an episode of dizziness. "**Dizziness is the antecedent of wind stroke**." It is imperative to treat and prevent dizziness and its underlying pathology in middle-aged adults and the elderly. Dizziness with severe headache occurring in a middle-aged person, accompanied by numbness or temporary unilateral weakness of the extremities, is a warning of impending wind stroke.

• **Recognize patterns with unfavorable prognoses.** A few cases of dizziness due to exhaustion of liver blood or kidney essence will advance to deafness and blindness. Dizziness due to liver yin deficiency, liver yang rising, or liver wind moving internally, accompanied by phlegm obstructing the channels, will progress to wind stroke. These two patterns have unfavorable prognoses.

CHAPTER 30

Tinnitus and Deafness

耳鳴 耳聾 *Er Ming Er Long*

Tinnitus and deafness refer to auditory impairment with varying degrees of diminished hearing. Tinnitus is the subjective sensation of hearing a ringing or buzzing sound in the ear. The noise may be high- or low-pitched, loud or soft, and heard in one or both ears. Tinnitus can interfere with auditory perception. Deafness is the partial or complete loss of hearing. Clinically, tinnitus and deafness may or may not present simultaneously. In some cases, tinnitus can induce deafness. Even though they have different manifestations, tinnitus and deafness share the same pathogenesis.

Relevant Diseases

- Otitis externa
- Otitis media
- Labyrinthitis
- Brain tumor
- Ototoxicity
- Hypertension
- Meniere's disease
- Acute or chronic renal failure
- Excessive cerumen in the ears

Etiology and Pathogenesis

Kidney essence deficiency: The ear, as one of the sensory orifices, relies on kidney essence for nourishment. Chronic disease, constitutional weakness or excessive sexual activity may injure kidney essence. Deficient kidney essence will not be able to generate marrow to fill the brain; thus, the ears are malnourished resulting in impaired hearing.

Spleen and stomach deficiency leads to deficiency of the qi and blood. Malnourishment due to deficiency of the qi and blood is compounded by the deficient spleen's failure to raise the clear yang to the sensory orifice.

Emotional stress: Emotional stress may lead to liver qi stagnation and further develop into liver fire. Fire due to stagnant qi can ascend through the gallbladder channel to the ear and disturb the auditory orifice.

Damp-heat accumulation: Improper diet can cause damp-heat or phlegm-fire accumulation in the middle burner. When phlegm-fire mists the sensory orifice, tinnitus or deafness will occur.

Wind-heat invasion: Exterior wind-heat enters and disturbs the channels around the ear causing tinnitus or deafness. Pathogenic factors trapped in the sensory orifice due to recurring episodes of common cold can also contribute to tinnitus or deafness.

Miscellaneous: Drug toxicity, prolonged or repetitive exposures to loud noise, and traumatic injury are precipitating factors for tinnitus and deafness.

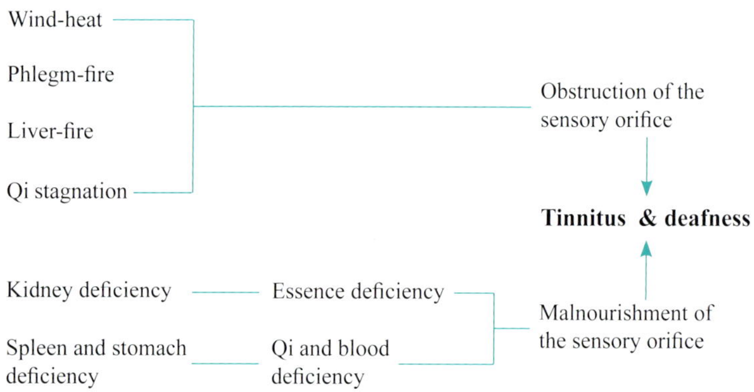

Diagnosis

A. Identification of etiology:

- Sudden onset of severe tinnitus or deafness accompanied by exterior signs and symptoms – Exterior wind-heat.
- Sudden tinnitus with a loud sound, aggravated by anger – Liver fire.
- Various degrees of tinnitus accompanied by dizziness and vertigo and a stifling sensation in the chest – Turbid phlegm.
- Gradual onset of constant, low-pitched tinnitus resembling running water that is worse in the evening, accompanied by soreness and weakness of the lower back and knees – Kidney essence deficiency.
- Gradual onset of tinnitus with a low volume relieved by rest and aggravated by exertion – Qi deficiency.

B. Identification of excess and deficiency patterns:

Tinnitus and deafness can have a transient occurrence or be permanent. Intensity and characteristics of symptoms may vary. The description of the ringing sounds can be very helpful in diagnosing tinnitus. High-pitched whistling, a sound like cicadas, and a low-pitched roar each suggest a different pathogenesis.

Excess patterns are characterized by acute onset, loud and high-pitched ringing, and sudden deafness.

Deficiency patterns are characterized by gradual onset, soft and low-pitched sounds, and gradual diminishment of hearing.

Basic Patterns

- Liver fire
- Wind-heat
- Spleen failing to raise the clear yang
- Phlegm-fire
- Kidney essence deficiency

Differentiation and Treatment

Treatment principle:

Excess: Dispel pathogenic factors by dispersing wind, clearing heat, draining fire and transforming phlegm.

Deficiency: Tonify the righteous qi by nourishing kidney essence, tonifying the qi and replenishing the blood.

Liver fire

Sudden onset of tinnitus and deafness, irritability, and short temper; aggravated by anger.

S: Headache, red face and eyes, bitter taste in the mouth, insomnia, distending pain in the hypochondriac region, dark scanty urine, and constipation.

T: Red tongue with yellow coating. **P:** Rapid and wiry.

- Clear liver heat and purge fire.
- *Long Dan Xie Gan Tang*
  - *Long Dan Cao*, *Zhi Zi* and *Huang Qin* clear and drain liver fire.
  - *Mu Tong*, *Che Qian Zi* and *Ze Xie* clear and drain damp-heat.
  - *Sheng Di Huang* and *Dang Gui* nourish liver blood and soften the liver.
  - *Chai Hu* spreads constrained liver qi.
- Constipation. + *Da Huang*
  Significant liver qi stagnation. + *Bai Shao, Chuan Lian Zi, Xia Ku Cao*
  Heat injuring kidney yin. + *Han Lian Cao, Nu Zhen Zi*
  Severe headache. + *Tian Ma, Gou Teng, Shi Jue Ming*

Phlegm-fire

Various degrees of tinnitus, even deafness, and distending pain in the ear.
S: Chest stuffiness, bitter taste in the mouth, nausea, copious sputum and irregular bowel movements.
T: Thin yellow greasy coating. **P:** Wiry and slippery.

- Transform phlegm, purge fire, harmonize the stomach and descend turbidity.
- *Wen Dan Tang*
  - *Ban Xia* and *Chen Pi* dry dampness, activate the qi and transform phlegm.
  - *Fu Ling* is a bland herb to leach out and drain dampness.
  - *Zhu Ru* and *Zhi Shi* clear heat, descend rebellious qi and expel phlegm.
- Enhance the effect to transform phlegm. + *Dan Nan Xing, Zhe Bei Mu, Tian Hua Fen*

  Heat accumulated in the diaphragm with irritability and restlessness. + *Zhi Zi, Dan Dou Chi*

  Insomnia. + *Yuan Zhi, Long Gu*

Wind-heat

Tinnitus and deafness with acute onset during an invasion of wind-heat, and pain or itchiness in the ears.
S: Aversion to wind, fever, headache, general body ache and sore throat.
T: Thin white coating. **P:** Floating and rapid, or wiry and rapid.

- Disperse wind and clear heat.
- *Yin Qiao San*
  - *Jin Yin Hua* and *Lian Qiao* are acrid and cool; as the chief ingredients in the formula, they disperse wind-heat and relieve toxicity.
  - *Bo He* and *Niu Bang Zi* assist the chief herbs to disperse wind-heat.
  - *Jing Jie* and *Dan Dou Chi* are acrid and warm; they strengthen the effect to release exterior pathogenic factors when combined with herbs above.
  - *Zhu Ye* and *Lu Gen* clear heat and generate the fluid.
- Enhance the effect to disperse wind. + *Ju Hua, Chan Tui, Bai Ji Li*

Kidney essence deficiency

Recurrent tinnitus or deafness accompanied by dizziness, vertigo, and soreness and weakness of the lower back and knees.
S: Tidal fever, malar flush, dry mouth, five-centers heat, nocturnal emission or irregular menstruation.
T: Red tongue with scanty coating. **P:** Thready and weak.

- Nourish the kidney, eliminate empty heat and restrain kidney essence.
- *Er Long Zuo Ci Wan*
  - *Liu Wei Di Huang Wan* tonifies kidney yin.
  - *Wu Wei Zi* astringes and binds the essence.
  - *Ci Shi* heavily anchors rebellious tubidity.
- To enhance the effects to nourish the yin and replenish the essence. + *Gui Ban, E Jiao, Nu Zhen Zi, Sang Shen Zi*

  Strengthen the sinews and bones. + *Niu Xi, Du Zhong*

Spleen failing to raise the clear yang

Recurrent tinnitus and deafness; temporarily relieved by rest and aggravated by exertion.

S: Fatigue, lassitude, dizziness, lack of appetite, heavy sensation in the lower abdomen, loose stool and diarrhea.

T: Thin white greasy coating. **P:** Thready and weak.

- Benefit the qi and raise the yang.
- *Yi Qi Cong Ming Tang*
  - *Ren Shen* and *Huang Qi* augment the qi and raise clear yang.
  - *Sheng Ma* and *Ge Gen* raise yang qi.
  - *Man Jing Zi* raises clear qi and unblocks the orifices.
- To enhance the effects of clearing the heart and unblocking the orifices. + *Shi Chang Pu, Fu Shen*

  Dizziness, heaviness of the head, stifling sensation in the chest, and greasy tongue coating. + *Bai Zhu, Ban Xia, Tian Ma*

Acupuncture Treatment

Excess:

- **Manipulation:** Reducing method.
- **Prescription:** TE17 Yifeng GB2 Tinghui TE3 Zhongzhu GB43 Xiaxi
- **Supplementary points:**
  - Liver fire. + LR2 Xingjian; GB41 Zulinqi
  - Phlegm-fire. + ST40 Fenglong; PC8 Laogong
  - Wind-heat. + TE5 Waiguan; LI4 Hegu

Deficiency:

- **Manipulation:** Reinforcing method.
- **Prescription:** TE17 Yifeng, GB2 Tinghui, BL23 Shenshu, CV4 Guanyuan, KI3 Taixi, GV4 Mingmen

Practical Hints

Even though the kidney opens into the ear and its essence and blood provide nourishment to the ear, **tinnitus and deafness can have other pathogeneses besides kidney deficiency**. In addition to kidney deficiency, the most common cause of tinnitus and deafness is wind-heat. Both wind and heat are yang pathogens that tend to affect the upper part of the body and attack the ear. Tinnitus due to inflammation of the eustachian tube is an example of wind-heat tinnitus. Phlegm accumulation obstructing the sensory orifice also may contribute to tinnitus and deafness, notably in labyrinthitis or Meniere's disease. The other common cause of tinnitus is liver fire blazing or hyperactive liver yang. Disturbed hearing due to liver fire or hyperactive liver yang occurs in hypertensive patients. Because there is more than one possible pathogenesis for tinnitus and deafness, treatment must not be limited to nourishing kidney essence. Accurate diagnosis is essential for effective treatment.

CHAPTER **31**

Painful Obstructive Syndrome

痺證 *Bi Zheng*

Painful obstructive syndrome, or *bi* syndrome, is caused by invasion of exterior pathogenic factors, such as wind, cold, dampness and heat, which obstruct the channels and collaterals, disturbing blood circulation and qi flow. The syndrome is characterized by localized discomforts in the muscles, joints and tendons. Major complaints include soreness and pain, numbness, heaviness, difficulty in movement, and/or red swollen joints that are warm to the touch. In some cases, deformity of the joints is apparent.

Relevant Diseases

- Rheumatic arthritis
- Rheumatoid arthritis
- Degenerative arthritis
- Osteoarthritis
- Gout
- Sciatica
- Subacromial bursitis
- Olecranal bursitis
- Carpal tunnel syndrome
- Fibromyalgia

Etiology and Pathogenesis

Deficient righteous qi accounts for the underlying etiology of painful obstructive syndrome. Unconsolidated interstitial layers between the muscles and skin are easily invaded by exterior wind, cold, dampness or heat. These pathogens obstruct the flow in the channels and vessels, leading to pain and difficulty in movement.

Exterior invasion: Invasion of exterior wind, cold and dampness is usually associated with conditions in the environment. Damp, cold living conditions, sudden cold or rainy weather, and working in the water for long periods of time can lead to wind, cold or dampness obstruction in the muscles, joints and channels.

Invasion of heat or other pathogenic influences transforming into heat: Heat painful obstructive syndrome can be caused by external heat or internal heat. Constitutional yang excess or constitutional yin deficiency contributes to excess or deficient heat. Individuals with constitutional internal heat are very susceptible to exterior pathogenic factors that accumulate and transform into heat.

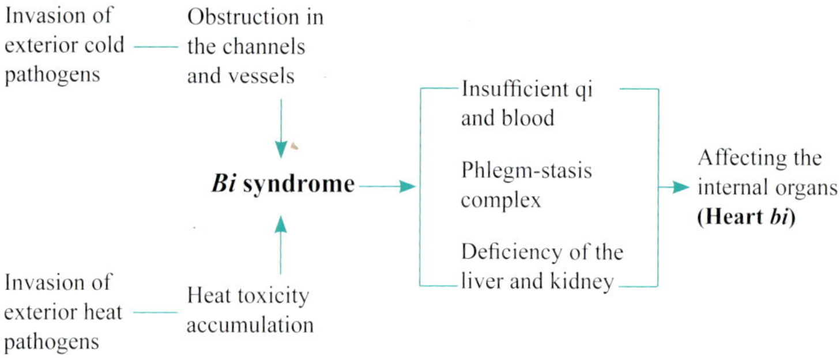

Diagnosis

A. Identification of wind, cold, damp and heat *bi*:

- Wind *bi* syndrome is characterized by pain that migrates from joint to joint. Other clinical manifestations include soreness and pain in the extremities.
- Cold *bi* syndrome is marked by severe, excruciating pain of the affected joints with limited range of motion.
- Damp *bi* syndrome is marked by swollen, numb and painful joints and limbs.
- Heat *bi* syndrome manifests as red, swollen, painful joints that are warm to the touch with erythema marginatum or circinatum.

B. Identification of complications:

Complications are usually seen in chronic painful obstructive syndrome.

- Phlegm accumulation and blood stasis: Longstanding *bi* syndrome affects the blood circulation and qi flow. Blood stasis forms obstruction and phlegm turbidity accumulates in the channels. Clinical presentations include erythema marginatum or circinatum, subcutaneous nodules, and swollen joints with limited range of motion.
- Qi and blood deficiency: Unremitting, intractable *bi* syndrome leads to the exhaustion of qi and blood. Various degrees of liver and kidney deficiency, or blood and essence deficiency, are common.
- *Zang-fu bi*, or *bi* in the internal organs: Chronic painful obstruction lingering in the channels will eventually affect the corresponding internal organs, especially the heart. According to an ancient text, "Heart *bi* syndrome is caused by obstruction in the heart's vessels, and manifests as irritability, palpitations, and over-expansion of the chest with an irregular heartbeat. In an acute episode, shortness of breath, wheezing and dyspnea are apparent."

C. Differential diagnosis of painful obstruction and atrophy syndromes:
Painful obstructive syndrome and atrophy syndrome share symptoms of pathology of the joints and extremities.

Painful obstructive syndrome is marked by soreness, pain, heaviness and difficult movement of the joints and muscles. Occasionally, numbness and swollen joints are present. Muscular atrophy can occur in *bi* syndrome if a painful extremity is not exercised normally, but flaccidity is not present.

Atrophy syndrome is characterized by weakness and flaccidity of the limbs and atrophy of the muscles, leading to loss of musculoskeletal function. Pain is not common in atrophy syndrome.

Basic Patterns

Acute episode:

- Wind bi
- Cold bi
- Damp bi
- Heat bi

Chronically active phase:

- Phlegm accumulation and blood stais
- Qi and blood deficiency
- Heart bi

Differentiation and Treatment

Treatment principle:
Expel wind, dispel cold, eliminate dampness, clear heat and unblock the channels.

Wind *bi*: Expel wind while tonifying the blood. "Treat the blood prior to expelling wind. As blood circulation is restored, wind is arrested inevitably."

Cold *bi*: Dispel cold while fortifying the yang. "Warmth can unblock the congealing cold."

Damp *bi*: Drying and draining dampness are the primary strategies, including tonifying the spleen. "Support the earth to defeat water."

Heat *bi*: Clear heat and include the other strategies accordingly.

Acute episode:

Wind bi

Soreness and pain that migrate from joint to joint.

S: Aversion to wind, fever and limited range of motion.

T: Thin white coating. **P:** Floating.

- Expel wind, unblock obstruction in the collaterals, disperse cold and eliminate dampness.
- *Fang Feng Tang*
  - *Fang Feng*, *Ma Huang* and *Qin Jiao* dispel wind, disperse cold and eliminate dampness.
  - *Dang Gui*, *Ge Gen* and *Rou Gui* invigorate the blood, warm the channels and unblock the obstruction in the collaterals.
  - *Fu Ling* strengthens the spleen and drains dampness.
- Mainly affecting the upper extremities. *+ Qiang Huo, Bai Zhi, Jiang Huang, Chuan Xiong*

  Mainly affecting the lower limbs. *+ Du Huo, Niu Xi, Mu Gua, Fang Ji*

  Mainly affecting the lower back or spine. *+ Du Zhong, Sang Ji Sheng, Ba Ji Tian, Xu Duan, Yin Yang Huo*

Cold bi

Excruciating pain in the affected joints and limbs. Pain is localized and aggravated by cold.

S: Stiffness of the joints with difficulty in movement.

T: Thin white or moist white coating. **P:** Floating and tight.

- Warm the channels, expel cold, dispel wind and eliminate dampness.
- *Wu Tou Tang*
  - *Wu Tou* and *Ma Huang* warm the channels, disperse cold, eliminate dampness and alleviate pain.
  - *Shao Yao* and *Gan Cao* moderate spasm and alleviate pain.
  - *Huang Qi* augments the qi and consolidates the surface of the body.
- Complicated by constitutional yang deficiency causing stubborn cold *bi*. *+ Rou Gui, Xi Xin*

Damp bi

Swollen, heavy, painful joints and numbness of the affected limbs.

S: General soreness and heaviness, fatigue and lack of strength with difficult movement.

T: White greasy coating. **P:** Soft and decelerating.

- Eliminate dampness, unblock obstruction in the channels, and dispel wind-cold.
- *Yi Yi Ren Tang*
  - *Yi Yi Ren* and *Cang Zhu* strengthen the spleen and eliminate dampness.
  - *Fang Feng*, *Qiang Huo* and *Du Huo* dispel wind-dampness.
  - *Chuan Wu*, *Ma Huang* and *Gui Zhi* warm the channels and disperse cold.

- *Dang Gui* and *Chuan Xiong* nourish and invigorate the blood.

- Significant swelling in the joints. + *Bi Xie, Mu Tong, Mu Gua, Fang Ji*
  Significant numbness. + *Hai Tong Pi, Xi Xian Cao*

Heat bi

Redness, swelling, and burning pain in joints that are warm to the touch, pain aggravated by pressure, and preference for cold.
S: Aversion to wind, fever, sweating, thirst, irritability and restlessness.
T: Red tongue with dry yellow coating. **P:** Slippery and rapid.

- Clear heat and unblock the collaterals, dispel wind and eliminate dampness.

- *Bai Hu Jia Gui Zhi Tang*
  - *Bai Hu Tang* clears heat and eliminates irritability.
  - *Gui Zhi* disperses wind and unblocks the collaterals.

- To reinforce the effects of clearing heat and relieving toxicity. + *Ren Dong Teng, Lian Qiao, Huang Bai*
  To enhance the effects of invigorating the blood, unblocking the collaterals, dispelling wind and eliminating dampness. + *Hai Tong Pi, Jiang Huang, Wei Ling Xian, Fang Ji, Sang Zhi*
  Erythema marginatum or circinatum. + *Mu Dan Pi, Sheng Di Huang*

Chronically active phase:

Phlegm accumulation and blood stasis

Swollen joints with intermittent pain, possibly deformity, stiffness, difficulty in movement, and subcutaneous nodules
T: Pulple tongue with white greasy coating. **P:** Thready and choppy.

- Transform phlegm, expel stasis and unblock the channels.

- *Tao Hong Yin*
  - *Tao Ren*, *Hong Hua* and *Dang Gui Wei* invigorate the blood and expel stasis.
  - *Chuan Xiong* dispels wind, alleviates pain, invigorates the blood and facilitates the movement of qi.
  - *Wei Ling Xian* dispels wind-dampness and unblocks the channels.

- Strengthen the effects of transforming phlegm and dissipating nodules. + *Bai Jie Zi, Dan Nan Xing*
  Enhance the effects of invigorating the blood, expelling stasis, and unblocking the collaterals. + *Chuan Shan Jia, Di Long*
  Reinforce the effects to gather wind and unblock the collaterals. + *Quan Xie, Wu Shao She*

Qi and blood deficiency

Intermittent joint pain with difficulty in movement, numbness of the limbs, soreness and weakness of the lower back and knees, cold intolerance, preference for warmth, fatigue, lassitude and shortness of breath.
T: Pale tongue with white coating. **P:** Thready and weak.

- Expel wind-dampness and unblock the obstruction to alleviate pain; tonify the qi and blood, and nourish the liver and kidney.
- *Du Huo Ji Sheng Tang*
  - *Du Huo*, the chief herb, dispels wind-dampness and unblocks the obstruction to alleviate pain.
  - *Xi Xin*, *Fang Feng* and *Qin Jiao* disperse wind and dispel cold-dampness.
  - *Du Zhong*, *Niu Xi* and *Sang Ji Sheng* strengthen the sinews and bones, and nourish the liver and kidney.
  - *Dang Gui*, *Chuan Xiong*, *Di Huang* and *Bai Shao* harmonize the blood.
  - *Ren Shen* and *Fu Ling* augment the qi and strengthen the spleen.
  - *Gui Zhi* warms and unblocks the blood circulation.
- Significant pain. + *Zhi Chuan Wu, Di Long, Hong Hua, Bai Hua She*
  Preponderance of cold. + *Fu Zi*
  Preponderance of dampness. + *Fang Ji*

Heart bi

Palpitations, shortness of breath aggravated by exertion, pale or purplish complexion, nails and lips.
T: Pale or purplish tongue. **P:** Intermittent and knotted.

- Augment the qi, nourish the heart, warm the yang and restore the regular pulse.
- *Zhi Gan Cao Tang*
  - *Zhi Gan Cao* is sweet and warm; it augments the qi and assists the yang.
  - *Gui Zhi* is acrid and warm; it warms and unblocks the flow of yang qi. When combines with *Gan Cao*, the acrid and sweet properties can transform into yang qi to restore the regular rhythm of the pulse.
  - *Ren Shen* and *Da Zao* augment the qi, and tonify the heart and spleen.
  - *Di Huang*, *E Jiao*, *Mai Men Dong* and *Huo Ma Ren* nourish the blood, replenish the yin and tonify the heart.
- To strengthen the effects of nourishing the heart and calming the spirit. + *Yuan Zhi, Wu Wei Zi*
  Significant palpitations and dyspnea. + *Huang Qi, Bai Zhu*
  Accompanied by chest congestion and chest pain. + *Dan Shen, Yu Jin*

Acupuncture Treatment

Acute episode

Wind bi:

- **Manipulation:** Reducing method.
- **Prescription:** BL12 Fengmen BL17 Geshu SP10 Xuehai

Cold bi:

- **Manipulation:** Moxibustion is primary. Reducing method with deep insertion and prolonged retention of needles.
- **Prescription:** BL23 Shenshu CV4 Guanyuan

Damp bi:

- **Manipulation:** Acupuncture and moxibustion.
- **Prescription:** ST36 Zusanli BL20 Pishu SP5 Shangqiu

Heat bi:

- **Manipulation:** Reducing method.
- **Prescription:** GV14 Dazhui LI11 Quchi

Local point selection:

- Add the following local points based on the affected joints, in addition to the primary prescriptions:

  - **Shoulder.** + TE14 Jianliao; LI15 Jianyu; SI10 Naoshu
  - **Elbow.** + LI11 Quchi; LI4 Hegu; TE10 Tianjing; TE5 Waiguan; LU5 Chize
  - **Wrist.** + TE4 Yangchi; TE5 Waiguan; LI5 Yangxi; SI5 Yanggu
  - **Hip.** + GB30 Huantiao; GB29 Juliao; GB39 Xuanzhong
  - **Knee.** + Extra38 Heding; Extra36 Xiyan; ST35 Dubi; SP9 Yinlingquan; GB34 Yanglingquan
  - **Ankle.** + ST41 Jiexi; SP5 Shangqiu; GB40 Qiuxu; BL60 Kunlun; KI3 Taixi
  - **Lower back and spine.** + GV26 Renzhong; GV3 Yaoyangguan; GV12 Shenzhu

Chronically active phase

Heart bi: Refer to Chapter 6, "Palpitations" (see page 45), and Chapter 7, "Chest Painful Obstruction" (see pages 53-54).

Practical Hints

• **Prevent intoxication from toxic herbs.** Herbs like *Fu Zi*, *Chuan Wu* and *Cao Wu* are often used to treat severe pain due to wind-cold-damp painful obstruction. These herbs have powerful effects to expel wind, cold and dampness, warm the channels and alleviate pain. However, they are toxic and hot in nature. Intoxication is frequently reported. Therefore, initiate therapy with a small dose and gradually increase the dosage, decoct these herbs for a long period of time, or decoct them with *Gan Cao*. These measures can reduce the toxicity of *Fu Zi*, *Chuan Wu* and *Cao Wu*. If symptoms of intoxication occur, such as numbness of the lips, tongue, hands and feet, palpitations, nausea, drooling or slow pulse, immediately discontinue the herbs and initiate emergency measures.

• **Modify the formulas according to the affected limbs.** Adding the following herbs will reinforce the therapeutic effect:

Shoulders, elbows or joints of the upper extremities. + *Qiang Huo, Bai Zhi, Gao Ben, Sang Zhi, Jiang Huang, Chuan Xiong*

Knees, ankles or joints of the lower extremities. + *Du Huo, Niu Xi, Fang Ji*

Lower back or lumbar intervertebral joints. + *Du Zhong, Sang Ji Sheng, Yin Yang Huo, Ba Ji Tian, Xu Duan*

Red, swollen and painful joints that are warm to the touch. + *Ren Dong Teng, Shi Gao, Zhi Mu, Lian Qiao, Qin Jiao*

CHAPTER 32

Atrophy Syndrome

痿 證 *Wei Zheng*

Atrophy syndrome, or *wei* syndrome, refers to a group of disorders whose symptoms range from flaccidity and weakness in the sinews and muscles to diminished muscle mass. Muscular atrophy may be localized or systemic. The lower extremities are most often affected resulting in weakness and difficulty ambulating. As the capacity for voluntary movement diminishes, unremitting *wei* syndrome progresses to a total loss of mobility of the extremities.

Relevant Diseases

- Multiple sclerosis
- Poliomyelitis
- Myasthenia gravis
- Progressive myodystrophy
- Periodic paralysis
- Polyneuritis
- Syringomyelia
- Myelitis
- Hysterical paralysis

Etiology and Pathogenesis

Atrophy syndrome is usually caused by injuries to the internal organs, especially insufficient essence and blood, and yin deficiency with excessive fire; therefore, symptoms pertaining to heat or deficiency are common.

Lung heat with fluid injury: Lung heat, from exterior attacks, injures the fluid and impairs the dispersing and descending functions of the lung. Moisture and nourishment are not disseminated to the sinews and muscles, which eventually impairs their normal functions. The extremities are affected, becoming weak and flaccid with decreased mobility.

Damp-heat accumulation results from exterior damp-heat invasion or from improper diet. Accumulation of damp-heat in the sinews and muscles obstructs the blood circulation and qi flow. The sinews become flaccid and weak and the muscles gradually lose mass and become atrophied.

Deficiency of the spleen and stomach: When the spleen and stomach are deficient they do not transform and transport or receive and ripen properly, thus the source of qi, blood, body fluid and essence is inadequate. Deficient qi fails to facilitate the circulation of blood and body fluid; deficient blood and body fluid fail to nourish and moisten the sinews, bones and muscles; pathology of the sinews, bones, joints and muscles ensues.

Deficiency of the liver and kidney: The liver governs the sinews and stores the blood to nourish the sinews, while the kidney governs the bones and stores the essence that produces marrow to nourish the bones. If the liver and kidney are deficient, they are unable to support their related tissues and there will be flaccidity and weakness of the sinews and bones.

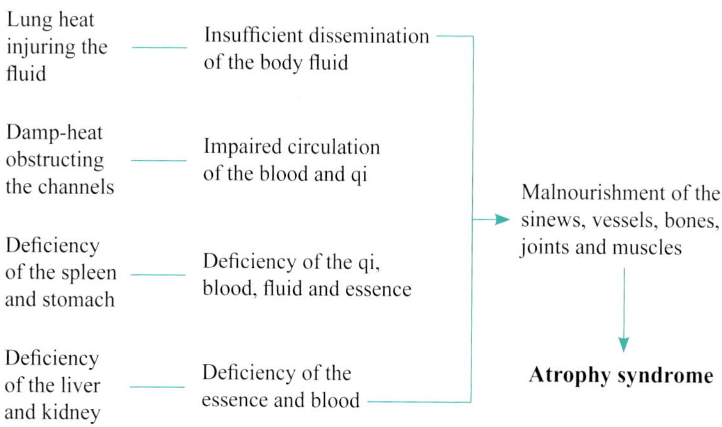

Diagnosis

A. Identification of excess and deficiency:

The most common patterns are those of deficiency and heat. Patterns of temporary excess or a combination of excess and deficiency are possible.

Excess patterns are caused by invasion of damp-heat. The onset is acute and there is rapid progression so that imobility and loss of muscle mass occur in a short period of time.

Deficient patterns are usually caused by deficiency of the spleen and stomach or liver and kidney. The onset is chronic followed by slow progression. In deficiency patterns, the lower extremities are most often affected. Weakness, flaccidity and muscular atrophy of the lower limbs are very common.

B. Differential diagnosis of similar disorders:

Painful obstructive syndrome, wind stroke and atrophy syndrome all involve pathology of the extremities.

Atrophy syndrome: Characterized by weakness and flaccidity of the extremities and atrophy of the muscles, atrophy syndrome leads to the loss of function of the skeletal muscles. The pattern of affected limbs can be random. Pain is not common in atrophy syndromes.

Painful obstruction syndrome: It is marked by soreness, pain, heaviness and difficulty in moving the joints and muscles. Numbness of the limbs and swollen joints are common. Although muscular atrophy may occur as a result of disuse and failure to exercise the affected limbs, flaccidity is not evident.

Wind stroke: Muscular flaccidity and atrophy are possible sequelae to wind stroke. However, these symptoms involve only one side of the body and are accompanied by numbness of the limbs and facial paralysis.

Basic Patterns

- Lung heat injuring the fluid
- Damp-heat accumulation
- Deficiency of the spleen and stomach
- Deficiency of the liver and kidney

Differentiation and Treatment

Treatment principle:

Excess: Clear heat, eliminate dampness, replenish the body fluid, nourish the yin and relax the sinews.

Deficiency: Augment the qi and harmonize the middle burner, tonify the spleen and stomach; nourish the liver and kidney, replenish the essence and blood, and strengthen the sinews and bones.

Lung heat injuring the fluid

Fever during the initial stage of the illness, or a fever followed by weakness, rapidly developing flaccidity and immobility of the extremities with muscular atrophy, and dry skin.

S: Irritability, thirst, cough, scanty sputum, scanty urine and dry stool.

T: Red tongue with yellow coating. **P:** Thready and rapid.

- Clear heat, moisten dryness, nourish the lung and generate the fluid.
- *Qing Zao Jiu Fei Tang*
  - *Sang Ye* and *Shi Gao* clear and disperse dry heat from the lung.
  - *Mai Dong*, *E Jiao* and *Hu Ma Ren* nourish the yin and moisten the lung.

- *Xing Ren* and *Pi Pa Ye* unblock the obstruction of lung qi.
- *Ren Shen* and *Gan Cao* tonify the qi and harmonize the middle burner.

- High fever, thirst and sweating. + *Zhi Mu, Jin Yin Hua, Lian Qiao*
  Dry cough with scanty sputum. + *Bei Mu, Gua Lou*

Damp-heat accumulation

Heaviness of the limbs, weak and flaccid extremities with numbness, and slight swelling in the affected extremities; most often affects the lower extremities.
S: Possibly fever, stifling sensation in the chest and epigastrium, and dark, scanty, painful and difficult urination.
T: Red tongue with yellow greasy coating. **P:** Slippery and rapid.

- Clear heat and drain dampness, unblock and facilitate circulation in the channels and vessels.

- *Si Miao Wan*
  - *Huang Bai*, bitter and cold, clears heat and dries dampness.
  - *Cang Zhu*, bitter and warm, dries dampness.
  - *Niu Xi* guides and carries the formula downwards.
  - *Yi Yi Ren* drains dampness and clears heat.

- To strengthen the effect of draining damp-heat via urination. + *Mu Tong, Fang Ji, Bi Xie*
  Excessive heat injuring the yin with irritability, red tongue and scanty coating. + *Sheng Di Huang, Gui Ban, Mai Men Dong*
  Numbness of the limbs with limited range of motion in the affected joints, purple tongue, and thready choppy pulse. + *Chi Shao, Dan Shen, Tao Ren*

Deficiency of the spleen and stomach

Flaccidity and weakness of the extremities aggravated by exertion, gradual loss of muscle mass, fatigue, lassitude and shortness of breath.
S: Poor appetite, loose stool, sallow complexion and abdominal distention.
T: Pale tongue with thin white coating. **P:** Thready and forceless.

- Strengthen the spleen and augment the qi.

- *Shen Ling Bai Zhu San*
  - *Dang Shen*, *Bai Zhu*, *Shan Yao*, *Bai Bian Dou* and *Lian Zi* benefit the qi and strengthen the spleen.
  - *Fu Ling* and *Yi Yi Ren* drain dampness and strengthen the spleen.
  - *Chen Pi* and *Sha Ren* harmonize the stomach and facilitate the flow of qi.

- Obesity with excessive phlegm, use *Liu Jun Zi Tang*.
  Significant qi deficiency or qi sinking, use *Bu Zhong Yi Qi Tang*.

Deficiency of the liver and kidney

Slow and gradual onset, weak and flaccid lower limbs, soreness and weakness of the lower back and spine, and inability to stand for a long time. Total loss of mobility and severe loss of muscle mass can result with exacerbation.

S: Dizziness, hair loss, dry throat, tinnitus, nocturnal emission, enuresis and irregular menstruation.

T: Red tongue with scanty coating. **P:** Thready and rapid.

- Tonify the liver and kidney, nourish the yin and clear heat.
- *Hu Qian Wan*
  - *Shu Di Huang* and *Gui Ban* nourish the blood, replenish the essence, and tonify the liver and kidney.
  - *Bai Shao* preserves the yin, generates the fluid and relaxes the sinews.
  - *Suo Yang* warms the yang and augments the essence.
  - *Zhi Mu* and *Huang Bai* nourish the yin and clear heat.
- To enhance the effects of nourishing the liver and kidney, strengthening the sinews and bones. *+ Zhu Gu Sui, Niu Xi*

  Sallow complexion, palpitations, pink tongue, and weak thready pulse. *+ Huang Qi, Dang Shen, Dang Gui, Ji Xue Teng*

Acupuncture Treatment

- **Manipulation:** Reducing method for heat patterns; reinforcing method for deficient patterns; puncture on the affected side.
- **Prescription:** Select the following primary points based on the affected limbs.

Upper limbs:	LI15 Jianyu	LI11 Quchi	LI4 Hegu
	TE5 Waiguan		
Lower limbs:	ST31 Biguan	ST34 Liangqiu	ST36 Zusanli
	ST41 Jiexi	GB39 Xuanzhong	GB34 Yanglingquan
	GB30 Huantiao	SP10 Xuehai	

- **Supplementary points:**
  - Lung heat. + LU5 Chize; BL13 Feishu
  - Damp-heat. + SP9 Yinlingquan; BL20 Pishu
  - Spleen and stomach deficiency. + CV6 Qihai; CV4 Guanyuan
  - Liver and kidney deficiency. + BL18 Ganshu; BL23 Shenshu

Practical Hints

To treat *wei* syndrome, strategies addressing the yang-brightness channels and organs should be adopted. The yang-brightness organs refer to the spleen and stomach because they generate and are the source of qi, blood, essence and body fluid. Located in the middle burner, they raise vital substances to the lung for dissemination to the entire body. They also supply the liver and kidney with blood and essence to nourish the sinews and bones. The spleen governs the muscles and provides them with nourishment. Strengthening the spleen and stomach will ensure their proper function and an adequate supply of vital substances. Sufficient nourishment and moistening significantly contribute to recovery from *wei* syndrome; therefore, when planning acupuncture or herbal treatment, yang-brightness should be the focus. Common treatment strategies include tonifying the spleen and stomach, clearing heat from the stomach, and clearing heat and draining dampness. The most commonly used acupuncture points include ST36, BL20, BL21, SP6, GB34 and GB39. Other strategies, such as clearing heat from the lung, moistening the lung, tonifying the liver and kidney, and tonifying the blood and essence, should be adopted according to the pattern.

CHAPTER 33

Emotional Disorder

鬱證 *Yu Zheng*

The simplest definition of *yu* in TCM refers to any obstruction resulting from stagnation, stasis, accumulation and retention. *Yu* syndrome is a general term for disorders of constraint caused by emotional frustration and qi stagnation. The name of this disorder indicates its etiology, pathogenesis, and complicated clinical presentation with various and mixed manifestaions.

The broad concept of *yu* syndrome encompasses all the clinical manifestations caused by stagnation of the qi, blood, phlegm, fire, dampness and food arising from the dysfunction of the internal organs or invasion by external pathogenic influences. In the narrow sense, *yu* syndrome refers to a specific set of psychological or affective presentations, such as depression, irritability, moodiness or anxiety, or a combination thereof, caused by qi stagnation associated with emotional stress. Examples include plum-pit syndrome and restless organ disorder.

Relevant diseases

- Somatoform disorders
- Hysteria
- Neurosis
- Depression
- Menopause

Etiology and Pathogenesis

Early stage of *yu* syndrome: Emotional stress such as frustration and anger may cause liver qi stagnation. Qi is the motive force of metabolism. In a condition of prolonged qi stagnation, other pathologies of blood stasis, accumulation of dampness or phlegm, and retention of food may arise consequently. These pathogenic derivatives may remain dormant internally and, after a long period of time, turn into fire, which is another source of stagnation.

Later stage of *yu* syndrome: In contrast to the early stage of *yu* syndrome in which the pathogenesis is relatively one of excess, the later stage is relatively deficient. Constrained liver qi inhibits the spleen's function. Impaired spleen function is not capable of generating sufficient qi and blood; malnourishment of the heart and spirit results from qi and blood deficiency. Therefore, deficiency of heart yin and blood will lead to kidney yin deficiency with empty fire.

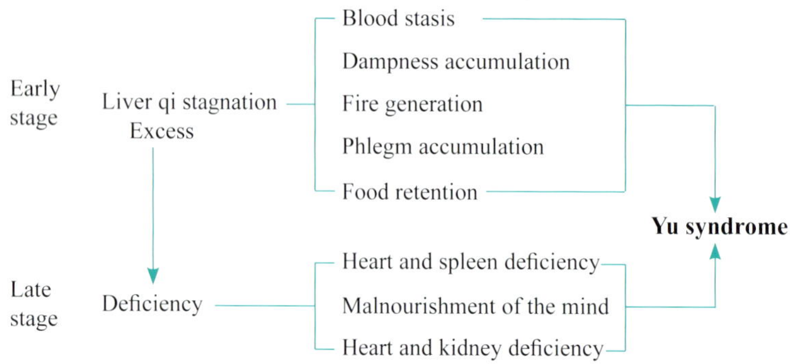

Diagnosis

A. Identification of emotional factors:

Mental or emotional factors trigger an episode of *yu* syndrome by aggravating the underlying qi stagnation. Explore the possibility of emotional stress to make an accurate diagnosis. Notice important cues, such as anger and frustration as well as other emotional factors such as overthinking, sadness, worry, shock or fear.

B. Identification of early and later stages of yu syndrome:

In its early stage, *yu* syndrome presents as an excess pattern, mainly liver qi stagnation that may or may not be accompanied by phlegm-dampness accumulation, food retention, heat accumulation and blood stasis. As the illness progresses, in its late stage, *yu* syndrome moves from the qi level into the blood level and from excess to deficiency. The clinical presentation, however, is a complicated pattern of excess and deficiency, such as spleen qi deficiency with dampness accumulation, heart blood deficiency with liver qi stagnation, and kidney yin deficiency with liver fire.

Basic Patterns

- Liver qi stagnation
- Qi stagnation turning into fire
- Obstruction of phlegm-qi complex (plum-pit syndrome)
- Heart deficiency and liver contraint (restless organ disorder)
- Heart and spleen deficiency
- Lack of communication between the heart and kidney

Differentiation and Treatment

Treatment principle:

Soothe the liver and facilitate the flow of qi.

Excess pattern: Primarily regulate the liver qi; invigorate the blood, transform phlegm, drain dampness, clear heat and eliminate food stagnation according to the patterns.

Deficiency pattern: Tonify the qi, nourish the blood, replenish the yin and calm the spirit.

Liver qi stagnation

Depression or mood swings, and distention and pain in the hypochondriac, chest, epigastric and abdominal regions with migrating locus.

S: Frequent sighing, crying spells, relief from belching or passing gas, poor appetite or irregular menstruation.

T: Thin white or thin greasy coating. **P:** Wiry or wiry and slippery.

- Soothe the liver and release constrained qi.
- *Chai Hu Shu Gan San*
  - *Chai Hu*, *Zhi Qiao* and *Xiang Fu* soothe the liver, facilitate the qi flow and release liver constraint.
  - *Chen Pi* promotes the movement of qi and harmonizes the middle burner.
  - *Chuan Xiong* and *Shao Yao* invigorate the blood and alleviate pain.
- Enhance the effect to release constrained qi. + *Yu Jin, Qing Pi, Fo Shou*

  Pacify the liver, descend rebellious qi and stop vomiting. +*Xuan Fu Hua, Dai Zhe Shi, Zi Su Geng*

  Fixed, distending hypochondriac pain or amenorrhea with a wiry and choppy pulse. + *Tao Ren, Hong Hua, Dang Gui, Yi Mu Cao, Dan Shen*

Qi stagnation turning into fire

Irritability, short temper, and distention and burning pain in the hypochondriac and chest regions.

S: Headache, tinnitus, red face and eyes, dry mouth, bitter taste in the mouth, upset stomach, acid regurgitation and constipation.

T: Red tongue with thin yellow coating. **P:** Wiry and rapid.

- Clear and drain liver fire; release constrained qi and harmonize the stomach.
- *Dan Zhi Xiao Yao San* and *Zuo Jin Wan*
  - *Dan Zhi Xiao Yao San* soothes constrained liver qi and clears heat.
  - *Zuo Jin Wan* clears heat from the liver, drains fire, descends rebellious qi and

harmonizes the stomach.

- Yellow tongue coating and constipation. + *Long Dan Cao, Da Huang*
  Liver fire flaring upwards with severe headache, irritability and constipation. + *Dang Gui Long Hui Wan*

Obstruction of phlegm-qi complex (plum-pit syndrome)

Discomfort in the throat, a sense of foreign body lodged in the throat that cannot be swallowed or expectorated.
S: A suffocating sensation in the chest, or distention and pain in the hypochondriac and chest regions.
T: Greasy coating. **P:** Wiry and slippery.

- Resolve phlegm to regulate the movement of qi and release constrained qi.
- *Ban Xia Hou Po Tang*
  - *Ban Xia* transforms phlegm, dissipates clumps and descends rebellious qi.
  - *Hou Po* facilitates the qi flow and dissipates clumps.
  - *Fu Ling* dries dampness and strengthens the spleen.
  - *Zi Su Ye*, an aromatic herb, facilitates the qi flow and spreads the constraint.
  - *Sheng Jiang* harmonizes the stomach and descends rebellious qi.
- To strengthen the effect of promoting the movement of qi. + *Xiang Fu, Zhi Qiao, Fo Shou*
  To enhance the effects to resolve phlegm and descend rebellious qi. + *Zi Su Geng, Su Zi, Xuan Fu Hua, Dai Zhe Shi*
  Dry and bitter taste in the mouth, nausea, vomiting and restlessness with a yellow greasy tongue coating, use *Huang Lian Wen Dan Tang*.

Heart deficiency and liver constraint (restless organ disorder)

Depression, frequent attacks of melancholy, crying spells, frequent bouts of yawning.
S: Disorientation and restlessness.
T: Pale tongue with thin white coating. **P:** Thready and wiry.

- Nourish the heart and calm the spirit.
- *Gan Mai Da Zao Tang*
  - *Gan Cao* and *Da Zao* are sweet and warm in nature; they harmonize the middle burner, strengthen the spleen and nourish the heart.
  - *Xiao Mai* is slightly cold; it nourishes the heart and calms the spirit.
- Enhance the effects to nourish the heart and calm the spirit. + *Bai Zi Ren, Suan Zao Ren, Fu Shen, Yuan Zhi*

Heart and spleen deficiency

Over-thinking, palpitations, timidity, insomnia and poor memory.
S: Pale complexion, dizziness, fatigue and poor appetite.
T: Pale tongue. **P:** Thready and weak.

- Benefit the qi and replenish the blood, nourish the heart and calm the spirit.
- *Gui Pi Tang*
  - *Dang Shen*, *Huang Qi* and *Bai Zhu* tonify the qi and augment the spleen.
  - *Dang Gui* nourishes the liver to generate heart blood.
  - *Suan Zao Ren* and *Long Yan Rou* tonify the blood and calm the spirit.
  - *Fu Shen* and *Yuan Zhi* quiet the heart and communicate the heart with kidney.
  - *Mu Xiang* facilitates the qi flow.
- To strengthen the effects to release constrained qi and calm the spirit. + *Yu Jin, Xiang Fu, He Huan Hua*

Lack of communication between the heart and kidney

Irritability and easily angered, dizziness, tinnitus, palpitations and insomnia.
S: Soreness of the lower back and knees, nocturnal emission or irregular menstruation.
T: Red tongue with scanty coating. **P:** Thready and rapid.

- Nourish the yin and clear heat; sedate the heart and calm the spirit.
- *Tian Wang Bu Xin Dan*
  - *Sheng Di Huang*, *Xuan Shen*, *Mai Men Dong* and *Tian Men Dong* nourish the yin and clear empty heat.
  - *Dan Shen* and *Dang Gui* nourish the blood and invigorate the blood.
  - *Ren Shen* and *Fu Ling* tonify the qi and quiet the heart.
  - *Suan Zao Ren*, *Bai Zi Ren*, *Yuan Zhi* and *Wu Wei Zi* nourish the heart and calm the spirit.
- Kidney yin deficiency with soreness of the lower back and nocturnal emission. + *Gui Ban, Zhi Mu, Qian Shi, Jin Ying Zi*

Acupuncture Treatment

Liver qi stagnation:

- **Manipulation:** Even method.
- **Prescription:** BL18 Ganshu, CV17 Tanzhong, CV12 Zhongwan, ST36 Zusanli, SP4 Gongsun, LR3 Taichong

Qi stagnation turning into fire:

- **Manipulation:** Reducing method.
- **Prescription:** CV13 Shangwan TE6 Zhigou GB34 Yanglingquan LR2 Xingjian GB43 Xiaxi

Obstruction of phlegm-qi complex (plum-pit syndrome):

- **Manipulation:** Even method.
- **Prescription:** CV22 Tiantu CV17 Tanzhong PC6 Neiguan ST40 Fenglong LR3 Taichong

Heart deficiency and liver constraint (restless organ disorder):

- **Manipulation:** Even method.
- **Prescription:** CV14 Juque HT7 Shenmen SP6 Sanyinjiao LR3 Taichong

Practical Hints

• In addition to having a complex pathology, ***yu* syndrome is characterized by numerous subjective complaints with lack of objective findings**, further complicating medical evaluation and treatment planning. Those who suffer from *yu* syndrome commonly seek medical evaluation and treatment from multiple practitioners. A variety of medical modalities for symptom management may mask significant cues that lead to an accurate diagnosis. In addition, medications taking for symptoms only and the misuse of medication due to inaccurate diagnosis will result in a poor response to therapy. When the therapeutic effect is not achieved after multiple trials, *yu* syndrome is regarded as intractable.

• Qi stagnation is the initial etiology and pathogenesis of *yu* syndrome, which also encompasses accumulation and obstruction by other pathogens that arise as qi stagnation progresses. **The formula *Yue Ju Wan* is an auxiliary remedy for *yu* syndrome** because it prevents formation of pathological derivatives. As long as liver qi stagnation is evident, *Yue Ju Wan* can be prescribed.

• Most herbs that soothe the liver and regulate the qi tend to be acrid, warm and drying in nature, thus may easily injure the yin. Prolonged stagnation of qi can transform into fire and injure the yin. Therefore, when treating *yu* syndrome, **select herbs that are acrid, neutral and moist,** such as *Xiang Yuan* and *Fo Shou*, or bitter and cold, such as *Yu Jin* and *Chuan Lian Zi*.

CHAPTER 34

Goiter

瘿瘤 *Ying Liu*

Goiter refers to a disorder manifested with enlargement or nodules by the thyroid cartilage at the neck. TCM theory believes that goiters are the result of qi stagnation, phlegm accumulation or blood stasis. The etiology of goiters may be related to emotional stress, improper diet and geographical environment.

Relevant Diseases

- Hyperthyroidism
- Thyroid tumor
- Thyroiditis
- Nodular goiter
- Simple goiter
- Exophthalmic goiter

Etiology and Pathogenesis

The basic pathogenesis of goiter is qi stagnation and phlegm accumulation; chronically, these factors precipitate blood stasis. In some cases, the stagnant qi and accumulated phlegm can turn into fire to injure the yin. Manifestations of heart and liver yin deficiency with empty fire may be present.

Emotional stress: Longstanding anger, frustration and worry will cause liver qi stagnation, which fails to properly circulate the body fluid and leads to phlegm accumulation. As qi stagnation combines with phlegm accumulation at the neck region, goiter will be formed. The extent, exacerbations and remissions of goiter are closely related to emotional activities. Unremitting, longstanding qi stagnation and phlegm accumulation will cause blood stasis. Once blood stasis is formed, the goiter will harden and nodules will be apparent.

Improper diet and environment: Spleen and stomach dysfunction may be caused by improper diet and environmental factors. Phlegm accumulates as the spleen and stomach fail to adequately transform and transport the body fluid. For the environmental factor, the incidence of goiter is greater in a population living in a place where there is deficiency of certain elements in the diet.

Constitutional factors: Females generally have a higher morbidity rate of goiters compare to their male counterparts. Many developmental stages of the female body are related to the qi and blood of liver channel. Normal menstruation, pregnancy, labor and delivery, and lactation all depend upon the adequate movement of liver qi and sufficient supply of liver blood. As the female body is closely related to the liver, women are more susceptible to emotional stress. In addition, those who have constitutional yin deficiency are more vulnerable to pathogenic fire generated from stagnant qi or accumulated phlegm.

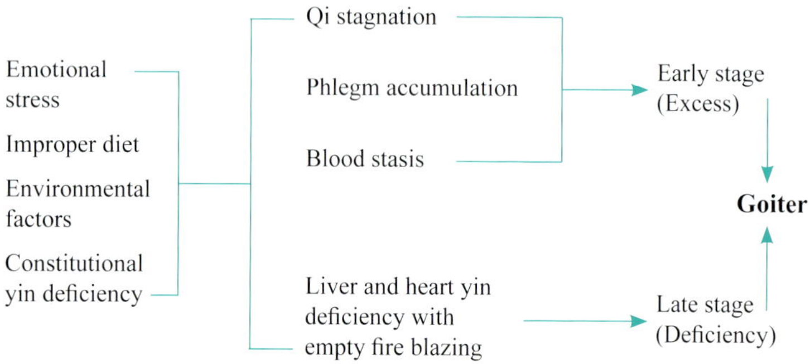

Diagnosis

Differential diagnosis of goiter and scrofula:

Goiter: It is commonly seen in female. It is manifested with nodules or enlargement by the thyroid cartilage at the neck. The mass fluctuates up and down as following the swallowing motion. It has a slow onset and grows gradually with various sizes. Goiter is usually soft and smooth under palpation. Unremitting, chronic goiter can become hard and nodular to the touch.

Scrofula: It is manifested by nodules palpated at bilateral side of the neck, along the sternocleidomastoid muscles from the post auricular region, inferior to the angle of the mandible, to the supraclavicular fossa. The multiple nodules are small in size, like beads.

Basic Patterns

- Qi stagnation and phlegm accumulation
- Phlegm accumulation and blood stasis
- Liver fire blazing upwards
- Heart and liver yin deficiency

Differentiation and Treatment

Treatment principle:

Facilitate the movement of qi, invigorate the blood, transform phlegm, soften hardness and dissipate clumps to eliminate goiters.

For hard mass or nodule, add herbs that invigorate the blood and dispel stasis.

For yin deficiency with empty heat, add herbs that nourish the yin and drain fire.

Qi stagnation and phlegm accumulation

Swelling surrounding the thyroid cartilage, soft and absent of pain upon palpation, and subjective distending sensation.

S: Stifling sensation in the chest, propensity to sighing, migrating distending pain in the chest and hypochondriac regions, and the conditions vary by emotional activities.

T: Thin white coating. **P:** Wiry.

- Facilitate the qi flow, relieve constraint, resolve phlegm and reduce goiters.
- *Si Hai Shu Yu Wan*
  - *Chen Pi* facilitates the qi flow, transforms phlegm and expels dampness.
  - *Mu Xiang*, aromatic in nature, facilitates the qi flow and revives the spleen.
  - *Kun Bu*, *Hai Dai*, *Hai Zao*, *Hai Piao Xiao* and *Hai Ge Ke* transform phlegm, soften hardness and dissipate accumulation.
- To reinforce the effects of facilitating the qi flow and relieving constraint. + *Chai Hu, Yu Jin, Xiang Fu*

  Benefit the throat and reduce swelling. + *Jie Geng, Niu Bang Zi, She Gan*

Phlegm accumulation and blood stasis

Mass surrounding the thyroid cartilage, hard or nodular to palpation, gradual onset and slow progress.

S: Stifling sensation in the chest and poor appetite.

T: Thin white or white greasy coating. **P:** Wiry or choppy.

- Invigorate the blood, resolve phlegm and reduce goiter.
- *Hai Zao Yu Hu Tang*
  - *Hai Zao*, *Kun Bu* and *Hai Dai*, salty and cold in nature, soften hardness, transform phlegm, and dissipate accumulation.
  - *Ban Xia* and *Bei Mu* transform phlegm and dissipate clumps.
  - *Qing Pi* and *Chen Pi* facilitate the qi flow and transform phlegm-dampness.
  - *Dang Gui* nourishes and invigorates the blood.
  - *Chuan Xiong* facilitates the qi flow and invigorates the blood to expel stasis.

- Hard nodules. + *San Leng, E Zhu, Dan Shen, Lu Feng Fang*
  Stifling sensation in the chest. + *Yu Jin, Xiang Fu*
  Stagnant qi transforming into fire with subjective hot sensation, irritability, red tongue with yellow coating and rapid pulse. + *Xia Ku Cao, Xuan Shen*

Liver fire blazing upwards

Swelling surrounding the thyroid cartilage, soft and smooth to palpation.
S: Irritability, hot sensation, profuse perspiration, short temper, exophthalmos, muscle tremors of the fingers and hands, hot flush and bitter taste in the mouth.
T: Red tongue with thin yellow coating. **P:** Wiry and rapid.

- Clear and drain liver fire.

- *Dan Zhi Xiao Yao San*
  - *Chai Hu* and *Bo He* soothe the liver to relieve liver constraint.
  - *Zhi Zi* and *Mu Dan Pi* clear and drain liver fire.
  - *Shao Yao* and *Dang Gui* preserve the yin, soften the liver, nourish the blood and invigorate the blood.

- To reinforce the effects of clearing the liver and draining fire. + *Long Dan Cao, Xia Ku Cao*
  To enhance the effects of dissipating accumulation and reducing the goiter. + *Hai Zao, Kun Bu*
  Severe tremors. + *Shi Jue Ming, Gou Teng, Bai Ji Li, Mu Li*
  Severe stomach fire with intense hunger and increased oral intake. + *Zhi Mu, Sheng Shi Gao*

Heart and liver yin deficiency

Soft swelling surrounding the thyroid cartilage, various sizes, gradual onset and slow progression.
S: Palpitation, irritability, insomnia, easily sweating, tremors of the hands and fingers, dry eyes and blurred vision, fatigue and lack of strength.
T: Red and quivering tongue. **P:** Wiry, thready and rapid.

- Nourish the yin, quiet the heart and soften the liver.

- *Tian Wang Bu Xin Dan*
  - *Sheng Di Huang*, *Xuan Shen*, *Mai Men Dong* and *Tian Men Dong* nourish the yin and clear heat.
  - *Dan Shen* and *Dang Gui* nourish and invigorate the blood.
  - *Suan Zao Ren* and *Wu Wei Zi* nourish heart blood, restrain heart qi, calm the spirit as well as reduce sweating.
  - *Bai Zi Ren* and *Yuan Zhi* nourish the heart and calm the spirit.

- *Ren Shen* and *Fu Ling* benefit the qi and quiet the heart.

- Liver yin deficiency with dull ache in the hypochondriac regions. + *Gou Qi Zi, Chuan Lian Zi*

  Liver wind swirling internally with trembling fingers and a quivering tongue. + *Gou Teng, Bai Ji Li, Bai Shao*

  Kidney yin deficiency with tinnitus, soreness and weakness of the lower back and knees. + *Gui Ban, Sang Ji Sheng, Niu Xi, Tu Si Zi*

  Essence and blood deficiency with scanty menstrual flow or amenorrhea in women or impotence in men. + *Huang Qi, Shan Zhu Yu, Shu Di Huang, Gou Qi Zi, He Shou Wu*

Acupuncture Treatment

- **Manipulation:** Reducing method.
- **Prescription:** TE13 Naohui; LI17 Tianding; SL17 Tianrong; CV22 Tiantu; BL4 Hegu; ST36 Zusanli; LR3 Taichong
- **Supplementary points:**
  - Palpitations. + PC6 Neiguan; HT7 Shenmen
  - Exophthalmos. + BL1 Jingming; BL2 Zanzhu; TE23 Sizhukong; GB20 Fengchi
  - Excessive sweating. + SP6 Sanyinjiao; KI7 Fuliu
  - Insomnia. + BL19 Danshu; BL15 Xinshu
  - Hunger and emaciation. + SP6 Sanyinjiao; ST36 Zusanli

Practical Hints

The use of incompatible herbs to obtain a greater therapeutic reaction for resolving goiters. *Hai Zao Yu Hu Tang*, the most common formula for treating goiters, contains two of the traditional eighteen herbal incompatibilities, *Gan Cao* and *Hai Zao*. This combination was purposely included in this formula. By utilizing two incompatible herbs to intensify the mutual herbal reactions, the goal of transforming phlegm, dissipating nodules and resolving goiters can be achieved. This formula has been utilized for thousands of years and there has not been a case of intoxication reported.

CHAPTER **35**

Aggregation and Accumulation Syndrome

積聚 *Ji Ju*

Ji ju, or aggregation and accumulation syndrome, refers to palpable or impalpable abdominal masses accompanied by pain or distention. *Ji*, or aggregation, signifies substantial masses with pain at a fixed location. *Ji* is a disorder of the blood level and yin organs. *Ju*, or accumulation, involves insubstantial masses with distention greater than pain. Distending pain migrates from site to site and the insubstantial mass appears intermittently and unpredictably. *Ju* is a disorder of the qi level and yang organs.

Relevant Diseases

- Hepatosplenomegaly
- Abdominal tumor
- Pyloric stenosis
- Partial bowel obstruction
- Intussusception
- Intestinal volvulus
- Intestinal disturbance

Etiology and Pathogenesis

Emotional stress results in liver qi constraint that impairs the circulation of the blood. Chronic qi stagnation leads to blood stasis. Emotional stress also disturbs the function of the spleen. Failure to transport and transform fluids causes phlegm accumulation. Phlegm obstructing the vessels complicates blood stasis, leading to *ji ju*.

Improper diet: Consuming too much greasy, sweet, rich food and alcohol can hinder the functions of the spleen and stomach. Phlegm turbidity forms when the spleen and stomach fail to properly metabolize fluids. Phlegm obstructs the flow of qi and leads to accumulation of stagnant qi and aggregation of stagnant blood and phlegm.

Exterior pathogenic factors: Cold-dampness or damp-heat can invade and linger in the abdomen. Unremitting and longstanding cold-dampness or damp-heat will accumulate and form *ju*, then aggregate to form *ji*.

Pathology of the liver, including jaundice, hypochondriac pain, malaria and schistosomiasis, is associated with turbid dampness accumulation and disharmony between the qi and blood. Stagnant qi, coagulated blood and phlegm accumulation may prolong and influence each other and fuse together in the abdomen.

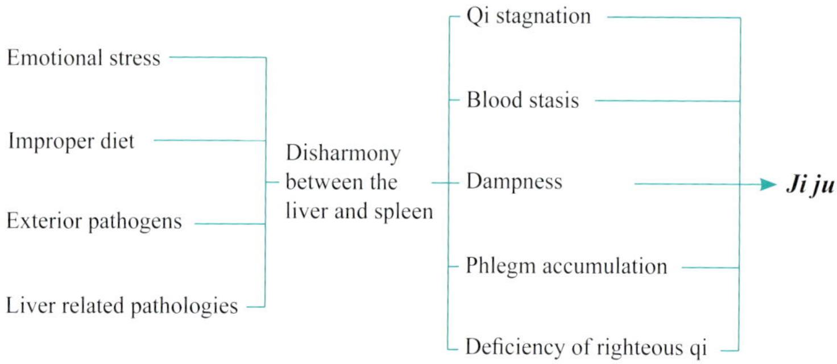

Diagnosis

A. Identification of qi stagnation, blood stasis, dampness or phlegm accumulation, and deficiency:

- At the initial stage, qi stagnation is most common and is characterized by distending pain. Masses are intermittently palpable with migrating locations and pain.
- Unremitting chronic conditions have an effect on the blood level. Blood stasis manifests with fixed pain and palpable hard masses.
- Dampness is elicited by spleen dysfunction; therefore, there will be secondary symptoms of spleen deficiency including poor appetite and loose stool.
- Phlegm is formed when longstanding unresolved dampness condenses. Symptoms include coughing up sputum and substantial masses that change shape upon palpation.
- Deficiency of righteous qi encompasses qi and yin deficiency, qi and blood deficiency, or yang qi deficiency, and results from chronic conditions consuming the vital energy. Symptoms will vary depending on the vital substances that are most deficient.

B. Identification of progressive stages:

Initial stage: The spleen and liver are affected simultaneously, presenting as qi stagnation, blood stasis and dampness obstruction. *Ji ju* located in the abdomen and related to qi stagnation, food retention and damp obstruction always involves dysfunction of the spleen and stomach. If there are masses in the hypochondriac region due to qi stagnation and blood stasis, the liver is affected.

Intermediate stage: In this stage, aggregation and accumulation syndrome forms a substantial mass as stagnant qi, stagnant blood and phlegm fuse together and concentrate.

Late stage: Righteous qi has been consumed as the condition lingers and progresses. Complications result from the deficiency of righteous qi and unresolved pathologies. Hemorrhages occur if the liver fails to store the blood and the spleen fails to control the blood; damp-heat obstruction in the middle burner inhibits bile drainage and causes jaundice; large amounts of accumulated fluids manifest as ascites or edema.

C. Differential diagnosis of similar disorders:

Aggregation and accumulation syndrome: Characterized by a localized enlargement of the abdomen having an irregular and asymmetrical shape.

Focal distention: A subjective sensation of fullness and distention in the epigastrium or abdomen. Despite the chief complaint of discomfort, palpable masses and enlargements are absent.

Tympanic abdominal distention: Characterized by drum-like abdominal distention, a pale-sallow skin tone, and distended veins on the abdominal wall. The abdominal enlargement is even and symmetrical. It is a result of retrogression following untreated or improperly treated *ji ju*.

Basic Patterns

Ju syndrome:

- Liver qi stagnation
- Food retention and phlegm obstruction

Ji syndrome:

- Qi stagnation disturbing blood circulation
- Blood stasis
- Deficient righteous qi with pathological aggregation

Differentiation and Treatment

Treatment principle:

Based on the pathogenesis and clinical manifestations, aggregation and accumulation syndrome is divided into two subtypes, *ji* and *ju*. Stagnant qi forming accumulation, or *ju*, precedes blood stasis forming aggregation, or *ji*.

Initial stage: Regulate the qi flow, reduce and guide out the accumulation, invigorate the blood and resolve dampness.

Intermediate stage: Promote the movement of qi, dispel blood stasis and expel phlegm.

Late stage: Support the righteous qi to expel pathogens by simultaneously tonifying the qi and blood, and eliminating aggregation and accumulation.

Ju syndrome:

Liver qi stagnation

Migrating abdominal flatulence with transient distending pain, aggravated by emotional stress.

S: Distention and fullness in the hypochondriac regions.

T: Thin coating. **P:** Wiry.

- Spread liver qi, relieve constraint, and reduce the accumulation.
- *Xiao Yao San*
  - *Chai Hu* spreads liver qi.
  - *Dang Gui* tonifies the blood and nourishes the liver.
  - *Bai Shao* preserves the yin, generates the fluid and comforts the liver.
  - *Bai Zhu*, *Fu Ling* and *Gan Cao* benefit the qi and strengthen the spleen.
  - *Bo He* is acrid to disperse constrained liver qi.
- To strengthen the effects of spreading liver qi and relieving constraint. + *Xiang Fu*, *Qing Pi*, *Mu Xiang*

  Signs of blood stasis. + *Yan Hu Suo*, *E Zhu*

Food retention and phlegm obstruction

Abdominal distention and pain with a rod-shaped abdominal prominence, pain elicited by pressure.

S: Constipation and poor appetite.

T: Greasy coating. **P:** Wiry and slippery.

- Guide out the accumulation and unblock the bowel, regulate the qi and transform phlegm.
- *Liu Mo Tang*
  - *Da Huang* drains downwards to reduce accumulation and unblock the bowel.
  - *Zhi Shi* and *Bing Lang* facilitate the qi flow and transform accumulation.
  - *Chen Xiang*, *Mu Xiang* and *Wu Yao* regulate the qi and resolve dampness.
- To enhance the effect of transforming phlegm-dampness. + *Chen Pi*, *Ban Xia*

  Recurrent episodes causing spleen qi injury, use *Xiang Sha Liu Jun Zi Tang*.

Ji syndrome:

Qi stagnation disturbing blood circulation

Abdominal masses, soft and fixed to palpation, with distention and pain.
T: Thin coating. **P:** Wiry.

- Regulate the qi, invigorate the blood, and reduce aggregation.
- *Jin Ling Zi San*
  - *Chuan Lian Zi* soothes the liver and regulates the qi.
  - *Yan Hu Suo* invigorates the blood and alleviates pain.
- To reinforce the effect of invigorating the blood. + *Shi Xiao San*

Blood stasis

Substantial abdominal masses, firm and tender to palpation, with a fixed location.
S: Dusky complexion, emaciation, dry and flaky skin, and amenorrhea.
T: Purple tongue with petechiae and thin coating. **P:** Thready and choppy.

- Expel stasis and soften hardness.
- *Ge Xia Zhu Yu Tang*
  - *Tao Ren*, *Hong Hua*, *Chuan Xiong*, *Chi Shao*, *Dang Gui*, *Wu Ling Zhi*, *Mu Dan Pi* and *Yan Hu Suo* invigorate the blood and transform stasis.
  - *Xiang Fu*, *Wu Yao* and *Zhi Qiao* facilitate the flow of qi to alleviate pain.
- To enhance the effects of breaking up and expelling stasis, and softening hardness. + *Chuan Lian Zi*, *San Leng*, *E Zhu*
  Large, firm masses with significant pain. + *Bei Jia Jian Wan*

Deficient righteous qi with pathological aggregation

Chronic, intractable hard masses with excruciating pain.
S: Sallow or dark complexion, reduction in food intake and emaciation.
T: Pale purple tongue without coating. **P:** Thready and rapid, or wiry and thready.

- Strongly tonify the qi and blood, invigorate the blood and transform stasis.
- *Ba Zhen Tang* and *Hua Ji Wan*
  - *Ba Zhen Tang* tonifies the qi and nourishes the blood.
  - *Hua Ji Wan* softens hardness, dissipates clumps, invigorates the blood and breaks up blood stasis.
- Severe yin injury with mirror tongue, and a rapid thready pulse. + *Sheng Di Huang*, *Sha Shen*, *Shi Hu*

Acupuncture Treatment

- **Manipulation:** Reducing method for excess patterns; reinforcing method for deficiency patterns.
- **Prescription:** CV12 Zhongwan PC6 Neiguan GB34 Yanglingquan BL18 Ganshu Extra20 Pigen
- **Supplementary points:**

  - Qi stagnation. + LR3 Taichong; TE5 Waiguan
  - Phlegm accumulation. + LU5 Chize; ST40 Fenglong
  - Blood stasis. + BL17 Geshu; SP10 Xuehai
  - Righteous qi deficiency. + CV6 Qihai; ST36 Zusanli

Practical Hints

Early diagnosis and treatment favors an optimistic prognosis. *Ji ju* refers to masses localized in the abdominal cavity with manifestations of pain or distention. This disorder very much resembles various benign or malignant abdominal tumors in modern medicine. *Ju*, pertaining to the qi level, occurs at the initial stage of the disorder when the condition is mild and manageable. As the condition becomes worse, *ji*, pertaining to the blood level, develops. *Ji* is the aggregation of phlegm and stagnant blood or occlusion of the vessels and is relatively severe. At the initial stage of *ji ju*, when pathogens are present and the righteous qi is intact, treatment should focus on attacking and expelling the pathogens. However, at the later stage, the pathogens are still present and the righteous qi has been exhausted. The treatment then should be modified to primarily tonify or support the righteous qi while auxiliary measures should be used to expel the pathogens. Auxiliary measures include transforming phlegm, softening hardness, expelling stasis, and dissipating nodules. It is necessary to closely monitor the development of the condition. Presence of jaundice and upper or lower gastrointestinal bleeding indicates worsening *ji ju*; tympanic abdominal distention is very likely to develop. These signs carry an unfavorable prognosis.

CHAPTER 36

Tympanic Abdominal Distention

臌脹 *Gu Zhang*

Named after its clinical presentation, tympanic abdominal distention is characterized by drum-like abdominal distention, pale-sallow skin tone, distended veins on the abdominal wall, hypochondriac or abdominal masses, and thin limbs. Pathological derivatives of the qi, blood and water, resulting from dysfunctions of the liver, spleen and kidney, accumulate in the abdominal cavity. This disorder is chronic, lingering, and intractable in nature. Critical symptoms, including hematemesis, hematochezia or melena, and comatose, may manifest at the end stage of the disorder.

Relevant Diseases

- Chronic hepatitis
- Cirrhosis with ascites
- Hepatic tumor
- Tuberculous peritonitis
- Metastatic cancer
- Schistosomiasis
- Systemic lupus erythematosus
- Tympanites

Etiology and Pathogenesis

Improper diet, including excessive consumption of alcohol and irregular eating patterns, directly damages the spleen. Dampness accumulates in the middle burner and obstructs the movement of qi, affecting the liver. The ensuing qi stagnation and blood stasis cause further injury to the spleen and involve the kidney, which has difficulty eliminating turbidity. As clear and turbid fuse and linger internally, water retention develops into tympanic abdominal distention.

Emotional stress primarily affects the liver by interfering with its function of regulating and distributing the qi, causing qi stagnation followed by blood stasis. Stagnant liver qi overacts on the spleen and stomach resulting in dampness. Water, dampness, stagnant qi and blood stasis fuse together and linger inside the abdomen. Eventually, the kidney's ability to eliminate water is impaired. Retarded elimination of pathological accumulation forms tympanic abdominal distention.

Infestation of schistosomes, as a precipitating factor, induces disharmony between the liver and spleen by obstructing the vessels and channels. Phlegm turbidity is generated and followed by chronic qi stagnation, blood stasis and phlegm accumulation. Unremitting, this condition progresses to tympanic abdominal distention as the pathological derivatives accumulate and fuse.

Chronic jaundice and abdominal masses: Jaundice results from accumulation of damp-heat or cold-dampness in the middle burner. Chronic damage occurs to the liver, spleen and kidney while qi and blood stagnate and the vessels and channels become obstructed. Abdominal masses form from qi stagnation, phlegm accumulation and blood stasis, growing progressively worse as time passes by. Consequently, localized or insignificant abdominal distention gradually grows into tympanic abdominal distention.

During the pathogenesis of this disorder, qi stagnation, blood stasis and water retention are in a cause-and-effect relationship and aggravate each other. They pertain to excess pathology. Deficiencies of righteous qi, specifically insufficiencies of the liver, spleen and kidney, result from pathological excess. The initial pathology involves the liver and spleen, chronically affecting the kidney. When kidney yang is deficient and fails to warm the spleen, pathology of spleen and kidney yang deficiency is apparent; on the other hand, when kidney yin is deficient and fails to nourish the liver, liver and kidney yin deficiency is evident. Tympanic abdominal distention is a complicated disorder with a deficient root and an excess branch.

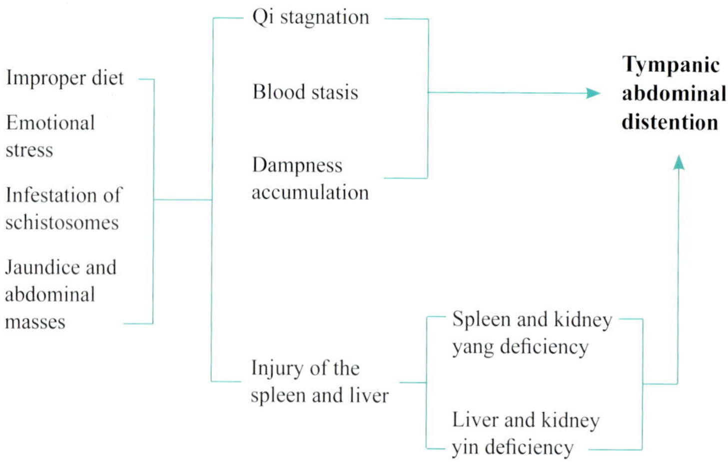

Diagnosis

A. Identification of qi stagnation, blood stasis and water retention:

In addition to the presence of drum-like abdominal distention, other manifestations may be present according to the contents in the distended abdominal cavity.

- Qi stagnation includes hypochondriac distention, a predilection for sighing, bitter taste in the mouth and wiry pulse; abdominal distention is momentarily alleviated by belching and passing flatus.
- Blood stasis is marked by distended veins on the abdominal wall, hypochondriac or abdominal masses, also spider angiomas on the face, neck, chest or arms, and palmar erythema, dry and flaky skin, dark red lips and nails, and petechiae on the tongue.
- Water retention manifests with abdominal distention and the sound of splashing water in the abdomen, shifting dullness on percussion, lassitude, fatigue and lack of strength, scanty urine and loose stool.

B. Identification of organ involvement:

Depending on the organs involved, clinical presentations will vary.

Spleen qi deficiency is characterized by a sallow complexion, lassitude, fatigue, poor appetite, a pale tongue and a decelerating pulse.

Spleen yang deficiency presents with cold intolerance, cold limbs, watery stool, a flabby pale tongue, and a deep, thready and forceless pulse.

Spleen and kidney yang deficiency is characterized by daybreak diarrhea, cold pain in the lower back and knees, impotence, and suppressed menstruation with pale, scanty menses.

Liver and kidney yin deficiency manifests as dizziness, tinnitus, soreness and weakness of the lower back and knees, irritability, insomnia, and hemorrhages.

C. Differential diagnosis of tympanic abdominal distention and edema:

As tympanic abdominal distention and edema progress to end stage, it becomes more difficult to identify and differentiate each disorder. Therefore, early diagnosis is necessary to guide the treatment.

	Tympanic Abdominal Distention	Edema
Affected Areas	Abdomen only.	Face, four extremities and entire body.
Accompanied Symptoms	Distended veins on the abdomen, spider angiomas, hematemesis, hematochezia or melena, jaundice, fever, agitation, and possible coma.	Stifling sensation in the chest, palpitations, dyspnea, nausea, vomiting, irritability and lethargy.

Basic Patterns

- Qi stagnation and dampness obstruction
- Cold-dampness hindering the spleen
- Damp-heat accumulation
- Liver and spleen blood stasis
- Spleen and kidney yang deficiency
- Liver and kidney yin deficiency

Differentiation and Treatment

Treatment principle:

Initial stage or excess pattern: Depending on the preponderance of qi stagnation, blood stasis, cold-dampness or damp-heat accumulation, treatment should regulate the qi and drain dampness, facilitate the qi movement and invigorate the blood circulation, strengthen the spleen and drain water, or aggressively force out the water accumulation with harsh expellants.

Late stage or deficiency pattern: Strengthen the spleen, warm the kidney, or nourish and replenish the liver and kidney yin.

Qi stagnation and dampness obstruction

Tympanic abdominal distention that is soft upon palpation, and a tympanic sound on percussion.

S: Distention and pain in the hypochondriac regions, poor appetite, increased distention after meals, distention alleviated by belching or passing flatus, bodily heaviness, fatigue and scanty urination.

T: White greasy coating. **P:** Wiry and slippery.

- Spread liver constraint and regulate the qi, eliminate dampness and reduce distention.
- *Chai Hu Shu Gan San*
  - *Chai Hu*, *Xiang Fu* and *Zhi Qiao* spread constrained liver qi.
  - *Chuan Xiong* and *Chi Shao* promote the movement of qi and invigorate the blood.
- To strengthen the effects of facilitating the qi flow and soothing the liver. + *Chuan Lian Zi*, *Qing Pi*

  To eliminate dampness and reduce distention. + *Wei Ling Tang*

Stabbing pain and masses in the hypochondriac regions. + *Yan Hu Suo, E Zhu, Dan Shen*

Lassitude, watery stool, flabby tongue and decelerating pulse. + *Gan Jiang, Sha Ren*

Cold-dampness hindering the spleen

Tympanic abdominal distention with baggy flanks that deform on palpation, a dull note on percussion, and a splashing sound on auscultation.

S: Swollen face and lower extremities, focal distention in the epigastrium and abdomen, distention relieved by warmth, lassitude, cold intolerance, scanty urine output and watery stool.

T: White greasy coating. **P:** Decelerating.

- Warm the middle burner, strengthen the spleen, facilitate the movement of qi, and promote urination.
- *Shi Pi Yin*
  - *Fu Zi*, *Gan Jiang*, *Bai Zhu* and *Gan Cao* warm the yang, strengthen the spleen and drain dampness.
  - *Mu Gua* and *Fu Ling* drain dampness.
  - *Hou Po*, *Da Fu Pi*, *Mu Xiang* and *Cao Guo* facilitate the flow of qi and dry dampness.
- To reinforce the function of qi transformation and promoting urination. + *Rou Gui, Zhu Ling, Ze Xie*

  Shortness of breath. + *Huang Qi, Dang Shen*

  Distention and pain in the hypochondrium and abdomen. + *Yu Jin, Qing Pi*

Damp-heat accumulation

Tympanic abdominal distention that is tense and firm to palpation, and excessive fullness limiting flexion at the waist.

S: Irritability, fever, bitter taste in the mouth, thirst with no desire to drink, dark scanty urination, constipation, and possible jaundice.

T: Red tongue with yellow greasy coating. **P:** Wiry and rapid.

- Clear heat, drain dampness, purge and force out accumulation.
- *Zhong Man Fen Xiao Wan*
  - *Huang Qin*, *Huang Lian* and *Zhi Mu* clear heat and dry dampness.
  - *Hou Po*, *Zhi Qiao*, *Ban Xia* and *Chen Pi* facilitate the qi flow and dry dampness.
  - *Fu Ling*, *Zhu Ling* and *Ze Xie* are bland and leach out dampness.
- Damp-heat jaundice, use *Yin Chen Hao Tang*.

Liver and spleen blood stasis

Tympanic abdominal distention that is tight and firm to palpation, visible distended veins on the abdomen, and stabbing pain in the hypochondriac regions and abdomen.

S: Spider angiomas on the face, neck, chest and arms, palmar erythema, tarry stool, dark purplish lips, thirst with desire to wet the mouth and inability to keep the water down.

T: Dark purplish tongue with petechiae. **P:** Thready and choppy.

- Invigorate the blood, transform blood stasis, facilitate the movement of qi, and promote urination.

- *Tiao Ying Yin*

  - *Dang Gui*, *Chuan Xiong*, *Chi Shao* and *Yan Hu Suo* invigorate the blood and transform stasis.

  - *Da Huang* and *E Zhu* break up and expel blood stasis.

  - *Bing Lang*, *Ting Li Zi* and *Sang Bai Pi* facilitate the movement of qi, reduce accumulation and drain water.

  - *Chi Fu Ling* and *Qu Mai* promote urination and reduce edema.

- Tarry stool. + *San Qi*, *Ce Bai Ye*

  Significant distention with a robust constitution, use *Zhou Che Wan* and *Shi Zao Tang* on a short-term basis to force out pathological fluids.

Spleen and kidney yang deficiency

Tympanic abdominal distention, which is better in the morning and worse in the evening.

S: Pale complexion, fullness in the epigastrium, poor appetite, cold intolerance, frigid extremities, swollen lower extremities and scanty urine.

T: Flabby and pale purple tongue. **P:** Deep, wiry and forceless.

- Warm and tonify the spleen and kidney yang, transform the qi and promote urination.

- *Fu Zi Li Zhong Wan* and *Wu Ling San* for spleen yang deficiency.

  - *Fu Zi Li Zhong Wan* warms and tonifies the yang of spleen and kidney and disperses cold.

  - *Wu Ling San* warms and unblocks the yang; it assists qi transformation and water metabolism.

- *Ji Sheng Shen Qi Wan* for kidney yang deficiency.

  - *Ji Sheng Shen Qi Wan*, a modified formula from *Jin Gui Shen Qi Wan*, warms and tonifies kidney yang, as well as promotes urination and reduces edema.

Liver and kidney yin deficiency

Tympanic abdominal distention, possibly distended veins on the abdomen.
S: Dusky complexion, purplish lips, dry throat, irritability, insomnia, subcutaneous and mucosal bleeding, and scanty urination.
T: Dry dark red tongue with scanty coating. **P:** Wiry, thready and rapid.

- Nourish the yin of liver and kidney, cool the blood and transform stasis.
- *Ge Xia Zhu Yu Tang* with either *Liu Wei Di Huang Wan* or *Yi Guan Jian*
  - *Ge Xia Zhu Yu Tang* invigorates the blood and transforms stasis; it is a basic formula for blood stasis located at hypochondriac regions, and for abdominal pain with masses.
  - *Liu Wei Di Huang Wan* tonifies kidney yin and replenishes the essence; it is the basic formula for kidney yin deficiency.
  - *Yi Guan Jian* nourishes liver yin, and softens and comforts the liver; it is a basic formula for liver yin deficiency.
- Significant yin deficiency with empty fire manifested by dry mouth, and dry and dark red tongue. + *Xuan Shen, Mai Men Dong, Shi Hu*
  Scanty urine. + *Zhu Ling, Hua Shi, Bai Mao Gen*
  Subcutaneous and mucosal bleeding with large dark purpura. + *Xian He Cao, Bai Mao Gen, Qian Cao Gen*
  Yin deficiency and yang rising with tinnitus. + *Gui Ban, Bie Jia, Mu Li*

Acupuncture Treatment

Qi stagnation:

- **Manipulation:** Reducing method.
- **Prescription:** CV17 Tanzhong, CV12 Zhongwan, CV6 Qihai, LR3 Taichong, ST36 Zusanli

Dampness accumulation:

- **Manipulation:** Reducing method. Moxibustion is applicable.
- **Prescription:** BL20 Pishu, BL23 Shenshu, CV9 Shuifen, KI7 Fuliu, SP4 Gongsun

Blood stasis:

- **Manipulation:** Reducing method.
- **Prescription:** LR14 Qimen, LR13 Zhangmen, CV5 Shimen, SP6 Sanyinjiao

Practical Hints

Temporary decompression with harsh expellants if righteous qi is intact. Most cases of tympanic abdominal distention are complicated conditions of excess and deficiency. When a patient has significant distention and his/her righteous qi is still intact, harsh expellant herbs and formulas may be used on a short-term basis. These herbs and formulas act aggressively to force out the pathological fluids via urination and bowel movements. The rationale for eliminating accumulated fluids from the abdominal cavity is supported by the modern medical measure of abdominal paracentesis, used to reduce the abdominal pressure in ascites. The classic formula, *Zhou Che Wan*, is formulated for this specific purpose. Because the ingredients in this formula are harsh and toxic, adverse effects should be monitored, such as nausea, vomiting, abdominal pain and headache. Fatigue is often seen as excessive unmetabolized fluid is removed. For those who have a bleeding tendency or cirrhosis with established collateral circulation, this formula may elicit upper and lower gastrointestinal hemorrhage. Because it has the potential to harm the righteous qi, this method and formula or class of herbs can only be used temporarily when the righteous qi remains intact.

CHAPTER 37

Hemorrhage

血證 *Xue Zheng*

Hemorrhage refers to emission of blood from its physiological reservoirs, such as the blood vessels and organs, with seepage into the surrounding tissues or discharge through the orifices. In internal medicine, the most common types of hemorrhage, or bleeding, are hemoptysis (coughing up blood); hematemesis (vomiting up blood); hematuria (blood in the urine); hematochezia and melena (blood in the stool); and subcutaneous and mucosal hemorrhages including epistaxis, bleeding gums, purpura and petechiae. Excessive bleeding can be critical and life-threatening if hemorrhagic shock or asphyxia occurs; asphyxia is caused by blood clots obstructing the airway.

Relevant Diseases

- Bronchiectasis
- Pulmonary tuberculosis
- Pulmonary abscess
- Lung cancer
- Acute gastritis
- Peptic ulcer
- Gastric cancer
- Liver cirrhosis
- Kidney stone
- Bladder, prostate and kidney tumor
- Thrombocytopenia purpura
- Hemophilia
- Hemopathy

Etiology and Pathogenesis

External pathogenic factors, particularly wind-heat, dryness and heat or fire, injure the blood vessels and make the blood run recklessly. External heat attacking the lung can cause hemoptysis or epistaxis; fire toxicity trapped in the nutritive or blood level can induce various types of hemorrhages; damp-heat accumulated in the intestines can lead to hematochezia; damp-heat infusing downwards to the bladder can cause hematuria.

Improper diet: Indulgence in hot spicy food or alcohol causes hemorrhages by producing internal damp-heat accumulation or by impairing the function of the spleen and stomach. Damp-heat accumulation in the middle burner can lead to hematemesis, hematochezia or melena, and bleeding gums. Improper diet impairs the spleen so that it fails to control the blood in the vessels resulting in hematemesis, hematochezia or melena, hematuria, and subcutaneous and mucosal bleeding.

Emotional stress: Excessive or prolonged emotional stimulations leads to qi stagnation that may transform into fire. Bleeding occurs when fire enters the vessels and causes the blood to move recklessly. Anger injures the liver and makes the liver qi stagnate. If the liver overacts on the stomach, there may be hematemesis; if liver qi stagnation transforms into liver fire and insults the lung, there may be hemoptysis or epistaxis; if pensiveness generates heart fire that moves downwards to the small intestine, there may be hematuria.

Overexertion: Mental or physical overexertion damages the qi and yin of the heart, spleen, and kidney. Deficient qi cannot control the blood, which leaks out of the vessels and results in hematemesis, blood in the stool, or subcutaneous and mucosal bleeding. Yin deficiency creates empty heat which forces blood out of the vessels leading to hematuria or subcutaneous and mucosal bleeding.

Chronic illness or the late stage of a febrile disease can lead to empty fire due to insufficiency of the body fluid and blood; empty fire induces bleeding. Qi may be consumed during a disease, weakening its function of holding the blood in the vessels. Lastly, the initial stage of disease affects the qi level or disturbs the movement of the qi; however, prolonged illness damages a deeper layer of the body, the blood level, and causes blood stasis in the minute collaterals and vessels. When the blood is unable to travel inside the vessels due to blood stasis obstruction, it will escape into the surrounding tissues.

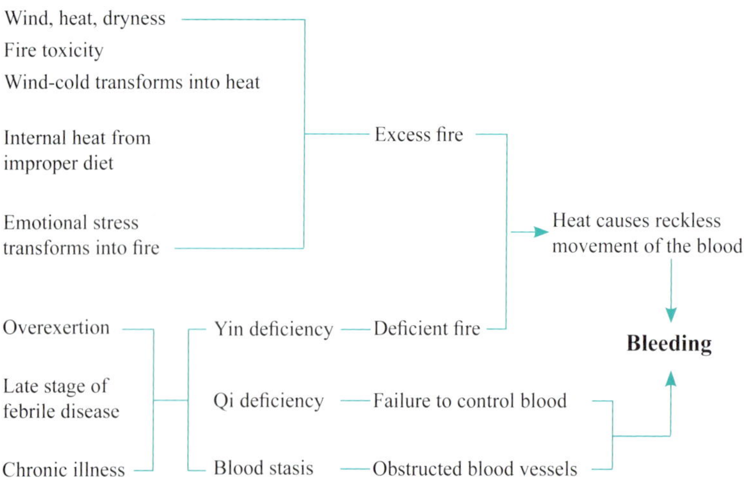

Diagnosis

A. Identification of associated pathogenic factors:

- Stomach fire manifests as hematemesis, blood in the stool or subcutaneous and mucosal bleeding with a fresh red color. Heat signs include a red face, irritability, bad breath, burning epigastric pain, a red tongue with yellow coating, and a slippery and rapid pulse.
- Liver fire flaring up can induce hematemesis, hemoptysis, and epistaxis with fresh red blood. Other symptoms include distending pain in the hypochondria, irritability, a red tongue with yellow coating, and a wiry and rapid pulse.
- Excessive heat causing reckless movement of the blood can manifest as hemoptysis, blood in the stool, or subcutaneous and mucosal bleeding with a fresh red color. Other symptoms include fever, thirst, irritability, constipation, scanty urine, a red tongue with yellow coating, and a slippery and rapid pulse.
- Yin deficiency with empty fire leads to hemoptysis, blood in the stool, or subcutaneous and mucosal bleeding, accompanied by dizziness, tinnitus, tidal fever, a red tongue with scanty coating, and a thready and rapid pulse.
- Qi failing to control the blood presents as bleeding with pale reddish blood. Common types of bleeding are hematemesis, blood in the stool, or subcutaneous and mucosal bleeding. Symptoms related to qi deficiency, such as fatigue, lassitude, dizziness, palpitations, a pale tongue with a thin white coating, and a thready and weak pulse, will be evident.
- Deficient cold of the spleen and stomach may result in blood in the stool and hematemesis with a scanty amount of dark red blood. Cold pain in the epigastrium and abdomen, cold limbs, a pale and flabby tongue, and a slow and forceless pulse are common manifestations of deficient cold.
- Qi collapse and blood depletion result from profuse and heavy bleeding. A pale face, nails and lips, profuse sweat and clammy skin, frigid extremities, lethargy and stupor, and a minute pulse indicate that the condition is life-threatening.

B. Identification of organ involvement by bleeding sites:

- Epistaxis – The lung, stomach or liver may be involved.
- Bleeding gums – The stomach or kidney may be involved.
- Hemoptysis – The lung or liver may be involved.
- Hematemesis – The spleen or stomach may be involved.
- Hematochezia or melena – The spleen, stomach or intestines may be involved.
- Hematuria – The kidney, spleen, heart or urinary bladder may be involved.
- Subcutaneous bleeding – The spleen, heart or kidney may be involved.

C. Identification of hemoptysis and hematemesis:

Hemoptysis: Blood is discharged from the respiratory system when coughing.

There could be blood-tinged sputum, mixed blood and sputum, or pure blood with a fresh red color and frothy appearance. Hemoptysis is preceded by coughing, itchy throat or chest congestion.

Hematemesis: Blood is discharged from the digestive system when vomiting. The blood can be fresh or dark red in color and undigested food may be apparent in the emesis. Hematemesis is preceded by stomachache or epigastric discomfort and nausea. Tarry stool can be seen after an episode of hematemesis.

Basic Patterns

Epistaxis (nosebleed):

- Heat attacking the lung
- Stomach heat
- Liver fire
- Qi and blood deficiency

Bleeding gums:

- Stomach fire
- Yin deficiency with empty fire

Hemoptysis (coughing blood):

- Dry-heat attacking the lung
- Liver fire
- Lung yin deficiency with empty fire

Hematemesis (vomiting blood):

- Stomach heat
- Liver fire
- Qi deficiency failing to control the blood

Hematochezia and melena (blood in the stool):

- Damp-heat in the intestines
- Spleen and stomach yang deficiency

Hematuria (blood in the urine):

- Heat in the lower burner
- Kidney yin deficiency with empty fire
- Spleen deficiency failing to control the blood
- Kidney deficiency failing to consolidate the lower burner

Subcutaneous bleeding:

- Heat in the blood
- Yin deficiency with empty fire
- Qi deficiency failing to control the blood

Differentiation and Treatment

Treatment principle:

Three primary treatment principles for treating hemorrhage address the three perspectives of fire, qi, and blood. Based on the principle of stopping bleeding by controlling fire, clear heat and drain fire for excess fire; nourish the yin and eliminate empty fire for deficient heat. Under the guideline of stopping bleeding by regulating the qi , facilitate and descend the qi flow for qi excess patterns, and tonify the qi for qi deficiency. The principle of harmonizing the blood to stop bleeding requires the careful selection of appropriate hemostatic herbs based on the pattern differentiation. Common methods to harmonize the blood include cooling the blood to stop bleeding, astringing to stop bleeding, invigorating the blood to stop bleeding, and warming the meridians to stop bleeding.

Epistaxis (nosebleed):

Heat attacking the lung

Nasal dryness and bleeding, dry mouth and throat.
S: Fever, coughing with scanty sputum.
T: Red tongue with thin yellow coating. **P:** Rapid.

- Clear heat from the lung, cool the blood and stop bleeding.
- *Sang Ju Yin*
  - *Sang Ye*, *Ju Hua*, *Bo He* and *Lian Qiao*, acrid and cool, disperse wind-heat.
  - *Jie Geng* and *Xing Ren* restore the dispersing and descending functions of lung qi, and benefit the throat.
  - *Lu Gen* clears heat and generates the fluid.
- To enhance the effects of cooling the blood and stopping bleeding. + *Mu Dan Pi, Bai Mao Gen, Ce Bai Ye, Han Lian Cao*
  Excessive lung heat. + *Huang Qin, Zhi Zi*
  Severe dryness of the mouth and nose. + *Xuan Shen, Mai Men Dong, Sheng Di Huang*

Stomach heat

Nasal bleeding or bleeding gums with fresh red blood.
S: Dry mouth, bad breath, desire for cold drink, irritability and constipation.
T: Red tongue with yellow coating. **P:** Rapid.

- Clear and drain stomach fire, cool the blood and stop bleeding.
- *Yu Nu Jian*
  - *Shi Gao* and *Zhi Mu* clear stomach heat and drain fire.

- *Di Huang* and *Mai Men Dong* nourish the yin and clear heat.
- *Niu Xi* guides the movement of blood downwards.

- To enhance the effects of cooling the blood and stopping bleeding. + *Bai Mao Gen, Da Ji, Ou Jie*
  Constipation. + *Sheng Da Huang*
  Damaged yin with a red tongue and scanty coating, and thready and rapid pulse. + *Tian Hua Fen, Shi Hu, Yu Zhu*

Liver fire

Nasal bleeding, headache, dizziness and a bitter taste in the mouth.
S: Red eyes, irritability, short temper and tinnitus.
T: Red tongue. **P:** Wiry and rapid.

- Clear and drain liver fire, cool the blood and stop bleeding.
- *Long Dan Xie Gan Tang*
  - *Long Dan Cao*, *Zhi Zi* and *Huang Qin* clear liver heat and drain fire.
  - *Sheng Di Huang* and *Dang Gui* nourish the yin and blood.
  - *Che Qian Zi*, *Mu Tong* and *Ze Xie* clear and drain damp-heat.
- Enhance the effect to stop bleeding. + *Bai Mao Gen, Pu Huang, Ou Jie*
  Damaged yin with dry mouth and nose. + *Xuan Shen, Mai Men Dong, Han Lian Cao*

Qi and blood deficiency

Nasal bleeding with a light red color, or bleeding gums, and subcutaneous and mucosal bleeding.
S: Pale complexion, insomnia, dizziness, palpitations, fatigue and lassitude.
T: Pale tongue. **P:** Thready and forceless.

- Tonify the qi to control the blood.
- *Gui Pi Tang*
  - *Gui Pi Tang* tonifies the qi to nourish the blood, as well as benefits the qi to restrain the blood.
- Enhance the effect to stop bleeding. + *Xian He Cao, E Jiao, Qian Cao*

Bleeding gums:

Stomach fire

Bleeding gums with fresh red blood, and red swollen painful gums.
S: Headache, bad breath and constipation.
T: Red tongue with yellow coating. **P:** Flooding and rapid.

- Clear stomach heat and drain fire, cool the blood and stop bleeding.
- *Qing Wei San*
  - *Huang Lian* clears stomach heat and drains fire.
  - *Sheng Di Huang* and *Mu Dan Pi* clear heat and cool the blood.
  - *Dang Gui* nourishes and invigorates the blood.
  - *Sheng Ma* vents heat and relieves toxicity.
- To enhance the effects of cooling the blood and stopping bleeding. + *Bai Mao Gen, Da Ji, Ou Jie*
  Red and swollen gums with purulent discharge. + *Jin Yin Hua, Pu Gong Ying*
  Severe thirst and constipation. + *Sheng Shi Gao, Zhi Mu, Da Huang*

Yin deficiency with empty fire

Bleeding gums with light red blood, swollen gums and loose teeth.
S: Chronic recurrent bleeding and five-centers heat.
T: Red tongue with scanty coating. **P:** Thready and rapid.

- Nourish the yin and eliminate fire, cool the blood and stop bleeding.
- *Zi Shui Qing Gan Yin*
  - *Zi Shui Qing Gan Yin*, a modified formula from *Liu Wei Di Huang Wan* and *Dan Zhi Xiao Yao San*, tonifies the liver and kidney, nourishes the yin and drains fire.
- To strengthen the effects of cooling the blood and stopping bleeding. + *Qian Cao Gen, E Jiao, Ce Bai Ye*

Hemoptysis (coughing blood):

Dry-heat attacking the lung

Cough, scratchy throat, blood-tinged sputum or coughing up pure blood.
S: Dry mouth and nose, fever, slight aversion to wind, and headache.
T: Dry red tongue with thin yellow coating. **P:** Rapid.

- Clear heat, moisten the lung and stop bleeding.
- *Sang Xing Tang*
  - *Sang Ye*, *Dan Dou Chi* and *Zhi Zi* clear and disperse lung heat.
  - *Sha Shen* and *Li Pi* nourish the yin and clear heat.
  - *Xing Ren* and *Bei Mu* moisten the lung and stop coughing.
- To enhance the effects of cooling the blood and stopping bleeding. + *Bai Mao Gen, Ce Bai Ye, Qian Cao*
  Exterior wind-heat. + *Jin Yin Hua, Lian Qiao, Ju Hua, Niu Bang Zi*
  Excessive heat in the lung. + *Sheng Shi Gao, Huang Qin, Sang Bai Pi*

Liver fire

Paroxysmal cough, blood-tinged sputum or coughing up pure blood, symptoms aggravated by emotions and stress.
S: Irritability, short temper, bitter taste in the mouth, dry throat, distending pain in the chest and hypochondriac regions.
T: Red tongue with thin yellow coating. **P:** Wiry and rapid.

- Clear heat from the liver and lung, cool the blood and stop bleeding.
- *Xie Bai San* and *Dai Ge San*
  - *Sang Bai Pi* and *Di Gu Pi* clear and drain lung heat.
  - *Qing Dai* clears liver heat and cools the blood.
  - *Hai Ge Ke* and *Gan Cao* clear lung heat and transform phlegm.
- To enhance the effects of cooling the blood and stopping bleeding. + *Sheng Di Huang, Han Lian Cao, Bai Mao Gen*
  Severe liver fire. + *Mu Dan Pi, Zhi Zi, Huang Qin*

Lung yin deficiency with empty fire

Dry cough with blood-tinged sputum or recurrent coughing of blood with fresh red color.
S: Dry mouth and throat, malar flush, tidal fever and night sweating.
T: Red tongue with scanty coating. **P:** Thready and rapid.

- Nourish the yin, moisten the lung and stop bleeding.
- *Bai He Gu Jin Wan*
  - *Bai He*, *Mai Men Dong*, *Xuan Shen* and *Di Huang* nourish the yin, generate the fluid and clear heat.
  - *Dang Gui* and *Bai Shao* replenish the yin and blood.
  - *Bei Mu* and *Gan Cao* transform phlegm and stop coughing.
- Enhance the effect to stop bleeding. + *Bai Ji, Ou Jie, Bai Mao Gen*
  Coughing blood constantly. + *E Jiao, San Qi*
  Tidal fever and hot flushes. + *Bie Jia, Di Gu Pi*
  Night sweating. + *Fu Xiao Mai, Wu Wei Zi*

Hematemesis (vomiting blood):

Stomach heat

Distending pain in the epigastrium and abdomen, vomiting red or dark purple blood. The vomitus often contains undigested food.
S: Bad breath, constipation or tarry stool.
T: Red tongue with yellow greasy coating. **P:** Slippery and rapid.

- Clear heat and drain fire, invigorate the blood and stop bleeding.
- *Xie Xin Tang*
  - *Huang Qin*, *Huang Lian* and *Da Huang* clear heat and drain fire.
- To enhance the effects of cooling and invigorating the blood to stop bleeding without leaving blood stasis. + *Shi Hui San*
  Nausea and vomiting. + *Xuan Fu Hua, Dai Zhe Shi, Zhu Ru*
  Distending epigastric and abdominal pain. + *Zhi Qiao, Chuan Lian Zi*

Liver fire

Vomiting fresh red or dark purple blood, bitter taste in the mouth and hypochondriac pain.
S: Irritability, short temper, insomnia or dream-disturbed sleep.
T: Dark red. **P:** Wiry and rapid.

- Clear liver and stomach fire, cool the blood and stop bleeding.
- *Long Dan Xie Gan Tang*
- To enhance the effects of cooling the blood and stopping bleeding. + *Bai Mao Gen, Han Lian Cao, Qian Cao, Ou Jie*

Qi deficiency failing to control the blood

Intermittent vomiting of light reddish-purple blood.
S: Pale complexion, palpitations, shortness of breath, fatigue and lassitude.
T: Pale. **P:** Thready and weak.

- Strengthen the spleen, tonify the qi and control the blood.
- *Gui Pi Tang*
- Enhance the channel warming and astringing effects to stop bleeding. + *Xian He Cao, Bai Ji, Hai Piao Xiao, Pao Jiang*
  Yang deficiency secondary to qi deficiency with cold intolerance and frigid extremities. + *Pao Jiang Tan, Ai Ye, Ce Bai Ye*
  Qi collapse due to severe bleeding with minute pulse, use *Du Shen Tang*.

Hematochezia and melena (blood in the stool):

Damp-heat in the intestines

Fresh red blood in the stool, uncomfortable sensation of incomplete defecation, and loose stool.
S: Burning sensation of the anus, distention and pain in the abdomen, and a bitter taste in the mouth.
T: Yellow greasy coating. **P:** Slippery and rapid.

- Clear heat, dry dampness, cool the blood and stop bleeding.
- *Di Yu San*
  - *Di Yu* and *Qian Cao Gen* cool the blood and stop bleeding.
  - *Huang Qin*, *Huang Lian* and *Zhi Zi* clear heat, dry dampness and relieve toxicity.
  - *Fu Ling* is bland to leach out and drain dampness.
- Severe bleeding. + *Huai Hua Mi, Bai Ji, San Qi, Ce Bai Ye*

Spleen and stomach yang deficiency

Dark red or tarry stool, dull abdominal pain and desire for warm beverages.
S: Pale and sallow complexion, fatigue, lethargy and loose stool.
T: Pale tongue with thin white coating. **P:** Thready and weak.

- Strengthen the spleen, warm the middle burner, nourish the blood and stop bleeding.
- *Huang Tu Tang*
  - *Zao Xin Tu* (*Fu Long Gan*) warms the middle burner and stops bleeding.
  - *Fu Zi* warms the yang and dipserses cold.
  - *Bai Zhu* and *Gan Cao* warm the middle burner and strengthen the spleen.
  - *E Jiao* and *Di Huang* nourish the blood and stop bleeding.
- Enhance the effect to astringe and stop bleeding. + *Bai Ji, Hai Piao Xiao*
  Enhance the effects of invigorating the blood and stopping bleeding. + *San Qi, Hua Rui Shi*
  Yang deficiency with cold limbs. + *Lu Jiao Shuan, Ai Ye, Pao Jiang*

Hematuria (blood in the urine):

Heat in the lower burner

Dark urination containing fresh blood, and burning sensation during urination.
S: Irritability, intense thirst, red face, sores in the mouth or on the tongue, insomnia or restless sleep.
T: Red. **P:** Rapid.

- Clear heat, drain fire, cool the blood and stop bleeding.
- *Xiao Ji Yin Zi*
  - *Xiao Ji*, *Sheng Di Huang*, *Ou Jie* and *Pu Huang* cool the blood and stop bleeding.
  - *Zhi Zi* and *Zhu Ye* clear heat and drain fire.
  - *Hua Shi* and *Mu Tong* drain dampness and clear heat.
- Enhance the effect to purge fire. + *Huang Lian, Huang Bai*

Kidney yin deficiency with empty fire

Scanty urine containing blood, dizziness, vertigo, tinnitus, hot flushes and tidal fever.
S: Fatigue, emaciation, nocturnal emission, soreness and weakness of the lower back and knees, and night sweating.
T: Red tongue with scanty coating. **P:** Thready and rapid.

- Nourish the yin, eliminate empty fire, cool the blood and stop bleeding.
- *Zhi Bai Di Huang Wan*
  - *Liu Wei Di Huang Wan* nourishes and tonifies kidney yin.
  - *Zhi Mu* and *Huang Bai* nourish the yin and drain fire.
- To strengthen the effect of nourishing the yin. + *Gui Ban*
  To strengthen the effects of cooling the blood and stopping bleeding. + *Da Ji, Bai Mao Gen, Pu Huang*

Spleen deficiency failing to control the blood

Blood in the urine and a history of chronic illness.
S: Sallow complexion, fatigue, lassitude, shortness of breath, possibly bleeding gums or subcutaneous bleeding.
T: Pale. **P:** Thready and weak.

- Tonify the spleen to stop bleeding.
- *Gui Pi Tang*
- To strengthen the effects of nourishing the blood and stopping bleeding. + *Shu Di Huang, E Jiao, Xian He Cao, Huai Hua Mi*
  Qi sinking with heavy sensation in the abdomen. + *Sheng Ma, Chai Hu*

Kidney deficiency failing to consolidate the lower burner

Light red blood in the urine and a history of chronic illness.
S: Dizziness, vertigo, fatigue, and soreness of the lower back and knees.
T: Pale. **P:** Deep and weak.

- Tonify the kidney, stabilize the lower burner and stop bleeding.
- *Wu Bi Shan Yao Wan*
  - *Shu Di Huang*, *Shan Yao* and *Shan Zhu Yu* augment kidney essence.
  - *Rou Cong Rong*, *Tu Si Zi*, *Ba Ji Tian*, *Du Zhong* and *Niu Xi* assist the yang and warm the kidney.
  - *Fu Ling* strengthens the spleen.
  - *Wu Wei Zi* and *Chi Shi Zhi* astringe.
- Enhance the hemostatic effect. + *Xian He Cao, Pu Huang, Huai Hua Mi*

Subcutaneous bleeding:

Heat in the blood

Fever and sudden appearance of purpura or petechiae on the skin.
S: Other types of bleeding, thirst and constipation.
T: Red tongue with yellow coating. **P:** Wiry and rapid.

- Clear heat, relieve toxicity, cool the blood and stop bleeding.
- *Xi Jiao Di Huang Tang*
  - *Shui Niu Jiao* (substitute for *Xi Jiao*) and *Sheng Di Huang* clear heat and cool the blood.
  - *Mu Dan Pi* and *Chi Shao* cool and invigorate the blood.
- To enhance the effects of cooling the blood and stopping bleeding. + *Shi Hui San*
  Severe bleeding due to heat toxicity. + *Sheng Shi Gao, Long Dan Cao*

Yin deficiency with empty fire

Intermittent purpura or petechiae, five-centers heat and tidal fever.
S: Other types of bleeding, hot flushes, irritability, thirst and night sweating.
T: Red tongue with scanty coating. **P:** Thready and rapid.

- Nourish the yin, eliminate empty fire and stop bleeding.
- *Qian Gen San*
  - *Qian Cao Gen*, *Ce Bai Ye* and *Huang Qin* clear heat, cool the blood and stop bleeding.
  - *Di Huang* and *E Jiao* nourish the yin, cool the blood and stop bleeding.
  - *Gan Cao* harmonizes the middle burner and relieves toxicity.
- Severe yin deficiency. + *Xuan Shen, Gui Ban, Nu Zhen Zi, Han Lian Cao*
  Kidney yin deficiency without excessive fire, use *Liu Wei Di Huang Wan*.

Qi deficiency failing to control the blood

Chronic and recurrent purpura or petechiae having a light red or dark red color, fatigue and lassitude.
S: Dizziness, vertigo, lack of appetite, pale or sallow complexion.
T: Pale and flabby tongue with thin white coating. **P:** Thready and weak.

- Tonify the qi to control the blood.
- *Gui Pi Tang*
- To strengthen the hemostatic effect. + *Xian He Cao, San Qi, Pu Huang Tan*
  Kidney qi deficiency. + *Shan Zhu Yu, Xu Duan, Tu Si Zi*
  Kidney yang deficiency. + *Xian Mao, Rou Gui*

Acupuncture Treatment

- **Manipulation:** Reducing method for all excess patterns; reinforcing or even method for all deficiency patterns.
- **Prescription:** Use the following primary points for specific types of hemorrhages; add auxiliary points based on the pattern differentiation.

Epistaxis:

- **Prescription:** LI20 Yingxiang LI4 Hegu GV23 Shangxing

Bleeding gums:

- **Prescription:** LI4 Hegu ST7 Xiaguan ST6 Jiache

Hemoptysis:

- **Prescription:** BL13 Feishu LU6 Kongzui LU5 Chize LU10 Yuji

Hematemesis:

- **Prescription:** CV13 Shangwan PC7 Daling PC4 Ximen HT7 Shenmen

Hematochezia and melena:

- **Prescription:** BL20 Pishu BL25 Dachangshu BL32 Ciliao GV1 Changqiang

Hematuria:

- **Prescription:** BL23 Shenshu CV4 Guanyuan

Subcutaneous bleeding:

- **Prescription:** BL17 Geshu BL20 Pishu SP10 Xuehai SP6 Sanyinjiao

Practical Hints

• **Hemorrhage can be caused by blood stasis**; this is a concept often being neglected when treating bleeding, especially chronic conditions. For instance, hematemesis as a result of peptic ulcer, purpura cased by thrombocytopenia, and persistent spotting of uterine blood are all closely related to blood stasis. Blood stasis not only obstructs the normal circulation of blood, but it also inhibits the regeneration of blood. In this case, even though bleeding is present, invigorating the blood to transform stasis remains the most appropriate treatment method. This is an application of the ancient treatment principle of unblocking the obstruction to treat an unremitting draining syndrome.

• **The substantial blood can not be generated immediately; therefore, adopt stabilizing the insubstantial qi at once as the principle.** In the case of excessive bleeding, qi collapse will follow blood loss. Clinical manifestations include pale complexion, clammy cold skin and extremities, abundant sweating and a minute pulse. This is a critical condition and the treatment principle is to strongly tonify the qi in order to save the patient from collapse. The imperial formula for first aid is *Du Shen Tang*.

CHAPTER 38

Abnormal Sweating

汗證 *Han Zheng*

Sweating, under normal circumstances, is a physiological function in which the body radiates heat and expels pathogenic factors from the superficial layer. Abnormal and excessive sweating that is not related to any environmental or physical influences is a pathological phenomenon.

Abnormal sweating is pathological perspiration due to disharmony between the yin and yang and an unconsolidated interstitial layer between the skin and muscle. Sweating during the day aggravated by mild activities is called spontaneous sweating. Sweating during the night ceased upon awakening is called night sweating. The focal sweating occuring unilaterally or on the head, hands or feet is called localized sweating.

Relevant Diseases:

- Hyperthyroidism
- Pulmonary tuberculosis
- Paroxysmal hypoglycemia
- Vegetative nerve functional disturbance
- Prostration
- Shock

Etiology and Pathogenesis

Deficiency of lung qi can result from constitutional lung deficiency or chronic cough consuming lung qi. Deficient lung qi fails to diffuse protective qi to the surface and interstitial layer between the skin and muscle. The pores in the unconsolidated protective layer open and abnormal sweating occurs.

Disharmony between protective qi and nutritive qi: When the equilibrium between the yin and yang is unstable, or when an exterior pathogen attacks a person with a pre-existing deficiency of protective qi, protective yang fails to restrain nutritive yin. As a result, abnormal sweating, pertaining to yin leakage, follows.

Yin deficiency with empty fire: Pathogenic heat injuring the yin, excessive blood or essence loss, and exhaustion of the yin due to excessive mental or physical exertion lead to yin deficiency with empty fire. Hyperactive empty fire may disturb the body fluid and force it to the surface where it leaks out of the pores as sweat.

Excess heat, including liver fire, stomach fire, and damp-heat, can disturb body fluid and force it out through the surface pores as sweat.

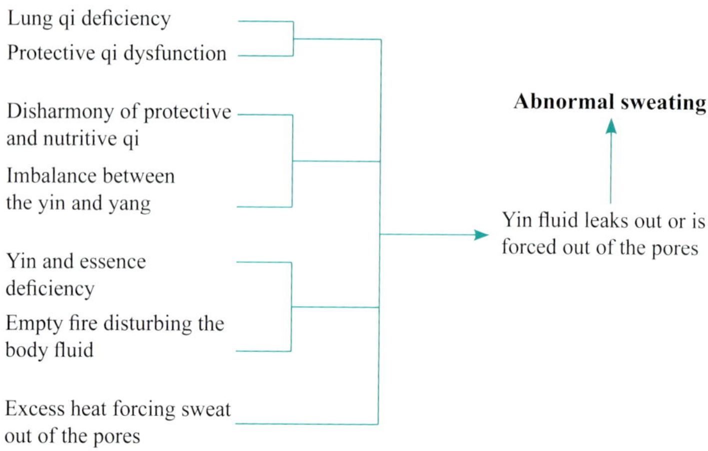

Diagnosis

A. Identification of types of abnormal sweating:

Spontaneous sweating: Associated with qi deficiency, spontaneous sweating occurs constantly throughout the day and is aggravated by mild activity.

Night sweating: Related to yin deficiency, night sweating occurs during sleep and ceases on awakening.

Collapse (*tuo*) sweating: Occurs in critical conditions when the righteous qi collapses and the yang can no longer restrain the yin. Clinical manifestations include profuse cold sweating, weak voice, shallow breathing, lassitude, frigid extremities and minute pulse. The prognosis is usually not favorable.

Shivering (*zhan*) sweating: Occurs during the acute stage of warm-febrile diseases. Shivering sweating occurs when the vigorous righteous qi attempts to expel pathogenic influences. Accompanying manifestations include high fever, irritability and intense thirst. After rigorous chills with profuse sweating, the fever will be reduced and systemic symptoms will be gradually relieved. Shivering sweating is a sign of sufficient righteous qi and the prognosis is usually favorable. Therefore, further treatment may not be required.

Yellow (*huang*) sweating: Characterized by sticky yellow sweat, yellow sweating may leave stains on the clothing. It is caused by damp-heat accumulation and it is associated with damp-heat jaundice.

Red (*hong*) sweating: Characterized by epistaxis that occurs during invasion of exterior wind-cold. Wind-cold congeals the surface of the body and closes the pores, preventing sweating. When a person's yang qi is vigorous, the robust righteous qi attempts to fight off the exterior pathogen. However, instead of perspiration, epistaxis occurs. This type of bleeding functions as perspiration, which releases the exterior; therefore, it is known as red sweating.

B. Identification of excess and deficiency:

- Spontaneous sweating is usually caused by qi deficiency.
- Night sweating is usually caused by yin deficiency.
- Liver fire and damp-heat induced sweating are excess conditions.
- Chronic abnormal sweating will injure the yin and lead to deficiency of both the qi and yin.
- Sweating due to internal accumulation of excess heat, which injures the yin, is a complex pattern of excess and deficiency.

Basic Patterns

- Lung qi deficiency
- Disharmony between protective and nutritive qi
- Yin deficiency with empty fire
- Excess heat flaring internally
- Damp-heat accumulation

Differentiation and Treatment

Treatment principle:

Deficient pattern: Benefit the qi, nourish the yin, consolidate the surface, and stop sweating.

Excess pattern: Clear and drain internal heat, resolve dampness and harmonize nutritive qi.

Because the pathogenesis of sweating is always related to an unconsolidated interstitial layer between the skin and muscle, herbs that stabilize and bind such as *Wu Wei Zi*, *Ma Huang Gen*, *Fu Xiao Mai* and *Mu Li* should be added to the selected formula.

In the case of profuse sweating that could deplete the yin and lead to the collapse of the yang, the treatment principle is to strongly tonify the qi, rescue the yang from collapse and restrain the remaining yin.

Lung qi deficiency

Aversion to wind, intermittent sweating aggravated by mild exertion, and susceptibility to catching cold.
S: Sallow complexion, poor appetite, fatigue and lassitude.
T: Thin white coating. **P:** Thready and weak.

- Tonify the qi and consolidate the exterior.
- *Yu Ping Feng San*
  - *Huang Qi* tonifies the qi, consolidates the surface and stops sweating.
  - *Bai Zhu* strengthens the spleen, dries dampness and assists *Huang Qi* to consolidate the surface.
  - *Fang Feng* disperses exterior wind; when used with *Huang Qi*, this combination will disperse as it tonifies.
- Excessive sweating. + *Ma Huang Gen, Fu Xiao Mai, Duan Mu Li*
  Severe qi deficiency. + *Dang Shen, Huang Jing*

Disharmony between protective and nutritive qi

Persistent sweating or localized sweating on the hands, feet, head, or half of the body, with persistent and recurrent episode of sweating.
S: Slight aversion to wind, low-grade fever, general body ache and headache.
T: Thin white coating. **P:** Floating and decelerating.

- Harmonize protective and nutritive qi.
- *Gui Zhi Tang*
  - *Gui Zhi*, acrid and warm, disperses exterior pathogens and acts on the protective qi.
  - *Bai Shao* is sour, preserves the yin and acts on the nutritive qi. When combined with *Gui Zhi*, one disperses and the other contains to harmonize the nutritive and protective qi.
  - *Sheng Jiang*, *Da Zao* and *Gan Cao* harmonize the middle burner.
- To strengthen the astringent effect. + *Duan Long Gu, Duan Mu Li*
  Significant qi deficiency. + *Huang Qi, Ren Shen*
  Significant yang deficiency. + *Fu Zi*

Yin deficiency with empty fire

Night sweating that ceases at the moment of awakening, insomnia, five-centers heat, and tidal fever.
S: Malar flush, dry mouth and throat, emaciation, irregular menstruation or nocturnal emission.
T: Tender red tongue with scanty coating. **P:** Thready and rapid.

- Nourish the yin, reduce empty fire and restrain sweating.
- *Dang Gui Liu Huang Tang*
  - *Sheng Di Huang*, *Shu Di Huang* and *Dang Gui* nourish the blood and yin.
  - *Huang Qin*, *Huang Lian* and *Huang Bai* clear heat.
  - *Huang Qi* augments the qi and consolidates the surface of the body.
- Steaming bone syndrome. + *Zhi Mu, Di Gu Pi, Qing Hao, Gui Ban, Bie Jia*
  Lung and kidney yin deficiency, use *Mai Wei Di Huang Wan*.

Excess heat flaring internally

Persistent profuse sweating or localized sweating on the head, irritability, restlessness, hot sensation in the chest, and thirst with desire to drink cold beverages.
S: Dark scanty urine or constipation.
T: Red tongue with thick yellow coating. **P:** Slippery and rapid.

- Clear heat and drain fire.
- *Bai Hu Tang*
  - *Shi Gao* clears heat, drains fire and eliminates irritability.
  - *Zhi Mu* clears heat, as well as nourishes the yin and generates the fluid.
  - *Gan Cao* and *Jing Mi* augment the stomach and generate the fluid.
- To enhance the effects of clearing heat and nourishing the yin. + *Sheng Di Huang, Mai Men Dong*
  Significant thirst and sweating. + *Xian Lu Gen, Tian Hua Fen, Shi Hu*
  Heat accumulation in the intestine with constipation. + *Xiao Cheng Qi Tang*

Damp-heat accumulation

Persistent perspiration with sticky sweat that leaves yellow stains on clothing, irritability and bitter taste in the mouth.
S: Fever, thirst without desire to drink, dark scanty urine and irregular bowel movements.
T: Red tongue with yellow greasy coating. **P:** Wiry and rapid.

- Clear heat and drain dampness.
- *Long Dan Xie Gan Tang*
  - *Long Dan Cao*, *Zhi Zi* and *Huang Qin* clear heat and drain fire.
  - *Che Qian Zi*, *Mu Tong* and *Ze Xie* clear and drain damp-heat.
  - *Dang Gui* and *Sheng Di Huang* nourish the yin and blood.
- Sticky yellow sweat. + *Yin Chen Hao*
  Damp-heat infusing downwards with excessive sweating in the external genital region or lower extremities, use *Si Miao Wan*.

Acupuncture Treatment

Excess:

- **Manipulation:** Reducing method.
- **Presciption:** GV14 Dazhui (cupping after needle removal)

Deficiency:

- **Manipulation:** Moxibustion.
- **Prescription:** GV14 Dazhui GV20 Baihui KI1 Yongquan

Practical Hints

• **"Sweat is the fluid of the heart."** Excessive sweating may deplete heart qi and yin and cause heart dysfunction. Iatrogenic causes of abnormal sweating, such as an overdose of diaphoretic herbs or the use of *Ma Huang Tang* in exterior deficiency pattern, should not be overlooked.

• **"The yang (function, ability) acting upon the yin (substance, liquid) creates the sweat."** Physiologically, when yang qi steams or evaporates the body fluid, sweat will be produced. Pathologically, any type of heat, including excess heat (liver fire, stomach fire or damp-heat) and deficient heat (yin deficiency with empty fire), can force out body fluid as abnormal sweating.

• **Harmonize protective and nutritive qi.** Normal perspiration relies on appropriate closing and opening of the interstitial layer between the skin and muscle, which is managed by the protective qi. When excess pathogens obstruct protective qi, or when there is disharmony between protective and nutritive qi, abnormal sweating will be evident.

• **Qi and body fluid are physiologically interdependent.** Qi is the commander of the blood as well as of the body fluid; on the other hand, body fluid is the carrier or transporter of the qi. Qi deficiency contributes to sweating because qi loses the ability to control the body fluid. Severe sweating may lead to qi depletion as qi loss follows the loss of body fluid. Sweating can be critical and life threatening if both qi depletion and yin exhaustion occur.

CHAPTER 39

Congested Fluids

痰 飲 *Tan Yin*

Congested fluids are a group of disorders characterized by retention of unmetabolized water in specific regions of the body. These disorders are most commonly caused by exterior cold-dampness, improper diet and deficient yang qi. Dysfunction of the three major water-metabolizing organs, the lung, spleen and kidney, plays an important role, especially spleen yang deficiency. Congested fluids are classified into four categories according to the location of the fluid accumulation. When there is accumulation in the stomach and intestines, known as phlegm-fluids (*tan yin*), a splashing sound can be heard in the abdomen. Suspended fluids (*xuan yin*), or fluid accumulation in the chest and hypochondria, manifests with chest and hypochondriac pain induced by coughing and spitting. Distal accumulation in the four extremities, known as diffused fluids (*yi yin*), is accompanied by systemic edema and general body ache. Congested fluids, which accumulates in and push against the lung is called propped fluids (*zhi yin*) and it causes coughing, shortness of breath and the need to sit upright to breathe.

Relevant Diseases

- Chronic bronchitis
- Bronchial asthma
- Pleurisy
- Gastrointestinal dysfunction
- Incomplete pyloric stenosis
- Bowel obstruction
- Intercostal neuralgia
- Nephritis
- Meniere's disease
- Chronic cor pulmonale

Etiology and Pathogenesis

Exterior cold-dampness: Cold-dampness damages the protective yang and lung qi, and lodges in the muscular layer. The lung and spleen cannot metabolize water efficiently, causing fluids to become congested.

Improper diet: Raw and cold foods injure the spleen yang, which then fails to metabolize water. Water, instead of being transformed into the body fluid, accumulates and turns into congested fluids.

Exhaustion, fatigue and chronic illness: In the case of chronic illness or any condition that exhausts spleen and kidney yang, metabolism of water is compromised and congested fluids accumulate.

Obstruction of the water passage in the triple burner: The triple burner is the passage for the qi and water. When the triple burner is obstructed, the flow of water is interrupted. Consequently, regional accumulation of water occurs and congested fluids develop.

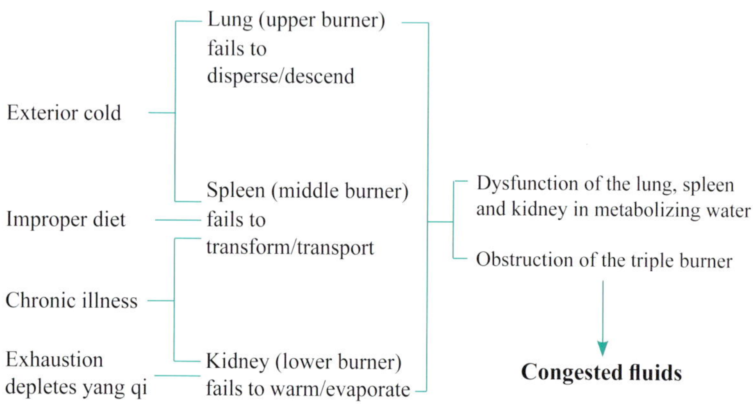

Diagnosis

A. Identification of phlegm, dampness, water and congested fluids:

These four pathological derivatives come from the same source; under certain conditions, they can transform into each other.

- Comparing consistency, congested fluids are thin; phlegm is thick and turbid; water is clear and flowing; dampness is sticky and stationary.
- Comparing manifestations, congested fluids are found in specific internal locations; phlegm and dampness can affect any part of the body and have various presentations; water diffuses and primarily affects the superficial layers of the body.
- Comparing pathogenesis, the formation of congested fluids is related to cold; heat consumes fluids and forms phlegm; water, according to its etiology, can be further classified as yang water or yin water; dampness, without a set form, combines with other pathogens to cause illness.

B. Identification of congested fluids and phlegm:

Congested fluids reside in specific regions and have localized symptoms. In the stomach and intestines, congested fluids cause splashing water sounds; diffusing into the interstitial layer of the body, they appear as edema; stagnated in the thoracic and hypochondriac regions, they trigger dull pain and cough; when congested fluids fill the chest, there will be breathlessness, wheezing and a congested sensation in the chest.

Phlegm follows the flow of qi and can reside in and affect any part of the body. Attacking the lung, it causes cough; ascending with liver wind, it induces dizziness; obstructing the channels, it leads to numbness, facial paralysis and hemiplegia; covering the heart's orifice, it triggers palpitations, disorientation and mania.

C. Differential diagnosis of diffused fluids and *feng shui*:

Both diffused fluids and *feng shui* (edema due to wind attack) share the common manifestation of general edema.

Diffused fluids: Closely related to exterior wind-cold, its manifestations include systemic edema, especially of the four extremities. Other symptoms include aversion to cold, absence of sweating, heavy and painful sensation of the body, wheezing, coughing with copious sputum and chest congestion.

Feng shui: A type of edema caused by invasion of exterior wind-heat and impaired dispersing and descending of lung qi, it has an acute and critical onset with edema starting from the eyelids then spreading to the extremities and entire body. Symptoms include aversion to wind, fever, sweating, and a red, swollen and sore throat.

Basic Patterns

Phlegm-fluids (tan yin):

- Spleen yang deficiency
- Fluids retention in the stomach and intestines

Suspended fluids (xuan yin):

- Fluids retention in the chest and hypochondria

Diffused fluids (yi yin):

- Fluids diffusion into the interstitial layer

Propped fluids (zhi yin):

- Cold congested fluids hidden in the lung
- Spleen and kidney yang deficiency

Differentiation and Treatment

Treatment principle:

Warming and transforming congested fluids is the primary principle. For those who suffer from congested fluids, warm herbs should be used in the treatment. Congested fluids are yin pathological influences; therefore, cold aggravates the condition and encourages its accumulation, while warmth transforms and resolves it.

In addition to warming and transforming, other treatment strategies should be applied based on the differentiations. For congested fluids diffused superficially, warming and dispersing to induce sweating is appropriate; for congested fluids accumulated internally, forcing fluids downwards and diuresis are preferable; for yang deficiency and insignificant congested fluids, the best method is to strengthen the spleen and warm the kidney.

Phlegm-fluids (tan yin):

Spleen yang deficiency

Fullness in the costal and hypochondriac regions, focal epigastric distention, splashing fluid sounds in the stomach, discomfort relieved by warmth, frequent nausea and vomiting of clear watery emesis.

S: Palpitations, shortness of breath, dizziness and vertigo, cold sensation on the back, puffy face in the morning and edema of the lower extremities in the afternoon.

T: Swollen tongue with white slippery coating. **P:** Wiry thready and slippery.

- Warm the spleen and transform congested fluids.
- *Ling Gui Zhu Gan Tang* and *Xiao Ban Xia Tang*
  - *Fu Ling* and *Bai Zhu* strengthen the spleen, drain dampness and eliminate phlegm-fluids.
  - *Gui Zhi* and *Gan Cao* warm and unblock the obstruction of yang qi.
  - *Ban Xia* and *Sheng Jiang* harmonize the stomach and descend rebellious qi.
- To enhance the effects of warming the middle burner and harmonizing the stomach to stop vomiting. + *Gan Jiang, Wu Zhu Yu, Chuan Jiao*
  Drain dampness. + *Ze Xie, Zhu Ling*
  Regulate the qi and reduce distention. + *Zhi Shi*

Fluids retention in the stomach and intestines

Stiffness, fullness and pain in the epigastrium and abdomen, hyperactive bowel sounds with splashing fluid sounds in the abdomen.

S: Abdominal distention and constipation, dry mouth and throat.

T: White or yellow greasy coating. **P:** Deep and wiry.

- Drain water and force out congested fluids.
- *Ji Jiao Li Huang Wan*
  - *Da Huang* and *Ting Li Zi* drain downwards to force out pathogenic fluids.
  - *Fang Ji* and *Jiao Mu* promote urination and eliminate pathogenic fluids.
- Congested fluids overflowing upwards with fullness of the chest. + *Zhi Shi, Hou Po*

Suspended fluids (xuan yin):

Fluids retention in the chest and hypochondria

Distending pain in the thoracic and hypochondriac regions induced by coughing and spitting, severe coughing and wheezing with inability to lie flat, intercostal fullness or a thoracic bulge on the affected side.
S: Dry heaves, shortness of breath, headache and dizziness.
T: White coating. **P:** Deep and wiry.

- Drain water, descend lung qi and force out congested fluids.
- *Shi Zao Tang*
  - *Yuan Hua*, *Gan Sui* and *Da Ji* aggressively expel congested fluids.
  - *Da Zao* is sweet to moderate the toxic and aggressive nature of the above herbs.
- Excessive phlegm with chest congestion. + *Xie Bai, Xing Ren*

Diffused fluids (yi yin):

Fluids diffusion into the interstitial layer

Heaviness and soreness of the body with systemic edema.
S: Aversion to cold, absence of sweating, or coughing and wheezing with abundant white frothy sputum, congested chest and no thirst.
T: White coating. **P:** Wiry and tight.

- Release the exterior and transform congested fluids.
- *Xiao Qing Long Tang*
  - *Ma Huang* and *Gui Zhi* disperse cold and release the exterior.
  - *Gan Jiang* and *Xi Xin* warm and transform cold congested fluids.
  - *Ban Xia* dries dampness and transforms phlegm.
  - *Wu Wei Zi* and *Bai Shao*, sour and binding in nature, enable the formula to restrain as well as disperse.
- Accompanied by oliguria or anuria. + *Fu Ling, Zhu Ling, Ze Xie*
  Accompanied by fever, irritability and yellow coating. + *Sheng Shi Gao*

Propped fluids (zhi yin):

Cold congested fluids hidden in the lung

Coughing and wheezing with chest fullness, difficulty breathing with the need to sit upright, copious white foamy sputum, year-round fluids congestion that is aggravated during cold weather.
S: Edema of the face and ankles in severe cases; or onset of symptoms only with exterior cold invasion, accompanied by aversion to cold, fever and back pain.
T: White, greasy or slippery coating. **P:** Wiry and tight.

- Warm the lung and transform congested fluids.
- *Ling Gan Wu Wei Jiang Xin Tang*
  - *Gan Jiang* and *Xi Xin* warm the lung and transform cold congested fluids.
  - *Fu Ling* strengthens the spleen and drains dampness.
  - *Wu Wei Zi* restrains lung qi and stops coughing.
- Significant symptoms of exterior wind-cold, use *Xiao Qing Long Tang*.
  Severe coughing and wheezing with dyspnea and copious sputum, use *Ting Li Da Zao Xie Fei Tang*.
  Excessive viscous sputum and chest congestion. + *Bai Jie Zi, Lai Fu Zi*
  Congested fluids turning into heat and injuring the yin with cough, breathlessness, thick viscous sputum and dry throat, use *Mai Men Dong Tang*.

Spleen and kidney yang deficiency

Rapid and shallow breathing aggravated by exertion, coughing with copious sputum, fullness of the chest, poor appetite, dysuria or oliguria, and pitting edema of the ankles.
S: Cold intolerance and cold limbs, lassitude, cold pain in the lower abdomen, dizziness and vertigo, and vomiting of clear watery emesis.
T: Swollen tongue with white greasy coating. **P:** Deep thready and slippery.

- Warm and tonify the spleen and kidney to transform congested fluids.
- *Jin Gui Shen Qi Wan* and *Ling Gui Zhu Gan Tang*
  - *Jin Gui Shen Qi Wan* warms the yang and tonifies the kidney to transform congested fluids.
  - *Ling Gui Zhu Gan Tang* tonifies the qi, strengthens the spleen and unblocks yang qi to transform congested fluids.
- Poor appetite and profuse sputum. + *Ban Xia, Chen Pi*
  Pulsating sensation in the lower abdomen with palpitations, dizziness and spitting clear fluids. + *Wu Ling San*
  Cold congested fluids overflowing against the heart, use *Zhen Wu Tang*.

Acupuncture Treatment

Phlegm-fluids:

- **Manipulation:** Even method and moxibustion.
- **Prescription:** CV12 Zhongwan, BL20 Pishu, ST25 Tianshu, PC6 Neiguan, ST40 Fenglong, ST36 Zusanli

Suspended fluids:

- **Manipulation:** Reducing method.
- **Prescription:** BL20 Pishu, CV9 Shuifen, KI7 Fuliu, SP4 Gongsun, GB40 Qiuxu, GB38 Yangfu

Diffused fluids:

- **Manipulation:** Reducing method.
- **Prescription:** LU7 Lieque, LI4 Hegu, LI6 Pianli, SP9 Yinlingquan, BL39 Weiyang, BL13 Feishu

Propped fluids:

- **Manipulation:** Even method and moxibustion.
- **Prescription:** LU7 Lieque, BL13 Feishu, LU5 Chize, LI4 Hegu, BL12 Fengmen, LU9 Taiyuan

Practical Hints

• **Congested fluids are pathological derivatives as well as pathogenic influences.** Congested fluids are disorders of deficient yang and excess yin, or that of righteous qi deficiency and pathogenic factor excess. When there is yang deficiency, dysfunction of water metabolism fails to properly transform water into body fluid. The pathological result is accumulation of cold congested fluids, which predominates at the initial stage of the disorder. Cold congested fluids act as a pathogenic influence to further damage the yang qi and result in yang deficiency. If the condition remains unresolved and the pathogen lingers, yang fails to carry out its normal functions and body fluid cannot be generated; yin deficiency therefore ensues.

• **Use bitter and cold herbs or acrid and warm herbs with caution.** At the initial stage, while the disorder presents as an excess condition, improper use of bitter and cold herbs to force out the congested fluids will injure both the yang and the yin. Later, when deficient cold becomes preponderant, overuse of aggressive acrid and warm herbs will complicate the condition, in which signs of both cold and heat co-exhibit, and increase the difficulty of rendering successful treatment.

• **Strengthen the spleen, augment the lung and tonify the kidney during the recovery stage.** The spleen, lung, and kidney are involved in congested fluid disorders. During the recovery stage, the treatment strategy should support these organs. Common formulas to augment the lung are *Yu Ping Feng San* and *Sheng Mai San*; *Liu Jun Zi Tang* is the formula of choice for strengthening the spleen; to tonify the kidney, both *Zuo Gui Wan* and *You Gui Wan* are recommended.

CHAPTER 40

Edema

水腫 *Shui Zhong*

Edema refers to the abnormal retention of fluid. Fluid can be retained peripherally in the interstitial spaces leading to puffiness around the eyelids, face and limbs. Excess fluid can also be retained systemically leading to swelling of the entire body. In severe cases, edema can develop in the thoracic or abdominal cavities. Complications range from mild to life-threatening.

Relevant Diseases

- Acute and chronic nephritis
- Nephrosis
- Primary hyperaldosteronism
- Hypoproteinemia
- Vitamin B1 deficiency
- Severe anemia
- Hypothyroidism
- Liver cirrhosis
- Heart failure

Etiology and Pathogenesis

Water metabolism depends on the movement of qi. Impairment of qi transformation may predispose a person to develop edema. The three organs accountable for water metabolism are the lung, spleen and kidney. Edema occurs when these three organs fail to disperse, transform, transport and eliminate water. Another important organ is the triple burner because it provides a patent passageway for the qi flow, and the metabolized fluid. In another word, the triple burner ensures that the metabolized fluid flows smoothly.

Exterior wind attacking the lung: The lung is the upper source of water metabolism. Its dispersing and descending functions are closely related to elimination of excessive fluid. The dispersing function of the lung ensures that metabolized water is evenly distributed on the surface of the body and eliminated as sweat. The descending function of the lung indirectly involves the elimination of water via urination. However, as the main organ dominating the exterior, the lung is highly susceptible to exterior wind invasion. If attacked, the lung's dispersing and descending functions will be impaired. Water metabolism will be disturbed and the fluid will not be eliminated via sweat or urine. Edema caused by exterior wind manifests as fluid accumulation in the superficial layer of the body.

Exterior dampness lingering around the spleen: Exterior dampness caused by a humid environment or a diet with excessive raw and cold food greatly hinders the spleen's function to transform and transport. Impairment of spleen's function is followed by water accumulation. The retained water will diffuse into the interstitial spaces and manifest as systemic edema.

Skin disorders contracted by exterior damp-heat toxicity affecting the lung and spleen: The skin is the extending exterior tissue of the lung whereas the muscle is the extending tissue of the spleen. Unremitting, prolonged skin disorders contracted through exterior damp-heat toxicity can affect these associated internal organs. Consequently, dysfunction of the lung and spleen limits their abilities to metabolize water and leads to edema.

Excessive damp-heat obstructing the triple burner: As a result of damp-heat obstructing the triple burner, the ascending and descending flow of fluid in the passage is interrupted. Sluggish water metabolism causes water retention.

Improper diet and overexertion injuring the spleen and stomach: By directly influencing the spleen and stomach organs, improper diet, physical exertion or stress can impair the functions of middle burner in transformation and transportation of fluid. Qi deficiency, following spleen deficiency, fails to properly transport and transform fluid. Indirectly, qi deficiency leads to fluid retention.

Excessive sexual activity or multiple deliveries directly consume the kidney. The exhausted kidney fails to properly evaporate the fluid and support the bladder in eliminating water.

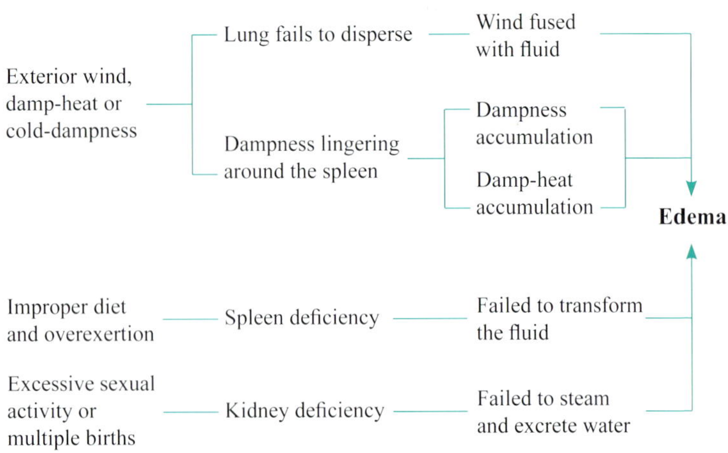

Diagnosis

A. Identification of yin and yang:

Yang edema begins from the upper body and is caused by exterior pathogens, including wind, dampness, damp-heat or damp-heat toxicity. It pertains to an exterior, excess and heat condition.

Yin edema starts from the lower body and is caused by miscellaneous factors, such as improper diet, overexertion, excessive sexual activity or multiple deliveries. It pertains to an interior, deficient and cold condition.

B. Identification of inter-transformation between yin and yang edema:

Yang edema pertains to an excess pattern whereas yin edema pertains to a deficient pattern or a complicated pattern of excess and deficiency. Under certain conditions, these two patterns undergo inter-transformation. Unremitting yang edema will eventually consume the righteous qi and deficiency will exacerbate water retention. The combination of both deficient qi and excessive water retention signifies the transformation into yin edema. Pre-existing yin edema complicated by repetitive invasions of exterior pathogens intensifies water retention. When excess preponderates, yang edema should be considered.

C. Identification of organ involvement:

Congested fluids, palpitations, wheezing, dyspnea, tympanic abdominal distention, oliguria-anuria, dysphagia and gagging syndrome will manifest during a crisis of edema. These symptoms indicate involvement of the internal organs.

- Edema accompanied by palpitations indicates heart involvement.
- Edema with hypochondriac or abdominal distention and a significantly enlarged abdomen limiting movement suggests complication of the liver.
- Edema with epigastric and abdominal distention, heaviness of the limbs or poor appetite indicates that the water retention has affected the spleen.
- Lung involvement is confirmed when there is coughing, breathlessness and chest congestion.
- If the kidney is affected, symptoms in addition to edema include soreness of the lower back and knees and a cold sensation in the external genitalia.

D. Differential diagnosis of edema and tympanic abdominal distention:

Edema: Water retention begins from either the head and face or the feet; gradually, it spreads to the entire body to become systemic edema. Distended veins are not noticeable on the abdomen.

Tympanic abdominal distention (*gu zhang*): Originates from the abdomen, *gu zhang* can develop further and affect the lower extremities and/or the entire body. It manifests with significant drum-shaped abdominal distention. Distended veins might also be apparent on the abdomen.

Basic Patterns

Yang edema:

- Water retention due to external wind
- Damp-heat toxicity affecting the lung and spleen
- Dampness accumulation
- Damp-heat accumulation

Yin edema:

- Spleen yang deficiency
- Kidney yang deficiency

Differentiation and Treatment

Treatment principle:

The focus of treatment is to eliminate pathogenic fluids by inducing sweating, promoting urination and draining downwards to force out the excessive fluids. Benefiting the qi, strengthening the spleen and warming the kidney are used to support the righteous qi. In addition, supportive measures, such as regulating the qi, invigorating the blood, relieving toxicity and eliminating turbidity, accelerate the therapeutic effects.

Yang edema:

Water retention due to external wind

Acute onset, edema starting from the eyelids and spreading to the limbs and the entire body, shiny thin skin tone, insignificant or no pitting on pressure, and oliguria.

S: Aversion to cold, fever, soreness or pain in the joints, coughing and wheezing, and possibly a swollen sore throat.

T: Thin white or thin yellow coating. **P:** Floating, slippery and tight, or floating, slippery and rapid.

- Dispel wind, clear heat, disperse lung qi and eliminate water retention.
- *Yue Bi Jia Zhu Tang*
  - *Ma Huang* disperses lung qi and induces sweating to release the exterior.
  - *Shi Gao* releases the pathogens from muscle and clears heat.
  - *Bai Zhu* and *Sheng Jiang* strengthen the spleen and transform dampness.
  - *Gan Cao* augments the qi and harmonizes the formula.

- To strengthen the effects of dispersing lung qi, promoting urination and reducing edema. + *Fu Ping, Fu Ling, Ze Xie*
  To strengthen the effects of clearing heat and promoting urination. + *Bai Mao Gen, Chi Xiao Dou*
  Swollen sore throat. + *Jie Geng, She Gan, Niu Bang Zi*
  Coughing and wheezing. + *Xing Ren, Jie Geng, Qian Hu*

Damp-heat toxicity affecting the lung and spleen

Acute onset, edema starting from the eyelids and spreading to the limbs and the entire body, dermal sores, rashes and ulcerations, and oliguria.
S: Aversion to wind, fever and severe itchiness of the skin.
T: Red tongue with thin yellow coating. **P:** Slippery or floating, and rapid.

- Disperse lung qi, relieve toxicity, drain dampness and reduce swelling.
- *Ma Huang Lian Qiao Chi Xiao Dou Tang* and *Wu Wei Xiao Du Yin*
  - *Ma Huang*, *Xing Ren* and *Sang Bai Pi* disperse and descend lung qi, and promote water metabolism.
  - *Lian Qiao* clears heat and relieves toxicity.
  - *Chi Xiao Dou* promotes urination and reduces edema.
  - *Jin Yin Hua*, *Ye Ju Hua*, *Pu Gong Ying* and *Zi Hua Di Ding* clear and relieve damp-heat toxicity.
- Excessive dampness with erosion. + *Ku Shen, Tu Fu Ling*
  Excessive wind with severe itchiness. + *Bai Xian Pi, Di Fu Zi*
  Constipation. + *Da Huang, Mang Xiao*

Dampness accumulation

Systemic pitting edema and oliguria.
S: Heavy sensation of the body, chest stuffiness, nausea and poor appetite.
T: White greasy coating. **P:** Deep and decelerating.

- Strengthen the spleen, resolve dampness, unblock yang qi and transform water.
- *Wu Pi San* and *Wei Ling Tang*
  - *Sang Bai Pi*, *Chen Pi*, *Da Fu Pi*, *Fu Ling Pi* and *Sheng Jiang Pi* transform dampness and promote water metabolism.
  - *Bai Zhu* and *Fu Ling* strengthen the spleen and dry dampness.
  - *Cang Zhu* and *Hou Po* dry dampness and facilitate the movement of qi.
  - *Zhu Ling* and *Ze Xie* promote urination and reduce edema.
  - *Gui Zhi* assists the bladder to transform the qi.
- Wheezing. + *Ma Huang, Xing Ren, Ting Li Zi*

*

Damp-heat accumulation

Systemic pitting edema and bright shiny skin tone.
S: Stuffy sensation in the chest and epigastrium, irritability, thirst, scanty urine, and constipation.
T: Yellow greasy coating. **P:** Deep and rapid, or soft and rapid.

- Clear heat and drain dampness.
- *Shu Zao Yin Zi*
  - *Qiang Huo* and *Qin Jiao* disperse wind and release the exterior pathogenic factors by way of sweating.
  - *Fu Ling Pi*, *Sheng Jiang* and *Da Fu Pi* assist *Qiang Huo* and *Qin Jiao* to eliminate the water from the skin.
  - *Shang Lu* drains downwards and forces out the fluids by ways of urination and bowel movements.
  - *Ze Xie*, *Mu Tong*, and *Chi Xiao Dou* assist Shang Lu to promote urination.
- Severe abdominal distention, urinary retention and constipation. + *Ji Jiao Li Huang Wan*
  Damp-heat injuring the yin, use *Zhu Ling Tang*.
  Damp-heat infusing downwards with dysuria and hematuria. + *Da Ji, Bai Mao Gen, Ou Jie*

Yin edema:

Spleen yang deficiency

Systemic pitting edema especially in the lower part of the body.
S: Distention of the epigastrium and abdomen, loose stool, poor appetite, sallow complexion, fatigue, cold limbs and oliguria.
T: Pale tongue with white greasy or white slippery coating. **P:** Deep and decelerating, or deep and weak.

- Warm and tonify spleen yang to resolve water retention.
- *Shi Pi Yin*
  - *Gan Jiang*, *Fu Zi* and *Cao Guo* warm the yang and disperse cold.
  - *Bai Zhu* and *Fu Ling* strengthen the spleen and dry dampness.
  - *Da Fu Pi* and *Mu Gua* drain dampness.
  - *Mu Xiang* and *Hou Po* regulate the qi to promote water metabolism.
- Severe qi deficiency. + *Ren Shen, Huang Qi*
  Impaired qi transformation with oliguria. + *Gui Zhi, Ze Xie*
  Severe edema with chest congestion, dyspnea and orthopnea, use *Wu Ling San* and *Ting Li Da Zao Xie Fei Tang*.

* Invigorate the blood in later stages.

Kidney yang deficiency

Puffiness of the face, systemic pitting edema especially in the lower part of the body, and possibly decreased or increased urine output.

S: Palpitations, shortness of breath, soreness, heaviness and cold sensation of the lower back and knees, frigid limbs, cold intolerance, lassitude and pale complexion.

T: Pale and flabby tongue with white coating. **P:** Deep and thready, or deep, slow and forceless.

- Tonify and warm kidney yang to resolve water retention.
- *Ji Sheng Shen Qi Wan* and *Zhen Wu Tang* - Strategy: Zuo Gui Wan
  - *Rou Gui* and *Fu Zi* warm and tonify kidney yang.
  - *Shu Di Huang*, *Shan Yao* and *Shan Zhu Yu* nourish and tonify kidney yin.
  - *Bai Zhu*, *Fu Ling*, *Ze Xie* and *Che Qian Zi* promote urination and reduce edema.
  - *Niu Xi* directs the action of the formula downwards.
- Shortness of breath with difficult inhalation aggravated by exertion, sweating and cold limbs. + *Ren Shen, Wu Wei Zi, Ge Jie*

  Palpitations, congested chest, cyanotic lips and tongue, and intermittent knotted pulse. + *Gui Zhi, Zhi Gan Cao, Dan Shen, Hong Hua*

  Headache, vomiting, trance, lethargy, loss of consciousness and ammonia breath. + *Da Huang, Huang Lian, Ban Xia*

Acupuncture Treatment

Yang edema:

- **Manipulation:** Even method.
- **Prescription:** LU7 Lieque, LI4 Hegu, LI6 Pianli, SP9 Yinlingquan, BL39 Weiyang

Yin edema:

- **Manipulation:** Reinforcing method and moxibustion.
- **Prescription:** BL20 Pishu, BL23 Shenshu, CV9 Shuifen, CV4 Guanyuan, KI7 Fuliu, ST36 Zusanli
- **Supplementary points:**
  - Facial edema. + GV26 Renzhong
  - Pedal edema. + GB41 Zulinqi; SP5 Shangqiu

Practical Hints

• **Strengthen the spleen to extract dietary essence.** When the spleen is deficient and fails to transform and transport, sufficient essence may not be extracted from food and water. In this case, puffiness of the face in the morning and swelling and distending sensation of the lower body in the evening will manifest along with symptoms of spleen qi deficiency, such as fatigue, loose stool, sallow complexion and increased urination. This is not considered a pattern of edema. Strengthening the spleen's function to extract the essence from diet should be the focus of the treatment; nutritional supplements are encouraged.

• **Integrate the method of promoting blood circulation.** The strategy of invigorating the blood to transform stasis is often used to address the need of unblocking obstruction in the triple burner. This method is especially useful in the treatment of ascites and end stage renal disease, in which, according to TCM, the water passage is no longer patent due to blood stasis and poor circulation. By using large doses of *Yi Mu Cao*, *Ze Lan*, *Tao Ren* and *Hong Hua*, obstruction in the water passage can be removed as blood stasis is resolved and the blood circulation is facilitated.

• **Control salt intake.** The recommendation is to avoid salt intake during the initial stage of edema. As edema is gradually reduced, a low-sodium diet can be resumed.

CHAPTER 41

Wasting and Thirsting Disorder

消 渴 *Xiao Ke*

Relevant Diseases

- Diabetes mellitus
- Diabetes insipidus

X*iao*, or wasting, signifies serious depletion of the vital substances despite excessive consumption of food and water. *Ke*, or thirsting, refers to excessive thirst that is not relieved by drinking.

Three excesses- excessive urine production or polyuria, excessive thirst or polydipsia, and increased food intake or polyphagia- together with emaciation characterize wasting and thirsting disorder. The other principal symptoms include turbid urine and sugar in the urine (glycosuria). Depending on which of the three excesses is dominant, the disorder is subcategorized into three patterns- upper *xiao*, middle *xiao* and lower *xiao*. The dominant symptom in upper *xiao* is intense thirst and frequent drinking; excessive hunger and increased food intake indicate middle *xiao*; and lower *xiao* is characterized by intense thirst and excessive urination.

Etiology and Pathogenesis

Improper diet: Excessive consumption of greasy, sweet, rich food and alcohol can hinder the function of the spleen and stomach. Impaired digestive function leads to food stagnation, which generates heat. Because heat is drying, it injures the yin and fluid and symptoms of wasting become apparent.

Emotional stress caused by longstanding emotional upset may disturb the flow of qi. Stagnant qi transforming into fire consumes the yin and fluid of the lung and stomach, inducing wasting and thirsting disorder.

Overexertion: Yin and essence can be exhausted when a yin deficient constitution is further depleted by excessive sexual activity. Yin deficiency with fire flaring upwards will consume lung and stomach yin and fluid. Kidney, lung and stomach yin becomes deficient and cause wasting and thirsting disorder.

The basic pathogenesis of wasting and thirsting disorder has yin deficiency as the root and heat-dryness as the branch. Yin deficiency and heat-dryness can mutually influence and aggravate each other. The major organs involved include the lung, stomach and kidney. Because the lung is the upper source of the body fluid, lung yin deficiency with heat-dryness will result in failure of the lung to disseminate the body fluid. When there is a lack of body fluid distributed by the lung, the stomach and kidney will suffer from yin deficiency. In a similar manner, excess stomach heat can injure stomach yin as well as consume lung and kidney yin. Kidney yin is the foundation that supplies the fluid for the entire body. Once kidney yin is deficient, lung and stomach yin will not have their source and eventually become diminished.

Yin and yang are interdependent. In chronic wasting and thirsting disorder, or longstanding yin deficiency, insufficient yin fails to support the functions of yang. As a result, yang becomes deficient, and deficiency of both yin and yang is evident.

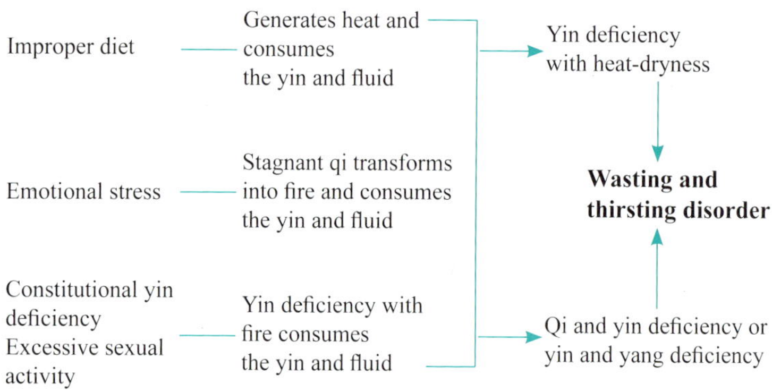

Diagnosis

A. Identification of organ involvement:

Clinically, the three excess symptoms can appear simultaneously; however, a preponderance of one symptom can be used to determine organ involvement.

- If intense thirst (polydipsia) and frequent drinking are the primary symptoms, lung involvement is certain. This is known as upper *xiao*.
- If excessive food intake (polyphagia) is the primary symptom, the stomach is the main organ affected. This is known as middle *xiao*.
- If the dominant symptom is excessive urination (polyuria), it indicates that kidney yin is deficient. This is known as lower *xiao*.

B. Identification of complications:

Consumptive lung disorder: Longstanding lung yin deficiency leads to consumptive lung disorder. The lung is severely damaged by inadequate moisture and nourishment and a dry cough develops accompanied by scanty sputum, blood-tinged sputum or hemoptysis, tidal fever, night sweating and emaciation.

Night blindness, cataract and deafness: Deficient kidney yin failing to nourish the liver will lead to deficiency of both the essence and blood. The eyes and ears will not receive adequate nourishment if the liver and kidney are deficient. There may be complications of visual and auditory impairments presenting as night blindness, cataract and/or deafness.

Abscesses, furuncles, sores and gangrene can result from heat-dryness. As heat-dryness consumes the nutritive qi and blood, obstruction and accumulation in the channels and vessels become apparent. Extreme heat may transform into toxicity. Toxic accumulation will lead to abscesses, furuncles, sores and gangrene in the affected area.

Edema: In the late stage, extremely deficient yin will no longer support the functions of yang. Consequently, the spleen and kidney will not be able to properly metabolize the fluids. Edema occurs when the fluids overflow and diffuse into the interstitial layer of the body.

Blood stasis: By the same mechanism as that of heat drying up the body fluid to form phlegm, when heat dries the fluid in the blood, the blood becomes concentrated and viscous. Blood stasis is the common result.

Wind stroke and hemiplegia: Yin deficiency with heat-dryness can consume the fluid to form phlegm. Obstruction of the channels and misting of the heart's orifice can result from phlegm accumulation.

Deficiency of both the yin and yang: When the yin is extremely deficient, it will fail to secure the yang and the yang will float upwards or outwards. The clinical presentation includes red face, headache, irritability, nausea and vomiting, enophthalmos, dry red lips and tongue, and breathing with deep, long breaths. If the condition progresses to loss of consciousness, frigid extremities and a minute pulse, it indicates the crisis of separation and disconnection of the yin and yang due to depleted yin or collapsed yang.

C. Differential diagnosis of similar disorders:

Goiter: In addition to excessive hunger with polyphagia and emaciation, patients suffering from goiter also have palpitations, a short temper, impatience, unilateral or bilateral palpable masses in the neck, and possibly exophthalmos. The early stage of goiter can be easily misdiagnosed as middle *xiao*.

True cold with false heat syndrome: With common manifestations of polydipsia, polyuria and emaciation, it should be differentiated from wasting and thirsting disorder. Although complaining of intense thirst, a patient suffering from true cold and false heat syndrome does not have a desire to drink or to eat. When frequent urination is a symptom, the total urine output does not match the output of wasting and thirsting disorder. The urine will be clear and pale. The patient will have a pale tongue and a decelerating pulse.

Basic Patterns

Upper xiao:

- Lung heat injuring the fluid

Middle xiao:

- Excess stomach heat

Lower xiao:

- Kidney yin deficiency
- Deficiency of both the yin and yang

Differentiation and Treatment

Treatment principle:

Upper *xiao*: Moisten the lung and clear heat from the stomach.

Middle *xiao*: Clear heat from the stomach in conjunction with nourishing the kidney.

Lower *xiao*: Replenish the kidney and tonify the lung.

Yin deficiency and heat-dryness easily induce blood stasis due to heat drying up the fluid and blood; therefore, herbs that invigorate the blood and transform stasis should be added to the treatment.

Upper xiao:

Lung-heat injuring the fluid

Irritability, frequent drinking, and dry mouth and tongue.

S: Polyuria and gradually developing emaciation.

T: Red edge of the tongue with thin yellow coating. **P:** Rapid and flooding.

- Clear heat, moisten the lung, generate the fluid and alleviate thirst.
- *Xiao Ke Fang*
  - *Tian Hua Fen* nourishes the yin, generates fluid and clears heat.
  - *Huang Lian* clears heat and drains fire.

- *Sheng Di Huang*, *Ou Zhi* and *Feng Mi* nourish and generate the yin.

- Reinforce the effects of generating the fluid to alleviate thirst and nourishing the yin to moisten dryness. + *Ge Gen, Mai Men Dong, Xuan Shen*
  Deficiency of the lung and kidney with rapid, flooding and forceless pulse, and unremitting intense thirst. + *Ren Shen, Mai Dong, Tian Dong, Zhi Mu*
  Flaring heat in the lung and stomach injuring the qi and yin with intense thirst, frequent drinking, and a flooding pulse, use *Bai Hu Jia Ren Shen Tang*.

Middle xiao:

Excess stomach heat

Propensity to hunger, polyphagia, and dry stool.
S: Emaciation.
T: Dry yellow coating. **P:** Slippery, full and forceful.

- Clear heat from the stomach, drain fire, nourish the yin and replenish the fluid.
- *Yu Nu Jian*
  - *Shi Gao* and *Zhi Mu* clear stomach heat and drain fire.
  - *Sheng Di Huang* and *Mai Dong* nourish the yin and generate body fluid.
  - *Niu Xi* guides and drains fire downwards.
- Enhance the effect to purge fire. + *Zhi Zi, Huang Lian*
  Constipation or fecal impaction. Use *Zeng Ye Cheng Qi Tang* temporarily until bowel movements occur, then resume the primary formula.

Lower xiao:

Kidney yin deficiency

Polyuria, and turbid, cloudy or sweet urine.
S: Dry mouth and lips, possibly five-centers heat.
T: Red tongue. **P:** Rapid, deep and thready.

- Nourish the yin and consolidate the kidney.
- *Liu Wei Di Huang Wan*
  - *Liu Wei Di Huang Wan* is a primary formula to nourish kidney yin, stabilize the kidney and fill the essence.
- Yin deficiency and empty fire with tidal fever, irritability, insomnia, nocturnal emission, red tongue and rapid thready pulse. + *Zhi Mu, Huang Bai, Long Gu, Mu Li, Gui Ban*
  Cloudy urine. + *Yi Zhi Ren, Sang Piao Xiao, Wu Wei Zi*
  Qi and yin deficiency with fatigue, lack of strength, shortness of breath, and reluctance to speak. + *Dang Shen, Huang Qi*

Deficiency of both the yin and yang

Polyuria, turbid and cloudy urine, greater urine output than fluid intake, cold intolerance and cold limbs.

S: The helix of the ear is dark and dry, dark complexion, soreness and weakness of the lower back and knees, and impotence.

T: Pale tongue with white coating. **P:** Deep, thready and forceless.

- Warm the yang, nourish the yin and consolidate the kidney.
- *Jin Gui Shen Qi Wan*
  - *Fu Zi* and *Rou Gui* warm and tonify kidney yang.
  - *Liu Wei Di Huang Wan* nourishes and tonifies kidney yin.
- Enhance the tonifying effect on the kidney to bind and restrain. + *Fu Peng Zi, Sang Piao Xiao, Jin Ying Zi*

Complications:

- Cataract, night blindness and deafness caused by kidney and liver essence and blood deficiency, use *Qi Ju Di Huang Wan*.
- Sores, abscesses and furuncles due to toxic heat accumulation, use *Wu Wei Xiao Du Yin*.
- Edema, wind stroke, painful urinary syndrome or syncope, refer to the relevant chapters for differentiation and treatment.

Acupuncture Treatment

Upper xiao:

- **Manipulation:** Even method.
- **Prescription:** HT8 Shaofu BL15 Xinshu LU9 Taiyuan BL13 Feishu
- **Supplementary points:**
  - Thirst and dry mouth. + CV23 Lianquan; CV24 Chengjiang

Middle xiao:

- **Manipulation:** Even method.
- **Prescription:** ST44 Neiting SP6 Sanyinjiao BL20 Pishu BL21 Weishu
- **Supplementary points:**
  - Hunger and stomach upset. + CV12 Zhongwan; PC6 Neiguan

Lower xiao:

- **Manipulation:** Even method.
- **Prescription:** KI3 Taixi LR3 Taichong BL18 Ganshu BL23 Shenshu
- **Supplementary points:**
  - Blurred vision. + GB37 Guangming
  - Dizziness. + GV23 Shangxing

Practical Hints

• Yin deficiency with heat-dryness is the primary pathogenesis of wasting and thirsting disorder. There will be clinical signs and symptoms of qi and yin deficiency or yin and yang deficiency. Therefore, in addition to prescribing the suggested formulas, **large doses of herbs that tonify both the yin and yang simultaneously are recommended,** such as *Shan Yao*, *Huang Qi*, *Xi Yang Shen* and *Tai Zi Shen*. The other commonly used herbs are those that clear heat and generate the fluid, such as *Ge Gen*, *Xuan Shen* and *Tian Hua Fen*.

• **Accurate diagnosis of wasting and thirsting disorder is indispensable for the treatment of complications.** A patient may seek assessment and treatment for the complications of wasting and thirsting disorder, such as recurrent intractable dermal ulcers, visual and auditory impairments, and recurrent urinary tract infections. Thorough physical examination and a detailed history are essential to find the underlying cause and to make an accurate diagnosis of the condition. Symptomatic management alone may not be therapeutically effective and may delay the appropriate treatment for wasting and thirsting disorder.

• **Pathological crisis may follow when prolonged wasting and thirsting disorder is neglected without proper treatment.** The presence of extreme fatigue, lack of appetite, nausea and vomiting, abdominal pain, headache, flushing, tachypnea and dyspnea indicate an exacerbation of the disorder. Without proper treatment, wasting and thirsting disorder can progress to lethargy, delirium, frigid limbs and sweet-smelling breath, analogous to the conditions of diabetic acidosis and diabetic coma.

CHAPTER 42

Fever of Internal Disequilibrium

内傷發熱 *Nei Shang Fa Re*

Fever includes both a subjective sensation of heat in the body and an objective elevation in body temperature. Fever can be caused by exterior pathogenic influences or by internal factors. This chapter introduces fevers due to the latter, fever of internal disequilibrium (FID).

FID includes any subjective heat sensation or objective elevation in body temperature due to malfunction of the internal organs and deficiency of vital substances. The onset is slow and gradual; the course is prolonged. FID usually manifests as a low-grade temperature, though it can also manifest as a high fever, five-centers heat or simply a subjective feverish sensation without a detectable elevation in body temperature. Clinical presentation will also include symptoms of internal deficiencies, liver constraint, blood stasis and accumulation of dampness.

Relevant Diseases

- Leukemia
- Systemic lupus erythematosus
- Menopause
- Hyperthyroidism
- Rheumatic fever
- Tuberculosis
- Chronic infections
- Fever of unknown origin

Etiology and Pathogenesis

Liver constraint: Liver qi stagnation secondary to emotional stress can transform into liver fire and cause fever. "Excessive qi may turn into fire." An excess of all the emotions, including anger, worry and pensiveness, grief, shock and fear, can strongly disturb the movement of qi, causing qi stagnation and leading to fever. This type of fever is known as liver constraint fever.

Blood stasis: Blood stasis can result from emotional stress, exhaustion and trauma. It obstructs the flow in the channels and produces heat, causing fever known as blood stasis fever.

Accumulation of dampness: Exteriorly-contracted or internally-generated dampness accumulates and transforms into heat. Damp-heat will induce an intractable fever known as dampness accumulation fever.

Spleen qi deficiency: Spleen qi is exhausted and becomes deficient through overexertion, improper diet or chronic illness. Equilibrium between the yin and yang cannot be maintained in a condition of extreme qi deficiency. Due to lack of connection with the yin, deficient qi or yang will float upwards and outwards to the surface of the body and induce fever. This type of fever is known as qi deficient fever, and it is not an uncommon disorder.

Blood deficiency occurs when not enough blood is generated because the spleen is deficient, or when there is excessive blood loss due to trauma, surgery or childbirth. Blood is yin in nature. When deficient yin and blood fail to bind the yang, yang qi floats upwards and outwards to the surface of the body, inducing fever. This type of fever is called blood deficient fever.

Essence and yin deficiency can be constitutional or a result of yin exhaustion during a warm-febrile disease. Chronic diarrhea, vomiting, and misuse of diaphoretics or other warm, drying and acrid herbs can also consume the yin. "Insufficient water fails to control fire." This relative excess of yang generates yin deficient fever.

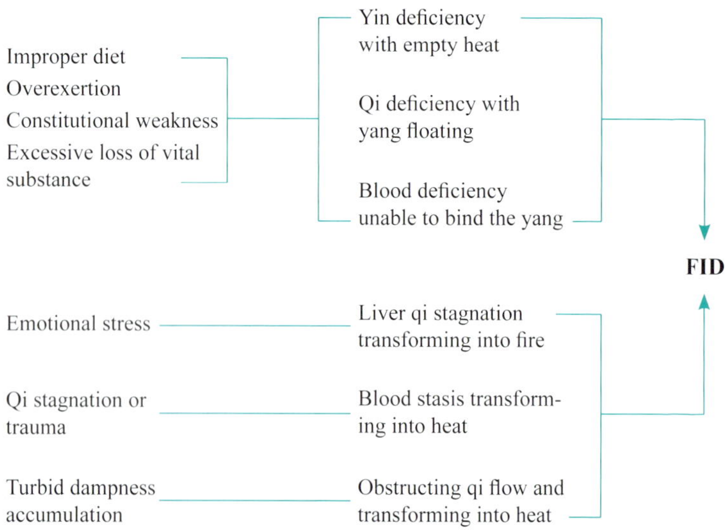

Diagnosis

Differential diagnosis of similar disorders:

Fever is a common symptom of various disorders. Distinguishing interior from exterior causes is important to guide diagnosis and treatment.

	Interior	Exterior
Etiology	Internal disequilibrium due to improper diet, emotional stress and overexertion.	Exterior pathogenic influences.
Onset	Gradual and slow.	Sudden and acute.
Course	Prolonged.	Short.
Characteristics of Fever	Primarily low-grade temperature or subjective sensation of heat, five-centers heat. Intermittent and unpredictable.	Primarily high fever. Constant.
Aversion to Cold	No aversion to cold. Cold intolerance, relieved by adding clothing or covers.	Aversion to cold. Chills, unrelieved after adding clothing or covers.
Secondary Symptoms	Pertaining to internal injury, such as dizziness, fatigue, reluctance to speack, spontaneous sweating and night sweating, and fever that is unrelieved by diaphoresis.	Pertaining to exterior conditions, such as headache, body ache, nasal congestion, rhinorrhea, and fever reduced by diaphoresis.
Tongue and Pulse	Scanty or no coating, thick greasy coating, red tongue or pale tongue with petechiae. Deficient and weak or wiry and choppy.	Thin white or thin yellow coating. Floating, rapid, slippery and tight.

Basic Patterns

- Liver constraint fever
- Dampness accumulation fever
- Blood deficient fever
- Blood stasis fever
- Qi deficient fever
- Yin deficient fever

Differentiation and Treatment

Treatment principle:

Excess: Spread the constrained liver qi to relieve qi stagnation, invigorate the blood to dispel stasis, eliminate dampness and clear heat. Modify the treatment strategy according to the dominant pathogenesis.

Deficiency: Replenish the yin and clear empty heat, augment the qi and strengthen the spleen, tonify the qi and nourish the blood.

Some clinical presentations are a combination of excess and deficiency. In the cases of qi deficiency with blood stasis, qi deficiency with dampness, yin deficiency with qi stagnation or yin deficiency with blood stasis, it is necessary to modify the treatment principle to support the righteous qi and eliminate the pathogens.

Liver constraint fever

Subjective or low-grade fever accompanied by irritability, fever that fluctuates with emotional status and stress, depression, agitation and short temper.

S: Stifling sensation in the chest and hypochondria, bitter taste and dry mouth, irregular menstruation, dysmenorrhea or distending breast pain.

T: Thin yellow coating. **P:** Wiry and rapid.

- Spread liver qi, relieve constraint and drain heat.
- *Dan Zhi Xiao Yao San*
  - *Mu Dan Pi* and *Zhi Zi* clear and drain liver heat.
  - *Chai Hu* and *Bo He* spread constrained liver qi and disperse heat.
  - *Dang Gui* and *Bai Shao* nourish the blood and soften the liver.
  - *Bai Zhu*, *Fu Ling* and *Gan Cao* augment the qi and strengthen the spleen.
- Red face and eyes, dark urine output and constipation. + *Long Dan Cao, Huang Qin, Xia Ku Cao, Sheng Di Huang*

  Significant pain in the hypochondria due to qi stagnation and blood stasis. + *Chuan Lian Zi, Yu Jin, Yan Hu Suo, Qing Pi*

  Irregular menstruation. + *Yi Mu Cao, Ze Lan*

  Yin deficiency complicated by liver constraint fever, use *Zi Shui Qing Gan Yin*.

Blood stasis fever

Fever in the afternoon or at night, possibly a subjective sensation of heat in certain areas of the body, and dry mouth and throat with a desire to wet the mouth but not to drink.

S: Fixed pain or possibly a palpable mass, dry and flaky skin, and a sallow or dusky complexion.

T: Bluish purple tongue with petechiae. **P:** Choppy.

- Invigorate the blood and transform stasis.
- *Xue Fu Zhu Yu Tang*
  - *Tao Ren*, *Hong Hua*, *Chuan Xiong*, *Chi Shao* and *Niu Xi* invigorate the blood and transform stasis.
  - *Dang Gui* and *Sheng Di Huang* nourish and invigorate the blood.
  - *Chai Hu*, *Zhi Qiao* and *Jie Geng* promote the movement of qi.
- Significant heat signs. + *Bai Wei*, *Mu Dan Pi*
  Complicated by qi deficiency. + *Huang Qi*
  Masses in the hypochondria or abdomen, use *Bie Jia Jian Wan*.
  History of significant trauma, use *Fu Yuan Huo Xue Tang*.

Dampness accumulation fever

Slow onset of low-grade fever that is worse in the afternoon, stifling sensation and fullness in the chest and abdomen.
S: Thirst without desire to drink, possibly vomiting, poor appetite, bodily heaviness, loose stool or a sensation of incomplete defecation.
T: White greasy or yellow greasy coating. **P:** Soft and rapid, or deep and slippery.

- Disperse and transform to expand the middle burner, drain dampness and clear heat.
- *San Ren Tang*
  - *Xing Ren* disperses lung qi in the upper burner.
  - *Bai Dou Kou* is aromatic to transform dampness, facilitate the qi flow and expand the middle burner.
  - *Yi Yi Ren* leaches and drains damp-heat.
  - *Hua Shi* and *Tong Cao* clear and drain damp-heat.
  - *Ban Xia* and *Hou Po* promote the qi flow, dry dampness, dispel clumps and eliminate focal distention.
- Stagnant dampness transforming into heat and obstructing the lesser-yang aspect with alternating chills and fever, bitter taste in the mouth, nausea and hiccough. + *Qing Hao*, *Huang Qin*

Qi deficient fever

Fever occurring with or aggravated by exertion and fatigue, fluctuating fever, lack of strength and spontaneous sweating.
S: Dizziness, reluctance to speak, propensity to catching cold, poor appetite and loose stool.
T: Pale tongue with thin white coating. **P:** Thready and weak.

- Augment the qi, strengthen the spleen, and use the sweetening and warming effects to eliminate heat.
- *Bu Zhong Yi Qi Tang*
  - *Bu Zhong Yi Qi Tang* is the imperial formula for augmenting the qi and raising the yang, as well as the imperial formula that eliminates heat by utilizing herbs with sweet and warm properties.
- Severe spontaneous sweating. + *Mu Li, Fu Xiao Mai, Nuo Dao Gen*
  Disharmony of nutritive and protective qi with sweating and aversion to wind. + *Gui Zhi, Bai Shao*
  Stifling sensation and focal distention in the chest and epigastrium with a greasy tongue coating. + *Cang Zhu, Hou Po, Huo Xiang*

Blood deficient fever

Low-grade fever, pale lips and nails, and sallow complexion.
S: Dizziness, blurred vision, fatigue, lack of strength and palpitations.
T: Pale tongue. **P:** Thready and weak.

- Augment the qi and nourish the blood.
- *Dang Gui Bu Xue Tang*
  - *Dang Gui Bu Xue Tang* is a formula that generates the blood by tonifying the qi; it is the imperial formula for blood deficient fever.
- For secondary symptoms related to blood deficiency. + *Gui Pi Tang*

Yin deficient fever

Fever in the afternoon or at night, possibly five-centers heat, sensation of heat hidden deep inside the body, tidal fever and malar flush.
S: Dry mouth, irritability, insomnia, dream-disturbed sleep, night sweating, dark scanty urine, and dry stool.
T: Dry red tongue with cracks and scanty coating. **P:** Thready and rapid.

- Nourish the yin and clear heat.
- *Zhi Bai Di Huang Wan*
  - *Zhi Mu* and *Huang Bai* nourish the yin and clear heat.
  - *Liu Wei Di Huang Wan* nourishes liver and kidney yin.
- To strengthen the effect of clearing deficient heat. + *Yin Chai Hu, Di Gu Pi, Hu Huang Lian, Qin Jiao*
  To reinforce the effect of nourishing the yin. + *Sheng Di Huang, Xuan Shen*
  Severe night sweating. + *Duan Mu Li, Fu Xiao Mai, Nuo Dao Gen*
  Insomnia. + *Suan Zao Ren, Bai Zi Ren, Ye Jiao Teng*

Acupuncture Treatment

Excess:

- **Manipulation:** Reducing method.
- **Prescription:** GV14 Dazhui LI4 Hegu
- **Supplementary points:**

  - Qi stagnation. + LR3 Taichong; GB34 Yanglingquan; TE5 Waiguan

  - Blood stasis. + BL17 Geshu; SP10 Xuehai; SP6 Sanyinjiao

Deficiency:

- **Manipulation:** Reinforcing method; moxibustion may be applicable.
- **Prescription:** SP6 Sanyinjiao ST36 Zusanli CV4 Guanyuan
- **Supplementary points:**

  - Qi deficiency. + BL20 Pishu; CV6 Qihai

  - Blood deficiency. + BL17 Geshu; BL18 Ganshu

  - Yin deficiency. + BL23 Shenshu; BL43 Gaohuangshu; KI1 Yongquan; KI3 Taixi

Practical Hints

• **Avoid bitter or dispersing herbs for fever of internal disequilibrium.** Before excluding internal causes of fever, using dispersing or bitter and cold herbs to treat fever is prohibited. Herbs with acrid and dispersing properties or herbs with bitter and cold nature are commonly indicated for fever induced by exterior causes. Acridity and dispersion tend to exhaust the qi and injure the body fluid while bitter and cold herbs are drying and injure the stomach. Both types of herbs tend to exacerbate the disequilibrium and aggravate FID.

• **Consider prophylactic measures to prevent fever in those with internal injury.** FID is a complicated pathology that involves various deficiencies of vital substances, dysfunction of internal organs, and multiple pathogeneses. Definite differentiation of the pattern is a great challenge. This type of fever tends to be persistent, recurrent, and chronically consumptive. Rapid and frequent modifications of treatments are often required based on the concurrent differentiation. Prophylactic measures, such as prompt supplementation of the body fluid, qi and blood, for those who suffer from high fever, hemorrhage, diarrhea, vomiting, severe sweating, and the late stage of warm-febrile disease are very important.

PART II

TCM Differentiation and Treatment for Western Medical Diseases

CHAPTER 43

Influenza

Influenza is a contagious respiratory tract infection caused by the influenza virus . It has an acute onset and is typically febrile, with elevated body temperature ranging as high as 102°F to 104°F. Pandemic outbreaks usually occur during winter and may begin as early as late September. Influenza infection induces both respiratory and non-specific systemic symptoms. Approximately 10 to 20 percent of the United States' population catches influenza annually, causing an estimated 36,000 deaths each year. A high prevalence of complications is found in the elderly (≥ 65 years old), those with chronic medical conditions, and pediatric populations. The influenza virus infects both the upper and lower respiratory tracts, being transmitted via hand-to-nose contact, aerosol particles or droplets. The disease course is partially dependent upon the generation of virus-specific antibodies. Definitive diagnosis is made by viral culture obtained by throat swab or nasal lavage. Imaging may detect diffuse bilateral pneumonia indicating pulmonary edema or respiratory distress syndrome associated with primary hemorrhagic viral pneumonia.

Influenza, as an infectious disease, has a relatively short incubation period of 1 to 3 days. Sudden occurrence of fever, chills, headache, myalgia and prostration composes the non-specific systemic symptoms, followed by various degrees of respiratory symptoms of rhinitis and pharyngitis, including nasal congestion, sore throat and dry cough. Even though the majority of patients have no complications and recover spontaneously, the rare complication of influenza viral pneumonia can be fatal. In influenza viral pneumonia, symptoms similar to those of respiratory distress syndrome manifest as severe dyspnea, cyanosis and scanty blood-tinged sputum. Other complications can be secondary to bacterial pneumonia, most often caused by *Streptococcus pneumoniae* and *Staphylococcus aureus.* Complications of bacterial trachitis can be life-threatening. Bacterial trachitis is characterized by obstructed airways, a barking cough, suffocative and difficult breathing, and laryngeal spasm. Occasionally myocarditis is associated with influenza A infection, while viral myositis of the calves is more common with influenza B. Reye's syndrome, related to infection with influenza A and B, is usually associated with administration of aspirin.

Treatment for influenza infection emphasizes supportive care by addressing patients' major complaints and providing comfort. Antipyretics other than aspirin are suggested to reduce fever and alleviate pain, because salicylates accelerate the occurrence of Reye's syndrome. Bed rest and hydration are important. Influenza vaccination is prophylactic, but efficacy is limited to 67 to 92 percent because of the rapid antigenic drift of the influenza virus.

References:

Brady, M. T. (2002). Viral respiratory infections. In A. M. Rudolph et. al. (Eds.), *Rudolph's Pediatrics* (21st ed, chap. 13). New York, NY: McGraw-Hill

Centers of Disease Control and Prevention. (2003). Influenza: The disease. Retrieved June 8, 2003 from http://www.cdc.gov/ncidod/diseass/flu/fluinfo.htm

Centers of Disease Control and Prevention. (2003). Laboratory diagnostic procedures for influenza. Retrieved June 8, 2003 from http://www.cdc.gov/ncidod/diseases/flu/flu_dx_table.htm

Based on the clinical manifestations, influenza can be referred to TCM differentiation and treatment for common cold and cough.

In TCM, influenza is viewed under the scope of epidemic cold disease due to its severity, high degree of contagiousness, and pandemic nature. Influenza is different from common cold; according to the season of occurrence and clinical manifestations, it may also be referred to wind-warm febrile disease, summer-warm febrile disease and fall dryness.

Influenza is caused by exterior wind attacking a person with deficient righteous qi and inadequate resistance to exterior pathogens; therefore, pathogenic wind invades through the skin and lodges in the interstitial layer between the skin and muscle. This kind of epidemic wind is more prevalent during non-seasonal changes of weather. Having a sudden and rapid course at the initial stage, influenza is characterized by high fever. In spite of the possibility of causations by wind-cold and wind-heat, influenza is most often caused by warm-febrile pathogens; therefore, the treatment principle is similar to that for common cold, but requires the addition of high dosages of herbs that clear heat and relieve toxicity.

In addition, constitutional strength plays an important role in the occurrence of influenza. A weak constitution with an unconsolidated surface increases susceptibility to epidemic wind; once the disease is contracted, the constitutional deficiency allows the pathogens to invade further and faster; therefore, the symptoms are more severe. Influenza is mostly an excess condition, though a pattern of deficient root with excess branch is apparent in those with deficient righteous qi.

Analysis of Primary Symptom

A. Fever:

Caused by epidemic toxicity, fever presents throughout the entire course. Through the observation of the characteristics of the fever and the accompanying symptoms, influenza's severity can be understood and predicted. Fever serves as an indicator for the progression of the disease:

- When fever begins, aversion to cold is common. If fever predominates over aversion to cold, contraction of a warm-febrile pathogenic factor is evident. The affected location is still superficial, at the protective qi level. Prompt treatment at this stage makes a difference in controlling the progression.
- When fever worsens and aversion to cold is not as pronounced, it is a condition of exterior wind-cold invasion transforming into heat or one of exterior wind-heat invasion. Pathogenic factors have affected the qi level and gradual worsening of influenza is foreseen.
- High fever without any aversion to cold, accompanied by thirst, chest congestion and productive cough results when heat accumulates in the lung and causes failure of lung qi to disperse.
- Intractable high fever, possibly with loss of consciousness, signifies that epidemic heat has invaded the nutritive level and covered the heart's orifice. This is a critical condition.
- There is a higher incidence of influenza during the winter and spring seasons. When it occurs during other seasons, seasonal pathogenic influences complicate the characteristics of fever. For instance, when catching influenza during late-summer or the rainy season, there will be recessive fever detectable by thermometer but not by touching the surface of the body. This is a manifestation of epidemic heat combining with seasonal dampness. If one contracts influenza during summer, there will be high fever, thirst, perspiration and shortness of breath; this is the result of epidemic heat combining with summer heat. If influenza occurs during the fall season, fever, dry mouth, dry throat, and nasal congestion will manifest as epidemic heat combines with dryness.

B. Productive cough, congested chest and dyspnea:

These are secondary symptoms; they are caused by pathogenic heat accumulating in the lung, leading to failure of lung qi to disperse and descend. When lung heat consumes the fluid, yellow viscous sputum is formed. If heat injures the vessels, cough with blood-tinged sputum will be evident. In the case of constitutional lung qi deficiency or constitutional excessive phlegm-dampness accumulation, there will be a severe productive cough accompanied by a congested chest and dyspnea, even in the early stage of the disease.

Basic Patterns

- Wind-heat attacking the protective level
- Pathogenic heat affecting both protective and qi levels
- Heat accumulation in the lung
- Heat lodged in the pericardium

Progression of Pattern

At the initial stage of influenza, the clinical manifestations of fever and slight aversion to cold result from pathogenic factors affecting the superficial layer. Prompt treatment may end the disease course at this stage. If the problem remains unresolved and the pathogenic factors continue their invasion, the condition progresses to pathogenic heat affecting both protective and qi levels, then to heat accumulation in the lung. The advanced stage manifests as a complication of influenza, a critical condition indicates that heat is trapped in the pericardium.

Treatment Principle

Influenza is caused by epidemic pathogenic influences and has severe symptoms. Therefore, it is as equally important to disperse the exterior pathogens as to utilize herbs that clear heat and relieve toxicity at the initial stage of the disease. Modify the formula according to the accompanying pathogenic factors. If pathogenic influences invade into the interior, the treatment should focus on clearing heat and relieving toxicity, accompanied by dispersing lung qi, clearing heat from the heart and opening the orifices.

Pattern and Suggested Measure

Wind-heat attacking the protective level

High fever, slight aversion to wind, headache, general body ache, nasal congestion, sore throat and thirst. Thin yellow coating, and floating rapid pulse.

- Release the exterior and disperse wind-heat.
- Modified *Yin Qiao San*

Jin Yin Hua 10g.	*Lian Qiao* 10g.	*Bo He* 6g.
Dan Dou Chi 10g.	*Jing Jie* 6g.	*Niu Bang Zi* 10g.
Jie Geng 6g.	*Zhu Ye* 6g.	*Lu Gen* 10g.

- Severely high fever. + *Ban Lan Gen* 10g., *Da Qing Ye* 10g.
  Fever during the summer that is not reduced by diaphoresis, accompanied by irritability, thirst and dark urine, use *Xin Jia Xiang Ru Yin*.
  Fever during the fall with aversion to cold, headache, nasal congestion, dry throat, and dry cough, or sticky sputum that is difficult to expectorate, use *Xing Su San* or *Sang Xing Tang*.

Pathogenic heat affecting both protective and qi levels

Fever worsening and aversion to cold lessening, red face, thirst, irritability, dark urine, ache in the lower back and spine, general body ache, and possibly coughing. Red tongue, and rapid floating and forceful pulse.

- Release the pathogenic factors from both protective and qi levels.
- Modified *Chai Ge Jie Ji Tang*

Chai Hu 10g.	*Ge Gen* 15g.	*Huang Qin* 10g.
Jie Geng 6g.	*Bai Shao* 10g.	*Qiang Huo* 10g.
Bai Zhi 10g.	*Shi Gao* 30g.	*Gan Cao* 6g.

- Swollen sore throat. + *Niu Bang Zi* 10g., *She Gan* 6g.
  Thirst, irritability and dark urine. + *Zhu Ye* 10g., *Tian Hua Fen* 20g.
  Cough with yellow sputum. + *Xing Ren* 10g., *Gua Lou Ren* 15g., *Zhe Bei Mu* 10g.

Heat accumulation in the lung

High fever, thirst, chest congestion, dyspnea, cough with sticky yellow sputum or blood-tinged sputum, irritability and restlessness, cyanotic lips, and dark scanty urination. Dark red tongue with yellow coating, and rapid pulse.

- Clear heat, relieve toxicity and disperse lung qi.
- Modified *Ma Xing Shi Gan Tang*

Shi Gao 30g.	*Ma Huang* 6g.	*Xing Ren* 10g.
Gan Cao 6g.	*Da Qing Ye* 10g.	*Jie Geng* 6g.
Zhi Mu 10g.	*Yu Xing Cao* 10g.	*Jin Yin Hua* 10g.

- Thirst and oliguria. + *Tian Hua Fen* 15g., *Lu Gen* 10g.
  Chest congestion and pain. + *Gua Lou* 30g., *Sang Bai Pi* 10g.
  Cough with sticky yellow sputum. + *Huang Qin* 10g., *Zhu Ru* 10g.

Heat lodged in the pericardium

Persistent high fever, general sensation of heat in the body, possibly frigid extremities, severe headache, irritability and restlessness, delirium and coma. Dark red tongue, rapid thready or rapid flooding pulse.

- Purge fire and relieve toxicity; clear the heart and open the orifice.

- Take *An Gong Niu Huang Wan* with *Qing Ying Tang*

Shui Niu Jiao 10g. (substitute for *Xi Jiao*)		*Sheng Di Huang* 10g.
Xuan Shen 10g.	*Dan Shen* 15g.	*Huang Lian* 10g.
Lian Qiao 10g.	*Jin Yin Hua* 10g.	*Zhu Ye* 10g.
Mai Men Dong 15g.		

- Accompanied by spasm and rigid extremities, take *Zi Xue Dan*.

Other Modality

A. Acupuncture:

- **Manipulation:** Reducing method.
- **Prescription:** LU10 Yuji; LU5 Chize; LI11 Quchi; ST44 Neiting; GV14 Dazhui; TE5 Waiguan
- **Supplementary points:**
  - Sore throat. + LU11 Shaoshang
  - High fever. + BL11 Dazhu; Extra24 Shixuan
  - Chest congestion and pain. + PC6 Neiguan; TE6 Zhigou
  - Copious yellow sputum. + LU7 Lieque; ST40 Fenglong
  - Significant breathlessness and cough. + CV22 Tiantu
- **Prophylactic points:**
  - Even method. GV14 Dazhui; BL12 Fengmen; ST36 Zusanli
  - Indirect moxibustion with ginger. BL12 Fengmen; BL13 Feishu

B. Herbs that have an antiviral effect against influenza are:

Bai Bu, *Mu Dan Pi*, *Di Yu*, *Pang Da Hai*, *Da Huang*, *She Gan*, *Jin Yin Hua*, *Ma Chi Xian*, *Qian Hu*, *Bai Tou Weng*, *Zhi Zi*, *Ban Lan Gen*, *Zi Cao*.

C. Prophylactic measures:

Use the following methods during the pandemic season of influenza for prevention:

❶ Diffusing vinegar steam in a confined room may disinfect the environment. Steam 5-8 ml. of vinegar (mixed with water at 1:1 ratio) per m^3 for 30 minutes.

❷ Experiential remedies:

Ban Lan Gen 15g.	*Ren Dong Teng* 30g.	*Chai Hu* 15g.
Su Geng 15g.	*Bai Zhi* 10g.	*Sheng Jiang* 10g.

Take the daily dose divided into three small doses for three days.

CHAPTER 44

Viral Hepatitis

Viral hepatitis is characterized by infectious inflammation of the liver cells; there are five subtypes caused by five distinctive viruses. Twenty years ago, the hepatitis B virus (HBV) was identified as the virus causing "serum hepatitis"; subsequently, research in advanced molecular biology differentiated the sequence of the two fecally-orally transmitted viruses, hepatitis A virus (HAV) and hepatitis E virus (HEV), and two additional parenterally transmitted viruses, hepatitis C virus (HCV) and hepatitis D virus (HDV).

Hepatitis A is transmitted by the fecal-oral route through ingesting contaminated food and water. There is a high incidence in developing countries. Hepatitis B is transmitted by blood, sexual contact and contaminated needles. Hepatitis B infects more than 50 percent of the world's population. Although the United States has a low prevalence of chronic carriers (< 2%), the CDC estimates that there are approximately 78,000 new infections annually. Currently, there are 1.25 million chronic carriers of HBV in the U.S. Hepatitis C is the most common blood-borne infection and it is the leading cause of chronic liver disease. An estimated 3.9 million people have been infected by HCV in the U.S., and 2.7 million people have chronic infections. It is projected that 20-30 percent of chronic hepatitis C patients develop cirrhosis after 10-20 years, making advanced hepatitis C the leading indicator for liver transplantation. Patients are at high risk of gastrointestinal bleeding, encephalopathy, life-threatening bacterial infections, and hepatorenal failure once liver cirrhosis develops. Moreover, cirrhosis secondary to hepatitis C puts patients at increased risk of hepatocellular carcinoma (HCC). Coinfection of HCV and HIV is very common. Hepatitis D infection is limited to the hepatocytes; there is no evidence of extracellular replication. Hepatitis D occurs only in association with HBV infection, never independently. Although the majority of cases are self-limited, HBV-HDV coinfection can result in severe hepatitis with hepatocellular necrosis. Hepatitis E is rare in the United States; it is self-limited and recovery takes place in 1-4 weeks. Its course is similar to HAV infection but with more severe manifestations.

Type	Hepatitis A	Hepatitis B	Hepatitis C	Hepatitis D	Hepatitis E
Transmission	Fecal-oral.	Blood and body fluids.	Blood and body fluids.	Blood and body fluids.	Fecal-oral.
Incubation	2-6 weeks.	6 weeks-6 months.	2-12 weeks.		2-10 weeks.
Essentials of Diagnosis	IgG for prior infection; IgM for recent infection.	HbsAg; Anti-HBc IgM for acute infection; Anti-HBc IgG for chronic infection; HbeAg for active HBV replication; Anti-HBe for inactive infection.	Enzyme-linked immunosorbent assay of anti-HCV for past exposure or ongoing infection; Serum HCV RNA.	Only in the presence of HBV infection. HbsAg; Anti-HDV IgM for acute infection; Anti-HDV IgG for chronic infection.	Anti-HEV.
Symptoms	Jaundice, fatigue, malaise.	Fatigue, anorexia, icterus, arthalgia, rash, angiodema, rarely proteinuria and hematuria.	84% asymptomatic; jaundice, fatigue, fever, vomiting and right upper quadrant discomfort.	Jaundice, fever, and black vomit.	Fever, abdominal pain, vomiting, dark urine, clay-colored stool, diarrhea, and macular skin rash.
Complications and Prognosis	Never chronic; Complete recovery.	15-25% chronically infected persons die from chronic liver disease; major risk for HCC and cirrhosis.	85% chronic infection; 20-30% cirrhosis in 10-20 years; HCC.	Chronic HBV-HDV coinfection; rapid development of cirrhosis; liver failure.	Self-limited.
Treatment	Supportive and bed rest, high caloric diet.	Interferon, lamivudine, and liver transplant.	interferon and ribavirin.	Clearance of HBV infection.	Supportive.
Prevention	Improved higene; vaccine with 94-100% efficacy.	Hepatitis B vaccine with > 90% efficacy.	Avoid high risk drug-related behavior.	Hepatitis B vaccine.	No effective vaccine.

Depending on subtype and length of time since onset, viral hepatitis can be subcategorized as acute or chronic. Severity of symptoms varies, ranging from asymptomatic or nonspecific to serious and complication-related. Acute hepatitis usually has nonspecific symptoms, including malaise, fatigue, nausea, anorexia, arthralgia, as well as low-grade fever; as the condition progresses, pruritus, dark-colored urine, scleral icterus and jaundice may follow. Persons suffering from chronic viral hepatitis are often asymptomatic, and are usually unaware of their diagnosis unless it is discovered as an incidental finding or the condition advances.

Treatment of viral hepatitis includes supportive measures and symptom management; pharmaceutical agents include interferon, lamivudine, and ribavirin. Interferon-α-2b was approved by the FDA in 1992 as the major treatment for hepatitis B. It utilizes direct antiviral mechanisms and also enhances immunologic response to viruses. Interferon can also be used for early cirrhosis. Liver transplant is reserved for end stage chronic hepatitis.

Viral hepatitis caused by HAV, HBV, HCV, HDV, and HEV is differentiated as in table on page 314.

References:

Centers of Disease Control and Prevention (2003). National Center for Infectious Diseases- Viral Hepatitis. Retrieved September 5, 2003, from http://www.cdc.gov/ncidod/diseases/hepatitis/index.htm.

Centers of Disease Control and Prevention (2003). National Center for Infectious Diseases-Viral Hepatitis A- Fact Sheet. Retrieved September 5, 2003, from http://www.cdc.gov/ncidod/diseases/hepatitis/a/fact.htm.

Centers of Disease Control and Prevention (2003). National Center for Infectious Diseases-Viral Hepatitis B- Fact Sheet. Retrieved September 5, 2003, from http://www.cdc.gov/ncidod/diseases/hepatitis/b/fact.htm.

Centers of Disease Control and Prevention (2003). National Center for Infectious Diseases-Viral Hepatitis C- Fact Sheet. Retrieved September 5, 2003, from http://www.cdc.gov/ncidod/diseases/hepatitis/c/fact.htm.

Fox, R. K. & Wright, T. L. (2003). Viral hepatitis. In S. L. Friedman, K. R. McQuaid, J. H. Grendell, & Lange Medical Books/McGraw-Hill (Eds.), *Current Diagnosis & Treatment in Gastroenterology* (2nd ed. chap. 35). New York, NY: The McGraw-Hill Companies, Inc.

Depending on the clinical manifestations, TCM differentiation and treatment of viral hepatitis can be referred under jaundice or hypochondriac pain.

Viral hepatitis, from the perspective of TCM, results from the interaction of both interior and exterior pathogenic influences. Interior factors include dampness secondary to spleen pathology and qi stagnation secondary to liver pathology; exterior pathogens include damp-heat or epidemic heat toxicity. Improper diet, such as greasy food and alcohol, injures the spleen, generating dampness which stagnates and turns into heat. When this internal damp-heat is complicated by exterior damp-heat or epidemic heat toxicity, internal and external pathogeneses combine. The pathogens cannot be dispelled or drained because the anti-pathogenic mechanism is weak and, for this reason, patients with internal deficiency are at higher risk of acquiring viral hepatitis.

Based on the etiology and the clinical manifestations, TCM classifies viral hepatitis into icterohepatitis (jaundice) and anicteric hepatitis (non-jaundice). Dampness causes jaundice. When damp-heat accumulates in the middle burner, it interferes with the liver's ability to ensure the smooth flow of qi and obstructs the drainage of bile. Consequently, bile overflows into the blood stream or body fluid, manifesting as a bright yellow discoloration of the sclera, skin and urine that is known as yang jaundice. If damp-heat is complicated by fire toxicity, acute epidemic jaundice (also yang type) manifests as an acute and sudden occurrence of golden-yellow discoloration. Some patients with epidemic jaundice experience hematemesis, subcutaneous and mucosal bleeding, or even loss of consciousness and delirium, reflecting the invasion of fire toxicity into the nutritive and blood levels. Patients with constitutional yang deficiency are susceptible to cold-dampness; cold-dampness accumulates in the middle burner and obstructs the drainage of bile. Jaundice secondary to cold-dampness, known as yin jaundice, manifests with a dusky and smoky yellow discoloration.

Pathogenic factors affect the qi level in anicteric hepatitis. Because bile drainage remains patent, no yellow discoloration is apparent; however, damp-heat and epidemic toxicity hinder spleen and liver functions. Spleen dysfunction is responsible for poor appetite, abdominal distention and loose stool; dysfunction of the liver causes distention and pain in the chest and hypochondriac regions. There will be nausea and vomiting if the stomach is involved.

The clinical presentation of chronic hepatitis can be attributed to the characteristics of the pathogens, dampness and heat. Dampness is a yin pathogen; dampness lingering in the middle burner hinders the function of the spleen, causing spleen deficiency. Because the earth element is deficient, the wood element overacts and liver qi stagnation follows. Therefore, persons with chronic hepatitis exhibit pathogeneses of liver qi stagnation, disharmony between the liver and stomach, or constrained liver qi with spleen deficiency. Heat is a yang pathogen and it tends to injure liver yin. Injury to the yin can also result from overusing bitter herbs to dry dampness; thus, liver yin deficiency is common in chronic hepatitis.

In summary, the spleen, stomach, liver and gallbladder are the affected organs in hepatitis. Acute hepatitis is an excess condition of damp-heat accumulation or epidemic toxicity trapped in the nutritive and blood levels. Chronic hepatitis is a combination of excess and deficiency or an exclusively deficient condition associated with liver qi stagnation or spleen and kidney deficiency.

Analysis of Primary Symptom

A. Jaundice:

Jaundice is characterized by yellow discoloration of the sclera, skin and urine; damp-heat or cold-dampness forces bile to detour from its physiological drainage route into the body fluid. According to the intensity of the yellow discoloration, jaundice can be subcategorized into yang jaundice or yin jaundice.

- Bright lustrous yellow pigmentation like an orange peel, accompanied by fever, thirst and constipation, is caused by the contest between heat and dampness, with a preponderance of heat. When heat rules the pathogenesis, the yellow pigmentation becomes bright and lustrous. This is a type of yang jaundice.
- When the yellow pigmentation is not as bright and is accompanied by heaviness of the head and body, distention and fullness of the epigastrium and abdomen, and loose stool, dampness predominates over heat. The yellow pigmentation is not as bright as in the previous pattern and there are also significant symptoms of dampness in this type of yang jaundice.
- If a golden-yellow discoloration manifests with sudden onset, high fever, irritability, delirium and loss of consciousness, the pathology is heat-toxin causing yang jaundice.
- When the yellow discoloration is dusky and smoky, and is accompanied by lassitude, cold intolerance, cold limbs, abdominal distention, and loose stool, the pattern is one of yin jaundice caused by cold-dampness accumulating in the middle burner.

In general, dampness is the major contributing factor to jaundice. When dampness is complicated by heat, resulting from constitutional yang excess or excessive stomach fire, damp-heat develops and causes yang jaundice. When dampness is accompanied by cold, secondary to excessive yin or spleen yang deficiency, cold-dampness results and causes yin jaundice.

B. Hypochondriac pain:

The liver is located beneath the diaphragm and its channels are distributed bilaterally around the hypochondria. The gallbladder is attached to the liver and its channels travel through the same regions. Therefore, the liver and gallbladder are responsible for the hypochondriac pain. Excess patterns are related to qi stagnation, blood stasis, and damp-heat accumulation; the deficient pattern is caused by liver yin and blood deficiency failing to nourish the organ.

- When the pain is distending in nature, migrating, and aggravated by emotional stress, a pattern of liver qi stagnation is established.
- If there is stabbing hypochondriac pain in a fixed location, blood stasis is the contributing factor. When the pain is excruciating and accompanied by hard,

palpable and immobile masses, it indicates a severe case of blood stasis, often seen in liver cirrhosis.

- Burning pain accompanied by a bitter taste in the mouth and jaundice indicates damp-heat accumulation in the liver and gallbladder, often seen in acute hepatitis.
- When constant hypochondriac pain has a vague and dull quality, is aggravated by exertion, and is accompanied by low-grade fever and fatigue, liver and kidney yin and essence deficiency failing to nourish the liver is the cause, often seen in chronic hepatitis.

C. Poor appetite and abdominal distention:

These symptoms are commonly accompanied by nausea, bitter taste in the mouth, and altered bowel movements. This group of symptoms signifies disharmony of the spleen and stomach.

- Poor appetite or anorexia, bitter taste in the mouth, nausea, abdominal distention, and yellow greasy tongue coating are symptoms of an excess pattern of damp-heat accumulation, most likely in acute hepatitis.
- Poor appetite, significant abdominal distention after meals or in the afternoon, dry mouth, and loose stool aggravated by greasy diet are the results of spleen and stomach qi deficiency with liver yin deficiency, most likely in the cases of chronic hepatitis.

D. Malaise and fatigue:

Malaise and fatigue are common complaints throughout the course of viral hepatitis. In the early stage, malaise and fatigue are usually accompanied by general heaviness caused by dampness accumulation. When the condition is prolonged, malaise and fatigue are accompanied by shortness of breath, spontaneous or night sweating, and low-grade fever, pertaining to either qi deficiency or yin deficiency.

Basic Patterns

Acute icterohepatitis:

- Yang jaundice
- Heat toxin jaundice
- Yin jaundice

Anicteric hepatitis:

- Liver qi stagnation
- Constrained liver qi with spleen deficiency
- Liver and kidney yin deficiency

Progression of Pattern

According to *zang-fu* theory, damp-heat accumulation in the liver and gallbladder and liver qi stagnation are common in the initial stage of active hepatitis. Liver constraint with spleen deficiency is apparent in the intermediate stage. As the condition progresses, liver and kidney yin deficiency becomes the major pathogenesis during the end stage.

From an etiological perspective, heat-toxicity is the major contributing factor in the initial and active stages. Dampness obstruction and impaired flow of yang qi predominates during the intermediate stage. In the end stage, qi stagnates and blood stasis forms in the collaterals.

Inter-transformation of patterns progresses from the excess patterns evident during the initial and active stages, to a combined pattern of excess and deficiency in the intermediate stage, and finally to a deficient pattern or pattern with a deficient root and excess branch in the end stage.

Treatment Principle

In the case of excess in the initial and active stages, clear and drain damp-heat from the liver and gallbladder, and soothe and spread liver qi. Address deficiency during the end stage by strengthening the spleen, tonifying the qi, and nourishing liver and kidney yin. For chronic hepatitis, invigorate the blood, transform stasis and unblock obstruction in the collaterals. In all stages of the disease, the essential principle is to soothe, nourish, comfort and soften the liver.

Pattern and Suggested Measure

Acute icterohepatitis:

Yang jaundice

Bright yellow sclera, skin and urine; fever, thirst, distention and pain in the right hypochondrium, bitter taste in the mouth, nausea, anorexia, dark and scanty urine output and constipation. Yellow greasy tongue coating, and wiry rapid pulse.

- Clear heat, eliminate dampness and drain downwards.
- Modified *Yin Chen Hao Tang*

Yin Chen Hao 15g.	*Zhi Zi* 10g.	*Da Huang* 6g.
Long Dan Cao 9g.	*Fu Ling* 15g.	*Zhu Ling* 10g.
Che Qian Zi 15g.	*Hua Shi* 15g.	

- Significant pain in the right hypochondrium. + *Chai Hu* 10g., *Yu Jin* 10g.
  Preponderance of dampness with lusterless yellow discoloration, accompanied by heavy sensation in the head and body, focal distention in the chest and hypochondria, and pasty stool, use *Yin Chen Wu Ling San*.

Heat toxin jaundice

Sudden and acute onset of golden-yellow discoloration of the sclera, skin and urine; high fever, intense thirst, hypochondriac pain, abdominal distention, irritability, agitation, unconsciousness and delirium; possibly subcutaneous and mucosal bleeding, and edema or ascites. Red tongue with yellow greasy coating, and wiry slippery pulse.

- Clear heat and relieve toxicity; cool the blood and open the orifices.
- Modified *Xi Jiao San*
  Shui Niu Jiao 10g. (powder, substitute for *Xi Jiao*) *Yin Chen Hao* 15g.
  Huang Lian 10g. *Zhi Zi* 10g. *Sheng Ma* 10g.
  Sheng Di Huang 10g. *Mu Dan Pi* 10g. *Xuan Shen* 10g.
  Lian Qiao 10g. *Ban Lan Gen* 6g.
- Subcutaneous and mucosal bleeding. + *Di Yu Tan* 10g., *Ce Bai Ye Tan* 10g.
  Oliguria and ascites. + *Da Fu Pi* 10g., *Ze Xie* 15g., *Che Qian Zi* 15g.
  Unconsciousness and delirium. + *An Gong Niu Huang Wan*

Yin jaundice

Dusky, smoky yellow discoloration of the sclera, skin and urine; lassitude, cold intolerance, poor appetite, epigastric fullness, abdominal distention, and pasty or loose stool. Pale tongue with greasy coating, and soft decelerating or deep slow pulse.

- Strengthen the spleen, harmonize the stomach and transform cold-dampness.
- Modified *Yin Chen Zhu Fu Tang*
  Yin Chen Hao 15g. *Fu Zi* 6g. *Gan Jiang* 10g.
  Bai Zhu 10g. *Fu Ling* 15g. *Ze Xie* 15g.
  Hou Po 10g. *Gan Cao* 6g.
- Distention and fullness in the epigastrium and abdomen. + *Cang Zhu* 10g., *Da Fu Pi* 10g.
  Persistent jaundice or dark yellow discoloration. + *Ze Lan* 10g., *Dan Shen* 10g.
  Pruritus. + *Qin Jiao* 10g., *Di Fu Zi* 15g.
  If yang jaundice is not treated promptly, or if bitter and cold herbs are overused, yang jaundice may transform into yin jaundice. When a diagnosis of yin jaundice is established, follow the treatment according to this pattern.

Anicteric hepatitis:

Liver qi stagnation

Distending and migrating pain in the right hypochondrium, distention of the chest and abdomen, poor appetite, fatigue, possibly irritability and dry mouth. Red tongue with thin yellow coating, wiry or wiry and rapid pulse.

- Soothe the liver and regulate the qi
- Modified *Chai Hu Shu Gan San*

Chai Hu 10g.	*Xiang Fu* 10g.	*Zhi Qiao* 10g.
Chen Pi 10g.	*Bai Shao* 15g.	*Chuan Xiong* 6g.
Zhi Zi 6g.	*Huang Qin* 10g.	Gan Cao 6g.

- Significant hypochondriac pain. + *Yan Hu Suo* 10g., *Chuan Lian Zi* 10g.
  Severe cases of qi stagnation and blood stasis with hard, palpable and immobile masses under the hypochondrium, use *Bie Jia Jian Wan*.

Constrained liver qi with spleen deficiency

Distention and pain in the chest and hypochondriac regions that is worse after meals, poor appetite, fatigue, abdominal pain with diarrhea, pain relieved by defecation. Pale and dusky tongue with thin white coating, and wiry pulse.

- Soothe the liver and strengthen the spleen.
- Modified *Xiao Yao San*

Chai Hu 10g.	*Dang Gui* 10g.	*Bai Shao* 15g.
Bai Zhu 10g.	*Fu Ling* 10g.	*Sheng Jiang* 6g.
Dang Shen 10g.	*Xiang Fu* 10g.	*Gan Cao* 6g.

- Poor appetite. + *Shen Qu* 10g., *Mai Ya* 10g., *Ji Nei Jin* 10g.
  Stomach upset, acid regurgitation, bitter taste in the mouth, and nausea; or signs of constrained liver qi overacting on the stomach. + *Zuo Jin Wan*

Liver and kidney yin deficiency

Chronic dull hypochondriac pain aggravated by exertion, dizziness, blurred vision, dry eyes, irritability, dry mouth and throat, soreness and weakness in the lower back and knees, insomnia and dream-disturbed sleep. Red tongue with scanty coating, and wiry thready and rapid pulse.

- Nourish the yin and tonify the liver and kidney.
- Modified *Yi Guan Jian*

Sheng Di Huang 15g.	*Sha Shen* 10g.	*Mai Men Dong* 10g.
Dang Gui 10g.	*Gou Qi Zi* 10g.	*Chuan Lian Zi* 10g.
Mai Ya 10g.	*Xiang Fu* 10g.	*Gan Cao* 6g.

- Low-grade fever in the afternoon or tidal fever. + *Mu Dan Pi* 10g., *Bai He* 10g. Irritability and insomnia. + *Zhi Zi* 10g., *Suan Zao Ren* 10g., *Mu Dan Pi* 10g.

Other Modality

A. Acupuncture:

Acute icterohepatitis:

- **Manipulation:** Reducing method for yang jaundice; even method and moxibustion for yin jaundice.
- **Prescription:** SP9 Yinlingquan BL18 Ganshu ST36 Zusanli BL19 Danshu GV9 Zhiyang
- **Supplementary points:**
  - Yang jaundice. + LR3 Taichong; GB34 Yanglingquan
  - Yin jaundice. + BL20 Pishu; BL48 Yanggang

Anicteric hepatitis:

- **Manipulation:** Reducing method for excess patterns; reinforcing or even method for deficient patterns.
- **Prescription:** LR14 Qimen TE6 Zhigou SP6 Sanyinjiao GB34 Yanglingquan
- **Supplementary points:**
  - Qi stagnation. + LR3 Taichong; GB40 Qiuxu
  - Blood stasis. + BL17 Geshu; BL18 Ganshu
  - Qi deficiency. + CV12 Zhongwan; BL20 Pishu
  - Yin deficiency. + BL23 Shenshu; KI3 Taixi; BL18 Ganshu

B. Experiential formula:

❶ For acute icterohepatitis:
Yin Chen Hao 30g. *Yu Mi Xu* 30g.
Decoction, daily.

❷ Eliminate jaundice:
Qing Dai *Ming Fan* *San Qi*
Powder, 1-1.5 g./each, twice per day.

❸ Single herbs that effectively reduce serum ALT:
Wu Wei Zi, *Tian Ji Huang*, *Ji Gu Cao*, *Chui Pen Cao*.

CHAPTER **45**

HIV Infection and AIDS

Acquired Immunodeficiency Syndrome (AIDS) is caused by the human immunodeficiency virus (HIV). Ever since the first case of AIDS reported in the United States in 1981, it has been a major challenge in the U.S. healthcare system. There are approximately 800,000 to 900,000 Americans living with HIV, and 40,000 new HIV infections occurring every year. Epidemiology reports indicate that men has higher morbidity rate than women; more than half of the new HIV infections occurs among African Americans. There are already 448,060 deaths reported through December 2000. HIV progressively destroys the defensive mechanism by killing or damaging the CD4 positive T cells (T4), which is accountable for fighting off infections. The latent period can be as long as one to two decades. While the infection progresses, AIDS eventually follows. According to the Centers of Disease Control and Prevention official criteria, the definition of AIDS encompasses two clinical presentations, 1) less than 200 T4 cells per cubic millimeter of blood, 2) 26 clinical presentations, mostly opportunistic infections, associated with advanced HIV infection. HIV can be transmitted via blood or body fluids. Higher morbidity is found associated with unprotected sex, exposure to infected blood, sharing needles, and maternal-fetal transmission.

HIV infection is a chronic, progressive illness and clinical manifestations may vary from asymptomatic to severe opportunistic infections. People with initial exposure to HIV are usually asymptomatic; however, some might experience flu-like illness, including fever, headache, tiredness and enlarged lymph nodes, within a month or two after exposure. When their immune system deteriorates, the first sign of enlarged lymph nodes or swollen glands manifests and may last for more than three months. Other symptoms before the onset of AIDS are lack of energy, weight loss, frequent fever and sweating, various infections, skin rashes or even herpes. As the onset of AIDS, the most severe stage of HIV infection, occurs, severe opportunistic infections will follow. Symptoms include fever, coughing and shortness of breath, difficult or painful swallowing, severe and persistent diarrhea, vision loss, seizures and lack of coordination, confusion and forgetfulness, severe headache or coma. In addition to opportunistic infection, AIDS is also found associated with morbidity of various cancers, especially those caused by viruses.

For the last ten years, many drugs have been approved by Food and Drug Administration (FDA) to treat HIV infection. In addition to the famous Cocktail Therapy, there are also nucleoside reverse transcriptase (RT) inhibitors, non-nucleoside reverse transcriptase inhibitors (NNRTIs), and protease inhibitors. RT inhibitors, including AZT, zalcitabine, dideoxyinosine, stavudine, lamivudine, ziagen and viread, interrupt an early stage of virus replication. NNRTIs, such as delvaridine, nevirapine and efravirenz, are usually prescribed together with other antiretroviral drugs. Protease inhibitors, such as norvir, invirase, crixivan, agenerase and viracept, are used to interrupt the later step of virus replication.

References:

Centers of Disease Control and Prevention (2001). HIV/AIDS update: A Glance at the HIV epidemic. Retrieved August 8, 2003 from http://www.cdc.gov/nchstp/od/news/At-a-Glance.pdf

National Institute of Allergy and Infectious Diseases (2000). HIV Infection and AIDS: An overview. Retrieved on August 8, 2003 from http://www.niaid.nih.gov/factsheets/hivinf.htm

U.S. Department of Health and Human Services (2003). AIDS info: Acquired immunodeficiency syndrome. Retrieved on August 8, 2003 from http://www.aidsinfo.nih.gov/ed_resoures/glossary/default.asp?id=4&letter=a

The clinical presentations of HIV infection and AIDS may be referred to the different progressive stages of warm-febrile disease for differentiation and treatment.

The etiology of HIV infection and AIDS are closely related to contraction of toxicity, according to TCM:

Excessive and unprotected sexual activities exhaust kidney essence. Instability of basal qi leading to deficiency increases the susceptibility to toxic pathogenic influences. Addiction to drugs, or toxin in TCM, is another major contributor to HIV infection and AIDS. Usually, the toxin is drying and hot in nature that it tends to deprive the yin and fluid, leading to yin depletion. The toxin acquired is hidden deep inside the body; the recent contraction from seasonal or epidemic pathogens may activate the latent toxin, leading to various manifestations. The toxic pathogenic influences may also enter the blood level directly via blood transfusion, another causal factor for the contraction of HIV.

The early and intermediate stages of HIV infection and AIDS can be referred to the four levels of warm-febrile disease for differentiations and treatments. The condition of righteous qi and the strengths of toxic pathogens determine the progression and prognosis. At the beginning of the infection, the battle is marked by deficient righteous qi and persistent toxic pathogens. The toxic pathogens continue to invade deeper into the nutritive and blood level and lodged thereof, and the deficient righteous qi is too weak to expel the pathogens. Exhaustion of righteous qi is inevitable as the pathogens rule. Separation and disconnection of yin and yang is forecast as the progression is inexorable; the prognosis is not favorable.

Analysis of Primary Symptom

A. Flu-like illness:

Including fever, sore throat and dry cough, these symptoms signify a pathogenic invasion to the lung and protective qi. The toxic warm-febrile pathogens attack the lung in the upper burner to dry up lung yin. When the lung vessels are injured, blood tinged sputum is likely. Dyspnea and chest pain develop if both lung qi and lung yin were destructed.

B. Abdominal pain and severe diarrhea with purulent blood in the stool:

These symptoms indicate the progression into qi level and accumulation of pathogens in the stomach and intestines. When the toxic pathogens become lodged in the middle burner, disturbance of ascending and descending functions may cause nausea and vomiting.

C. Seizures, lack of coordination, confusion or coma:

When toxic pathogens continue to invade into the nutritive and blood levels, or pathogens are trapped in the pericardium, disturbance of the spirit will manifest as alteration of mentality. At this stage, the toxic pathogens directly and rapidly deprive the yin and trigger liver wind. This is a critical phase.

The above mentioned symptoms follow the progressive order of the infection; however, fever, night sweating, enlarged lymph nodes, emaciation and lassitude are observable throughout the course, pertaining to a presentation of toxic pathogenic excess and righteous qi deficiency.

Basic Patterns

- Febrile pathogens depriving lung and stomach yin
- Qi sinking and heat accumulation in the stomach and intestines
- Phlegm-heat misting the orifices and lodging in the terminal yin
- Separation and disconnection of the yin and yang

Progression of Pattern

The progression of HIV infection and AIDS matches that of warm-febrile disease, from protective to qi level, from nutritive to blood level. The toxic pathogens rule the entire course, while the righteous qi has always been deficient throughout. The progression of the illness ends in a state of depletion of basal qi, and separation and disconnection between the yin and yang.

Treatment Principle

Deficient righteous qi and lingering toxic pathogens constitute the major pathogenesis; therefore, the treatment principle aims to support the righteous qi and expel the toxic pathogenic influences.

Pattern and Suggested Measure

Febrile pathogens depriving lung and stomach yin

Fever, sore throat, dry cough with scanty sputum or blood tinged sputum, chest congestion and pain, dyspnea, pruritus, rashes, night sweating and emaciation. Dry red tongue with thin yellow coating, and rapid thready pulse.

- Nourish the yin, clear heat and moisten the lung.
- Modified *Bai He Gu Jin Wan*

Sheng Di Huang 10g.	*Shu Di Huang* 10g.	*Mai Men Dong* 10g.
Bai He 15g.	*Chuan Bei Mu* 10g.	*Xuan Shen* 10g.
Dang Gui 10g.	*Bai Shao* 15g.	*Ren Shen* 6g.
Jie Geng 6g.	*Gan Cao* 6g.	*Xing Ren* 10g.

- Cough with dyspnea. + *Wu Wei Zi* 10g., *He Zi* 10g.
  Blood tinged sputum. + *Zhi Mu* 10g., *Mu Dan Pi* 10g., *Ou Jie* 10g.
  Unremitting night sweating. + *Wu Mei* 10g., *Fu Xiao Mai* 15g., *Wu Wei Zi* 10g.

Qi sinking and heat accumulation in the stomach and intestines

Recurrent fever, emaciation and lassitude, nausea and vomiting, abdominal pain and diarrhea with purulent blood and tenesmus. Greasy tongue coating and soft thready pulse.

- Benefit the qi and lift the yang, eliminate dampness and relieve toxicity.
- Modified *Bu Zhong Yi Qi Tang* and *Bai Tou Weng Tang*

Huang Qi 15g.	*Dang Shen* 10g.	*Bai Zhu* 10g.
Sheng Ma 10g.	*Chai Hu* 10g.	*Bai Tou Weng* 10g.

Qin Pi 10g.	*Huang Lian* 10g.	*Huang Bai* 10g.
Guan Zhong 10g.	*Bai Shao* 10g.	*Mu Xiang* 10g.

- Persistent vomiting. + *Ban Xia* 10g., *Sheng Jiang* 6g.
  Constant diarrhea. + *Hong Teng* 10g., *Xian He Cao* 10g.

Phlegm-heat misting the orifices and lodging in the terminal yin

Fever, headache, nausea and vomiting, irritability, delirium or loss of consciousness, stiff neck, convulsions or spasms of the extremities. Yellow greasy tongue coating and rapid slippery pulse.

- Clear the heart and open its orifice, cool the liver and arrest wind.
- Modified *Niu Huang Zhi Bao Dan*
  Taking *Niu Huang Zhi Bao Dan* with the decoction of *Shui Niu Jiao* 30g. and *Ling Yang Jiao* 3g.

Separation and disconnection of the yin and yang

Severe diarrhea or fecal incontinence, severe vomiting and unable to ingest food, emaciation, lethargy, spontaneous or night sweating, pale nails, dry and lusterless hair. Flabby pale tongue with petechiae or purpura, and deep thready forceless pulse.

- This is a critical stage of the righteous qi failure, and separation and disconnection of the yin and yang. The emergency approach includes restoring devastated yang, restraining the yin, warming the kidney, binding the intestine, tonifying the qi and lifting the collapse.

CHAPTER 46

Acute Bronchitis

Acute bronchitis occurs with sudden onset of inflammation in the tracheobronchial tree. Extrinsic factors, including infectious microorganisms and allergens, are responsible for the occurrence of acute bronchitis. Acute infectious bronchitis as a result of viral or secondary bacterial infection usually follows an acute respiratory infection in winter. Other contributing factors include malnutrition and exposure to polluted air. Recurrent bronchitis is common in respiratory-compromised patients due to poor clearance of the bronchi, and is seen with conditions such as chronic sinusitis, bronchiectasis, bronchopulmonary allergy or chronic obstructive pulmonary disease (COPD). Bronchoconstriction resulting from inhalation of allergens is responsible for the occurrence of cough-variant asthma, especially in atopic persons or those with longstanding exposure to air irritants. In the initial stage of acute bronchitis, the respiratory mucosa is hyperemic, desquamated, and edematous; this is followed by leukocytic infiltration of the submucosa and production of sticky or mucopurulent exudates. As respiratory cilia, phagocytes and lymphatics are not able to defend the bronchi, susceptibility to bacterial infection increases, and the cough of acute bronchitis becomes a major defensive factor to clear the airway. When the condition progresses, edema of the airway, secretions and bronchial spasm may cause obstruction.

Since it is preceded by upper respiratory infection, the initial symptoms of acute infectious bronchitis reflect the antecedent disease, including chills, slight fever, body ache, sore throat and malaise. Onset of a distressing cough signifies the emergence of bronchitis. Usually, a dry and nonproductive cough will rapidly develop to scanty then to copious sputum production; abundant mucoid or mucopurulent sputum indicates bacterial infection. Burning substernal pain is possible, especially when coughing. Fever usually ranges between 101°F and 102°F; however, if fever persists when other acute symptoms disappear after three to five days, consider pneumonia, which is a critical complication of acute bronchitis. If the airway is obstructed, dyspnea will be obvious.

Although acute bronchitis is self-limiting and recovery is spontaneous, it may become very serious in debilitated patients and those with chronic pulmonary and cardiac pathologies. A clear history at intake of symptoms and signs is the basis for diagnosis; chest x-ray can be utilized to eliminate other possible diagnoses. Arterial blood gases (ABG) should be monitored if the condition is complicated by serious chronic respiratory disease. Sputum culture is indicated when antibiotics produce unfavorable results. Bed rest is recommended while there is fever and fluid supplements are important. Antipyretic analgesics are helpful for symptom management. When a sputum culture confirms the microorganisms, appropriate antibiotics may be selected.

When acute bronchitis extends its course and involves airway obstruction, chronic bronchitis as well as COPD follows.

Reference:

Beers, M. H. & Berkow, R. et. Al. (Eds.). (1999). Acute bronchitis. *The Merck Manual of Diagnosis and Therapy* (17th ed. chap. 69). West Point, PA: Merck & Co., Inc.

Based on the clinical manifestations, acute bronchitis is categorized according to TCM differentiation and treatment in the chapter on cough.

TCM perceives acute bronchitis as an exterior condition. Because cough is the primary symptom, acute bronchitis is categorized as exterior cough. Sudden weather changes and poor adaptation of the host to drastic alterations of climate predispose to acute bronchitis. Poor defense against the exterior pathogenic inlfuences by the righteous qi allows the pathogens to attack the lung via the mouth, nose or skin. These exterior pathogens impair the ascending and descending function of lung qi, leading to cough.

Dominant pathogens of the four seasons: As stated in the Chapter on Discussion of Cough in *He Jian Liu Shu*, "All six pathogenic factors, including cold, summer heat, dryness, dampness, wind and fire, may induce cough." However, the dominant pathogen varies with each of the four seasons; therefore, patterns of wind-cold, wind-heat and dry-heat can be distinguished. Based on his clinical experience, the ancient TCM scholar Jingyue Zhang summarized, "All six pathogenic factors can cause cough, especially wind-cold."

Wind as the leading pathogen: Wind is the leading pathogen of all six exterior influences; it migrates and is characterized by rapid progression and alteration. Wind leads or carries other pathogens with it to invade the lung.

Lung as the primary affected organ: The lung dominates the qi and controls respiration; it connects the airway and throat, and extends to the nose. The lung is located on top of all the other organs. Known as the "delicate and fragile organ," the lung has a direct connection to the external environment via the airway, nose and skin. It is the organ that is most vulnerable to exterior pathogenic invasions. Failure of lung qi to disperse leads to cough, and failure to metabolize fluid of the lung causes fluids to accumulate to form phlegm.

In general, when the pathogens stay at the superficial layers during the initial stage, a pattern of excess is apparent. However, people with constitutional lung deficiency are susceptible to exterior attacks. When acute bronchitis occurs in this population, a mixed pattern of excess with deficiency is common. If prompt treatment is not provided or the treatment provided is not appropriate, acute bronchitis will extend its course and manifest as a chronic cough, which further injures lung qi and leads to chronic pulmonary pathology, or COPD.

Analysis of Primary Symptom

A. Cough, dry or productive:

Cough is the primary symptom of acute bronchitis, which is categorized under the scope of exterior cough. Because cough results from impaired dispersion of lung qi due to exterior pathogenic influences, symptoms pertaining to an exterior condition must be present, including aversion to cold and fever. Cough is a defense mechanism to clear the airway and expel pathogens. Clinically, it has various presentations corresponding to the nature of the pathogenic factors:

- Barking cough with thin white sputum, accompanied by significant aversion to cold, slight fever, nasal congestion and watery nasal discharge, indicates an exterior wind-cold condition, mostly seen in winter season. When wind-cold obstructs lung qi so that it cannot disperse and descend, cough follows.
- Hoarse cough with heavy respiration, yellow sputum that is difficult to expectorate, fever, aversion to wind, and nasal congestion with turbid discharge are symptoms of a wind-heat pattern, especially during spring season. Wind-heat attacking the lung will impair the dispersion and descent of lung qi and induce coughing.
- Dry cough with scanty and sticky sputum that is difficult to expectorate, aversion to wind, fever, dry mouth and throat, chest pain elicited by coughing, and a dry thin yellow tongue coating are the manifestations of a pattern of dry-heat. Impairment of lung qi dispersion is caused by dry-heat injuring the lung fluid, leading to cough.
- Persistent cough, accompanied by dyspnea, increasing production of sticky yellow sputum, and worsening fever and diminishing aversion to cold, or persistent high fever with no chills, indicates a pattern of excessive heat accumulating in the lung; this may be caused by exterior pathogens invading

the interior or cold turning into heat. Increasing production of sputum signifies a severe infection, and persistent fever suggests the possibility of pneumonia.

B. Chills, or aversion to cold, and fever:

These two symptoms are common in the initial stage of acute bronchitis. Attacking exterior pathogenic factors injure the protective yang, which then fails to warm the superficial layers of the body, manifesting as aversion to cold. Attacks by exterior pathogens engage the righteous qi in a contest against the pathogens, manifesting as fever. Therefore, aversion to cold and fever are typical symptoms of exterior patterns, and they usually exist simultaneously. The preponderance of aversion to cold or fever, as well as the accompanying symptoms, suggest the nature of the pathogenic factor.

C. Dyspnea:

Unremitting cough injures lung qi, extending the course of the disease to chronic pulmonary pathology. Mild cases present as exertional dyspnea or wheezing, whereas severe cases manifest with orthopnea, puffy face and swollen feet. When a pattern of lung and kidney deficiency is apparent, the deficient lung fails to descend the qi and the deficient kidney fails to receive the qi, resulting in dyspnea. Dyspnea signifies a progression of acute bronchitis into chronic bronchitis.

Basic Patterns

- Wind-cold attacking the lung
- Wind-heat attacking the lung
- Dry-heat injuring the lung
- Exterior cold with internal heat
- Lung qi failing to disperse due to residual pathogens

Progression of Pattern

Acute bronchitis is caused by exterior pathogenic factors attacking the lung and protective qi level; it is categorized as exterior cough. The nature of the progression of the disease is two-fold: progression between the patterns, and progression from exterior to interior cough. The common pattern at the initial stage of acute bronchitis is wind-cold attacking the lung, which can develop into exterior cold with interior heat when lung qi is stagnant and turns into heat. When symptoms of an exterior condition are not as significant, yet pathogens remain trapped in the lung, the pattern is failure of lung qi to disperse due to residual pathogens. In addition to progression between patterns, exterior cough may also develop into interior cough. This is caused by secondary lung fluid injury due to chronic cough or heat, progressing into patterns of lung qi deficiency or lung yin deficiency. If the condition is complicated by unresolved phlegm-dampness or stagnant heat in the lung, patterns of phlegm-dampness accumulating in the lung and phlegm-heat accumulating in the lung follow, indicating progression into chronic pulmonary disease.

Treatment Principle

The essential pathogenesis of acute bronchitis includes contraction of exterior pathogens and failure of dispersion of lung qi; therefore, the treatment principles focus on dispelling pathogens to release the exterior, and dispersing lung qi to stop coughing. Adjuvant approaches are recommended based on the nature of the pathogens, such as dispersing cold, clearing heat, moistening dryness and transforming phlegm.

When the disease course is extended and injures righteous qi, a chronic pulmonary disease is foreseen; refer to the chapter on Chronic Obstructive Pulmonary Disease for differentiation and treatment.

Pattern and Suggested Measure

Wind-cold attacking the lung

Barking cough with heavy breathing, thin white sputum and itchy throat, accompanied by nasal congestion with clear discharge, sneezing, aversion to cold, fever, absence of sweating, headache or general body ache. Thin white tongue coating, and floating or floating tight pulse.

- Expel cold, disperse lung qi and stop coughing.
- Modified *San Ao Tang*

Ma Huang 6g.	*Xing Ren* 10g.	*Jie Geng* 6g.
Zi Su Ye 6g.	*Jing Jie* 6g.	*Qian Hu* 10g.
Zi Su Zi 10g.	*Gan Cao* 6g.	

- Copious, thin white sputum. + *Ban Xia* 10g., *Chen Pi* 10g., *Fu Ling* 15g.
  Headache and general body ache. + *Fang Feng* 10g., *Qiang Huo* 10g.
  Accompanied by aversion to wind, fever, sweating and floating decelerating pulse, use *Gui Zhi Jia Hou Po Xing Zi Tang*.

Wind-heat attacking the lung

Barking cough with dyspnea or hoarseness, viscous yellow sputum that is difficult to expectorate, accompanied by nasal congestion with yellow discharge, fever, aversion to wind, sore throat, general body soreness and aching, and slight thirst. Red tip and edge of the tongue, and rapid floating pulse.

- Expel wind, clear heat and disperse lung qi.
- Modified *Sang Ju Yin*

Sang Ye 10g.	*Ju Hua* 10g.	*Bo He* 6g.
Lian Qiao 10g.	*Jie Geng* 6g.	*Xing Ren* 10g.
Lu Gen 10g.	*Qian Hu* 10g.	*Niu Bang Zi* 10g.
Gan Cao 6g.		

- Viscous yellow sputum that is difficult to expectorate. + *Huang Qin* 10g., *Zhi Mu* 6g.

  Dry mouth and thirst. + *Tian Hua Fen* 10g., *Nan Sha Shen* 10g.

  Red swollen sore throat and hoarseness. + *Chan Tui* 6g., *She Gan* 6g.

  Significant phlegm-heat causing chest congestion, shortness of breath, yellow sticky sputum, thirst and desire to drink cold beverages, fever or constipation, use *Qin Jin Hua Tang Tang*.

Dry-heat injuring the lung

Dry cough or cough with scanty sputum that is difficult to expectorate, chest pain when coughing, dry nose and throat or mouth, possibly fever, slight aversion to wind or cold. Red tip and edge of the tongue with thin yellow coating, lack of moisture, and floating rapid pulse.

- Clear the lung and moisten dryness.
- Modified *Sang Xing Tang*

Sang Ye 10g.	*Xing Ren* 10g.	*Sha Shen* 10g.
Zhe Bei Mu 10g.	*Dan Dou Chi* 10g.	*Zhi Zi* 6g.
Li Pi 6g.	*Yu Zhu* 10g.	*Jie Geng* 6g.
Gan Cao 6g.		

- Significant heat signs. + *Zhi Mu* 10g., *Huang Qin* 6g.

  Significant dryness or yin injury. + *Mai Men Dong* 10g., *Xuan Shen* 10g.

  In severe cases of warm-dryness with dry cough, dyspnea, headache, fever, irritability and intense thirst, use *Qing Zao Jiu Fei Tang*.

  In the cases of cold-dryness with cough, thin sputum and white tongue coating, use *Xing Su San*.

Exterior cold with interior heat

Barking cough with sticky yellow sputum that is difficult to expectorate, tachypnea, possibly fever and dyspnea. Thin yellow tongue coating, and floating, slippery and rapid pulse.

- Dispel cold and clear heat.
- Modified *Ma Xing Shi Gan Tang*

Ma Huang 6g. *Xing Ren* 10g. *Shi Gao* 30g.
Gan Cao 6g. *Sang Bai Pi* 10g. *Huang Qin* 6g.
Jie Geng 6g. *Zi Su Ye* 10g. *Qian Hu* 10g.

- Significant aversion to wind and body ache. + *Fang Feng* 10g., *Jing Jie* 6g.
  Significant interior heat with red swollen sore throat. + *Niu Bang Zi* 10g., *Tian Hua Fen* 10g.
  Unremitting fever with intense thirst, constipation, greasy tongue coating and slippery pulse. + *Gua Lou Ren* 30g., *Da Huang* 3g.

Lung qi failing to disperse due to residual pathogens

Chronic productive cough with white or yellow sputum, itchy throat, possibly slight aversion to cold and fever, accompanied by chest congestion, and poor appetite. Thin white or thin yellow tongue coating.

- Disperse lung qi, transform phlegm and stop coughing.
- Modified *Zhi Sou San*

Zi Wan 10g. *Bai Qian* 10g. *Bai Bu* 10g.
Jie Geng 6g. *Ju Hong* 10g. *Xing Ren* 10g.
Zhi Qiao 10g. *Dang Shen* 6g. *Jing Jie* 6g.
Gan Cao 6g.

- Copious white sputum that is easy to expectorate and greasy tongue coating. + *Cang Zhu* 10g., *Hou Po* 10g., *Ban Xia* 6g.
  Itchy throat or sore throat. + *Chan Tui* 6g., *Mu Hu Die* 3g.

Other Modality

Acupuncture:

Wind-cold attacking the lung:

- **Manipulation:** Reducing method, combine acupuncture and moxibustion.
- **Prescription:** LU7 Lieque LI4 Hegu BL13 Feishu TE5 Waiguan

Wind-heat attacking the lung:

- **Manipulation:** Reducing method.
- **Prescription:** LU5 Chize BL13 Feishu LI11 Quchi GV14 Dazhui

Dry-heat injuring the lung:

- **Manipulation:** Reducing method.

- **Prescription:** LI1 Shangyang, KI7 Fuliu, BL13 Feishu, LU5 Chize

Exterior cold with interior heat:

- **Manipulation:** Reducing method.
- **Prescription:** BL12 Fengmen, BL13 Feishu, CV22 Tiantu, LU5 Chize, ST40 Fenglong, LU11 Shaoshang

Lung qi failing to disperse due to residual pathogens:

- **Manipulation:** Even method.
- **Prescription:** BL13 Feishu, LU9 Taiyuan, LR13 Zhangmen, SP3 Taibai, ST40 Fenglong

CHAPTER 47

Asthma

Affecting five percent of the U.S. population, asthma is a chronic inflammatory disorder of the airway. In 2000, there were an estimated 465,000 hospital admissions and 4487 deaths due to asthma attacks. Both men and women have an equal chance of being affected by asthma; however, African Americans and children are at higher risk for hospitalization, and African American adolescents and young adults have a higher mortality rate. For the last twenty years, the prevalence of asthma, and asthma-related hospitalizations and deaths have been increasing. Major contributing factors to asthma include atopy and exposure to allergens, such as animal dander, polluted air, tobacco smoke and seasonal pollens. Non-specific precipitating factors are upper respiratory tract infections, rhinitis, sinusitis, postnasal drip, aspiration, gastroesophageal reflux, weather changes, and stress. Pharmacological contributors are aspirin, NSAIDs, and tartrazine dyes.

Histopathologic findings include denudation of respiratory epithelium, collagen deposition under the basement membrane, airway edema, mast cell activation, and inflammatory cellular infiltration of neutrophils, eosinophils, and lymphocytes. Hypertrophy of bronchial smooth muscle and mucous glands causes obstruction in the airway with copious viscous mucus. Asthma is characterized by episodic and recurrent airway obstruction, manifesting as breathlessness, wheezing, cough, and chest tightness. The characteristic symptoms worsen at night or in the early morning hours. Complications of asthma are exhaustion, dehydration, respiratory infections, cor pulmonale, and tussive syncope. Diagnostic examinations and tests include pulmonary function tests, routine chest x-ray, laboratory tests for cell counts and mediator titers, and skin tests for sensitivity to allergens.

Treatment for acute asthma attack involves first aid to maintain airway patency. Considering the chronic nature of asthma, long-term management is essential to avoid acute attacks and hospitalizations. Treatments integrate anti-inflammatory medications, antimicrobials, and respiratory therapies. Prophylactic measures include avoiding exposure to allergens and annual influenza and pneumococcal vaccinations.

References:

Centers of Disease Control and Prevention (2003). Asthma prevalence, health care use and mortality, 2000-2001. Retrieved on July 24, 2003 from http://www/cdc.gov/nchs/products/pubs/pubd/hestats/asthma/asthma.htm

Chesnutt, M. S. & Prendergast, T. J. Disorders of the airways. In L. M. Tierney, et. al. (Eds.), *Current Medical Diagnosis & Treatment* (42nd ed. chap. 9). New York, NY: McGraw-Hill Companies, Inc.

Practitioners of TCM perceive asthma as a disease of exterior pathogenic influences triggering latent phlegm in the lung. Phlegm is the primary etiology of asthma; it results from failure of the lung to distribute and disseminate fluids adequately, or from failure of the spleen to transform and transport fluids, or from failure of the kidney to steam and transform fluids. Phlegm forms, accumulates and lies in the lung; latent phlegm can be stirred by weather changes (exterior wind carrying allergens), improper diet, emotional stress, and exertion. Airway obstruction by latent phlegm causes impaired dispersion and descent of lung qi, manifesting as wheezing, breathlessness, chest congestion, and productive cough.

Based on the clinical manifestations, asthma can be subcategorized into two phases, acute episode and chronic remission.

Acute episodes are characterized by phlegm obstruction in the lung, and can be further classified into cold and heat patterns. The primary symptoms are wheezing, breathlessness, cough, hunched shoulders and use of accessory muscles for labored breathing. These symptoms are caused by difficulty passing air through a narrowing airway. When air passes through the latent phlegm, a wheezing sound is heard.

The chronic remission phase is characterized by recurrent longstanding asthma that transforms from an excess to a deficient pattern. The remission phase involves deficient lung qi failing to distribute fluids and consolidate the surface, resulting in phlegm formation and increased risk of acute episodes due to increased susceptibility to exterior pathogens. Spleen or kidney deficiency also plays an important role during remission. The deficient spleen generates phlegm, adding to the latent phlegm in the lung. Phlegm formation is also related to kidney deficiency. Kidney yang deficiency fails to metabolize fluids while empty fire secondary to kidney yin deficiency consumes the body fluid; both pathologies lead to phlegm formation. Symptoms in this phase are not as pronounced, but include shortness of breath, fatigue, and constant mild wheezing. When the condition relapses and is exacerbated by contributing factors, the crisis of an asthma attack occurs with severe constant wheezing; if heart yang is affected, qi collapse follows as tussive syncope.

Refer to "Wheezing" in Chapter 4 for comprehensive TCM differentiation and treatment of asthma (see page 19-24).

CHAPTER 48

Bronchiectasis

Bronchiectasis refers to irreversible focal bronchial dilation affecting a single segment, a single lobe or multiple lobes of the lung. Most commonly occurring in the lower lobes, it is often accompanied by chronic respiratory infection. Congenital bronchiectasis is rarely seen; secondary to maldevelopment of the lung, it is characterized by cystic dilation of developed bronchi. Acquired bronchiectasis results from direct destruction of the bronchial wall or mechanical alterations. Infections, inhalation of noxious chemicals, immunologic reactions or vascular abnormalities directly damage the bronchial wall by depriving the bronchial tissue of nutrition. Increased traction of the bronchial wall can be mechanically induced by atelectasis and loss of parenchymal volume, leading to secondary infection and bronchial dilation. Pathologically, bronchiectasis has characteristics of extensive inflammatory destruction of the bronchial walls, increased mucous secretion and loss of cilia. Depending on the degrees and features of pathological changes, functional and hemodynamic abnormalities vary, including reduced lung volumes and airflow rates, ventilation/perfusion defects, and hypoxemia. A chest X-ray may show bronchiectasis if there is notable peribronchial fibrosis, intrabronchial secretions, pulmonary atelectasis, and cystic dilation. High-resolution CT (HRCT) of the chest has been widely adopted to provide more accurate imaging, in which the dilated airway is clearly illustrated by tram lines, a signet ring appearance, or grapelike clusters in more severely affected areas. Fiberoptic bronchoscopy is indicated for bronchiectasis with recent onset to rule out substantial obstruction related to a tumor, foreign body or other endobronchial abnormalities.

Conditions predisposing to bronchiectasis include severe pneumonia, necrotizing pulmonary infections, substantial bronchial obstruction, and chronic fibrosing lung diseases. Immunologic deficits, whether acquired, congenital or hereditary, increase the susceptibility to infection.

Most patients suffer from chronic cough and sputum production, often elicited by a respiratory infection. The symptoms worsen gradually over time and the cough becomes more productive as the course advances. The characteristic cough has a unique pattern, in which a productive cough occurs in the morning on arising, in the late afternoon, and on retiring. The copious sputum can be separated into three layers, frothy at the top, greenish and turbid in the middle, and thick with pus at the bottom. Other symptoms, such as hemoptysis that can be the first or only complaint, recurrent fever and pleuritic pain, are also common. When the condition advances and becomes complicated by chronic obstructive pulmonary disease, symptoms of wheezing and shortness of breath pertaining to cor pulmonale may occur. Treatments for bronchiectasis are designed to address infection, mucous secretion, airway obstruction, and prevention of complications. Avoid cigarette smoking, exposure to irritants and administration of sedatives and antitussives. Compliance with childhood immunization, improved living conditions, and adequate nutrition serve a prophylactic function in reducing prevalence, morbidity and mortality.

Reference:

Beers, M. H. & Berkow, R. et. Al. (Eds.). (1999). Bronchiectasis. *The Merck Manual of Diagnosis and Therapy* (17th ed. chap. 70). West Point, PA: Merck & Co., Inc.

Based on the clinical manifestations, bronchiectasis can be referred to TCM differentiation and treatment for cough, lung abscess, and hemorrhage.

From the perspective of TCM, bronchiectasis is a disorder of phlegm-dampness and warm-febrile pathogens acting on an existing deficiency of the lung.

Pre-existing spleen and lung deficiency, the root of bronchiectasis, is closely related to congenital insufficiency. Higher risk of pathogenic invasion and the inability to expel exterior pathogens result from deficiency of the spleen and lung; therefore, recurrent upper respiratory infections characterize this disease.

Exterior pathogenic influences, the primary extrinsic etiology, attack the deficient lung, especially wind-cold, wind-heat and epidemic toxicity. Congested heat, secondary to pathogens trapped in the lung, can injure the lung vessels and exhaust the lung fluids, leading to hemoptysis and coughing up purulent sputum.

Emotional stresses, primarily anger and frustration injuring the liver, indirectly cause cough and hemoptysis when liver fire insults the lung and injures the vessels.

Yin deficiency with empty fire results from chronic medical conditions that consume the yin, leading to empty fire. Empty fire injures the lung vessels.

Blood stasis obstructing in the lung may be due to secondary circulatory disturbances caused by the previously mentioned pathogens obstructing lung qi, or by emission of blood from the lung vessels.

The entire disease course, from contraction of exterior pathogens to injury of lung vessels, is chronic, progressive and irreversible. The root deficiency of lung and spleen is evident throughout the course, and the excess branch of attacks by exterior pathogens is recurrent. Bronchiectasis is initiated by pathology of the lung and gradually involves the spleen and liver; at its advanced stage, the heart and kidney are affected. Injury to the lung vessels is the major pathogenesis of bronchiectasis, and the recurrent nature of the disease reflects repetitive insults to the vessels from various pathogenic factors, including exterior pathogens and pathogenic heat from relevant organs.

Analysis of Primary Symptom

A. Cough and production of sputum:

Cough becomes more productive and intense as the disease advances, primarily elicited by respiratory tract infections.

- A loud cough with sticky sputum that is more pronounced in the morning when arising or after meals indicates phlegm-dampness accumulating in the lung. "The spleen is the origin of phlegm formation," and "The lung is the container of phlegm storage." Therefore, productive cough is commonly accompanied by poor appetite and loose stool, symptoms pertaining to spleen deficiency.
- When a cough with heavy respiration, tachypnea and breathlessness, and foul sticky sputum is also accompanied by fever, thirst and irritability, congested phlegm-heat is forming an abscess. This group of symptoms is common in bronchiectasis complicated by severe pulmonary infections.
- Coughing up scanty sputum or a dry cough accompanied by malar flush, tidal fever and night sweating signifies a secondary lung yin deficiency due to excessive heat. This group of symptoms appears in the later stage of bronchiectasis when exterior conditions are no longer significant factors. If yin deficiency generates empty fire, dry cough and hemoptysis are possible.

B. Hemoptysis:

As another primary symptom, sometimes hemoptysis is the first and only complaint; it may accompany a productive cough. Hemoptysis results from heat, deficient or excess, injuring the lung vessels.

- If blood-tinged sputum or foul, purulent sputum is accompanied by fever and thirst, phlegm-heat congestion in the lung should be suspected. As phlegm-heat congests in the lung, it decomposes the tissue and forms pus and abscesses, an excess pattern. If coughing yields excessive bright-red blood, or persistent hemoptysis, is accompanied by short temper, bitter taste in the mouth, and hypochondriac pain, there is a pattern of liver qi stagnation turning into fire, another excess pattern pertaining to liver fire insulting the lung and injuring lung vessels.

- Recurrent hemoptysis with fresh red blood accompanied by five-centers heat and night sweating is precipitated by yin deficiency with empty fire that injures the lung vessels.
- Intractable, excessive hemoptysis with palpitations, shallow breathing, pallor, and abundant sweating indicates a critical condition of qi deficiency failing to keep the blood in the vessels. This is an advanced stage of yang devastation secondary to yin depletion, therefore one of insufficient qi and yin.

Basic Patterns

- Phlegm-dampness accumulation in the lung
- Phlegm-heat accumulation in the lung
- Liver fire insulting the lung
- Yin deficiency with empty fire

Progression of Pattern

The initial stage of bronchiectasis presents as recurrent cough and increased production of sputum. If phlegm stagnates and transforms into heat, or if the condition is complicated by toxic pathogenic influences, there is the characteristic pattern of phlegm-heat accumulation in the lung. Longstanding lung heat compromises the state of the lung and involves the liver; as the metal element is weakened, relatively hyperactive liver fire exacerbates the pathology and a pattern of liver fire insulting the lung is inevitable, manifesting as hemoptysis with abundant bright-red blood due to heat forcing the reckless movement of the blood. Both phlegm-heat and liver fire consume the yin, leading to yin deficiency with empty fire, thus the end stage of bronchiectasis becomes yin depletion and qi exhaustion, a condition of qi loss secondary to blood loss.

Treatment Principle

The treatment principle is built upon the essential pathogenesis of phlegm-heat accumulation in the lung and heat-toxicity injuring the lung vessels: clear lung heat and transform phlegm, and cool the blood and stop bleeding. In respect to the inevitable pathology of lung vessel injury, lung qi rebellion and blood stasis, adjuvant approaches to descend lung qi and invigorate the blood are equally important.

Pattern and Suggested Measure

Phlegm-dampness accumulation in the lung

Recurrent cough with a loud sound and viscous sputum that is worse in the morning on arising or after meals and aggravated by greasy or sweet food, chest congestion, nausea and vomiting, poor appetite, abdominal distention and loose stool. White greasy tongue coating, and soft slippery pulse.

- Dry dampness, transform phlegm, benefit the qi and strengthen the spleen.
- Modified *Liu Jun Zi Tang* and *San Zi Yang Qin Tang*

Ban Xia 10g.	*Chen Pi* 10g.	*Fu Ling* 15g.
Dang Shen 10g.	*Bai Zhu* 10g.	*Bai Jie Zi* 10g.
Su Zi 10g.	*Lai Fu Zi* 10g.	*Gan Cao* 6g.

- White frothy sputum with cold intolerance. + *Gan Jiang* 6g., *Xi Xin* 3g.
  Focal distention in the epigastrium and abdomen with thick and greasy tongue coating. + *Cang Zhu* 10g., *Hou Po* 10g.

Phlegm-heat accumulation in the lung

Cough with purulent and viscous yellow sputum, possibly foul-smelling and difficult to expectorate or blood-tinged, tachypnea, heavy breathing, distention and fullness in the chest and hypochondriac regions, chest pain elicited by cough, thirst, subjective sensation of a foul odor in the throat, irritability, possibly fever or swollen painful gums, and dry stool. Red tongue with yellow greasy coating, and rapid slippery pulse.

- Clear heat and transform phlegm.
- Modified *Qian Jin Wei Jing Tang* and *Jia Wei Jie Geng Tang*

Dong Gua Ren 30g.	*Yi Yi Ren* 30g.	*Tao Ren* 10g.
Lu Gen 10g.	*Jin Yin Hua* 10g.	*Jie Geng* 6g.
Bei Mu 10g.	*Ju Hong* 6g.	*Ting Li Zi* 10g.
Bai Ji 6g.	*Gan Cao* 6g.	

- Copious sputum production that is purulent and foul-smelling. + *Yu Xing Cao* 10g., *Bai Jiang Cao* 10g., *Lian Qiao* 10g.
  Thirst, irritability and constipation. + *Tian Hua Fen* 15g., *Da Huang* 6g.
  Blood-tinged sputum or hemoptysis. + *Bai Mao Gen* 10g., *Zhi Zi* 10g., *Ou Jie* 6g.

Liver fire insulting the lung

Coughing up pure blood or sputum with abundant blood, intractable hemoptysis, irritability, restlessness, bitter taste in the mouth, and pain in the chest and hypochondriac regions. Red tongue with yellow coating, and rapid wiry pulse.

- Clear and purge liver heat, cool the blood and stop bleeding.
- Modified *Xie Bai San* and *Dai Ge San*

Sang Bai Pi 10g.	*Di Gu Pi* 10g.	*Qing Dai* 2g.
Hai Ge Ke 15g.	*Sheng Di Huang* 10g.	*Bai Mao Gen* 10g.
Da Xiao Ji 10g.	*Ce Bai Ye* 10g.	*Gan Cao* 6g.

- Excessive liver fire with dizziness, red eyes, irritability and short temper. + *Zhi Zi* 10g., *Mu Dan Pi* 10g., *Huang Qin* 10g.
  Severe cough. + *Xing Ren* 10g., *Jie Geng* 6g., *Huang Qin* 10g.
  Cough with excessive sputum. + *Yu Xing Cao* 10g., *Gua Lou Ren* 15g.

Yin deficiency with empty fire

Cough with scanty sputum or blood-tinged sputum or recurrent hemoptysis with bright-red blood, dry mouth and throat, five-centers heat and night sweating. Dry red tongue with scanty coating or no coating, and rapid thready pulse.

- Nourish the yin, clear heat, moisten the lung and stop coughing.
- Modified *Bai He Gu Jin Wan*

Bai He 10g.	*Chuan Bei Mu* 10g.	*Mai Men Dong* 10g.
Xuan Shen 10g.	*Sheng Di Huang* 10g.	*Bai Shao* 10g.
Dang Gui 10g.	*Zhi Mu* 10g.	*Bai Ji* 10g.
Bai Mao Gen 10g.	*Gan Cao* 6g.	

- Severe deficient fire with tidal fever and night sweating. + *Di Gu Pi* 10g., *Bai Wei* 6g., *Wu Wei Zi* 10g., *Mu Li* 30g.
  Recurrent hemoptysis with abundant blood. + *E Jiao* 10g., *San Qi* 6g.
  Critical condition due to qi loss following blood loss with abundant hemoptysis, profuse perspiration and pallor, use *Du Shen Tang* in conjunction with first aid intervention and strict bed rest.

Other Modality

A. Acupuncture:

Phlegm-dampness accumulation in the lung:

- **Manipulation:** Even method.
- **Prescription:** BL13 Feishu, BL20 Pishu, ST36 Zusanli, ST40 Fenglong, CV12 Zhongwan, LU5 Chize

Phlegm-heat accumulation in the lung:

- **Manipulation:** Reducing method.

- **Prescription:** CV22 Tiantu, LU5 Chize, ST40 Fenglong, LU7 Lieque, LU11 Shaoshang, BL13 Feishu

Liver fire insulting the lung:

- **Manipulation:** Reducing method.
- **Prescription:** BL13 Feishu, BL18 Ganshu, LU8 Jingqu, LR3 Taichong, LR2 Xingjian

Yin deficiency with empty fire:

- **Manipulation:** Even method.
- **Prescription:** BL13 Feishu, LU1 Zhongfu, LU7 Lieque, KI6 Zhaohai, KI3 Taixi, SP6 Sanyinjiao
- **Supplementary points:**
  - Hemoptysis. + LU6 Kongzui; LU5 Chize; LU10 Yuji

B. Experiential remedies:

1. Single herbs:

❶ Fresh *Zhu Li Shui* 15-20 ml. (three times per day).

❷ *Tian Zhu Huang* 0.5-1 g. (powder, three times per day).

2. Formulas:

❶ For recurrent cough with purulent sputum.
Yu Xing Cao 30g. *Jin Yin Hua* 30g. *Dong Gua Ren* 30g.
Yi Yi Ren 30g. *Jie Geng* 15g. *Huang Lian* 5g.
Huang Qin 10g. *Bei Mu* 10g. *Tao Ren* 10g.
Gan Cao 5g.
Decoction, once per day.

❷ For recurrent hemoptysis.
Da Ji, *Bai Ji* and *Da Huang*
Powder, routine dosage in the ratio of 3:2:1; 3-5 g, once per day.

CHAPTER 49

Chronic Obstructive Pulmonary Disease

Chronic obstructive pulmonary disease (COPD) is the fourth leading cause of death in the United States with over 100,000 deaths reported annually. The median survival time for severe COPD patients is approximately four years. Counting merely the home oxygen therapy cost is already about 300 to 500 dollars per month. According to the estimation from the National Heart, Lung and Blood Institute, there are fourteen millions Americans diagnosed with COPD and equal numbers remained undiagnosed. COPD is characterized by obstruction in the airway secondary to chronic bronchitis or emphysema; such airway obstruction progresses gradually, and airway hyperreactivity is possible. Patients diagnosed with COPD usually have both conditions of chronic bronchitis and emphysema. The former is manifested by excessive secretion of bronchial mucus and productive cough for a minimum of three months in at least two consecutive years; diagnosis of chronic bronchitis should include ruling out other possible pathological causes contributing to the symptoms. Emphysema is the condition of abnormal, permanent enlargement of distal air spaces of the terminal bronchiole with destruction of the walls; however, fibrosis is not significant. Cigarette smoking is thought to be the major contributing factor to COPD. In addition, air pollution, respiratory infection, familial factors or heredity, and allergy may also elicit COPD.

The chief complaints of patients who suffer COPD are excessive cough, sputum production and shortness of breath. These symptoms usually last for ten years or more, and they progressively worsen. Dyspnea may be initiated only on heavy exertion, then on mild physical activities, finally even at rest. Frequent exacerbations of COPD are common and they lead to sick leaves and eventually disability from work. Death secondary to acute respiratory failure occurs during exacerbation.

Conditions including acute bronchitis, pneumonia, pulmonary thromboembolism, and concomitant left ventricular failure may worsen COPD; however, advanced COPD may be accompanied by pulmonary hypertension, cor pulmonale and chronic pulmonary failure. Be alert if hemoptysis presents, which may indicate chronic bronchitis or bronchogenic carcinoma. Cessation of smoking is considered the most important intervention in both COPD prevention and treatment. Comprehensive treatment includes low flow oxygen therapy, bronchodilators, corticosteroids, antibiotics and respiratory treatment.

Reference:

Chesnutt, M. S. & Predergast, T. J. (2003). Lung-Disorders of the airway: Chronic obstructive pulmonary disease. In L. M. Tierney, Jr., et. al. (Eds.), *Current Medical Diagnosis & Treatment* (42nd ed. chap 9). New York, NY: McGraw-Hill Companies Inc.

Based on the clinical manifestations, COPD can be referred to TCM differentiation and treatment of cough, breathlessness, wheezing and congested fluids.

COPD is a consequence from the progression of various pulmonary dysfunctions and diseases. It has a slow onset and progressive nature; therefore, it is primarily characterized by deficiency, which increases the susceptibility of the patient to contraction of exterior pathogens that exacerbate the condition. In general, COPD is a progressive irreversible pathology. The following intrinsic and extrinsic factors implicate the occurrence of COPD:

Extrinsic factors consist of both exterior pathogenic factors and lifestyle factors. Exterior pathogenic factors invading through the skin, mouth or nose to attack the lung and disturb the function of the lung to properly disperse and descend. Lifestyle factors, such as overindulgence in tobacco, alcohol or spicy food, may elicit an obstruction in the airway, leading to lung qi rebelling upwards manifested by coughing, wheezing and breathlessness. Clinical presentations of cold, heat and dryness are determined by the combination of different characteristics of extrinsic factors and various constitutions.

Intrinsic dysfunctions: Dysfunction of the lung results from disharmony of other organs. Spleen dysfunction leads to phlegm accumulation, which obstructs in the lung. Qi rebelling upwards to cause stagnation in the lung can be a consequence from the kidney failing to receive the qi. Kidney yin deficiency with empty fire, which injures lung fluid, results in lung qi failing to descend. These factors contribute to the lung's dysfunction by impairing the dispersing and descending function, manifested by cough, dyspnea and production of sputum.

COPD results from the interactions between the intrinsic and extrinsic factors. Extrinsic factors injure the lung, causing lung qi deficiency; deficient lung qi increases the susceptibility to extrinsic factors. Mutual aggravation by each other, extrinsic and intrinsic factors create a chronically progressive irreversible COPD.

During remission, deficiency predominates in the condition, while exacerbation is caused by contraction of extrinsic factors, bringing on a complicated condition of deficiency and excess.

Analysis of Primary Symptom

A. Excessive cough and sputum production:

Excessive cough and sputum production usually manifest simultaneously; this group of symptoms can be used to differentiate pathogeneses of either exterior-contraction or internal injury. Such criteria differentiate acute exacerbation from remission, or distinguish the pathology of deficient root with excess branch from pure deficiency. Differentiations can be determined based on the characteristics of phlegm and cough:

- Productive cough with excessive sputum, tachypnea, and symptoms of aversion to cold and fever indicates acute exacerbation. In addition to the above symptoms, white frothy sputum signifies the condition of exterior wind-cold with interior cold congested fluids; yellow viscous sputum that is difficult to expectorate signifies a condition of exterior wind-cold with interior phlegm-heat.
- Weak cough with thin sputum, aversion to wind and spontaneous sweating are symptoms of lung qi deficiency. Dry cough with scanty sputum, tidal fever and night sweating are symptoms of lung yin deficiency or lung and kidney yin deficiency.

B. Shortness of breath and dyspnea:

- Tachypnea, dyspnea, heavy breathing, flaring nostrils, yellow viscous sputum and fever manifest phlegm-heat accumulation in the lung.
- Tachypnea, dyspnea, elevated shoulder and opened mouth to breathe, orthopnea, copious white sputum and nausea manifest phlegm-dampness obstruction in the lung.
- Tachypnea, dyspnea and difficulty with inhalation than exhalation that are aggravated by exertion, shortness of breath, and lack of strength are classic presentations of kidney failing to receive the qi. These symptoms are commonly seen in kidney deficiency or lung and kidney deficiency.
- Tachypnea, dyspnea, palpitations, dysuria and edema indicate a complicated condition of yang deficiency of both the spleen and kidney with water overflowing towards the heart and lung.
- When pulmonary symptoms, such as tachypnea, dyspnea, elevated shoulder and opened mouth to breathe, productive cough with excessive sputum, condition occurring year round especially during cold weather, are accompanied by symptoms of exterior wind-cold, the patient has a condition of exterior wind-

cold triggering the latent congested fluids in the lung. This condition is very common during acute exacerbation.

C. Blood-tinged sputum or hemoptysis:

These are secondary symptoms manifesting complications, commonly in the advanced stage. Presence of blood indicates the damage of lung vessels by heat, excess heat in the lung or empty fire secondary to lung yin deficiency or to lung and kidney yin deficiency.

D. Edema:

Edema signifies presence of complication in advanced stage of COPD. Spleen and kidney yang deficiency is accountable for failure of fluid metabolism. Advanced complication is apparent when edema is accompanied by dysuria, tachypnea and dyspnea, palpitations, possible cyanotic lips; heart involvement is certain, namely cor pulmonale in Western medicine.

Basic Patterns

Acute exacerbation episode:

- Exterior wind-cold triggering the latent congested fluids
- Exterior wind-cold with phlegm-heat accumulation

Remission:

- Phlegm-dampness accumulation in the lung
- Phlegm-heat obstruction in the lung
- Lung deficiency
- Kidney deficiency
- Spleen and kidney yang deficiency

Progression of Pattern

COPD is a result from other pulmonary pathology; chronic and progressive, COPD is primarily dominated by deficiency. During acute exacerbation, a complicated combination of deficient root and excess branch is apparent. Cough and productive cough are the primary symptoms in early stage of COPD in which the lung is the primary organ involved. When the kidney is involved, the primary symptoms shift to shortness of breath and breathlessness. In the advanced stage, palpitations and edema manifest spleen and kidney yang deficiency.

Treatment Principle

Deficient root and excess branch dominate the primary pathogenesis of COPD. Tonify the lung, strengthen the spleen, and warm the kidney to address the deficient root. Transform phlegm, eliminate dampness, release the exterior, disperse lung qi, clear heat and promote urination to address the excess branch.

Pattern and Suggested Measure

Acute exacerbation episode:

Exterior wind-cold triggering the latent cold congested fluids

Productive cough with copious white frothy sputum, breathlessness, orthopnea, unremitting condition aggravated by cold weather; aversion to cold, fever, no sweating, general body ache during acute exacerbation by cold. White slippery tongue coating, and wiry tight pulse.

- Disperse cold, release the exterior, warm the lung and transform congested fluids.
- Modified *Xiao Qing Long Tang*

Ma Huang 10g.	*Gui Zhi* 6g.	*Xi Xin* 3g.
Gan Jiang 10g.	*Ban Xia* 10g.	*Bai Shao* 10g.
Wu Wei Zi 10g.	*Gan Cao* 6g.	*Xing Ren* 10g.

- Copious viscous sputum and stifling sensation in the chest. + *Bai Jie Zi* 10g., *Lai Fu Zi* 10g.

  If exterior wind-cold is released, yet productive cough with excessive sputum and breathlessness remain, use *Ting Li Da Zao Xie Fei Tang*.

Exterior wind-cold with phlegm-heat accumulation

Productive cough, tachypnea, copious sputum that is yellow viscous or blood-tinged and is difficult to expectorate; accompanying symptoms include aversion to cold, fever, body ache, perspiration or sluggish sweating, and thirst. Thin yellow or yellow greasy tongue coating, and rapid floating or rapid slippery pulse.

- Disperse lung qi, release the pathogenic influences, clear heat and transform phlegm.
- Modified *Ding Chuan Tang*

Ma Huang 10g.	*Bai Guo* 10g.	*Su Zi* 6g.
Xing Ren 10g.	*Kuan Dong Hua* 10g.	*Ban Xia* 6g.
Sang Bai Pi 10g.	*Huang Qin* 10g.	*Gan Cao* 6g.

- Significant exterior wind-cold with aversion to cold and fever. + *Fang Feng* 10g., *Qian Hu* 10g.
  Significant internal heat with fever and thirst. + *Shi Gao* 30g., *Tian Hua Feng* 10g.
  Yellow sticky sputum that is difficult to expectorate. + *Zhu Ru* 10g., *Jie Geng* 6g., *Gua Lou Ren* 15g.

Remission:

Phlegm-dampness accumulation in the lung

Productive cough with copious sputum that is white and viscous, stifling sensation in the chest, possibly breathlessness, poor appetite, focal distention and fullness in the epigastrium and abdomen, and loose stool. White greasy tongue coating, and soft slippery pulse.

- Strengthen the spleen, dry dampness and transform phlegm.
- Modified *Liu Jun Zi Tang* and *San Zi Yang Qin Tang*

Dang Shen 10g.	*Bai Zhu* 10g.	*Fu Ling* 15g.
Ban Xia 10g.	*Chen Pi* 10g.	*Su Zi* 10g.
Bai Jie Zi 10g.	*Lai Fu Zi* 10g.	*Gan Cao* 3g.

- Significant focal distention and fullness in the epigastrium and abdomen with thick greasy tongue coating. + *Cang Zhu* 10g., *Hou Po* 10g.

Phlegm-heat obstruction in the lung

Productive cough with copious sputum that is yellow and viscous or blood-tinged, possibly foul smelling, intense heat and irritable sensation or distention and pain in the chest, thirst with preference for cold beverages, scanty urination and dry stool. Red tongue with yellow or greasy coating, and rapid slippery pulse.

- Clear heat from the lung and transform phlegm.
- Modified *Sang Bai Pi Tang*

Sang Bai Pi 10g.	*Zhi Zi* 10g.	*Huang Qin* 10g.
Huang Lian 6g.	*Su Zi* 10g.	*Xing Ren* 10g.
Bei Mu 10g.	*Ban Xia* 6g.	*Lu Gen* 10g.

- Significant heat. + *Shi Gao* 30g., *Zhi Mu* 10g.
  Suffocating sensation, and distention and pain in the chest. + *Jie Geng* 6g., *Ting Li Zi* 10g., *Gua Lou Ren* 15g.
  Viscous sputum or foul smelling sputum. + *Yu Xing Cao* 10g., *Yi Yi Ren* 15g., *Dong Gua Ren* 10g.
  Thirst and dry throat. + *Tian Hua Fen* 15g.

Lung deficiency

Weak cough with thin sputum, shallow and rapid respirations and shortness of breath, spontaneous sweating, aversion to wind and propensity to catching cold; dry cough with scanty viscous sputum, thirst, dry throat and malar flush. Pale tongue or dry red tongue, and thready weak or rapid thready pulse.

- Augment the qi, nourish the yin and tonify the lung.
- Modified *Bu Fei Tang* and *Sheng Mai San*

Ren Shen 6g.	*Huang Qi* 15g.	*Shan Yao* 15g.
Mai Men Dong 10g.	*Shu Di Huang* 10g.	*Wu Wei Zi* 10g.
Zi Wan 10g.	*Sang Bai Pi* 10g.	

- Significant lung qi deficiency. + *Bai Zhu* 10g., *Jie Geng* 6g.
  Significant lung yin deficiency. + *Sha Shen* 10g., *Bai He* 10g.
  Complicated by spleen qi deficiency with poor appetite, abdominal distention and loose stool, use *Bu Zhong Yi Qi Tang*.

Kidney deficiency

Primary symptoms of dyspnea characterized by breathlessness and tachypnea, more difficulty with inhalation than exhalation, and condition aggravated by exertion; possibly secondary symptoms include lassitude, fatigue, cold intolerance, cold limbs, and cyanotic or dusky complexion; pale tongue with moist white coating, and weak thready pulse. Or possibly secondary symptoms of irritability, restlessness, red face, dry mouth and throat, blood-tinged sputum and oily perspirations; dry red tongue, and rapid thready pulse.

- Tonify and assist the kidney to receive the qi.
- Modified *Jin Gui Shen Qi Wan* and *Shen Ge San* for kidney yang deficiency.

Fu Zi 6g.	*Rou Gui* 10g.	*Shu Di Huang* 10g.
Shan Zhu Yu 15g.	*Shan Yao* 15g.	*Fu Ling* 15g.
Ze Xie 10g.	*Ren Shen* 6g.	*Ge Jie* 2g.
Ci Shi 30g.	*Hu Tao Rou* 15g.	

- Significant malaise and lack of strength. + *Huang Qi* 15g., *Bai Zhu* 10g.
- Modified *Qi Wei Du Qi Wan* and *Sheng Mai San* for kidney yin deficiency.

Ren Shen 10g.	*Mai Men Dong* 15g.	*Wu Wei Zi* 10g.
Shu Di Huang 15g.	*Shan Zhu Yu* 10g.	*Shan Yao* 15g.
Fu Ling 15g.	*Mu Dan Pi* 10g.	*Ze Xie* 10g.

- Dry mouth and throat. + *Zhi Mu* 10g., *Sha Shen* 10g., *Bai He* 10g.
  Hemoptysis. + *Bai Mao Gen* 10g., *E Jiao* 10g.
  Five-centers heat and night sweating. + *Di Gu Pi* 10g., *Zhi Mu* 10g.

Spleen and kidney yang deficiency

Stifling and suffocating sensation in the chest, tachypnea or breathlessness, palpitations, dysuria, thirst without desire to drink, and general edema, especially the lower extremities. Flabby pale tongue, and deep thready pulse.

- Warm the yang and promote urination.
- Modified *Zhen Wu Tang*

Fu Zi 10g.	*Bai Zhu* 15g.	*Fu Ling* 15g.
Sheng Jiang 10g.	*Bai Shao* 10g.	*Gui Zhi* 6g.
Fang Ji 15g.	*Ting Li Zi* 10g.	*Gan Cao* 6g.

- Cyanotic complexion or lips. + *Dan Shen* 15g., *Chuan Xiong* 6g., *Tao Ren* 10g.

Other Modality

A. Acupuncture:

For those with significant productive cough with copious sputum, refer to "Cough" in Chapter 2 for differentiation and treatment (see pages 17-18).

For those with significant breathlessness with rapid perspirations, refer to "Breathlessness" in Chapter 4 for differentiation and treatment (see page 31).

B. Experiential remedies:

❶ *Zi He Che* 1.5g. (powdered form, twice per day).

❷ *Ge Jie* 0.5 g. (scorched and powdered, twice per day).

❸ *Hu Tao Rou* 3 pieces (once per day).

CHAPTER **50**

Pulmonary Abscess

Since effective antibiotic therapy was introduced in the 1940's and 1950's, the mortality rate from pulmonary abscess decreased from 30-50 percent to 5-20 percent. With the recent resurgence in immunologically compromised populations, the mortality rate for intensive care and immunosuppressed patients is currently as high as 28 percent. Pulmonary abscess occurs when pus collects in a cavity formed by disintegrated tissue. It is considered acute if the condition lasts less than six weeks or chronic if the condition lasts longer than six weeks. Two major types of pulmonary abscess are classified according to etiology. Aspiration of oropharyngeal contents is the most common predisposing factor to primary pulmonary abscess, followed by necrotic pneumonia, chronic pneumonia, and opportunistic infection. Secondary pulmonary abscess usually follows bronchial obstruction, cavitating lesions, direct extension, and hematogenous dissemination. Suppurative microorganisms inducing pulmonary abscess include *S. aureus, Streptococcus pyogenes, K. pneumoniae, E. coli* and *pseudomonas*. However, uncommon organisms, such as *Candida albicans, Legionella micdadei, L. pneumophila* and *Pneumocystis carinii*, are the leading causes of opportunistic infection in immunocompromised patients.

Typical complaints with pulmonary abscess are an insidious onset of cough, fever, dyspnea, and pleuritic chest pain. Patients suffering from chronic pulmonary abscess also complain of malaise and weight loss. There is hemoptysis at the initial stage, followed by a productive cough with foul-smelling, purulent sputum indicating rupture of the abscess into the bronchus. If the abscess ruptures into the pleural cavity, pyopneumothorax, sepsis and empyema necessitatis occur. Diagnosis is based on laboratory and imaging findings. The non-specific laboratory finding of an increased number of white blood cells indicates infection. Chest X-ray can show an intensely consolidated area or rounded density with or without an air-fluid level. Sometimes, CT scan provides a better image. Bronchoscopy is required for bronchial obstruction. Fine needle aspiration provides more accurate culture and sensitivity compared to a sputum specimen and bronchoalveolar lavage; it is especially indicated for immunodeficient patients. Antibiotics, chiefly penicillin and clindamycin, are effective treatments for pulmonary abscess. However, pyopneumothorax due to an abscess rupturing into the pleural cavity requires surgery, usually lobectomy.

Reference:

Jablons, D., Cameron, R. B., & Turley, K. (2003). Thoracic wall, pleural, mediastinum, & lung: Diseases of the lungs. In L. W. Way (Ed.), *Current Surgical Diagnosis & Treatment* (11th ed. chap. 19). Norwalk, Connecticut: McGraw-Hill Companies, Inc.

From the perspective of TCM, pulmonary abscess is one of the internal abscesses. The lung is responsible for the pathogenesis, and the pathology pertains to heat excess, or excessive heat accumulation in the lung. From the initial invasion of exterior pathogens to formation and perforation of the abscess, there are four stages, each one with significant pathological markers.

The initial stage is the exterior stage, in which the exterior pathogens, especially wind-heat, attack the lung and affect both the protective layer and lung organ. Symptoms at this stage are insidious with aversion to wind, fever, cough and sweating.

The second stage is the suppurative stage, in which the cavity of pus is formed as a result of the interaction of phlegm-heat, heat toxicity and blood stasis. When phlegm-heat and blood stasis are obstructed in the lung, they start to decompose the tissues. Dead tissues and these two pathogens fuse and form pus. Clinical manifestations in this stage include high fever, chills, cough, tachypnea and pleuritic chest pain.

When the suppurative stage is not treated promptly, complications develop in the perforating stage. As the phlegm-heat, blood stasis, heat toxicity and dead tissues continue to damage the lung and lung vessels, the abscess ruptures into the bronchus or pleural cavity and a productive cough with foul-smelling, purulent and bloody sputum follows.

If the condition lasts longer than six weeks, a chronic recurrent lung abscess will result, manifesting as low-grade fever, malaise, weight loss, and intermittent expectoration of purulent bloody sputum. However, if proper treatment is rendered and the patient responds well, a recovery stage ensues. During this stage, the accumulated pathogens are discharged along with the sputum. Systemic symptoms are decreased as fever is reduced, cough is relieved and sputum becomes clear, indicating the recovery of righteous qi and the healing of lung tissue.

Refer to "Lung Abscess" in Chapter 5 for comprehensive TCM differentiation and treatment of pulmonary abscess (see pages 33-38).

CHAPTER 51

Arrhythmias

Arrhythmia is a broad category that encompasses disturbances of cardiac rhythm and conduction; it can be mild and asymptomatic, symptomatic (syncope, near syncope, dizziness or palpitations) or even fatal.

Predisposition to cardiac arrhythmias can be due to hereditary or acquired structural heart diseases. Electrolyte abnormalities, hormonal imbalances, hypoxia, pharmaceutical adverse effects and myocardial ischemia all can increase the risk. Cardiac arrhythmias can be categorized into four major types: 1) Disorders of automaticity are closely related to S-A node arrest, premature beats, and initiation of reentry arrhythmias. 2) Abnormal impulse conduction can occur at any point in the pacemaking or conduction system; it may occur within the atria or ventricles, resulting in sinoatrial exit block, atrioventricular block, or reentry circuits. 3) Reentry accounts for many arrhythmias; it induces premature beats, most paroxysmal supraventricular tachycardias, and atrial flutter. 4) Triggered activity (depolarization triggered by abnormal electrical impulses) may be associated with ventricular tachycardia in cases of digitalis toxicity or long QT syndrome.

Diagnosis is made by establishing a causal relationship between the disturbed rhythm and symptoms; however, due to their sporadic nature, cardiac arrhythmias can be easily missed, especially when there is no significant discomfort. A 24-hour Holter monitor is used to record the heart rhythm and establish a correlation with the symptoms. Exercise testing is especially helpful if symptoms are related to exertion and stress. When symptomatic bradyarrhythmias or supraventricular tachyarrhythmias are detected, therapy can be started promptly and further studies might not be necessary. On the other hand, if ventricular tachyarrhythmias are noted, a electrocardiogram is recommended.

Supraventricular and ventricular arrhythmias are the two major types of arrhythmias. Supraventricular arrhythmias include sinus arrhythmia, bradycardia and tachycardia, premature atrial contraction, paroxysmal supraventricular tachycardia, atrial fibrillation, atrial flutter and multifocal atrial tachycardia. Ventricular arrhythmias include premature ventricular contraction, ventricular tachycardia, ventricular fibrillation, accelerated idioventricular rhythm, and long QT syndrome.

Pharmaceutical agents form the major treatment for arrhythmias. Membrane sodium channel blockers slow down conduction and increase refractoriness; beta-blockers decrease automaticity and prolong atrioventricular conduction and refractoriness; potassium channel blockers decrease automaticity and conduction as well as prolong refractoriness; calcium channel blockers decrease automaticity and atrioventricular conduction.

References:

American College of Cardiology Foundation (2002). Cardiac arrhythmias. Retrieved on July 24, 2003 from http://www.acc.org/media/patient/chd/cardiac_arrhythmias.htm

Massie, B. M. & Amidon, T. M. (2003). Disturbances of rate and rhythm. In L. M. Tierney Jr. et. Al. (Eds.), *Current Medical Diagnosis & Treatment* (42nd ed. chap. 10). New York, NY: McGraw-Hill Companies, Inc.

In TCM, arrhythmia occurs as a result of heart pathology, primary or secondary. Some arrhythmias are due to the primary conditions of deficient qi and blood failing to nourish the heart and/or deficient yang failing to warm the heart. The primary condition of heart yin deficiency with empty fire disturbing the heart will also lead to arrhythmia. Arrhythmias can also result from secondary conditions caused by blood stasis in the heart vessels or cold congested fluids overflowing towards the heart.

In addition to a chief complaint of palpitations, pulse analysis is essential to diagnose arrhythmias:

1. Slow pulse signifies excessive yin-cold pathogens obstructing the conduction of the pulse and/or deficient yang failing to initiate the pulse, commonly seen in class II and III atrioventricular block, sinus arrhythmias and digitalis toxicity.

2. Rapid pulse implies excessive yang and deficient yin, commonly seen in various tachyarrhythmias.

3. Hasty pulse is a sign of extremely hyperactive yang with depleted yin, or a sign of heat accumulation in the triple burner with deteriorated yin and blood; commonly seen in atrial and ventricular fibrillation, and in frequent attacks of premature atrial and ventricular contractions.

4. Knotted pulse results from excessive yin-cold pathogens with declining yang qi; this irregular pulse is associated with various bradyarrhythmias, such as sinoatrial block or atrioventricular block.

5. Intermittent pulse signifies exhaustion and debility of the vital organs. Intermittent pulse can manifest as bigeminal pulse, trigeminal pulse and S-A node arrest, and it is detectible in premature atrial and ventricular contractions.

Refer to "Palpitations" in Chapter 6 for comprehensive TCM differentiation and treatment of arrhythmias (see pages 39-46).

CHAPTER 52

Hypertension

Detected by sphygmomanometer, an exhibition of elevated blood pressure (systolic blood pressure equal to or exceed 140 mmHg or diastolic blood pressure equal to or exceed 90 mmHg) in three separate occasions constitutes hypertension. Incidence of hypertension increases with age and is more common in African Americans than Caucasian Americans. Its diagnosis is based on the objective finding of elevations of either the systolic or diastolic blood pressure, and its treatment objectives aim to achieve the normalization of both. Diagnosis of essential or primary hypertension is applied if the cause is not identifiable, whereas that of secondary hypertension is established if a specific cause is related. Estrogen usage, renal disease, renal vascular pathology, Cushing's syndrome, and other vascular or endocrine dysfunctions are highly associated with secondary hypertension. In addition, heredity and environmental factors are believed to be closely related to morbidity of hypertension.

The most common complications of hypertension are stroke and coronary heart disease. Hypertension also plays a causative factor to end stage renal disease and heart failure. These complications are related either to persistent elevations of blood pressure or to atherosclerosis. For the past thirty years, although the mortality rates for stroke and coronary heart disease have decreased and leveled off, the morbidity of end stage renal disease and heart failure continues to increase.

After years of asymptomatic period, patients with mild to moderate essential hypertension may exhibit headache or dizziness. However, if hypertensive encephalopathy evolved as hypertension is accelerated, confusion, auditory and visual disturbances, and nausea and vomiting may occur. Patients with episodic hypertension might experience anxiety attacks, palpitations, profuse perspiration, pallor, tremors or chest pain. Other symptoms related to causative pathologies may accompany elevated blood pressure in those with secondary hypertension. Medication composes the major strategy for treatments. Initiation of medication should be built upon a thorough consideration of the entire cardiovascular system, not merely blood pressure. Common antihypertensive agents include diuretics, beta-adrenergic blocking agents, angiotensin-converting enzyme inhibitors and calcium channel blockers. A comprehensive measure, integrating management in diet and exercises, improving life style, and avoiding high risk behaviors, is preferable.

Reference:

Massie, B. M. (2003). Systemic Hypertension. In L. M. Tierney, Jr. et. Al. (Eds.), *Current Medical Diagnosis & Treatment* (42nd ed. chap. 11). New York, NY: McGraw-Hill Companies, Inc.

Based on the clinical manifestations, hypertensive disease can be referred toTCM differentiation and treatment of headache, dizziness, tinnitus and palpitations.

The incidence of hypertension is closely related to the following contributing factors:

Emotional stresses, such as excessive anger and frustration, are the predisposing factors for liver qi stagnation, and rising of liver wind-yang complex. Stagnant liver qi may turn into fire and exhaust liver yin. When insufficient yin fails to restrain the yang, hyperactive liver yang occurs.

Improper diet: Overindulgence in rich, greasy and sweet diet injures the spleen and stomach, leading to generation of damp-turbidity. Accumulated damp-turbidity can further stagnate and transform into heat, rising to disturb the clear orifices. The mechanism of ascending clear yang and descending turbidity is interrupted.

Kidney essence deficiency fails to generate the marrow, leading to emptiness of the sea of the marrow.

Caused by contributing factors stated above, disequilibrium of the yin and yang results. A pathology of excess above and deficiency below is indicated by liver and kidney yin deficiency and hyperactive liver yang rising. Hyperactive yang may transform into wind and generate fire. When wind and fire mutually aggravate each other, blood follows the rebellious qi upwards to disturb the mind and cover the orifices. As a result, wind-stroke or syncope will likely develop.

Analysis of Primary Symptom

A. Headache and dizziness:

Headache and dizziness may come about as the primary symptoms simultaneously or independently in hypertensive disease.

- Sudden onset, distending or explosive headache accompanied by dizziness, red face and eyes, irritability and short temper is related to pathology of liver qi stagnation turning into fire. Fire flaring upwards disturbs the clear orifice. This is an excess pattern.

- Headache and dizziness together with distending sensation of the eyes, heaviness of the head and weakness of the lower extremities, and soreness and weakness of the lower back indicate a complicated pathology. As liver and kidney yin are deficient, or water failing to nurture the wood, and hyperactive liver yang rises to disturb the orifices, this condition pertains to a pattern of excess above and deficiency below.
- Dizziness, blurred vision, dry eyes, and numbness and tingling of the extremities are symptoms of liver and kidney yin deficiency. Lacking dissemination of essence upwards leads to malnourishment of the clear orifices, as well as deficit of moistening to the sinews and vessels. This is a deficiency pattern.
- Dizziness and headache with an empty sensation, complicated by weak and numb extremities or heel pain, signify yang deficiency due to consumption of the yin, or deficiency of both the yin and yang, leading to emptiness of the sea of the marrow.
- Headache characterized by heaviness and cloudiness, dizziness, stifling sensation in the chest, nausea and poor appetite are related to damp-turbidity. As damp-turbidity obstructs the middle burner and covers the orifices, clear yang becomes inactive and fails to thrive.

B. Tinnitus:

Tinnitus or auditory disturbance may present in hypertensive disease when complications developed. Tinnitus is often a result of pathogenic heat covering the orifices or malnourishment from deficient kidney essence.

- Sudden onset of tinnitus or loud high-pitched buzzing, aggravated by anger or emotional excitement, signifies an excess heat pattern or hyperactive yang pattern, such as liver fire blazing or hyperactive liver yang.
- Constant tinnitus with soft noise like cicadas, relieved by rest and aggravated by mild physical exertion, is caused by deficient kidney essence failing to provide nourishment. Liver and kidney yin deficiency, and both kidney yin and yang deficiency are examples of this pattern.
- Tinnitus or decreased auditory acuity with a stuffy sensation in the ear is most likely a result of phlegm-heat disturbing upwards and misting the orifices.

C. Palpitations:

Palpitations occur during the later stage of hypertension; it usually indicates complications of cardiovascular pathologies. Palpitations can be excess or deficient pattern. When hyperactive yang with heat disturbs the mind, symptoms of palpitations, irritability, restlessness, and difficulty falling into sleep will follow. If yin and blood deficiency fail to nourish the mind, palpitations, forgetfulness and restless sleep will manifest. Results from inactive chest yang caused by phlegm-dampness obstruction are palpitations, stifling sensation in the chest, nausea and vomiting.

Basic Patterns

- Liver fire excess
- Yin deficiency with hyperactive yang
- Liver and kidney yin deficiency
- Deficiency of both the yin and yang
- Damp-turbidity obstruction

Progression of Pattern

The presentation during the initial stage is mostly an excess pattern, gradually turning into deficiency or the combination of excess and deficiency patterns at the later stage. Longstanding excessive liver fire consumes the yin, leading to liver and kidney yin deficiency; gradually, consumption of the yin causes yang deficiency, deficiency of both the yin and yang then follows. Hyperactive yang may rise from liver and kidney yin deficiency. A complicated condition of deficient root with excess branch, or yin deficiency with hyperactive yang, is indicated.

Treatment Principle

The major pathogeneses of hypertensive disease are hyperactive liver yang, and liver and kidney yin deficiency. Treatment principles should address the need to pacify the liver, subdue the yang, and nourish the liver and kidney. At the initial stage, the focus is on pacifying the liver and subduing the yang, as well as extinguishing wind and transforming phlegm. At the later stage or when the condition stabilizes, the focus should shift to nourishing the yin of the liver and kidney.

Pattern and Suggested Measure

Liver fire excess

Headache, dizziness, tinnitus, red face and eyes, irritability, short temper, bitter taste in the mouth, dark scanty urination, and constipation. Dry red tongue with yellow coating, and rapid wiry and forceful pulse.

- Clear and purge liver fire, pacify the liver and subdue the yang.
- Modified *Long Dan Xie Gan Tang*

Long Dan Cao 10g.	*Zhi Zi* 10g.	*Huang Qin* 10g.
Sheng Di Huang 15g.	*Ju Hua* 10g.	*Jue Ming Zi* 15g.
Gou Teng 15g.	*Ze Xie* 15g.	*Chuan Niu Xi* 10g.

- Severe headache and dizziness. + *Shi Jue Ming* 30g., *Zhen Zhu Mu* 30g.

Yin deficiency with hyperactive yang

Dizziness and headache, heavy sensation in the head and weak lower extremities, soreness and weakness of the lower back, tinnitus, palpitations, insomnia and five-centers heat. Red tongue with thin coating, and wiry thready pulse.

- Nourish the yin and subdue the yang.
- Modified *Tian Ma Gou Teng Yin*

Tian Ma 10g.	*Gou Teng* 15g.	*Shi Jue Ming* 30g.
Huang Qin 10g.	*Sheng Di Huang* 10g.	*Ju Hua* 10g.
Du Zhong 10g.	*Huai Niu Xi* 15g.	*Sang Ji Sheng* 15g.
Ye Jiao Teng 10g.	*Fu Shen* 10g.	*Nu Zhen Zi* 10g.

- During the maintenance phase, use *Qi Ju Di Huang Wan*.

Liver and kidney yin deficiency

Dizziness, dry eyes, tinnitus with soft tone like cicada, soreness and weakness of the lower back and knees, dream-disturbed sleep, night sweating and numb limbs. Red tongue with scanty coating, and deep thready or rapid thready pulse.

- Nourish and tonify the yin of both the liver and kidney.
- Modified *Zuo Gui Wan*

Shu Di Huang 10g.	*Shan Zhu Yu* 10g.	*Shan Yao* 15g.
Mu Dan Pi 10g.	*Ze Xie* 10g.	*Fu Ling* 15g.
Du Zhong 10g.	*Gui Ban Jiao* 6g.	*Gou Qi Zi* 10g.
Huai Niu Xi 10g.		

- Severe dizziness. + *Tian Ma* 6g., *Gou Teng* 15g.

Deficiency of both the yin and yang

Dizziness, headache with empty sensation in the head, cold weak and numb limbs, heel pain, possibly edema of the lower extremities, palpitations and shortness of breath, seminal emission and amenorrhea. Pale or red tongue with thin coating, and weak deep and thready pulse, especially at bilateral rear positions.

- Replenish the yin and assist the yang.
- Modified *Er Xian Tang*

Xian Mao 10g.	*Yin Yang Huo* 10g.	*Dang Gui* 10g.
Zhi Mu 10g.	*Huang Bai* 10g.	*Ba Ji Tian* 10g.

- Preponderance of yin deficiency. + *Shu Di Huang* 10g., *Shan Zhu Yu* 10g.
  Preponderance of yang deficiency. + *Rou Gui* 6g., *Tu Si Zi* 10g., *Du Zhong* 10g.

Damp-turbidity obstruction

Dizziness, headache with heavy and cloudy sensations in the head, possibly stuffy sensation in the ear, stifling sensation in the chest, palpitations, poor appetite and nausea. Pale and flabby tongue with thick white greasy coating, and wiry slippery pulse.

- Dry dampness, transform phlegm and extinguish wind.
- Modified *Ban Xia Bai Zhu Tian Ma Tang*

Ban Xia 10g.	*Fu Ling* 20g.	*Bai Zhu* 10g.
Tian Ma 6g.	*Shi Chang Pu* 10g.	*Chen Pi* 6g.
Zhi Shi 6g.	*Gou Teng* 10g.	

- Phlegm-dampness transforming into heat with yellow greasy coating. + *Zhu Ru* 10g., *Huang Lian* 6g.
  Severe dizziness and nausea. + *Xuan Fu Hua* 10g., *Zhu Ru* 10g., *Dai Zhe Shi* 20g.

Other Modality

A. Acupuncture:

- **Common points:** GB20 Fengchi, GV20 Baihui, LI4 Hegu, GB34 Yanglingquan, SP6 Sanyinjiao, ST36 Zusanli

Modify point selections based on differentiation and manifestation in chapters on headache and dizziness (see pages 191, 199).

B. Experiential remedies:

❶ *Ku Ding Cha* 10g. *Xia Ku Cao* 30g. *Ye Ju Hua* 15 g.
Decoction, daily.

❷ Black and white *Mu Er* 50g. each
Slowly cook with crystal sugar for minimum of 2 hours.
Take the full dose in 10 days

❸ Peanuts with peel 5-10 pcs.
Soaked with vinegar for 5-7 days, three times per day.

C. Single anti-hypertensive herbs:

Luo Bu Ma, *Xi Xian Cao*, *Han Fang Ji*, *Chou Wu Tong*, *Xia Tian Wu*, *Gou Teng*, *Di Long*, *Ye Ju Hua*.

CHAPTER 53

Coronary Artery Disease

Coronary artery disease (CAD) is a chronic medical condition most commonly caused by atheromatous plaques obstructing the coronary arteries. Affecting more than 12 million people and costing roughly $118 billion dollars in the year 2000, CAD leads other diseases as the cause of cardiovascular disability and death in the United States. Men are overall four times more likely than women to develop CAD; taking age into consideration, the ratio of men to women is even higher at 8:1 before age 40. CAD is most prevalent in men aged 50 to 60 and in women aged 60 to 70. Risk factors contributing to the occurrence of CAD include demographic traits (family history, age and male gender), other medical conditions (hyperlipoproteinemia, diabetes mellitus and hypertension), and lifestyle (physical inactivity and cigarette smoking). Among all the risk factors, abnormal lipid metabolism is the one directly implicated in the pathology of CAD. The higher the LDL cholesterol level, the higher the risk of CAD; the higher the HDL cholesterol level, the lower the risk. Being a chronic disorder, CAD develops in several stages until occlusion of the coronary arteries occurs. The initial step is the formation of "fatty streaks", the subendothelial accumulations of lipids and macrophages along the inner layer of the vessel walls. As macrophages continue migrating to the lesion, persistent atheromatous plaques are formed. In spite of insignificant hemodynamic alteration, the endothelial function to resist entry of lipoproteins into the vessel wall is limited. As the condition advances, a fibrous cap forms on the base of stable plaque, leading to calcification and narrowing of the vessel.

The extent of vascular occlusion determines the severity and consequences of CAD. Clinical symptoms range from an asymptomatic state to angina pectoris, or even myocardial infarction. Post-exertional dyspnea could be an early indicator of CAD. Patients may complain of vague chest pain, described as mild pressure-like discomfort or a burning and numb sensation, or more specific chest pain that is suffocating, crushing, heavy and squeezing. Sudden onset of strangling anxiety may be remarkable. Retrosternal pain that radiates down the ulnar aspect of the left arm is typical. Other accompanying symptoms include dyspnea, faintness, fatigue or eructation. Electrocardiogram (ECG) and echocardiography are non-invasive diagnostic measures; however, definite diagnosis and the extent of vessel occlusion are established based on more thorough assessment by cardiac catheterization, coronary arteriography and left ventricular angiography.

Medical treatment for CAD is built on a comprehensive approach that integrates treatment for underlying medical conditions, pharmaceutical measures and improvement of lifestyle. Surgical approaches via percutaneous catheter-based techniques or coronary bypass effectively resuppply the blood to the heart.

References:

Centers of Disease Control and Prevention (2003). Preventing heart Disease and stroke: Addressing the nation's leading killers; at a glance 2003. Retrieved on August 7, 2003 from http://www.cdc.gov/nccdphp/aag/aag_cvd.htm

Gersh, B. J., Braunwald, E., & Bonow, R. O. (2001). Chronic coronary artery disease. In E. Braunwald, D. P. Zipes, & P. Libby (Eds.), *Heart Disease: A Textbook of Cardiovascular Medicine* (6th ed. chap. 37). St. Louis, MO: W. B. Saunders Company.

Massie, B. M. & Amidon, T. M. (2003). Coronary heart disease. In L. M. Tierney, Jr. et. Al. (Eds.), *Current Medical Diagnosis & Treatment* (42nd ed. chap. 10). New York, NY: McGraw-Hill Companies, Inc.

From the perspective of TCM, CAD is always a combination of deficiency and excess. The root is usually a deficiency of the spleen, heart, and kidney or a combined deficiency of these three organs. The manifestations are related to an excess of blood stasis, congealed cold, qi stagnation and/or phlegm accumulation.

Congealed cold, qi stagnation, blood stasis and phlegm accumulation are attributed to inactivity of heart yang and obstruction in the heart vessels, inducing a sudden onset of excruciating throbbing, stabbing and crushing chest pain.

Of all deficiencies, kidney deficiency is the primary causal factor; kidney yang deficiency can lead to heart yang deficiency failing to warm and circulate the heart blood. Kidney yin deficiency leads to insufficient heart yin, causing blood to become viscous and retarding circulation. Poor circulation of the blood and increased risk of blood stasis directly affect the heart and cause CAD.

The consequences of CAD extend to its severe complications. A complete occlusion of the heart vessels manifests in true cardiac pain, or myocardial infarction. Obstruction of the flow of heart yang results in disturbances of heart rhythm, manifesting as palpitations, strangling anxiety and knotted or intermittent pulse, known as arrhythmias. Yang deficiency of both the heart and kidney causes cold fluids to congeal internally and overflow towards the heart, presenting as dyspnea, palpitations and systemic edema, known as heart failure.

Refer to "Chest Painful Obstruction" in Chapter 7 for comprehensive TCM differentiation and treatment of CAD (see pages 47-54).

CHAPTER 54

Cor Pulmonale

Cor pulmonale refers to right ventricular hypertrophy and dilatation secondary to pulmonary hypertension from lung disorder. It is not related to left ventricular failure, congenital cardiac diseases and acquired valvular cardiac diseases. Acute cor pulmonale is caused by acute episode of pulmonary embolism or acute exacerbation of chronic cor pulmonale, which is usually caused by COPD. Alveolar hypoxia, hypoxemia and hypercapnic acidosis all contribute to pulmonary hypertension. Alveolar hypoxia induces pulmonary vasoconstriction and promotes hypertrophy of smooth muscles in the pulmonary arterioles; chronic hypoxemia contributes to pulmonary hypertension by increasing polycythemia, blood viscosity and cardiac output; hypercapnic acidosis induces pulmonary hypertension by stimulating vasoconstriction.

Arterial blood gases (ABG) help determine hypercapnic acidosis and hypoxemia; chest X-Ray may indicate enlargement of the right ventricle and proximal pulmonary artery; electrocardiogram (ECG) can provide evidence of various degrees of pulmonary hypertension as well as right ventricular hypertrophy; echocardiograph and radionuclide ventriculography are valuable tools for assessing functions of the right and left ventricles. Confirmation of the diagnosis can be obtained via right heart catheterization or echocardiograph; the former measures the pressure of pulmonary artery while the latter measures the systolic pressure in the right ventricle. History of COPD is certain in majority of cor pulmonale cases.

The most common symptom for pulmonary hypertension is cough and exertional dyspnea; syncope and fatigue after exertion, and substernal anginal pain are also common. A left substernal systolic lift and a loud pulmonic second sound are possible; however, murmurs indicate deficits of tricuspid and pulmonic valves. When cor pulmonale progresses into right heart failure, signs of distended jugular veins, hepatomegaly and edema will be apparent. Treatment for cor pulmonale consists of medications and surgeries. Phlebotomy has been suggested for acute cor pulmonale caused by pulmonary embolism. Long-term anticoagulants may be necessary to reduce the risk of venous thromboembolism, constant oxygen administration may decrease pulmonary hypertention and mortality by reducing blood viscosity caused by polycythemia. Many other drugs, such as digitalis, hydralazine, calcium blockers, nitrous oxide and prostacyclin are still not proven effective. Monitoring and replacement for electrolytes during diuresis are important. Among all, treatment and prevention of the underlying diseases are essential.

References:

Beers, M. H. & Berkow, R., et. al. (Eds.). (1999). Heart failure: Cor pulmonale. *The Merck Manual of Diagnosis and Therapy* (17th ed. chap 203). West Point, PA: Merck & Co., Inc.

Massie, B. M. & Amidon, T. M. (2003). Heart- Pulmonary hypertension & heart disease: Cor pulmonale. In L. M. Tierney, Jr., et. al. (Eds.), *Current Medical Diagnosis & Treatment* (42nd ed. chap 10). New York, NY: McGraw-Hill.

McLaughlin, V. V. & Rich, S. (2001). Cor pulmonale. In E. Braunwald, et. al. (Eds.), *Heart Disease: A textbook of Cardiovascular Medicine* (6th ed. chap 54). Philadelphia, PA: W. B. Saunders.

The clinical manifestations of cor pulmonale can be referred to chapters on breathlessness, cough, congested fluids, palpitations and edema for TCM differentiation and treatment.

Cor pulmonale is one of the common cardiac diseases. This is a chronic condition characterized by recurrent pulmonary infections; resistance to antibiotics develops after frequent administrations of antibiotics. During exacerbation complicated by pulmonary infection, the combination of herbal remedy and antibiotics may enhance the antimicrobial effects and reduce the frequent usage of antibiotics.

According to TCM theory, "Invasion of pathogenic factors must be precipitated by a deficiency of righteous qi". Cor pulmonale results from an interaction of deficient root and excess branch; as the disease originates from the lung, it progresses and involves the spleen and kidney, finally the heart.

Recurrent lung diseases weaken lung qi, arising the deficient protective qi and unconsolidated surface. Exterior pathogenic factors may easily invade through the weakened defensive layers and exacerbate the deficiency of lung qi. Unremitting condition manifests with coughing and spitting out sputum. Chronic lung disease involves the spleen; when deficient spleen fails to properly metabolize water, dampness and phlegm will be generated internally and they will be accumulated in the lung. Once exterior pathogenic factors invade, latent phlegm can be triggered, resulting in severe wet cough with copious sputum. Complication of phlegm-heat accumulation in the lung may be caused by phlegm turning into heat or by wind-heat attacking the lung. Manifestation of productive cough with yellow sticky sputum and fever indicates an exacerbating episode.

"The blood flow of the entire body has to circulate through the lung". Lack of force to move the blood from deficient spleen and lung can easily induce blood stasis, presenting with cyanotic lips and palpitations. Chronic condition of lung and spleen deficiency affects the kidney, which fails to accomplish its two physiological functions. Failure of receiving qi leads to deficient wheezing with more difficulty in inhalation than exhalation and having exertional dyspnea. Failure of metabolizing fluids leads to accumulation of water and dampness with oliguria and edema. To its severe extent, the heart is also affected as the water overflow towards the heart, with symptoms of palpitations and shortness of breath.

Dysfunction of internal organs and contraction of exterior pathogens form the fundamental pathology of this complicated condition, which is characterized by recurrences and progression. Deficient root manifests the remission phase and excess pathogens manifest the relapse phase.

Analysis of Primary Symptom

A. Exertional dyspnea, cough and copious sputum:

- Cough indicates a fault of the lung, exertional dyspnea is a fault of the kidney, and copious sputum should be blamed on the spleen, which generates the phlegm and store it in the lung. These three symptoms usually occur simultaneously throughout the course as the major presentations during remission, a deficiency of the internal organs; however, exacerbation of these three symptoms occurs during relapse. This group of symptoms has characteristics of aggravation with exertion during cold seasons, and increased amount of sputum in the morning.
- During relapse, exacerbated symptoms, including aggravated cough, dyspnea, increased amount of sputum, tachypnea, stifling sensation in the chest and orthopnea accompanied by aversion to cold and fever, result from invasion of the exterior pathogens, which trigger the latent phlegm in the lung. Thin white or frothy sputum and significant aversion to cold are results of lung and kidney qi deficiency with exterior wind-cold. Sticky yellow sputum with fever is caused by lung and kidney qi deficiency with exterior wind-heat.

B. Palpitations, shortness of breath and congested chest:

The chest is where the heart and lung reside. This group of symptoms, including palpitations, shortness of breath and congested chest, may be a result from deficiency or a complex of deficiency and excess. Lung qi deficiency affects the heart, leading to heart and lung qi deficiency and manifesting with deficient patterns of palpitations, shortness of breath and congested chest. On the other hand, when the qi is deficient and the blood is static in the heart, or when spleen and kidney yang is deficient with cold water overflowing towards the heart, a complex of deficiency and excess occurs.

C. Cyanosis, distended jugular veins and hepatomegaly:

"The blood flow of the entire body has to circulate through the lung" and "The heart governs the blood and blood vessels". Chronic lung qi deficiency leads to failure of adequate circulation of the blood, inhibits the blood flow from returning back to the heart. Severity of the cyanosis and distended jugular veins indicate the extent of the condition; rapid recovery of cyanosis and extended jugular veins after rest or treatments indicate a mild condition, while constant cyanosis and extended jugular veins signify a severe blood stasis and a complicated condition.

D. Edema:

The statements, "Spleen governs the transformation and transportation of fluids" and "Kidney governs fluids", clearly illustrate the important roles that the spleen and kidney play in water metabolism. Spleen and kidney yang deficiency fails to distribute fluid adequately, leading to edema and dysuria. Worsening of these two symptoms warns the progression of cor pulmonale into an exacerbation.

Basic Patterns

Remission:

- Lung and kidney qi deficiency

Acute exacerbation episode:

- Lung and kidney qi deficiency with exterior wind-cold
- Lung and kidney qi deficiency with exterior wind-heat
- Cold water overflowing towards the heart
- Devastated and collapsed basal yang

Progression of Pattern

The early stage of cor pulmonale indicates a lung and kidney qi deficiency pattern, mainly manifested by pulmonary dysfunction. When this condition is complicated by exterior wind-cold or wind-heat, clinical manifestations will be presented as multifaceted pulmonary dysfunction with respiratory tract infection. When the condition reoccurs and progresses, the pattern of spleen and kidney yang deficiency with cold water overflowing against the heart will then follow. At this stage, cardiac dysfunction becomes the primary presentation. Once the basal qi is greatly damaged, manifestations of devastated and collapsed basal yang resemble cardiogenic shock and heart failure.

Treatment Principle

Deficient root and excess branch dominate the primary pathogenesis of cor pulmonale. Tonify lung qi, and warm the spleen and kidney to address the deficient root during remission accordingly. Based on the presence of exterior pathogens, heat excess, water retention, excessive phlegm and blood stasis, expel the excess pathogenic influences during relapse.

In addition to excessive phlegm throughout the course, it seems like blood stasis plays a part in pathogenesis as well during the entire course; such rationale is supported by improvement of therapeutic effects with integrating treatment methods of transforming phlegm and expelling blood stasis. Therefore, invigorating the blood to expel stasis becomes a common strategy for cor pulmonale.

Pattern and Suggested Measure

Remission:

Lung and kidney qi deficiency

Cough with frothy sputum, shortness of breath, exertional dyspnea, soreness and weakness of the lower back and knees, and poor appetite. Pale tongue with thin white coating, and deep thready pulse.

- Tonify the lung, assist the kidney to receive the qi and calm wheezing.
- Modified *Bu Fei Tang* and *Shen Ge San*

Ren Shen 6g.	*Huang Qi* 10g.	*Shu Di Huang* 10g.
Wu Wei Zi 15g.	*Zi Wan* 10g.	*Sang Bai Pi* 10g.
Ge Jie 6g.	*Hu Tao Rou* 15g.	*Ju Hong* 10g.

- Spleen deficiency with copious sputum, abdominal distention and loose stool. + *Bai Zhu* 10g., *Fu Ling* 15g., *Ban Xia* 10g.

  Kidney yang deficiency with soreness and weakness of the lower back and knees, cold intolerance and cold limbs. + *Zhi Fu Zi* 6g., *Bu Gu Zhi* 10g.

  Yin deficiency. + *Sha Shen* 10g., *Mai Men Dong* 10g., *Sheng Di Huang* 10g.

  Qi deficiency and blood stasis with cyanotic lips and distended jugular veins. + *Dan Shen* 15g., *Chi Shao* 10g., *Chuan Xiong* 6g.

Acute exacerbation episode:

Lung and kidney qi deficiency with exterior wind-cold

Severe cough and breathlessness, shortness of breath, copious frothy white or clear sputum, aversion to cold, fever, nasal congestion with clear or watery discharge, and general body ache. Thin white coating and floating tight pulse.

- Disperse lung qi, expel cold, transform phlegm and calm wheezing.
- Modified *Xiao Qing Long Tang*

Ma Huang 6g.	*Gui Zhi* 10g.	*Xi Xin* 3g.
Gan Jiang 6g.	*Wu Wei Zi* 10g.	*Ban Xia* 10g.
Bai Shao 10g.	*Xing Ren* 10g.	*Gan Cao* 6g.

- Excessive sputum. + *Su Zi* 10g., *Qian Hu* 10g., *Bai Jie Zi* 10g.
  Breathlessness and spontaneous sweating. + *Fang Feng* 10g., *Bai Zhu* 10g.

Lung and kidney qi deficiency with exterior wind-heat

Severe cough and breathlessness necessitating a sitting upright position to breath, yellow viscous sputum that is difficult to expectorate, fever, aversion to wind, nasal congestion with yellow or turbid discharge, sore throat and thirst. Yellow tongue coating and rapid slippery pulse.

- Clear heat, transform phlegm and calm wheezing.
- Modified *Ma Xing Shi Gan Tang*

Ma Huang 6g.	*Shi Gao* 30g.	*Xing Ren* 10g.
Huang Qin 10g.	*Jin Yin Hua* 10g.	*Lian Qiao* 10g.
Sang Bai Pi 10g.	*Gua Lou* 15g.	

- High fever with insignificant aversion to cold. + *Zhi Zi* 6g., *Zhi Mu* 10g.
  Dry throat and thirst. + *Tian Hua Fen* 15g., *Lu Gen* 10g.
  Copious sputum and breathlessness that necessitates sitting upright. + *Yu Xing Cao* 10g., *Dong Gua Ren* 10g., *Ting Li Zi* 10g.

Cold water overflowing towards the heart

Systemic edema especially worse in the lower extremities, palpitations, shortness of breath, exertional dyspnea and orthopnea, scanty urination, cold limbs and cyanotic lips. Dark purple tongue with white greasy coating, and deep thready or knotted intermittent pulse.

- Warm the yang and drain water.
- Modified *Zhen Wu Tang*

Fu Zi 10g.	*Bai Zhu* 10g.	*Fu Ling* 15g.
Sheng Jiang 10g.	*Shao Yao* 10g.	*Gui Zhi* 6g.
Zhu Ling 15g.	*Ze Xie* 10g.	

- Blood stasis with significant cyanosis and distended jugular veins. + *Tao Ren* 10g., *Dan Shen* 10g., *Yi Mu Cao* 10g.
  Severe pitting edema. + *Che Qian Zi* 10g., *Da Fu Pi* 10g.
  Severe asthmatic respiration. + *Ting Li Zi* 10g., *Ma Huang* 6g., *Bai Guo* 10g.

Devastated and collapsed basal yang

Systemic edema especially worse in the lower extremities, palpitations, shortness of breath, exertional dyspnea and orthopnea, scanty urination, cold limbs and cyanotic lips, dark and dusky complexion, profuse sweating and clammy cold limbs. Pale tongue and deep thready or minute pulse.

- Restore devastated yang, reverse peripheral frigidity, and benefit the qi to rescue qi collapse.
- Modified *Si Ni Tang* and *Sheng Mai San*

Fu Zi 10g.	*Gan Jiang* 10g.	*Zhi Gan Cao* 15g.
Ren Shen 10g.	*Huang Qi* 15g.	*Mai Men Dong* 15g.
Wu Wei Zi 15g.	*Huang Jing* 10g.	*Dan Shen* 10g.

- Persistent dyspnea or orthponea. + *Ge Jie* 2g.

Other Modality

A. Acupuncture:

Remission:

- **Manipulation:** Reinforcing method, may combine with moxibustion.
- **Prescription:**

BL13 Feishu	BL23 Shenshu	ST36 Zusanli
CV6 Qihai	PC6 Neiguan	HT7 Shenmen

Acute exacerbation episode:

Refer to "Cough" in Chapter 2 (see page 17), "Breathlessness" in Chapter 4 (see page 31), and "Edema" in Chapter 40 (see page 285) accordingly.

B. Experiential remedies:

❶ The following formula is used for chronic yet stable condition:

Tai Zi Shen 10g.	*Huang Qi* 15g.	*Bu Gu Zhi* 6g.
Dan Shen 15g.	*Chi Shao* 10g.	*Zhi Fu Zi* 3g.
Yu Zhu 15g.	*Yin Yang Huo* 10g.	*Hong Hua* 6g.

Make into the concentrated granular powder; 3g. twice per day.

❷ The following formula is used for elderly with deficiency type of breathlessness.

Hu Tao Rou 500g. *Xing Ren* 150g.

Mixed with honey to make honey pills of 10g. each; 2 pills per day.

CHAPTER **55**

Gastritis

The mucosal layer in the stomach is normally protected by several mechanisms, namely a mucus barrier, removal of excess hydrogen ions by epithelial cells, and removal of excessive acid by mucosal blood flow. When these defense mechanisms fail, the gastric mucosa becomes inflamed, resulting in gastritis. Gastritis can be categorized by the affected site (cardia, corpus or antrum), and by the inflammatory cell type (acute or chronic).

Polymorphonuclear cell infiltration of the mucosa characterizes acute gastritis, most commonly at the antrum and corpus. Acute erosive gastritis is caused by medications, especially nonsteroidal anti-inflammatory drugs (NSAIDs), alcohol and acute stress. It is commonly accompanied by a certain degree of bleeding manifesting as submucosal petechiae that are visible on endoscopic examination. Severely ill patients have a higher risk of acute stress gastritis; upper gastrointestinal bleeding in this population is very common. Predisposing factors include severe burns, central nervous system trauma, sepsis, shock, respiratory failure, and hepatic and renal failure. In contrast to acute gastritis, chronic gastritis is characterized by some degree of atrophy with loss of functional capacity of the mucosa, or by metaplasia. The antrum is the most commonly affected site with loss of G cells and decreased gastrin secretion; when the corpus and oxyntic glands are affected, acid, pepsin and intrinsic factor will be reduced. Chronic erosive gastritis is diagnosed endoscopically by the presence of multiple punctate or aphthous ulcers. Chronic erosive gastritis can be idiopathic or caused by drugs (NSAIDs), Crohn's disease or viral infections; it is not caused by *Helicobacter pylori (H. pylori)*. Symptoms related to chronic erosive gastritis are usually nonspecific, such as nausea, vomiting, and epigastric discomfort. Treatment for chronic erosive gastritis involves symptom management and is not considered curative.

There is also nonerosive gastritis, which is caused by *H. pylori* infection and characterized by various degrees of inflammation. Superficial gastritis occurs at the surface layer of the mucosa and affects the antrum and corpus. Atrophy and metaplasia are not present. Deep gastritis involves mononuclear cells and neutrophils infiltrating the entire mucosal layer as deep as the muscularis. Superficial gastritis, atrophy and metaplasia may accompany deep gastritis; symptoms are usually vague and dyspeptic. Gastric atrophy is predisposed by various injuries, especially longstanding antral (type B) gastritis. Atrophy and antibodies to parietal cells can be found in corpus (type A) gastritis, which is related to pernicious anemia. There are two major types of metaplasia in chronic nonerosive gastritis: mucous gland and intestinal. Mucous gland metaplasia is associated with severe atrophy of the gastric glands. Intestinal metaplasia is precipitated by chronic mucosal injury, and is marked by gastric mucosa which resembles small intestinal mucosa. Intestinal metaplasia is closely related to gastric cancer. Metaplasia is detected by histological studies.

Reference:

Beers, M. H. & Berkow, R. et. al. (Eds.) (1999). Gastritis and peptic ulcer disease. *The Merck Manual of Diagnosis and Therapy* (17th ed. chap. 23). West Point, PA: Merck & Co., Inc.

From the perspective of TCM, the stomach is responsible for the pathology of gastritis; however, the liver and spleen also play a role in its pathogenesis.

The stomach is in charge of receiving and ripening ingested food; in the normal physiological state, the qi of the stomach descends. Any precipitating factor disturbing the harmonious state of the stomach can cause epigastric discomfort and contribute to the pathogenesis of gastritis.

Cold congeals the qi flow in the stomach, resulting in epigastric discomfort. Dietary overindulgence leads to food retention and interrupts the normal qi flow in the digestive system. Greasy, spicy food and alcohol consume stomach yin, leading to malnourishment of the stomach. Excessive amounts of cold, raw food or cold natured herbs will injure stomach yang; inadequate warming of the stomach results in epigastric pain. The liver plays a role in pathogenesis when stagnant liver qi overacts on the stomach; the stomach qi rebels, presenting as pain, nausea and vomiting. When a chronic liver-stomach disharmony progresses from qi stagnation to blood stasis, complications of gastrointestinal bleeding follow as hematemesis and malena. The stomach and spleen are physiologically-pathologically related; spleen qi ascends and stomach qi descends, maintaining proper digestive and absorptive functions. When spleen yang is deficient, it fails to warm the stomach, leading to a deficient cold pattern of both organs; spleen yang deficiency can also lead to a pattern of secondary blood stasis due to the congealing effect of internal cold.

With epigastric discomfort as the primary symptom, comprehensive TCM differentiation and treatment of gastritits is presented in Chapter 9 on "Epigastric Pain" (see pages 63-69).

CHAPTER 56

Peptic Ulcers

Peptic ulcers are excoriated lesions formed in the mucosal membrane of the digestive system, most commonly seen in the stomach (gastric ulcer) and the beginning segment of the duodenum (duodenal ulcer). For almost a century, lifestyle factors, such as stress and diet, were thought to be the major causal factors for the formation of peptic ulcers until the discovery of imbalance between the hydrochloric acid and pepsin. However, recent research indicates that infection caused by *Helicobacter pylori* (*H. pylori*) accounts for the primary cause. *H. pylori* is a spiral-shaped bacterium, first found in the stomach in 1982. Numerous studies also indicate that using antibiotics to eliminate *H. pylori* can effectively treat peptic ulcers. Nonsteroidal anti-inflammatory drugs (NSAIDs) are another contributing factor. NSAIDs are weak acid; they can inhibit production of prostaglandin, leading to microenvironmental alterations in the stomach. Secondary reduced gastric blood flow and HCO_3 secretion, and decreased cell repair and replication further cause mucosal defense mechanisms impairment.

History taking as well as endoscopy exam consist the major approaches for diagnosis. Via fiberoptic endoscopy, the actual lesion and its nature can be assessed directly. Double-contrast barium X-ray serves as an alternative for detecting ulcers. However, to differentiate ulcer from malignancy, cytology and biopsy are more reliable.

The major discomfort associated with peptic ulcers is described as a dull, gnawing ache in the epigastric region. The pain has a nature of rhythmicity and periodicity. Secondary symptoms include poor appetite, bloating and acid regurgitation. When the ulcer heals, as the cicatricial contracture is formed, partial or complete pyloric obstruction follows, manifesting with nausea and vomiting. If peptic ulcers remained untreated, ulcers may burrow through the gastric or duodenal wall and cause gastrointestinal bleeding and perforation. Sudden sharp and persistent stomach pain accompanied by hematemesis, hematochezia or melena, and systemic prostration indicate a critical complication may arise. Previous focus of treatment for peptic ulcers was aimed to neutralize and decrease gastric acidity. However, ever since the discovery of

H. pylori, antibiotic treatments have been adopted as the primary modality for those with peptic ulcer secondary to *H. pylori*.

References:

Health on the Net Foundation (2002). Stomach and duodenum ulcer. Retrieved June 24, 2003, from http://www.helioshealth.com/digestive/ulcers/ulcers_who.html

Health on the Net Foundation (2002). Stomach and duodenum ulcer. Retrieved June 24, 2003, from http://www.helioshealth.com/digestive/ulcers/what_causes.html

Health on the Net Foundation (2002). Stomach and duodenum ulcer. Retrieved June 24, 2003, from http://www.helioshealth.com/digestive/ulcers/symptoms.html

Beers, M. H. & Bowker, R., et. al. (Eds.). (1999). Gastritis and peptic ulcer disease. *The Merck Manual of Diagnosis and Therapy* (17th ed. chap. 23). West Point, PA: Merck & Co., Inc.

Peptic ulcer can be categorized into TCM differentiation and treatment of epigastric pain and stomach upset; it can also be referred to acid regurgitation and melena.

The incidence of peptic ulcers is closely related to the following contributing factors:

Emotional stresses: Liver is highly susceptible to emotional stresses, which can cause liver qi stagnation. Stagnant liver qi overacts on the stomach, inhibiting the stomach qi from descending. Stagnant liver qi can further develop into liver fire, which consumes stomach yin and scorches the stomach vessels.

Improper diet, such as crapulence and irregular diet habits, hinders the functions of the spleen and stomach. The ascending and descending flow of qi in the middle burner is obstructed and stomach qi is not harmonized.

Spleen and stomach deficiency results from improper diet or constitutional insufficiency. There is inadequate warmth and support to the stomach when spleen yang is deficient; or lack of moistening effect and nourishment of the stomach if stomach yin is insufficient.

Analysis of the Primary Symptom

A. Stomachache:

Both obstruction and malnourishment of the stomach may cause stomachache. Below are different Characteristics of pain:

- Distending pain: A discomfort feeling of fullness, relieved by belching and passing flatus, and aggravated by emotional stresses. This type of pain results from liver qi stagnation overacting on the stomach or the obstruction of qi flow in the middle burner.
- Burning pain: Manifested with urgent excruciating pain and burning sensa-

tion in the stomach, aggravated after meal, aversion to pressure, dry mouth and bitter taste in the mouth. This type of pain is caused by stagnant liver qi transforming into fire, which flares upwards and disturbs the stomach, leading to rebellious stomach qi.

- Stabbing pain: Sharp and pricking in nature with fixed location and aversion to pressure. Blood stasis secondary to qi stagnation in the stomach vessels contributes to blockage and disturbances in the stomach.
- Dull pain: Resulting from stomach yin deficiency failing to nourish and moisten the stomach, dull stomachache is accompanied by dry mouth and throat, dry stool or constipation. Also resulting from spleen yang deficiency failing to warm and support the stomach, this type of pain prefers warm compression, is alleviated after meals and aggravated by cold or exertion.

B. Acid regurgitation and stomach upset:

Spleen and stomach disharmony will cause damp-heat to accumulate in the stomach. Stagnant liver qi transforming into fire will overact on the stomach and prevent stomach qi from descending. Stomach qi rebelling upwards will cause acid regurgitation whereas damp-heat disturbing internally may lead to stomach upset.

C. Hematemesis and melena:

Excessive heat causing the blood to move recklessly may result from stomach excess heat or liver fire overacting on the stomach. Deficient middle burner failing to control the blood may cause the blood to escape from its reservoirs. When the condition is prolonged, blood stasis will occlude in the minute collaterals, creating a detour of the blood circulation. The emission of blood, when following the rebellious stomach qi upwards, will result in hematemesis; when following the digestive tract downwards, will result in hematochezia or melena in the stool.

Basic Patterns

- Qi stagnation
- Yin deficiency
- Blood stasis
- Constrained heat
- Deficient cold

Progression of Pattern

At the initial stage, peptic ulcers are very much excess in nature, and qi stagnation is the major pathogenesis. Qi stagnation may progress and involve other pathogenesis. For example, qi stagnation may transform into fire, known as constrained heat. Stagnant qi failing to circulate the blood will cause blood stasis. When dampness accumulation results from obstructed qi flow, symptoms of damp-heat or cold-dampness may manifest. During the course, a complicated pattern is possible. Spleen and stomach deficiency may follow when stomachache is unremitting and prolonged. Spleen and stomach deficiency may also be a result of constitutional spleen deficiency further complicated by improper diet. Two major pathogeneses in later stage of peptic ulcers are spleen yang deficiency and stomach yin insufficiency.

Treatment Principle

Qi stagnation and blood stasis are the basic pathology; spleen and stomach deficiency is the underpinning triggers for the onset of peptic ulcers. Therefore, promoting the qi flow, transforming stasis, strengthening the spleen and nourishing the stomach should be the major principle. According to various patterns, such as constrained heat, empty cold and yin deficiency, also adopt clearing stomach heat, warming the middle burner and dispersing cold, and nourishing stomach yin.

Pattern and Suggested Measure

Qi stagnation

Distending stomachache radiating to the hypopchondria, aggravated by emotional stress, belching and sighing. White tongue coating and wiry pulse.

- Spread liver qi, harmonize the stomach and alleviate pain.
- Modified *Chai Hu Shu Gan San*

Chai Hu 10g.	*Xiang Fu* 10g.	*Zhi Qiao* 10g.
Chen Pi 10g.	*Chuan Xiong* 10g.	*Bai Shao* 15g.
Gan Cao 6g.	*Mu Gua* 10g.	*Sha Ren* 6g.

- Severe focal distention of the epigastrium and abdomen and thick greasy tongue coating. + *Cang Zhu* 10g., *Hou Po* 10g.

Constrained heat

Burning stomachache aggravated after meals, bitter taste in the mouth, acid regurgitation, irritability, short temper, possible hematemesis, scanty urination and dry stool. Red tongue with yellow coating, and rapid wiry pulse.

- Drain heat and harmonize the stomach.
- Modified *Hua Gan Jian* and *Zuo Jin Wan*

Zhi Zi 10g.	*Mu Dan Pi* 10g.	*Qing Pi* 10g.
Bai Shao 15g.	*Zhe Bei Mu* 6g.	*Huang Lian* 10g.
Wu Zhu Yu 1.5g.	*Pu Gong Ying* 10g.	*Chuan Lian Zi* 6g.

- Hematemesis, use *Xie Xin Tang*.

Yin deficiency

Dull and burning stomachache, dry mouth, poor appetite, dry heaves, dry stool, and emaciation. Red tongue with scanty coating, and rapid thready pulse.

- Nourish the yin and augment the stomach.
- Modified *Yi Wei Tang*

Sha Shen 10g.	*Mai Men Dong* 10g.	*Sheng Di Huang* 10g.
Yu Zhu 10g.	*Huang Jing* 10g.	*Bai Shao* 10g.
Gan Cao 6g.		

- Shortness of breath and weakness of the extremities. + *Tai Zi Shen* 10g.
  Dry stool. + *Gua Lou Ren* 15g., *Huo Ma Ren* 10g.

Deficient cold

Dull pain aggravated by cold or exertion and alleviated by warm compress and pressure, vomiting clear fluid emesis, pale complexion, lassitude, cold limbs, loose stool or melena. Pale tongue with white coating, deep and weak pulse.

- Strengthen the spleen and stomach, warm the middle burner and disperse cold.
- Modified *Huang Qi Jian Zhong Tang*

Huang Qi 15g.	*Dang Shen* 10g.	*Gui Zhi* 6g.
Bai Shao 15g.	*Zhi Gan Cao* 6g.	*Chen Pi* 10g.
Yi Tang 15g.		

- Melena, use *Huang Tu Tang*.
  Vomiting up clear watery emesis. + *Ban Xia* 10g., *Sheng Jiang* 6g.

Blood stasis

Stabbing or prickling stomachache, fixed location and aversion to pressure, excruciating pain radiating to corresponding point at the back when exacerbated, recurrent hematemesis and melena. Dark purple tongue with petechiae, and wiry thready and choppy pulse.

- Invigorate the blood and transform stasis, facilitate the qi flow and harmonize the stomach.
- Modified *Shi Xiao San* and *Dan Shen Yin*

Pu Huang 10g.	*Wu Ling Zhi* 10g.	*Dan Shen* 30g.
Tan Xiang 6g.	*Sha Ren* 6g.	*Zhi Da Huang* 3g.
Gan Cao 3g.		

- Hematemesis or melena. + *Bai Ji* 10g., *San Qi* 3g.
  Severe stomachache. + *Yan Hu Suo* 10g.

Other Modality

A. Acupuncture:

Point selections based on differentiation and manifestation are found on "Epigastric Pain" in Chapter 9 (see page 69).

B. Experiential remedy:

San He Tang:

Gao Liang Jiang 10g.	*Xiang Fu* 10g.	*Bai He* 30g.
Wu Yao 10g.	*Dan Shen* 30g.	*Tan Xiang* 6g.
Sha Ren 3g.		

The formula above is effectively used in treating longstanding unmerited peptic ulcers that has a mixed pattern of cold-heat and excess-deficiency.

Complicated by blood stasis with fixed stabbing stomachache. + *Wu Ling Zhi* 10g., *Pu Huang* 10g. This modified *San He Tang* is also known as *Si He Tang*.

C. Single effective herbs in treating peptic ulcer:

❶ Anti-acid: *Hai Piao Xiao*, *Wa Leng Zi*, *Chuan Bei Mu*, *Hai Ge Ke*.

❷ Hemostatics: *Bai Ji*, *Bai Lian*, *Qing Dai*, *Da Huang*, *San Qi*.

❸ Promote the healing of ulcerations: *San Qi*, *Zhen Zhu*, *Xue Jie*, *Er Cha*.

CHAPTER 57

Inflammatory Bowel Disease

Inflammatory bowel disease (IBD) consists of two related conditions: ulcerative colitis (UC) and Crohn's disease (CD). Ulcerative colitis is a chronic disease of unknown etiology causing inflammation limited to the rectum and colon. Most patients are diagnosed when they are between the age of 15 and 30 years, then a second peak of incidence appears between 55 and 65 years of age. It has been speculated that the etiology of UC are from infection, food allergy, environmental factors, immune response to bacteria and others. Crohn's disease, on the other hand, is a chronic inflammatory condition that may affect any part of the digestive tract, from the lips to the anus. The onset of disease is greatest in people in the teens and 20s, and there may be a second peak in the 70s. Smokers have a 2- to 5-fold increased risk of developing the disease. The etiology of CD remains unclear, and environment and heredity have been implicated but are unproven.

Persistent bloody diarrhea is the most common symptom of UC, often associated with rectal urgency or tenesmus. The history prior to diagnosis of CD is chronic diarrhea, abdominal pain, anorexia, weight loss, unexplained fever, aphthous ulcers in the mouth, and arthralgias. Extraintestinal manifestations of UC include erythema nodosum (tender and inflamed nodules, most often on the anterior surface of the lower legs), oral aphthous ulcers (found in at least 10% of patients with active colitis and resolve with disease remission), acute arthropathy (seen in 10-15% of patients with acute UC, affects larger joints and usually resolves with improvement in colitis), ankylosing spondylitis (1-2%), primary sclerosing cholangitis (occurs in 3% of UC patients resulting in cholestatic liver disease), cirrhosis may develop over a period of years.

For CD, sinus tracts can result from disease extending through the serosa. If the sinus tracts end in a blind area, this results in an abscess, causing abdominal pain, fever, a tender palpable mass. Inflamed serosal surfaces may become adherent and disease may penetrate into other loops of intestine, resulting in a fistula (internal). External fistulas such as vaginal fistulas may cause feculent vaginal discharge. Perforation (1-2% of CD patients) occurs more in the ileum compared to the colon. If perforation occurs in the colon, the resulting peritonitis may be fatal. Other extraintestinal manifestations of CD are erythema nodosum, clubbing, amyloidosis (rare but can be life threatening), thromboembolic complications, fatty liver and primary sclerosing cholangitis. Infections may exacerbate CD, particularly respiratory tract infections and C. difficile colitis. Cigarette smoking, nonsteroidal anti-inflammatory drugs (NSAIDs), and stress may cause symptoms to appear or can aggravate IBD.

Reference:

Engstrom, P. F. & Gooseberg, E. B. (1999). Inflammatory bowel disease. *Diagnosis and Management of bowel Diseases* (1st ed. pp. 123-196). Philadelphia, PA: Professional Communication, Inc.

Based on the primary clinical manifestations, IBD can be categorized into TCM differentiation and treatment of abdominal pain, diarrhea and dysentery disorder.

IBD is a chronic, recurrent and progressive disease that involves complicated symptoms. Perceptions of IBD pathology are not yet consistent among TCM practitioners. In general, IBD can be referred to as diarrhea or dysentery disorders.

Damp-heat plays a significant role in the formation of IBD. Damp-heat can be a result from either exterior contraction or interior spleen deficiency. Damp-heat accumulates in the large intestine further obstructing the circulation of qi and blood. When blood stasis combines with damp-heat, they may injure the intestinal vessels. This is an excess pathology; its clinical manifestations are abdominal pain, severe diarrhea with pus, blood and mucous, and tenesmus. Usually, this pattern is identical to and categorized into dysentery disorder.

Deficient spleen fails to transform and transport dampness, resulting in dampness accumulation. Hyperactive liver overacting on the spleen leads to malfunction of the spleen to transform and transport dampness, resulting dampness accumulation. This is a deficient pathology; its clinical presentations include abdominal distention and fullness, loose stool or watery diarrhea, stool mixed with mucous. Usually, this pattern is similar to and categorized into diarrhea disorder.

As indicated, exterior pathogenic factors, improper diet and spleen deficiency are the contributing factors to occurrence of IBD.

Analysis of Primary Symptom

Diarrhea is the key symptom to IBD; together with the characteristics of abdominal pain, tenesmus, and bowel movements, the diagnosis and treatment plan can be formulated.

A. Diarrhea, abdominal pain and tenesmus:

- When abdominal pain and tenesmus are relieved after diarrhea, this is most likely an excess pattern. When damp-heat accumulation is eliminated by defecation, the blockage is removed, therefore pain is relieved. When urgency in diarrhea manifests, heat predominates over dampness. If severe heavy sensation is felt at the anus, dampness predominates over heat.
- If abdominal pain and tenesmus are not relieved or insignificantly relieved after diarrhea, it indicates a deficient pattern, such as spleen and stomach qi deficiency, spleen qi sinking or spleen and kidney yang deficiency.
- When abdominal pain and diarrhea are elicited or triggered by emotional stresses, and temporary relief of pain is followed by recurrent severe painful diarrhea, a hyperactive liver qi overacting on the spleen is evident.
- Unremitting diarrhea or even incontinence, condition worsens before dawn, is a typical symptom of spleen and kidney yang deficiency.

B. Diarrhea with mucous, pus or blood:

- In diarrhea with mixed mucous and purulent blood, excessive mucous indicates preponderance of dampness, and excessive purulent blood signifies preponderance of heat.
- When excessive mucous is seen in the stool or the stool is loose and watery, and the stool is mixed with undigested food, pattern of spleen qi deficiency or kidney yang deficiency failing to digest food is certain.
- Diarrhea with mucous, accompanied by thirst and irritability is seen in pattern of stomach heat with intestinal cold. It is a complicated pattern of mixed heat and cold.
- When the stool contains blood clots or the stool is black, and abdominal pain aggravated by pressure, this is a pattern of blood stasis obstructing in the intestinal vessels.

Basic Patterns

- Damp-heat accumulation
- Combination of cold and heat
- Hyperactive liver with deficient spleen
- Spleen and stomach qi deficiency
- Spleen and kidney yang deficiency
- Qi stagnation and blood stasis

Progression of Pattern

During the initial stage, the presentation of IBD is a pattern of excess pathogens, or damp-heat accumulation. When severe diarrhea injures the qi or dampness hinders the spleen, spleen and stomach qi deficiency follows. Spleen and stomach qi deficiency signifies the remission phase of IBD; in this phase, disease continues to progress and further involves the kidney. When spleen and kidney yang deficiency manifests, the pathology becomes primarily deficiency. If damp-heat continues to linger, qi stagnation and blood stasis follow, or blood stasis will cause obstruction in the intestinal vessels. This is a relative excess pattern because of the presence of qi stagnation and blood stasis, resembling persistent intestinal ulcerations.

The acute episode in chronic IBD presents to be a complicated pattern of both heat and cold or hyperactive liver with deficient spleen. In advanced aged or weak patients, spleen and kidney yang deficient pattern occurs even in early stage. A combination or inter-transformation among patterns stated above is also possible.

Treatment Principle

The pathology of IBD surrounds the pathogenesis of spleen deficiency with dampness accumulation and disharmony of qi and blood in the intestines. To address the root, tonify the spleen and augment the qi; to address the branch, eliminate dampness and transform stasis. Combine auxiliary strategies of regulating the qi to invigorate the stagnation; clearing heat for heat accumulation; pacifying the liver for hyperactive liver; stopping bleeding for excessive hematochezia; tonifying the kidney and binding the intestine for chronic diarrhea and incontinence.

Pattern and Suggested Measure

Damp-heat accumulation

Fever, abdominal pain, diarrhea with purulent blood and mucus, tenesmus and scanty urination. Yellow greasy tongue coating, and rapid slippery pulse.

- Clear and drain damp-heat.
- Modified *Bai Tou Weng Tang*
  Bai Tou Weng 15g. *Qin Pi* 10g. *Huang Lian* 6g.
  Huang Bai 10g. *Che Qian Zi* 10g. *Mu Xiang* 10g.
  Zhi Qiao 10g.
- Complicated by exterior heat. + *Ge Gen* 15g., *Sheng Ma* 10g., *Fang Feng* 10g.
  Preponderance of heat. + *Jin Yin Hua* 10g., *Huang Qin* 10g.

Preponderance of dampness. + *Cang Zhu* 10g., *Hou Po* 10g.

Combination of cold and heat

Dull abdominal pain, diarrhea with mucous and blood, symptoms aggravated by cold, bitter taste in the mouth and poor appetite. Pale tongue with white greasy coating, and deep rapid pulse.

- Warm the organs and clear heat.
- Modified *Wu Mei Wan*

Wu Mei 15g.	*Gan Jiang* 10g.	*Chuan Jiao* 6g.
Zhi Fu Zi 6g.	*Dang Shen* 10g.	*Bai Zhu* 10g.
Huang Lian 10g.	*Huang Bai* 6g.	*Mu Xiang* 10g.
Che Qian Zi 10g.		

- Stool with dark red blood. + *San Qi* 10g., *Bai Ji* 10g.

Hyperactive liver with deficient spleen

Abdominal pain and diarrhea, temporary relief after defecation, followed by a cycle of recurrent severe abdominal pain and diarrhea, distention and fullness in the chest, hypochondria, epigastrium and abdominal regions, and frequent passing of flatus. Thin white tongue coating and wiry thready pulse.

- Pacify the liver and strengthen the spleen.
- Modified *Tong Xie Yao Fang*

Bai Shao 15g.	*Bai Zhu* 15g.	*Fang Feng* 10g.
Chen Pi 10g.	*Chai Hu* 10g.	*Yi Yi Ren* 15g.
Jiao Shan Zha 10g.		

- Significant spleen deficiency with fatigue and poor appetite. + *Dang Shen* 10g., *Zhi Gan Cao* 6g.

  Significant liver qi stagnation. + *Dang Gui* 10g., *Mu Gua* 10g., *Zhi Gan Cao* 6g.

Spleen and stomach qi deficiency

Borborygmus and diarrhea, increased frequency of bowel movements following indulgence of greasy diet, stool containing undigested food, abdominal distention, poor appetite and fatigue. Pale tongue with white coating, soft and decelerating pulse.

- Strengthen the spleen and augment the stomach.
- Modified *Shen Ling Bai Zhu San*

Dang Shen 12g.	*Bai Zhu* 10g.	*Fu Ling* 15g.
Shan Yao 12g.	*Bian Dou* 10g.	*Sha Ren* 6g.

Lian Zi 10g. *Chen Pi* 6g. *Ban Xia* 10g.
Ge Gen 15g.

- Significant deficient cold, use *Li Zhong Wan*.
  Spleen qi sinking, use *Bu Zhong Yi Qi Tang*.

Spleen and kidney yang deficiency

Borborygmus and diarrhea, mostly occurring before dawn, accompanied by cold intolerance, pale complexion, coldness, soreness and weakness of the lower back and knees. Thick white or thick slippery tongue coating, and deep thready and forceless pulse.

- Warm and tonify the spleen and kidney, bind the intestines and stop diarrhea.
- Modified *Si Shen Wan*
  Bu Gu Zhi 10g. *Wu Wei Zi* 10g. *Rou Dou Kou* 10g.
  Wu Zhu Yu 10g. *Fu Zi* 6g. *Gan Jiang* 6g.
  Chi Shi Zhi 30g.

Qi stagnation and blood stasis

Discomfort sensation of incomplete defecation after diarrhea or blood clots in the stool, black stool, severe abdominal pain aggravated by pressure, and dusky complexion. Petechiae on the tongue, and choppy pulse.

- Facilitate the qi flow and invigorate the blood, together with auxiliary strategy to strengthen the spleen and eliminate dampness.
- Modified *Tao Hong Si Wu Tang*
  Tao Ren 10g. *Hong Hua* 10g. *Chuan Xiong* 6g.
  Chi Shao 10g. *Dang Gui* 10g. *Wu Yao* 10g.
  Xiang Fu 10g. *Yan Hu Suo* 10g. *Wu Ling Zhi* 6g.
  Fu Ling 15g. *Bai Zhu* 10g. *Gan Cao* 3g.
- Excessive blood in the stool. + *San Qi* 3g. (powder), *Xue Jie* 3g. (powder)
  Cold pain in the abdomen. + *Gan Jiang* 6g., *Xiao Hui Xiang* 10g.

Other Modality

A. Acupuncture:

Refer to Chapter 13 on "Diarrhea" for differentiation and treatment if deficient patterns are identified (see page 97).

Refer to Chapter 14 on "Dysentery Disorder" for differentiation and treatment if excess patterns are identified (see pages 103-104).

B. Herbal enema:

Retention enema with herbal formula effectively improves the symptoms of IBD. By directly acting on the lesions in the intestines, various therapeutic effects are achieved on the congested and edematous intestinal mucosa, the bleeding sites or lesions of the blood vessels, and ulcers.

1. Bowel preparation with cleansing enema is needed prior to introducing therapeutic enema.

2. Administer enema of 200 ml., 98.6 to 102°F herbal formula.

3. Retain herbal enema for 3 hours.

4. Continue the therapy on a daily basis for a full course of 2 to 3 weeks.

5. Select formula prescriptions based on differentiations. May use the herbs in routine dosage or higher.

❶ For effects of debridement and granulation (a basic formula for all patterns):

Dang Gui	*Hu Po*	*Xue Jie*	*Lu Gan Shi*
Hua Shi	*Bing Pian*	*Bai Zhi*	*Gan Cao*

❷ For effects of clearing heat and draining dampness (pattern of damp-heat accumulation):

Huang Qin	*Huang Lian*	*Bai Jiang Cao*	*Huai Hua Mi*
Bai Zhi	*Hai Piao Xiao*	*Gan Cao*	

❸ For effect to promote the movement of qi (pattern of hyperactive liver with deficient spleen):

Bai Shao	*Bai Zhu*	*Fang Feng*	*Chai Hu*
Wu Yao	*Chen Pi*	*Yu Jin*	*Gan Cao*

❹ For effects of augmenting the qi and strengthening the spleen (pattern of spleen and stomach deficiency):

Huang Qi	*Dang Shen*	*Bai Zhu*	*Chen Pi*
Dang Gui	*Chai Hu*	*Zhi Ru Xiang*	*Zhi Mo Yao*
Gan Cao			

❺ For warming effect on the kidney to restrain essence (pattern of spleen and kidney yang deficiency):

Fu Zi	*Liu Huang*	*Yin Yang Huo*	*Bu Gu Zhi*
Shi Liu Pi	*Bai Zhi*	*Gan Cao*	

CHAPTER 58

Irritable Bowel Syndrome

Irritable bowel syndrome (IBS) is the best known functional gastrointestinal disorder. It is characterized by absence of detectible organic disease plus symptoms of dysfunction in any part of the gastrointestinal tract, including the oropharynx, esophagus, stomach, small or large intestine, anorectum or biliary tract. IBS accounts for approximately half of all outpatient referrals to gastroenterologists in the United States; it is estimated that a minimum of one-third of the adult population has been experienced functional gastrointestinal syndrome, with an international prevalence of IBS as high as 10-20 percent. The cost of IBS is not limited to medical services, but also includes loss of productivity due to absenteeism from work. An environmental etiology has been proposed due to a higher incidence in socioeconomically disadvantaged groups. In addition, women tend to report IBS-related symptoms more frequently than men. Research has not established a clear etiology and pathogenesis for IBS. Proposed theories include abnormal visceral nociperception, abnormal colonic myoelectric activities, altered small intestinal motor activities, general smooth muscle or nervous system disturbances, psychological factors, and diet.

Patients with IBS often complain of abdominal pain which is poorly localized, varying in nature and migrating around the abdomen, accompanied by alteration in bowel movements. Both constipation and diarrhea are common, along with rectal urgency, a feeling of incomplete evacuation, and passage of mucus. Constipation consists of decreased frequency of bowel movements and straining or incomplete defecation; diarrhea usually does not involve loose or watery stool, presenting as increased frequency of bowel movements. Based on a classic study done in the United Kingdom, out of fifteen valuable diagnostic symptoms, the following six symptoms associated with bowel movements and pain are the most important criteria, known as the Manning criteria, for diagnosis: 1) pain relief after bowel movements, 2) increased frequency of bowel movements with onset of pain, 3) looser stool at onset of pain, 4) visible abdominal distention, 5) a sensation of incomplete evacuation after bowel movements, and 6) passage of mucus per rectum.

Diagnostic tests or examinations, such as colonoscopy and blood tests, are used to exclude organic pathology. It is observed that most patients with IBS experience psychosocial disturbances; therefore, current treatment provides reassurance, education and dietary modification; medication or behavioral therapy is not necessary for most patients. Avoiding exposure to predisposing factors is recommended, and placebo therapy is widely used; some patients may require psychotherapy.

Reference:

Talley, N. J. (2003). Functional gastrointestinal disorders: Irritable bowel syndrome. In S. L. Friedman, et. al., (Eds.), *Current Diagnosis & Treatment in Gastroenterology* (2nd ed. chap. 6). New York, NY: McGraw-Hill Companies, Inc.

Based on the clinical manifestations, IBS can be referred to chapters on abdominal pain, diarrhea and constipation for TCM differentiation and treatment.

Abdominal pain and alteration in bowel movements are the two major symptoms of IBS. From the perspective of *zang-fu* theory, the organs affected are the stomach and intestines stemming from the root pattern of disharmony between the liver and spleen. Prolonged impairment of the spleen's function to transform and transport, along with disturbance of the large intestine's function in moving the bowel, injures the kidney, ultimately leading to dysfunction of the liver, spleen, stomach, intestines and kidney. Common etiologies follow:

Emotional stress is the most common factor inducing IBS. Anger, frustration, and emotional suppression hinder the liver's function to ensure smooth flow of the qi. Liver qi stagnation results in abdominal pain; when stagnant liver qi overacts on the spleen, secondary spleen deficiency produces diarrhea; when stagnant liver qi transforms into heat, it consumes the fluid in the stomach and intestines and causes constipation.

Improper diet is directly implicated in malabsorption and altered bowel movements. Food retention results from overindulgence; damp-heat is generated by a diet of greasy and sweet food; secondary spleen and stomach injury is caused by eating raw and cold food. Food retention, damp-heat accumulation and impaired function of spleen and stomach all contribute to IBS.

Spleen and stomach qi deficiency is the existing intrinsic factor. Constitutional spleen and stomach deficiency increases the host's susceptibility to exterior pathogens or extrinsic influences, which impair the ascending and descending functions of the spleen and stomach, leading to abdominal pain, diarrhea and constipation.

IBS is initiated by pathology of the spleen, stomach and liver; chronic cases affect the kidney, resulting in spleen and kidney deficiency.

Analysis of Primary Symptom

A. Abdominal pain:

This is the principle symptom of IBS. It commonly presents in conjunction with altered bowel movements. The extent of the pain changes with alterations in bowel movements:

- Distending, migrating abdominal pain that is difficult to localize and is relieved by passing flatus suggests a pathogenesis of qi stagnation. If emotional stress aggravates the pain, increases bowel movements or diarrhea, and pain is alleviated after bowel movements, a diagnosis of liver qi stagnation overacting on the spleen is established. Abdominal pain results from liver hyperactivity, an excess pathogenesis; diarrhea results from insufficient spleen, a deficient pathogenesis.
- If abdominal distending pain is accompanied by fullness, visible abdominal distention and a palpable rod-like prominence in the abdomen, dry stool, decreased bowel movements, and dry mouth and throat, consider insufficient fluid in the stomach and intestines. Lack of moisture in the intestines leads to retention of bowel contents.
- Constant dull abdominal pain that is relieved by warmth and pressure, and is accompanied by poor appetite, lassitude and weakness, indicates a pattern of spleen and stomach qi deficiency failing to warm and nourish the vital organs.

B. Diarrhea:

Diarrhea is reported by patients with increased bowel movements, but not necessarily loose or watery stool. Diarrhea is closely related to the following organs.

- Spleen dominates the function of transformation and transportation; its function of extracting essence from food is known as ascending the clear qi. A deficient spleen will not be able to lift the clear qi, nor can it disseminate food essence to the entire body, resulting in diarrhea. Diarrhea secondary to spleen deficiency usually is accompanied by poor appetite, lassitude, epigastric and abdominal distention and fullness after meals, all reflecting the pathogenesis of a deficient spleen.
- Diarrhea related to the liver, also known as painful diarrhea, is characterized by abdominal pain, increased frequency of bowel movements, looser stool with the onset of pain, and pain relieved after bowel movements; symptoms follow a repetitive cycle.
- The kidney is affected in chronic IBS; diarrhea related to the kidney has the

unique features of abdominal cold pain, borborygmus, and diarrhea before dawn, known as daybreak diarrhea.

C. Constipation:

Constipation in IBS usually does not manifest with hard dry stool, but with less frequent bowel movements. It can result from various pathogeneses. Yin deficiency failing to moisten the intestines and failure of the large intestine to move the bowel manifest with dry stool, decreased bowel movements and dry mouth, tongue and throat. Spleen qi deficiency and failure to facilitate the qi flow in the intestines manifest as passage of dry stool initially, followed by progressively looser stools, and possibly difficulty moving the bowels, even with great effort.

Basic Patterns

- Stagnant liver qi overacting on the spleen
- Combination of cold and heat
- Stomach and intestine fluid deficiency
- Spleen and stomach qi deficiency

Progression of Pattern

The core pathogenesis is stagnant liver qi overacting on the spleen during the initial stage of IBS. If the condition is complicated by cold, heat or phlegm-dampness, a pattern of disharmony of the liver and spleen with a combination of cold and heat is manifested. Longstanding liver qi stagnation turning into heat may further injure the yin and exhaust the fluid, progressing to a pattern of stomach and intestine fluid deficiency. A constitutionally deficient spleen and stomach and secondary spleen deficiency due to liver qi overacting lead to a pattern of spleen and stomach qi deficiency. Chronic spleen pathology eventually involves the kidney; therefore, progression to spleen and kidney deficiency is possible.

Treatment Principle

IBS is characterized by liver qi stagnation and spleen qi deficiency; the treatment principles are to soothe the liver, strengthen the spleen, and augment the qi. Address the complication of cold and heat patterns by adding the appropriate herbs. In the case of stomach and intestine fluid deficiency, nourish the yin and replenish the fluid to moisten dryness.

Pattern and Suggested Measure

Stagnant liver qi overacting on the spleen

Emotional stress elicits symptoms of abdominal distention and pain, borborygmus, and diarrhea. Pain is relieved by bowel movements. Secondary symptoms include distention and fullness in the epigastrium and abdomen, belching, poor appetite, and irritability. Red edge of the tongue with thin coating, and wiry pulse.

- Soothe the liver and support the spleen.
- Modified *Tong Xie Yao Fang*

  Bai Shao 15g. *Bai Zhu* 10g. *Fang Feng* 10g.
  Chen Pi 10g. *Chai Hu* 10g. *Zhi Qiao* 10g.
  Mu Xiang 6g. *Gan Cao* 6g.

- Hypochondriac distention and abdominal pain. + *Chuan Lian Zi* 10g., *Xiang Fu* 10g., *Yan Hu Suo* 10g.

  Irritability, agitation, and red tongue, double the dosage of *Bai Shao*, + *Wu Mei* 10g., *Mu Gua* 10g.

  Chronic diarrhea with significant spleen deficiency. + *Dang Shen* 10g., *Huang Qi* 10g., *Lian Zi* 10g.

Combination of cold and heat

Distention and pain in the abdomen, borborygmus, diarrhea with sensation of incomplete defecation or alternating diarrhea and constipation, distention and fullness in the epigastrium and abdomen, poor appetite, and dry mouth. Red tongue with greasy coating, and wiry slippery pulse.

- Harmonize the stomach and intestine.
- Modified *Wu Mei Wan*

  Wu Mei 15g. *Dang Shen* 15g. *Gan Jiang* 6g.
  Gui Zhi 6g. *Fu Zi* 3g. *Chuan Jiao* 3g.
  Huang Lian 10g. *Huang Bai* 6g. *Dang Gui* 10g.
  Gan Cao 6g.

- Significant cold signs with abdominal distention and pain, remove *Huang Lian*, + *Xiao Hui Xiang* 10g., *Li Zhi He* 10g.

  Burning pain in the epigastrium and abdomen with thirst and bitter taste in the mouth, remove *Gan Jiang*, *Fu Zi* and *Chuan Jiao*, + *Zhi Zi* 10g., *Wu Zhu Yu* 6g.

  Dampness accumulation with abdominal distention and incomplete defecation. + *Hou Po* 10g., *Zhi Shi* 10g.

Stomach and intestine fluid deficiency

Dry stool, decreased frequency of bowel movements, straining to defecate, abdominal distention and fullness, and a detectible rod-like abdominal prominence in severe cases; thirst, headache and irritability. Red tongue with scanty or dry coating, and wiry pulse.

- Nourish the yin, moisten the intestines and unblock the bowel.
- Modified *Zeng Ye Tang* and *Ma Zi Ren Wan*

Xuan Shen 15g.	*Mai Men Dong* 15g.	*Sheng Di Huang* 10g.
Ma Zi Ren 15g.	*Xing Ren* 10g.	*Bai Shao* 10g.
Zhi Shi 6g.	*Hou Po* 10g.	*Da Huang* 3g.

- Qi deficiency with stool that is initially dry followed by loose bowel movements. + *Huang Qi* 10g., *Tai Zi Shen* 10g.
  Complicated by qi stagnation with frequent belching and abdominal distention. + *Mu Xiang* 10g., *Bing Lang* 10g.

Spleen and stomach qi deficiency

Loose stool or diarrhea containing undigested food, poor appetite, focal distention in the epigastrium, especially after meals, increased bowel movements due to improper diet, dull epigastric and abdominal pain, lassitude and weakness. Pale tongue with white coating, and weak pulse.

- Strengthen the spleen and augment the qi.
- Modified *Shen Ling Bai Zhu San*

Dang Shen 10g.	*Bai Zhu* 10g.	*Fu Ling* 15g.
Shan Yao 10g.	*Bian Dou* 10g.	*Lian Zi* 10g.
Yi Yi Ren 15g.	*Sha Ren* 6g.	*Chen Pi* 10g.

- Spleen qi sinking with unremitting diarrhea. + *Huang Qi* 10g., *Sheng Ma* 10g.
  Daybreak diarrhea with soreness and weakness of the lower back and knees, cold intolerance and cold limbs, use *Si Shen Wan*.

Other Modality

Acupuncture:

Refer to Chapter 13, "Diarrhea", for patients with abdominal pain and diarrhea (see page 97).

Refer to Chapter 16, "Constipation", for patients with abdominal pain and constipation (see page 116).

CHAPTER 59

Cholelithiasis and Cholecystitis

As one of the most common gastrointestinal diseases, cholelithiasis, or gallstones, affects any age group, particularly women in their reproductive years. The higher gender and age specific prevalence can be explained partly by endogenous estrogens. Estrogen increases the saturation of cholesterol in bile by inhibiting enzymatic conversion of cholesterol to bile acids. Other attributing factors include pregnancy, history of ileal pathology and obesity; ethnic traits seem to be associated with prevalence and types of gallstones. There are two major types of gallstones, cholesterol and pigment stones. The former is cholesterol rich and it is the popular kind among Americans and Europeans, whereas pigment stones are more common among Asians and Africans. However, in westernized Asian countries like Japan, the prevalence of cholesterol stones has been increasing. Most patients with gallstones are asymptomatic until the onset of acute cholecystitis, which is inflammation of the gallbladder. Its clinical manifestations are consistent with cholecystitis.

Acute cholecystitis is closely related to gallstones, which accounts for more than 90% of the cases. When the stone impacts the cystic duct, inflammation of the gallbladder behind the blockage follows. Large meals and greasy diet usually precipitate an acute attack. Acute cholecystitis manifests with sudden onset of severe steady epigastric or hypochondriac pain that may subside within 12-18 hours, fever and possible vomiting. Physical examination reveals muscle tenderness over the right upper quadrant with muscle guarding and rebound pain; in some cases, the enlarged gallbladder may be palpable. Depending on the degree of obstruction, jaundice may appear; in another word, persistent or severe jaundice suggests a possibility of gallstones.

Cholelithiasis and cholecystitis rely on laboratory and imaging evidences to make a diagnosis. Laboratory findings with elevated white blood cell count, serum bilirubin, serum aminotransferase and alkaline phosphatase all can be present during acute cholecystitis. The diagnosis of cholelithiasis can be confirmed with the presence of gallstones in imaging examination, such as ultrasonography, computed tomography (CT scan), magnetic resonance imaging (MRI), and endoscopic retrograde cholangiopancreatography (ERCP). Advanced technology, ^{99m}Tc hepatobiliary imaging (HIDA scan), is very useful in showing an obstructed cystic duct; therefore, it is a valuable diagnostic tool for both cholecystitis and cholelithiasis. Cholecystitis usually responds well to conservative therapy, incorporating resting the gastrointestinal system, administering intravenous fluids, analgesic and antibiotics. However, due to its high recurrent rate, surgical removal of the gallbladder is usually the choice of treatment for gallstone. Antibiotic therapy is required before surgery if symptom of acute pancreatitis is present. Modern technology, namely laparoscopic cholecystectomy, has greatly reduced the mortality risk of surgery to less than 1%. Non-surgical procedure, like extracorporeal shock wave lithotripsy (ESWL), can break the stone size to allow for oral bile acid dissolution therapy.

References:

Friedman, L. S. (2003). Liver, biliary tract & pancreas: Diseases of the biliary tract. In L. M. Tierney, Jr., et al. (Eds.), *Current Medical Diagnosis & Treatment* (42nd ed. chap. 15). New York, NY: McGraw-Hill Companies, Inc.

Jacobson, I. M. (2003). Gallstones. In S. L. Friedman, et. al. (Eds.), *Current Diagnosis and Treatment in Gastroenterology* (2nd ed. chap. 50). New York, NY: McGraw-Hill Companies, Inc.

Based on the clinical manifestations, cholelithiasis and cholecystitis can be referred to chapters on hypochondriac pain and jaundice for TCM differentiation and treatment.

Recently, a group of experts in Integration of TCM and Western Medicine has successfully intervened to come up with a conservative approach as an alternative to invasive therapy. Instead of surgeries, these experts have adopted the administration of herbal formula to treat acute abdomen, disorders that primarily manifest with acute abdominal pain, including acute cholecystitis and acute attack of gallstone. Based on TCM theory, "The yang organs function when they remain patent" and "Any obstruction induces pain". They use approaches to invigorate the blood, relieve toxicity and purge out accumulations with very good effect and surgical procedures may be avoided. For instance, the formula mentioned later in this chapter, *Pai Shi Tang*, or stone-eliminating decoction, has proven to be effective in pharmacological studies. This formula can alleviate spasm of Oddi's sphincter and promote the drainage and excretion of bile, eliminating the small gallstones and preventing formation of new ones. It is therapeutically effective in stabilizing the condition and disease prevention.

The primary organ involved is the gallbladder and its related channels, which may further involve the liver and its related channels. The spleen and stomach, to a certain degree, contribute to the occurrence of these disorders. The following are primary etiologies:

Improper diet: Overindulgence of alcohol or greasy rich diet results in damp-heat accumulation in the stomach and intestines. An insult from earth to wood leads to stagnant liver and gallbladder qi, and poor drainage and excretion of the bile.

Emotional stress: Liver and gallbladder have an internal-external relationship. Once the liver is affected by emotional stresses, the effect on the gallbladder is obvious, manifesting in sluggish excretion of bile.

Exterior pathogenic factors: Stagnant heat transformed from wind-cold can be trapped in the lesser-yang aspect. Warm-febrile pathogens or damp-heat attacking the liver and gallbladder may lead to sluggish qi flow and dysfunction of the lesser-yang organs, and blockage in the yang-brightness aspect. As a result, bile is stagnated inside the gallbladder, and it may form stones to obstruct the bile duct.

"Gallbladder is an organ that store purified substance", located in the hypochondriac region and attached to the liver. The major function of the gallbladder is to excrete bile; its proper function relies on smooth descent and patency. The liver dominates free flow of the qi; it prefers a liberal environment and dislikes suppression. These etiologies can hinder the qi flow of the liver and gallbladder, resulting in stagnant bile, blockage in the collaterals and hypochondriac pain. When the bile seeps into the skin, yellow discoloration of the skin is apparent; when the bile infuses into body fluids, yellow discoloration of the urine is evident; being steamed by the liver fire, retention of bile in the gallbladder forms stones.

Analysis of Primary Symptom

A. Right hypochondriac pain:

Pain in the right upper quadrant is the earliest and the most important sign. Hypochondriac regions are where the liver and gallbladder channels travel through. Disturbance in the qi flow of the liver and gallbladder, and failure of patent descent of the gallbladder qi may lead to pain secondary to obstruction. Predisposing factors to obstruction include qi stagnation, blood stasis, excessive toxicity and damp-heat.

- Migrating and distending hypochondriac pain, which is aggravated by emotional stress, is secondary to liver and gallbladder qi stagnation.
- Fixed stabbing pain that worsens at night and possibly palpable mass at the hypochondriac region are most likely an implication of blood stasis in the liver and gallbladder channels and collaterals.
- Burning pain in the hypochondriac regions with muscle guarding, alteration of chills and fever or high fever and bitter taste in the mouth, results from excess

fire in liver and gallbladder channels. Another possible pathogenesis is pathogenic factors invading the lesser-yang aspect, causing disturbance on the qi flow with excessive heat-toxicity.

- Severe hypochondriac pain or constant low grade fever, and thick yellow greasy tongue coating are symptoms and signs of damp-heat accumulation, which obstruct inside the liver and gallbladder channels and collaterals.
- Intermittent dull pain in the hypochondriac regions that is aggravated by exertion is caused by insufficiency of the yin and fluid failing to nourish the channels of the liver and gallbladder. This is a deficient pattern.

B. Jaundice:

Dampness is the primary predisposing factor to jaundice. When stagnant dampness turning into heat obstructs the drainage and excretion of bile, bile diffuses into the skin, causing yellow discoloration of the skin. In addition, jaundice secondary to cholelithiasis and cholecystitis can be contributed by fire toxicity and obstruction of the stones. Different types of jaundice are based on the nature of yin and yang.

- Yang jaundice is characterized by bright, lustrous, yellow pigmentation like an orange peel. Excessive damp-heat is the major contributing factor to this type; it is often seen in the acute stage. Clinically, differentiations can be further subcategorized based on the preponderance of dampness or heat.
- Yin jaundice is characterized by dusky and smoky yellow pigmentation. It commonly manifests after the acute stage, when prompt treatment was not initiated during the acute stage, and when there is an overuse of bitter and cold herbs that can injure spleen and stomach yang.
- Heat toxin jaundice has a sudden onset and is a rapid progressive type of jaundice as evidence by a discoloration of golden-yellow. This is due to excessive fire toxicity in the liver and gallbladder. During critical progression of yang jaundice, acute jaundice may develop into fire-toxicity trapping inside the pericardium with coma.

C. Fever:

There may be high fever or low grade fever.

- High fever usually manifests during the acute stage. It is commonly accompanied by symptoms of sweating, red face, thirst, irritability and restlessness. These are symptoms and signs of fire-toxicity secondary to excessive fire of the liver and gallbladder. If the fever remains high after sweating, or if there is thirst but no desire to drink, damp-heat obstruction in the liver and gallbladder is evident.
- Low grade fever is mostly common in yin deficiency; it has various clinical presentations, including tidal fever and five-centers heat with night sweating. When disease progresses to involve the spleen and stomach, low grade fever

secondary to qi deficient is also possible, manifesting in low grade fever aggravated on exertion accompanied by spontaneous sweating and aversion to wind. Low grade fever is commonly seen during remission phase or when righteous qi is exhausted.

- Alteration of chills and fever are seen occasionally. This is a classic presentation of pathogenic factors trapped in the aspect of lesser-yang, and it is caused by the contest of righteous qi and pathogenic factors.

D. Digestive symptoms:

Digestive symptoms, including epigastric pain, hypochondriac pain, bitter taste in the mouth, nausea and vomiting, and constipation, are indications of stagnant earth with constrained wood. Constrained liver and gallbladder qi overacts on the stomach causing nausea and vomiting. Disturbance in qi flow of the lesser-yang and obstructed qi in the yang-brightness organs manifest as constipation.

Basic Patterns

- Liver and gallbladder qi stagnation
- Liver and gallbladder fire excess
- Liver and gallbladder damp-heat
- Yin deficiency accompanied by dampness
- Blood stasis obstruction in the collaterals

Progression of Pattern

Pathogenic excess dominates the early stage of cholecystitis and cholelithiasis, and a complicated condition of deficiency with excess dominates the later stage. Liver and gallbladder qi stagnation may transform into fire, leading to the pattern of liver and gallbladder fire excess. Liver and gallbladder qi stagnation or heat consuming the fluid in the blood may also lead to blood stasis obstruction in the collaterals due to poor blood circulation. Longstanding liver and gallbladder damp-heat injures the yin, complicating the condition to yin deficiency accompanied by dampness. These patterns may present in isolation or in combination.

The presentations during the disease progression indicate the dominant involvement of lesser-yang channels and yang-brightness organs, that is, the obstruction in either lesser-yang channels or in yang-brightness organs.

Treatment Principle

The key element to the occurrence of cholelithiasis and cholecystitis is the obstruction from qi stagnation, damp-heat accumulation and fire toxicity; therefore, the treatment principle is based on the guideline to "Unblock the obstruction to alleviate pain". For excess patterns, regulate the qi, invigorate the blood, clear heat and expel dampness; for deficient patterns, nourish the yin, and soften and comfort the liver. During remission or after surgery, strengthen the spleen and soothe the liver to eliminate any remaining dampness and heat, and to prevent yin and blood injury that may lead to unremitting recurrent condition.

Pattern and Suggested Measure

Liver and gallbladder qi stagnation

Right upper quadrant distention and pain, possible paroxysmal colic pain, possibly focal distention and fullness in the epigastrium, belching, retching, poor appetite, irregular bowel movements, bitter taste in the mouth and dry throat. Slightly red tongue with thin white or thin yellow coating, and wiry thready or wiry tight pulse.

- Soothe the liver, regulate the qi flow and alleviate pain.
- Modified *Chai Hu Shu Gan San*

Chai Hu 10g.	*Bai Shao* 15g.	*Zhi Shi* 10g.
Xiang Fu 10g.	*Chuan Xiong* 6g.	*Sheng Gan Cao* 6g.
Yu Jin 10g.	*Qing Pi* 10g.	*Chi Shao* 15g.

- Severe hypochondriac pain. + *Fo Shou* 10g., *Yan Hu Suo* 10g.
  Stagnant qi transforming into fire with bitter taste in the mouth, dry throat and red tongue. + *Zhi Zi* 10g., *Huang Qin* 10g., *Mu Dan Pi* 10g.
  Focal distention and fullness in the epigastrium and abdomen, poor appetite and loose stool. + *Fu Ling* 15g., *Bai Zhu* 10g.
  Distention and pain in the abdomen, and constipation. + *Hou Po* 10g., *Da Huang* 6g., *Mang Xiao* 6g.

Liver and gallbladder fire excess

Burning pain at the right upper quadrant with muscle guarding, distention and fullness in the epigastrium and abdomen, alteration of chills and fever, bitter taste in the mouth, red face, irritability, retching, poor appetite, constipation and dark urination, and yellow discoloration of the sclera and the skin. Red tongue with dry yellow coating, and rapid soft or rapid flooding pulse.

- Clear heat, drain fire, soothe the liver and drain dampness.
- Modified *Huang Lian Jie Du Tang* and *Da Chai Hu Tang*

Huang Lian 10g.	*Huang Qin* 10g.	*Huang Bai* 10g.
Zhi Zi 10g.	*Chai Hu* 10g.	*Da Huang* 6g.
Ban Xia 10g.	*Zhi Shi* 10g.	*Bai Shao* 15g.
Mu Xiang 10g.	*Gan Cao* 6g.	

- Severe hypochondriac pain. + *Chuan Lian Zi* 10g., *Yan Hu Suo* 10g., *Xiang Fu* 10g.
  Significant heat signs. + *Long Dan Cao* 10g., *Mu Dan Pi* 10g., *Xuan Shen* 10g.
  Constipation. + *Hou Po* 10g., *Mang Xiao* 10g.
  Jaundice. + *Yin Chen Hao* 10g., *Jin Qian Cao* 10g.
  Gallstones. + *Jin Qian Cao* 10g., *Ji Nei Jin* 10g., *Hai Jin Sha* 30g.

Liver and gallbladder damp-heat

Right hypochondriac pain that is paroxysmal and progressively intensified, possibly a palpable mass at the hypochondriac region, high fever, chills, focal distention and fullness of the epigastrium and abdomen, nausea, vomiting with yellow bitter emesis, thirst without desire to drink, dark yellow and scanty urination, constipation, and yellow discoloration on the sclera and skin. Red tongue with yellow greasy coating, and rapid slippery pulse.

- Clear heat, drain dampness, soothe the liver and promote drainage of the bile.
- Modified *Yin Chen Hao Tang* and *Long Dan Xie Gan Tang*

Yin Chen Hao 15g.	*Zhi Zi* 10g.	*Da Huang* 6g.
Long Dan Cao 6g.	*Chai Hu* 10g.	*Huang Qin* 10g.
Mu Tong 10g.	*Ze Xie* 15g.	*Che Qian Zi* 15g.
Yu Jin 10g.	*Gan Cao* 6g.	

- Excessive heat. + *Mu Dan Pi* 10g., *Huang Lian* 10g.
  Excessive dampness. + *Cang Zhu* 10g., *Hou Po* 10g.
  Vomiting with yellow bitter emesis. + *Huang Lian* 6g., *Wu Zhu Yu* 3g.
  Severe jaundice or gallstones. + *Jin Qian Cao* 10g., *Hu Zhang* 10g., *Hai Jin Sha* 30g., *Ji Nei Jin* 10g.

Yin deficiency accompanied by dampness

Intermittent dull pain in the right hypochondriac region that is aggravated by exertion, five-centers heat, dry mouth and throat, dark yellow urination and constipation. Red tongue with thin yellow greasy coating, and rapid wiry thready pulse.

- Nourish the yin and clear heat primarily, and drain dampness.
- Modified *Yi Guan Jian* and *Gan Lu Xiao Du Dan*

Sheng Di Huang 15g.	*Mai Men Dong* 10g.	*Sha Shen* 10g.
Dang Gui 10g.	*Gou Qi Zi* 10g.	*Chuan Lian Zi* 10g.
Yin Chen Hao 6g.	*Huang Qin* 10g.	*Hua Shi* 20g.
Mu Tong 10g.	*Bai Dou Kou* 6g.	*Huo Xiang* 6g.
Shi Chang Pu 6g.		

- To enhance the effects of soothing constrained qi and comforting the liver for significant hypochondriac pain. + *Mei Gui Hua* 10g., *Chai Hu* 10g., *Bai Shao* 10g. Five-centers heat. + *Qing Hao* 10g., *Bie Jia* 20g., *Zhi Mu* 10g.

Blood stasis obstruction in the collaterals

Stabbing pain at a fix location in the right hypochondrium that is worse at night, palpable masses at the hypochondriac regions, distention and fullness in the abdomen, and dry stool. Dark purple tongue, and choppy pulse.

- Regulate the qi flow, invigorate the blood and expel stasis.
- Modified *Fu Yuan Huo Xue Tang*

Chai Hu 10g.	*Tao Ren* 10g.	*Hong Hua* 10g.
Dang Gui 10g.	*Gua Lou Gen* 15g.	*Da Huang* 6g.
Chi Shao 15g.	*E Zhu* 10g.	*Yu Jin* 10g.
Xiang Fu 10g.		

- To enhance the effects of invigorating the blood and facilitating the qi flow for significant hypochondriac pain. + *Yan Hu Suo* 10g., *San Leng* 10g., *Fo Shou* 10g. Hypochondriac pain with palpable masses, use *Bie Jia Jian Wan*.

Other Modality

A. Acupuncture:

- **Manipulation:** Reducing method.
- **Prescription:** BL19 Danshu; BL18 Ganshu; GB24 Riyue; LR14 Qimen; GB34 Yanglingquan; Extra39 Dannangxue; LR3 Taichong
- **Supplementary points per patterns:**
  - Qi stagnation. + LR2 Xingjian; GB40 Qiuxu
  - Blood stasis. + BL17 Geshu
  - Excessive heat. + GV26 Renzhong; GV14 Dazhui; PC6 Neiguan; GB41 Zulinqi
  - Damp-heat. + ST36 Zusanli; SP9 Yinlingquan

- **Supplementary points per symptoms:**
  - Colic pain. + LI4 Hegu; PC4 Ximen
  - Jaundice. + GV9 Zhiyang; BL48 Yanggang
  - Vomiting. + PC6 Neiguan
  - Fever. + LI11 Quchi; GV14 Dazhui

B. Topical paste:

Ingredients:

Sheng Da Huang 60g. (powder), *Mang Xiao* 30g. (powder), Garlic 1 clove, Vinegar

Procedure:

Crush 1 clove of garlic and mix it with *Sheng Da Huang* 30g. and *Mang Xiao* 30g. Apply the mixed paste topically at the gallbladder area for 10 minutes.

Mix the rest of *Sheng Da Huang* 30g. with vinegar to make another paste.

Apply the second paste on the gallbladder region topically after removal of the first paste.

Use the pastes twice per day.

C. Experiential remedy:

Pai Shi Tang:

Hu Zhang 30g.	*Mu Xiang* 15g.	*Zhi Qiao* 15g.
Da Huang 10g.	*Jin Qian Cao* 30g.	*Zhi Zi* 12g.
Yan Hu Suo 15g.		

This formula, stone-eliminating decoction, can facilitate the excretion of bile and eliminate gallstones.

CHAPTER 60

Acute Glomerulonephritis

Acute glomerulonephritis (AGN) is an acute inflammatory renal disease, in which the diffuse proliferative renal glomerular lesions cause sudden decrease in glomerular filtration rate. The clinical manifestations of AGN are edema, hematuria, proteinuria, oliguria and hypertension. The defected glomerular basement membrane allows the excretion of serum red blood cells and proteins; decreased glomerular filtration rate results in sodium retention and therefore follows the manifestations of edema and hypertension. Current scientific evidence chooses the theory of immunologically mediated response as the cause for AGN; antigen-antibody complexes are detected in both blood sample and real biopsy specimen. Some AGN might progress and continue its course to acute renal failure, chronic nephritis and chronic renal failure.

Varied in etiologies and pathological progressions, AGN is clinically categorized into two major types, post-streptococcal acute glomerulonephritis and rapidly progressive glomerulonephritis (RPGN). The former accounts for the majority of post-infectious cases; the occurrence of post-streptococcal AGN follows pharyngitis, tonsillitis or pyoderma by a nephritogenic streptococcal strains. Children of age 2-10 years have higher prevalence of classic streptococcal sore throat, especially during winter and spring seasons; while pyoderma occurs primarily in children at age 2-6 years in seasons of summer and early fall. The first sign of hematuria follows 7 days to 12 weeks after streptococcal infection. Post-streptococcal AGN is an acute reversible disease; most cases recover spontaneously. Within one to two weeks after onset, normal urination will be resumed; it takes approximately four weeks for serum creatinine level to return to normal; hematuria may resolved in six months; however, 15% of patients might still experience mild proteinuria for as long as three years and 2% of patients have mild proteinuria up to ten years. Although the majority of patients suffer from post-streptococcal AGN have fully recovered; few cases might still suffer various degrees of residual symptoms, such as hypertension, recurrent or persistent proteinuria, and chronic renal insufficiency. Treatment for post-streptococcal AGN focuses on acute symptom managements, by integrating antibiotics, corticosteroids, intravenous gamma globulin, antihypertensive agents, diuresis and electrolyte replacements.

RPGN, on the other hand, is a rapid progressive renal disease that causes renal function to decline rapidly and critically, and it develops into acute renal failure or end stage renal disease within days to weeks. It accounts for 2-4% of all glomerulonephritis cases. Its diagnosis relies on renal biopsy, which demonstrates cellular crescents surrounding majority of the glomeruli. Unlike post-streptococcal AGN, RPGN requires aggressive medical treatments. In acute healthcare facility, glucocorticoids and cyclophosphamide are the main agents; plasma exchange may be intervened to remove circulating autoantibodies.

References:

Bisno, A. L. (2000). Nonsuppurative post-streptococcal sequelae: Rheumatic Fever and Glomerulonephritis- Glomerulonephritis. In G. L. Mandell, J. E. Bennett, & R. Dolin (Eds.), *Mandell: Principles and Practice of Infectious Diseases* (5th ed. pp. 2123-2126). Philadelphia, PA: Churchill Livingstone.

Hricik, D. E., Chung-Park, M., & Sedor, J. R. (1998). Medical progress: Glomerulonephritis. *The New England Journal of Medicine, 339*(13), 888-899.

Based on the clinical manifestations, AGN can be categorized into TCM differentiation and treatment of edema; it may also be referred to the disorder of hemorrhage.

The occurrence of AGN is induced by exterior wind, cold, dampness, heat and toxicity, and it is associated with the dysfunctions of the lung, spleen and kidney.

Exterior wind impairs the function of the lung to regulate the water passage. Wind-water complex diffuses into the interstitial layers between the skin and muscles, manifesting as edema, or *feng shui*.

Exterior dampness invasion is usually associated with an excessively damp environment, and it can directly affect the spleen. Water accumulation and edema occur following the failure of the spleen to transport and transform fluids. Damp-heat or damp-toxicity obstructs the triple burner, leading to poor circulation in the water passage. Edema results.

Qi deficiency of the lung, spleen and kidney composes the intrinsic etiology of AGN, particularly kidney qi deficiency. According to Chapter 61 in Su Wen, "*Feng shui* roots from the kidney." The internal deficiency increases the susceptibility to exterior pathogenic attacks.

The hallmark of pathogenesis of AGN is the invasion of exterior pathogens. Sudden and acute onset, and rapid progression indicates the invasion of wind; relatively gradual onset and slower progress signify the invasion of dampness.

Analysis of Primary Symptom

A. Edema:

Edema is the primary symptom of AGN. The rapid onset is first noticeable on the eyelid, face and upper body:

- Lung disperses and descends; it regulates the water passage and dominates the surface of the body, namely the skin layer. Therefore, during invasion of exterior wind, the lung and its extended tissue are affected, leading to impairment of water metabolism. Unmetabolized fluids diffuse into the interstitial layer and fuse with exterior wind, presented as edema, also known as *feng shui*. The fact that the lung is located in the upper burner determines the edema initiating from the eyelid, face and upper body. When the upper burner affects the middle and lower burners, gradual development of systemic edema occurs. Since the AGN is induced by exterior pathogens, symptoms of exterior condition manifest as aversion to wind or cold, fever and sore throat. Thin white tongue coating and floating tight pulse help diagnose preponderance of cold of *feng shui*. Red tip and edge of the tongue and floating rapid pulse help diagnose preponderance of heat of *feng shui*. Excess wind-water complex pertains to the scope of yang edema.
- Invading and lingering dampness hinders the spleen's functions, follows edema secondary to impairment of fluid transformation and transportation. This type of edema also pertains to yang edema. The onset and progression of edema secondary to spleen dysfunction are relatively slower and edema can gradually affect the entire body. As the spleen governs the muscles, fatigue, weak and heavy limbs are common.

B. Hematuria or dark tea color urine output:

Hematuria and dark tea color urine output result from wind-heat invasion with heat infusing downwards to the lower burner or excessive damp-heat injuring the vessels.

Basic Patterns

- Wind-heat attacking
- Wind-cold attacking
- Damp-heat toxicity attacking
- Dampness accumulation
- Damp-heat accumulation
- Excessive heat in the lower burner

Progression of Pattern

Initial stage of AGN is mostly caused by exterior pathogens, inducing *feng shui*. When the disease progresses, symptoms pertaining to exterior condition will be resolved and the condition turns into pattern of dampness accumulation. Excessive dampness further injures the spleen and kidney qi or turns into heat, damp-heat accumulation or excessive heat in the lower burner follows. Since heat injures the yin, kidney yin deficiency may manifest during recovery stage as damp-heat reduces.

Treatment Principle

The primary etiologies are wind and damp-toxicity. The treatment principle should be dispersing wind, transforming dampness, clearing heat and relieving toxicity. Adjuvant treatments to promote urination and reduce edema, cool the blood and stop bleeding, and cultivate the basal qi and tonify the kidney should be added accordingly.

Pattern and Suggested Measure

Wind-heat attacking

Aversion to wind, fever, sore throat, systemic edema starting from the eyelids to the lower extremities and then the entire body, general body ache and dysuria. Red edge and tip of the tongue, and floating rapid pulse.

- Disperse wind-heat, promote urination and reduce edema.
- Modified *Yin Qiao San* and *Wu Pi San*
  Jin Yin Hua 10g. *Lian Qiao* 10g. *Bo He* 6g.
  Jing Jie 6g. *Niu Bang Zi* 10g. *Jie Geng* 6g.
  Zhu Ye 10g. *Fu Ping* 10g. *Sang Bai Pi* 10g.
  Fu Ling Pi 15g. *Da Fu Pi* 10g. *Chen Pi* 10g.
- Severe sore throat. + *Shan Dou Gen* 6g., *She Gan* 6g.
  Excessive heat, use *Yue Bi Jia Zhu Tang*.

Wind-cold attacking

Aversion to cold, fever, no sweating, systemic edema starting from the eyelids to the lower extremities and then the entire body, general body ache, cough and dysuria. Thin white tongue coating, and floating tight pulse.

- Dispel wind-cold, disperse lung qi and promote urination.
- Modified *Ma Huang Tang* and *Wu Pi San*

Ma Huang 6g.	*Gui Zhi* 10g.	*Xing Ren* 10g.
Zi Su Ye 10g.	*Sheng Jiang Pi* 10g.	*Fu Ling Pi* 10g.
Da Fu Pi 10g.	*Sang Bai Pi* 10g.	*Chen Pi* 10g.
Niu Xi 15g.	*Che Qian Zi* 10g.	

Damp-heat toxicity attacking

Pyoderma followed by edema starting from the eyelids spreading to the limbs and the entire body, and dysuria. Possible aversion to wind and fever. Red tongue with thin yellow coating, and rapid slippery pulse.

- Relieve toxicity, disperse lung qi, drain dampness and reduce edema.
- Modified *Ma Huang Lian Qiao Chi Xiao Dou Tang* and *Wu Wei Xiao Du Yin*

Ma Huang 6g.	*Xing Ren* 10g.	*Lian Qiao* 10g.
Sang Bai Pi 10g.	*Chi Xiao Dou* 20g.	*Jin Yin Hua* 10g.
Ye Ju Hua 15g.	*Pu Gong Ying* 10g.	*Zi Hua Di Ding* 10g.

- Dermal sores with excessive discharge. + *Ku Shen* 10g., *Tu Fu Ling* 10g.
  Dermal sores with severe itchiness. + *Bai Xian Pi* 10g., *Di Fu Zi* 10g.

Dampness accumulation

Systemic edema, oliguria, heavy extremities, poor appetite, abdominal distention and loose stool. White greasy tongue coating, and deep decelerating pulse.

- Strengthen the spleen, drain dampness, unblock the obstruction of yang qi and promote urination.
- Modified *Wei Ling Tang*

Cang Zhu 10g.	*Hou Po* 10g.	*Chen Pi* 10g.
Fu Ling 15g.	*Ze Xie* 15g.	*Zhu Ling* 15g.
Rou Gui 6g.	*Da Fu Pi* 10g.	*Sha Ren* 6g.

- Severe edema with dyspnea. + *Ma Huang* 6g., *Xing Ren* 10g., *Ting Li Zi* 10g.

Damp-heat accumulation

Systemic edema, dark scanty urine with tea color, bitter taste and sticky sensation in the mouth, focal distention and fullness in the epigastrium and abdomen, and constipation or incomplete defecation. Thick greasy tongue coating and rapid slippery pulse.

- Clear and drain damp-heat.
- Modified *Cheng Shi Bi Xie Fen Qing Yin*

Bi Xie 10g.	*Che Qian Zi* 15g.	*Fu Ling* 15g.
Huang Bai 10g.	*Shi Chang Pu* 10g.	*Lian Zi Xin* 10g.
Bai Zhu 10g.	*Dan Shen* 15g.	

- For severe edema, the treatment principle should be draining and forcing out damp-heat through bowel movements and urination, use *Ji Jiao Li Huang Wan*.

Excessive heat in the lower burner

Dark and scanty urination or bright red hematuria, irritability, thirst, possible sores in the mouth and on the tongue, and insomnia. Red tongue with scanty coating, and rapid deep pulse.

- Clear heat, drain fire, cool the blood and stop bleeding.
- Modified *Xiao Ji Yin Zi*

Xiao Ji 10g.	*Sheng Di Huang* 10g.	*Ou Jie* 10g.
Pu Huang 10g.	*Zhi Zi* 10g.	*Zhu Ye* 10g.
Hua Shi 20g.	*Dang Gui* 10g.	*Han Lian Cao* 10g.

Patterns above are seen in acute episodes, which are characterized by edema and observable hematuria under the naked eyes. Once these two symptoms resolve, AGN progresses into recovery stage and the treatment should be modified based on the clinical presentations. Treat spleen deficiency with *Shen Ling Bai Zhu San*, and yin deficiency with *Liu Wei Di Huang Wan*, and qi and yin deficiency with *Da Bu Yuan Jian*.

Other Modality

A. Acupuncture:

- **Manipulation:** Reducing method.
- **Prescription:** BL13 Feishu, LU7 Lieque, LI4 Hegu, SP9 Yinlingquan, CV9 Shuifen, BL22 Sanjiaoshu
- **Supplementary points:**
  - Sore throat. + LU11 Shaoshang
  - Facial edema. + GV20 Renzhong
  - Hypertension. + LI11 Quchi; LR3 Taichong

B. Experiential remedies:

❶ *Bai Mao Gen* 250g. (take the decoction in frequent multiple doses daily).

❷ *Yu Mi Xu* 60 g. (take the decoction in frequent multiple doses daily).

❸ Herbs with anti-proteinuria effect: *Huang Qi*, *Yi Yi Ren*, *Bai Hua She She Cao*, *Yu Mi Xu*, *Lei Gong Teng*, *Kun Ming Shan Hai Tang*.

CHAPTER **61**

Urinary Tract Infections

Urinary tract infection (UTI) is a disease of the urinary tract caused by various infectious microorganisms, including bacteria, fungi and parasites. Bacteria cause most urinary tract infections. The prevalence of UTI changes according to demographics. Male infants have more UTIs than female infants, possibly due to congenital variances; the incidence in boys aged 1 to 5 years is 0.03 percent, compared to 1-2 percent for girls of the same age. Adult women aged 20 to 50 years are fifty times more likely to develop a UTI than their male counterparts; however, risk increases in men after age 50 due to prostate pathology. *Escherichia coli (E. coli)* is the leading cause of bacterial infectious UTI; it is responsible for 80 percent of community-acquired infections, followed by *Staphylococcus saprophyticus*, which accounts for an additional 10 percent. Ninety-five percent of cases occur as retrograde infection when bacteria ascend and colonize the urethra, bladder, and renal pelvis. *Candida albicans* accounts for the majority of fungal infections and is associated with indwelling urinary catheterization and nosocomial infection following antibiotic therapy. Although parasites can cause UTI, these cases are rarely seen.

Diagnosis of UTI is based on urinary tract symptoms. Microbiologic laboratory findings based on urine culture and sensitivity testing can accurately identify infectious microorganisms as well as the most effective antibiotics.

While some patients are asymptomatic, others have symptoms specific to the affected regions of the urinary tract. Bacterial infectious urethritis has a gradual onset and mild symptoms of a purulent or whitish urethral discharge in men, and dysuria, frequency and pyuria in women. Bacterial infectious cystitis has an acute onset and more pronounced symptoms, such as frequency, urgency, burning or painful urination with scanty output, nocturia, and suprapubic or lower back pain. Urine output tends to be turbid and sometimes there will be gross hematuria. Men with prostatitis experience chills, fever, urinary frequency and urgency, perineal and lower back pain, as well as obstructed urination, dysuria, nocturia or gross hematuria. As retrograde infection reaches the higher part of the urinary tract, acute or chronic pyelonephritis is possible. Symptoms associated with acute pyelonephritis include rapid onset of chills, fever, flank pain, nausea and vomiting, and possibly urinary frequency and dysuria. Symptoms related to chronic pyelonephritis occur gradually and they may be vague and inconsistent. Antimicrobials are the essential treatment for all UTI cases, though surgical correction may be required to address anatomical anomalies in some patients. Prevention of UTI can be achieved by voiding immediately after sexual intercourse, by not using a diaphragm, and by scrupulous personal hygiene. Cranberry juice has been found very helpful in UTI prevention. Fungal infectious UTI should not be overlooked when there is a history of indwelling urinary catheterization and misuse or overuse of antibiotics.

Reference:

Beers, M. H. & Berkow, R. et. al. (Eds.). (1999). Urinary tract infections. *The Merck Manual of Diagnosis and Therapy* (17th ed. chap. 227). West Point, PA: Merck & Co., Inc.

Based on clinical manifestations, UTI is categorized for TCM differenitiation and treatment in the chapters on painful urinary syndrome and lower back pain.

The urinary bladder and kidney are the primary organs responsible for UTI according to TCM theory. When damp-heat infuses downwards and accumulates in the bladder, or when the kidney is deficient and unable to transform qi, obstructed elimination in the urinary tract is evident along with urinary discomfort.

Damp-heat accumulation in the bladder results from exterior damp-heat invasion or internally generated damp-heat. Poor personal hygiene creates susceptibility to exterior damp-heat attacks that develop into retrograde infection. Interior damp-heat is generated when the spleen is deficient or from excessive consumption of sweet and greasy food; interior damp-heat infuses downwards and accumulates in the bladder. Damp-heat accumulation in the bladder leads to impaired qi transformation and causes obstructed elimination, manifesting as urgency, frequency and painful urination.

Kidney qi deficiency results from congenital insufficiency, excessive sexual activity, accumulation of urinary sand and calculi, and advanced age. When these predisposing factors deplete kidney qi, the kidney fails to transform qi and assist the bladder in eliminating fluids, leading to distending pain in the suprapubic region, dysuria, increased frequency of and painful urination. Deficient kidney qi can also fail to consolidate the lower burner, resulting in leakage of vital substances via urination, manifesting with turbid urine, nocturia or hematuria.

The kidney and bladder are internally-externally related. The water passage connects these two organs, and they are interdependent physiologically and pathologically. Deficient kidney failing to transform the qi will cause disturbances in fluid elimination and accumulation of damp-heat in the bladder. Bladder damp-heat can also harass upwards to injure the kidney.

The disease course can be divided into acute and chronic phases depending on recent or gradual onset, the relative strength of the righteous qi and pathogenic factors, and the extent of organ involvement. The initial stage of UTI, the acute phase, is characterized by the pathogenic influence of excess damp-heat. Lingering damp-heat injures the body fluid, causing symptoms of kidney yin deficiency or kidney and spleen deficiency; therefore, deficient righteous qi with lingering damp-heat characterizes the chronic phase.

Analysis of Primary Symptom

A. Changes in urination:

These are the primary symptoms of UTI, especially during the acute phase.

- Acute onset of urinary urgency, frequency, burning sensation and pricking pain during urination, dark yellow, red or turbid urine output, and hematuria are symptoms of heat or damp-heat accumulation in the bladder.
- Unremitting disease gradually progresses to the chronic phase. Frequent and obstructed urination with scanty output, accompanied by signs of yin deficiency, is evidence of kidney yin deficiency with residual damp-heat. Frequent and obstructed urination aggravated by exertion and accompanied by signs of qi deficiency, indicates spleen and kidney deficiency with impairment of qi transformation.

B. Lower back pain:

During the acute phase, heat excess causes distending and burning lower back pain that is aggravated by pressure or percussion. In contrast, lower back pain during the chronic phase of UTI is usually vague and persistent, with soreness aggravated by exertion and alleviated by pressure and percussion, typifying pain due to deficiency.

C. Fever:

Fever, during the acute phase, occurs with sudden and rapid onset. It is a high fever accompanied by chills, reflecting acute infection. Fever in the acute phase is related to damp-heat and attributable to the contest between the righteous qi and pathogenic influences. However, during the chronic phase, the fever tends to be low-grade and may present as five-centers heat, indicating liver and kidney deficiency with empty heat.

Basic Patterns

- Damp-heat accumulation in the bladder
- Stagnant heat in the liver and gallbladder
- Kidney yin deficiency with residual damp-heat
- Spleen and kidney deficiency with residual heat

Progression of Pattern

Damp-heat accumulation in the bladder characterizes the initial stage. Prompt treatment at this stage can greatly speed recovery. A few cases become recurrent and retrogressive due to iatrogenic factors or constitutional weakness. Damp-heat injures the qi and yin, leading to patterns of kidney yin deficiency or spleen and kidney deficiency with residual heat; both patterns have a deficient root and an excess branch. Unremitting excess patterns gradually turn into deficient patterns.

Treatment Principle

Kidney deficiency and damp-heat accumulation in the bladder are the basic pathogeneses. A damp-heat pathogenic factor is present throughout the entire disease course; therefore, clearing and draining damp-heat is the essential treatment principle in UTI, whether treating the acute or chronic phase. However, when the condition becomes chronic and there is kidney yin deficiency or spleen and kidney deficiency, treatment must address both the root and the branch. Nourishing kidney yin and draining damp-heat is applicable to the former pattern, whereas tonifying the spleen and kidney and draining damp-heat is appropriate for the latter pattern.

Pattern and Suggested Measure

Damp-heat accumulation in the bladder

Urgent and frequent urination with burning and pricking pain, dark yellow, red and turbid urination, suprapubic pain, possibly accompanied by fever and sore throat. Red tongue with yellow greasy coating, and rapid slippery pulse.

- Clear heat, drain dampness and unblock obstruction in the urinary tract.
- Modified *Ba Zheng San*

Bian Xu 10g.	*Qu Mai* 10g.	*Che Qian Zi* 10g.
Hua Shi 20g.	*Deng Xin Cao* 6g.	*Zhi Zi* 10g.
Da Huang 6g.	*Wu Yao* 6g.	*Gan Cao* 6g.

- Preponderance of dampness. + *Cang Zhu* 10g., *Hou Po* 10g., *Bai Dou Kou* 10g.
  Preponderance of heat. + *Shi Gao* 30g., *Tian Hua Fen* 10g., *Zhu Ye* 10g.

Stagnant heat in the liver and gallbladder

Urgent and frequent urination with burning sensation, dark yellow urine output or hematuria, alternating chills and fever, irritability, nausea, poor appetite, fullness and distention in the flank or hypochondria, bitter taste in the mouth and red face. Red tongue with yellow coating, and rapid wiry pulse.

- Clear heat from the liver and gallbladder.
- Modified *Long Dan Xie Gan Tang*

Long Dan Cao 10g.	*Zhi Zi* 10g.	*Huang Qin* 10g.
Sheng Di Huang 15g.	*Ze Xie* 15g.	*Che Qian Zi* 20g.
Qing Pi 10g.	*Chai Hu* 6g.	*Gan Cao* 6g.

- Alternating chills and fever, irritability and nausea. + *Xiao Chai Hu Tang*
  Fullness and distending pain in the flank or hypochondria. + *Qing Pi* 10g.
  Abdominal distention and constipation. + *Da Huang* 6g., *Zhi Shi* 10g., *Hou Po* 10g.

Kidney yin deficiency with residual damp-heat

Frequent but scanty urination, obstructed urination, dysuria with pricking pain, and low-grade fever, dizziness, tinnitus, soreness of the lower back, and dry throat and lips. Red tongue with scanty coating, and rapid thready pulse.

- Nourish kidney yin and eliminate damp-heat.
- Modified *Zhi Bai Di Huang Wan*

Mu Dan Pi 10g.	*Fu Ling* 15g.	*Ze Xie* 15g.
Shan Yao 10g.	*Sheng Di Huang* 15g.	*Shan Zhu Yu* 10g.
Huang Bai 10g.	*Zhi Mu* 10g.	*Che Qian Zi* 20g.

- Dizziness and tinnitus. + *Ju Hua* 10g., *Gou Teng* 10g., *Gou Qi Zi* 10g.
  Bright red hematuria. + *Han Lian Cao* 10g., *Bai Mao Gen* 10g., *Da Ji* 6g.

Spleen and kidney deficiency with residual heat

Frequent and dribbling urination aggravated by exertion, possibly turbid urine or nocturia, systemic edema, fatigue, soreness and weakness of the lower back and knees. Pale tongue with moist white coating, and deep thready and forceless pulse.

- Tonify the spleen and kidney, and eliminate turbid dampness.
- Modified *Wu Bi Shan Yao Wan*

Shan Yao 10g.	*Fu Ling* 15g.	*Ze Xie* 15g.
Shu Di Huang 10g.	*Ba Ji Tian* 10g.	*Tu Si Zi* 10g.
Du Zhong 10g.	*Niu Xi* 15g.	*Pu Gong Ying* 10g.
Huang Qin 10g.		

- Scanty urination and edema. + *Zhu Ling* 10g., *Che Qian Zi* 10g.
  Spleen qi sinking with heavy sensation in the lower abdomen and hesitant urination. + *Bu Zhong Yi Qi Tang*
  Kidney yang deficiency with cold intolerance and cold limbs. + *You Gui Wan*

Other Modality

A. Acupuncture:

Acute phase:

- **Manipulation:** Reducing method.
- **Prescription:** CV3 Zhongji SP9 Yinlingquan BL39 Weiyang BL28 Pangguangshu
- **Supplementary points:**
  - High fever. + LI4 Hegu; LI11 Quchi
  - Liver/Gallbladder stagnant heat. + LR2 Xingjian

Chronic phase:

- **Manipulation:** Even method.
- **Prescription:** BL23 Shenshu CV3 Zhongji BL28 Pangguangshu
- **Supplementary points:**
  - Kidney yin deficiency. + KI3 Taixi; KI6 Zhaohai; SP6 Sanyinjiao
  - Spleen and kidney deficiency. + BL20 Pishu; ST36 Zusanli; CV6 Qihai

B. Single herbs that have antibacterial effects:

❶ Herbs with an antibacterial effect against *E. Coli*:
Yu Xing Cao, *Bai Hua She She Cao*, *Pu Gong Ying*, *Xu Chang Qing*.

❷ Herbs with an antibacterial effect against *Staphylococcus* and *pseudomonas*:
Ban Zhi Lian, *Jin Yin Hua*, *Lian Qiao*, *Huang Qin*.

❸ Herbs with broad-spectrum antibacterial effects:
Da Qing Ye, *Ban Lan Gen*, *Zhi Zi*, *Zi Hua Di Ding*.

CHAPTER 62

Chronic Renal Failure

When acute renal failure is not resolved within months, chronic renal failure will develop. Chronic renal failure is characterized by progressively declining renal function with azotemia over months to years; it is rarely reversible. Diabetes mellitus and hypertension accounts for over 50% of the cases; 20-25% of the cases are caused by other urological diseases, including glomerulonephritis and cystic diseases; 16% of the cases have unknown etiology.

Some patients who suffered from chronic renal failure are asymptomatic until the disease is far advanced. The slowly developed and nonspecific symptoms are fatigue, weakness and malaise. As the disease progresses, laboratory changes of glomerular filtration rate (GFR) will be < 10-15 ml per minute; elevated blood urea nitrogen and serum creatinine mark uremia; multiple systems will be affected. Anorexia, nausea and vomiting indicate the involvement of gastrointestinal complication, and hiccough is very common. When the neurologic system is complicated, irritability, difficulty in concentration, insomnia, restless legs and twitching are apparent. Depositions of urea on the skin result in pruritus. Chest pain is possible if pericarditis develops. Secondary edema may result from cardiovascular insufficiency, and sodium and water retention. Hemodynamic disturbances, such as anemia and platelet dysfunction, are common. As uremia progresses to end stage renal disease, irregular menstruation, paresthesia, stupor, confusion and coma occur. Hypertension is very common in patients with chronic renal failure. Secondary hypertension may result from sodium and water retention; pre-existing hypertension and diabetes mellitus can be complicated and become difficult to manage.

In addition to the laboratory findings of elevated blood urea nitrogen and creatinine, the diagnosis of chronic renal failure can be supported by ultrasonography, in which bilateral kidneys are small (< 10 cm). The treatment of chronic renal failure addresses the management of complications, including approaches to balance the electrolytes and fluid, balance the acid with the base, manage symptoms, and monitor the progression. Patients are usually put on a renal diet which restricts the intake of protein, potassium, sodium and fluid.

Regular and routine dialysis is usually a permanent treatment to sustain life for end stage renal disease unless a kidney transplant is performed. The mortality rate for dialysis patients is as high as 22.4 deaths per 100 patient years. The remaining life expectancy for patients in the age group of 55-64 is merely 5 years. Cardiac dysfunction accounts for 48% of the mortality. Kidney transplant is a curative measure for end stage renal disease. Nearly half of the cases are qualified for a transplant. With proper medication use, patients undergone successful kidney transplant with a higher degree of HLA-type matching has a nearly normal life span.

Reference:

Watnick, S. & Morrison, G. (2003). Kidney: Chronic renal disease. In L. M. Tierney, Jr., et. al. (Eds.), *Current Medical Diagnosis & Treatment* (42nd ed. chap. 22). New York, NY: McGraw-Hill Companies, Inc.

Depending on the clinical manifestations, chronic renal failure can be referred to TCM differentiation and treatment of oliguria-anuria, hiccough, and edema.

Chronic renal failure is subsequent to a combination of spleen and kidney deficiency and turbid dampness accumulation, and these conditions are usually complicated by recurrent exterior attacks, leading to a serious pathology of nearly total loss of the kidney's function.

Chronic renal failure is precipitated by various renal diseases. Its progression is relatively gradual despite some factors accelerating the speeds and degrees of the process.

Exterior pathogenic factors deplete lung qi and cause failure of water metabolism, leading to subsequent dampness accumulation, and aggravating the existing deficiency.

Interior injury results from overexertion and excessive sexual activities, further depriving the deficiency of the spleen and kidney.

Improper diet injures the spleen and increases the vulnerability of the spleen to damp environment, further complicating the condition of spleen and kidney deficiency.

Spleen and kidney are the acquired and congenital vital sources. The kidney dominates water metabolism and the spleen is in charge of transportation and transformation. Once kidney qi is depleted, the process of qi transformation is disturbed, aggravating the accumulation of dampness. Oliguria and edema manifest. Deficient spleen fails to perform its task in generating the qi and blood, follows anemia and prostration. Implications of failure of the spleen and kidney manifest on multiple systems. Dampness obstructing the qi flow leads to secondary nausea and vomiting; dampness obstructing the ascent of clear yang causes dizziness and irritability; dampness misting the heart's orifice manifests with trance, disorientation or altered consciousness. Complications that involve all of the five internal organs are apparent at end stage renal disease.

Analysis of Primary Symptom

Chronic renal failure is a gradually progressive disease, and it can be asymptomatic at the initial stage until it is far advanced. Advanced chronic renal failure, in addition to its primary presentations of oliguria and secondary edema, have other multiple systemic symptoms:

A. Nausea, vomiting and hiccough:

These can be the first group of symptoms, and a result of secondary rebellious stomach qi from turbid dampness accumulating in the middle burner. Heaviness, fatigue, weakness, malaise and anorexia are nonspecific but also common. Irregular bowel movements are related to dampness as well; damp-heat causes constipation and cold-dampness together with spleen yang injury leads to loose stool.

B. Anemia:

Anemia is secondary to spleen deficiency, which fails to extract the essence from food and water ingested. Because essence and blood share the common source and they are interdependent, anemia can also be related to kidney essence deficiency.

C. Subcutaneous and mucosal hemorrhage:

Including epistaxis, bleeding gums, petechiae and purpura, and hematemesis, hemorrhage is due to excessive heat forcing the blood to move recklessly. Heat is generated from congested dampness, pertaining to excess. Hemorrhage can also be related to spleen and kidney deficiency, in which deficient qi fails to control the blood flow, pertaining to deficiency and cold.

D. Irritability and insomnia:

Irritability and insomnia are caused by disturbance of the mind from turbidity. Once the disease advances, turbid-dampness and toxicity obstructing the heart's orifice will follow, manifesting in trance, disorientation or even coma.

E. Pruritus and muscle twitching:

Yin depletion secondary to yang deficiency results in malnourishment of the liver, leading to liver wind swirling internally. Mild cases manifest with pruritus and muscle twitching. If the condition remains unresolved, contractions and shaking of the extremities, together with restless leg, irritability, anuria, edema and frigid limbs will also follow. Condition is far advanced; both yin and yang are depleted, and separation and disconnection of the yin and yang is foreseen.

Basic Patterns

- Kidney yang deficiency with turbid-dampness accumulation
- Qi and yin deficiency with excessive heat-toxicity

Progression of Pattern

The basic pattern is yang deficiency of the spleen and kidney; deficiency of the qi and yin is also common. Chronic renal failure involves multiple systems as it advances; therefore, patterns alter as the organs involved vary. At the end stage, yin depletion secondary to yang deficiency leads to a pattern of depletion of both the yin and yang.

Treatment Principle

Primary treatment principle is based on the differentiations; however, symptom management should also be planned based on the multiple systems involved. Depletion and deficiency of both the spleen and kidney are the fundamental pathogenesis, with the root of the various degrees and types of deficiency from internal organs' yin and yang. The excess branch of chronic renal failure falls on the secondary accumulation of the pathological derivatives, such as turbid-dampness, heat-toxicity, liver wind, and blood stasis. Therefore, a holistic treatment plan should address the root and branch, and integrate strategies of supporting the righteous qi and expelling the pathogens.

Pattern and Suggested Measure

Differentiation and treatment

Kidney yang deficiency with turbid-dampness accumulation

Dusky complexion, pale lips and nails, shortness of breath, fatigue, soreness and weakness of the extremities, facial edema, cold intolerance and cold limbs, foul breath of smell of ammonia, oliguria, nausea and vomiting, and diarrhea. Flabby tongue with teeth marks and white greasy coating, and deep thready and weak pulse.

- Warm and tonify spleen and kidney yang, promote urination and reduce edema.

- Modified *Jin Gui Shen Qi Wan* and *Shi Pi Yin*

Fu Zi 6g.	*Rou Gui* 10g.	*Shu Di Huang* 10g.
Shan Yao 10g.	*Shan Zhu Yu* 10g.	*Ze Xie* 15g.
Fu Ling 15g.	*Mu Dan Pi* 10g.	*Gan Jiang* 10g.
Bai Zhu 10g.	*Mu Gua* 10g.	*Hou Po* 6g.

Qi and yin deficiency with excessive heat-toxicity

Sallow complexion, weakness, malaise, dry mouth, bitter taste in the mouth or foul breath of smell of ammonia, nausea and vomiting, five-centers heat, tinnitus, spasmodic pain in the lower abdomen, scanty dark urine and constipation. Red tongue with yellow greasy coating, and rapid slippery pulse.

- Benefit the qi, nourish the yin, eliminate turbid dampness and harmonize the stomach.
- Modified *Da Bu Yuan Jian* and *Wen Dan Tang*

Ren Shen 10g.	*Shan Yao* 10g.	*Shu Di Huang* 10g.
Du Zhong 10g.	*Gou Qi Zi* 10g.	*Dang Gui* 10g.
Mai Men Dong 15g.	*Huang Qi* 10g.	*Ban Xia* 10g.
Huang Lian 6g.	*Chen Pi* 10g.	*Zhu Ru* 10g.
Zhi Qiao 10g.	*Fu Ling* 15g.	

Symptom management

Nausea and vomiting:

- Stomach qi rebelling due to spleen and stomach qi deficiency or turbid-dampness hindering the spleen and stomach, use *Xiao Ban Xia Tang*.
- Stomach qi fails to descend due to heat-toxicity accumulating and obstructing the qi flow with constipation, use *Xiao Cheng Qi Tang*.

Hemorrhage:

- Bleeding due to deficient qi failing to control the blood, use *Gui Pi Tang*.
- Bleeding due to heat in the blood causing reckless movement of the blood, *use* *Xi Jiao Di Huang Tang*.
  Modify the selected formulas by adding hemostatic herbs for location and nature of bleeding.

Anemia:

- Mostly caused by insufficiency of the liver and kidney, or essence and blood deficiency, use *Dang Gui Bu Xue Tang* or *Ba Zhen Tang*; modify these formulas by adding blood tonics.

Hypertension:

- Qi deficiency and blood stasis with dampness accumulation, manifesting as weakness, lassitude, headache, tinnitus and pitting edema, use *Ban Xia Bai Zhu Tian Ma Tang*, and add qi tonics.
- Yin deficiency with yang rising manifests as headache, tinnitus, numbness of the limbs, and soreness and weakness of the lower back and knees, use *Tian Ma Gou Teng Yin*.

Pruritus:

- Mainly related to yin and blood deficiency with wind swirling internally, use *Si Wu Tang* and *Er Zhi Wan*.

Other Modality

A. Acupuncture:

Acupuncture is used as an adjuvant modality; moxibustion is commonly used to warm and tonify the spleen and kidney.

Refer to yin edema in Chapter 40, "Edema", for basic pattern (see page 285).

Refer to the following chapters for relevant symptom managements.
- Chapter 10, "Vomiting" (see page 78).
- Chapter 37, "Hemorrhage" (see page 263).
- Chapter 52, "Hypertension" (see page 362).

B. Application of *Da Huang* in chronic renal failure:

Recent studies have shown that *Da Huang* has a reliable therapeutic effect on chronic renal failure. Its effects of clearing heat and relieving toxicity are successful in reducing azotemia. Clinically *Da Huang* is administered via various routes depending on the presentations. Its oral administration can be widely applicable by taking the powdered form alone or taking the formulas containing *Da Huang*, such as *Wen Pi Tang* and *Da Cheng Qi Tang*. It also can be administered via retention enema with formulas that contain *Da Huang* as the primary ingredient.

❶ Oral administration of *Sheng Da Huang*:
Orally taking the powdered form in a dosage of 3-9 g. daily. This prescription is used adjunctively to formula that supports the righteous qi.

❷ Retention enema with *Sheng Da Huang*:
Sheng Da Huang 15g. *Mu Li* 30g. *Huai Hua Mi* 30g.
(may add *Fu Zi* 15g. for deficient cold pattern).

C. Application of herbs in hemodialysis:

Hemodialysis is the major treatment for uremia; it prolongs the life span for patients suffering from chronic renal failure. However, this measure can provoke other acute or gradual complications, and it has no therapeutic effect on improving nephrogenic anemia. Some patients, especially the elderly, might experience dry stool, poor appetite and malnourishment. Based on differentiations, using herbal remedies in conjunction to hemodialysis is proven effective in decreasing the occurrences of complications and in improving quality of life.

1. Hypotension:

Symptomatic hypotension accounts for the primary acute complication in hemodialysis; this secondary symptom is caused by rapid and great amount of fluid removal or anaphylactic reaction. In addition, hymodialysis can further aggravate pre-existing hypotension. Manifestations of hypotension include palpitations, sweating, dizziness and fatigue, pertaining to pattern of heart qi and yin deficiency. Treatment principle should be to augment the qi and nourish the yin; the formula of choice is *Sheng Mai San*.

2. Dialysis disequilibrium:

Dialysis disequilibrium occurs near the end or soon after completion of hemodialysis. Its clinical presentations are headache, nausea and vomiting, pertaining to spleen and kidney deficiency and phlegm-dampness accumulation. The following herbs are commonly used to to prevent this complication:

Huang Qi, Gou Qi Zi, Sheng Di Huang, Shan Zhu Yu, Shan Yao, Fu Ling, Chen Pi, Ban Xia, Zhu Ru, Shi Chang Pu.

3. Anorexia:

Most patients will regain their appetite after hemodialysis; however, some patients experience anorexia. Anorexia is caused by spleen and stomach qi deficiency with dampness accumulation. The following herbs are commonly used for symptom management:

Tai Zi Shen, Bai Zhu, Fu Ling, Sha Ren, Chen Pi, Mu Xiang, Shen Qu, Shan Zha, Huang Lian.

4. Constipation:

Constipation is caused by rapid and excessive fluid removal during hemodialysis, and it is aggravated by limited fluid intake. Constipation can further inhibit a route for eliminating toxins, therefore, increasing risk for autointoxication. It is a pattern of yin deficiency with intestinal dryness; syrup form of the following herbs can be administered to improve this condition:

Sheng Di Huang, Dang Gui, He Shou Wu, Rou Cong Rong, Huo Ma Ren, Yu Li Ren, Gua Lou Ren.

5. Thrombosis:

Thrombosis is a complication that is relatively difficult to manage. When platelet dysfunction with tendency to bleeding is common in chronic renal failure, heparin drip for treating thrombosis secondary to hemodialysis might further exacerbate hemorrhage. Application of herbal remedy that augments the qi and invigorates the blood can be therapeutically effective in reducing thrombosis. Commonly used herbs consist of:

Huang Qi, *Sheng Di Huang*, *Dang Gui*, *Chuan Xiong*, *Chi Shao*, *Tao Ren*, *Hong Hua*, *Niu Xi*, *Dan Shen*.

CHAPTER 63

Aplastic Anemia

Aplastic anemia is a rapidly fatal disease, if left untreated. All blood cells, including red blood cells, white blood cells and platelets, arise from a common root, the pluripotent stem cells. Pluripotent stem cells are generated in the bone marrow. If the bone marrow is injured or the expression of the stem cells is abnormal, hypoplastic marrow results and pancytopenia follows. Aplastic anemia is caused by defected or hypoplastic bone marrow that fails to produce adequate amount of red blood cells. Radiation, chemotherapy, toxins or pharmacological agents may injure the stem cells directly; however, autoimmune suppression of hematopoiesis by T cell-mediated cellular mechanism seems to be the most common pathogenesis of aplastic anemia.

The diagnosis of aplastic anemia relies on confirmation of pancytopenia, absence of abnormal cells and hypocellular bone marrow. Although pancytopenia is the key to diagnosing aplastic anemia, it is not uncommon that only one or two cell lines are reduced during the early stage.

Resulting from pancytopenia, anemia is marked by weakness and fatigue; neutropenia leads to increased susceptibility to infections; thrombocytopenia is signified by subcutaneous and mucosal hemorrhage. Fever indicates infections. If hepatosplenomegaly, lymphadenopathy, and bone tenderness are present, consider other diagnoses. Differential diagnosis from myelodysplastic disorders and acute leukemia is important. Bone marrow aspiration and biopsy may help establishing the diagnosis. Mild cases of aplastic anemia may require only supportive measures, such as transfusion of packed red blood cell and platelet pheresis, and administration of antibiotics. The median survival rate of severe cases (three of the following signs: neutrophills < 500/uL; platelets < 20,000/uL; reticulocytes < 1%; bone marrow cellularity < 20%) without any treatment is about three months; only 20% of patients make it to a year after their diagnosis.

The most effective treatment is bone marrow transplant. Adults (under age 50) can benefit from bone marrow transplant of HLA-matched siblings, whereas children or young adults under age 30 may benefit from a HLA-matched unrelated donor. For those who are older than age 50 or when there is no HLA-matched sibling available, immunosuppression with antithymocyte globulin (ATG) in conjunction with cyclosporine is the choice of treatment.

Reference:

Linker, C. A. (2003). Blood- Anemia: Aplastic anemia. In L. M. Tierney, Jr., et. al. (Eds.), *Current Medical Diagnosis & Treatment* (42nd ed. chap. 13). New York, NY: McGraw-Hill Companies, Inc.

Based on the clinical manifestations, aplastic anemia can be referred to TCM differentiation and treatment on hemorrhage and consumptive deficiency.

Pathogenesis of aplastic anemia is depletion of the marrow and blood. It involves deficiency of both the spleen and kidney, especially kidney essence and qi deficiency. The following factors may elicit aplastic anemia via causing kidney essence deficiency and spleen deficiency, resulting in a deficient source for blood generation:

Kidney qi deprivation: Kidney stores the essence, governs the bones and generates the marrow. It is the congenital source of pre-heaven qi. The essence and blood are interdependent. Kidney essence deficiency results from congenital insufficiency or acquired deprivation caused by excessive sexual activities, leading to presentations of blood deficiency. According to the ancient medical document, Xu Lao Xin Zhuan (Collection of Experiences on Consumptive Deficiency), "Juvenile morbidity is caused by congenital deficiency, especially maternal heredity." Aplastic anemia occurs in all ages, predominately young adults. This phenomenon seems to agree with the ancient theory.

Injury of the spleen and stomach: Improper diet or irregular diet habit has a direct impact on the spleen and stomach. Anger injures the liver, leading to stagnant qi, which overacts on the spleen. Pensiveness and worry injure the spleen qi. The injured spleen fails to transform and transport the food and fluids for the extraction of their nutritional essence, which bring about insufficient generation of the qi and blood.

Environmental influences, including hazardous chemicals or toxins, and exterior warm-febrile toxicity, easily infect a person with deficient righteous qi. The chemicals and toxins are harmful to the kidney; they can exhaust the essence and qi of the kidney. Exterior warm-febrile toxicity, on the other hand, invades through the protective barrier of the nutritive and blood levels. By consuming and injuring the marrow, they elicit aplastic anemia.

The five internal organs are inter-dependent. Kidney deficiency may influence the integrity of the spleen, and vise versa. The yin, yang, qi and blood deficiency of the organs increases the vulnerability to environmental influences. However, environmental influences also contribute to the exacerbation of aplastic anemia by weakening righteous qi. These complicated pathogeneses lead to the complex symptoms.

Analysis of Primary Symptom

A. Weakness and fatigue, along with abnormal hematological findings, and other presentation of anemia:

These symptoms are consistent with the concept of blood deficiency in TCM. The following organs contribute to the production and circulation of the blood:

- Spleen generates the blood. The middle burner is the generating source for the qi and blood. The intact digestive function abstracts the essence from the food and fluids and transforms the essence into nutritive qi and body fluid. After advanced metabolism, the essence turns into blood. This process plays a key role in blood formation.
- Kidney stores the essence, which generates the marrow. Marrow is stored in the bones. The modern medical belief that bone marrow is the major organ in blood production somehow matches the TCM concept that the essence and blood share common origin.
- The phrase, "The liver stores the blood", implies the function of liver to store and regulate the flow of blood.
- Heart governs the blood and vessels. The blood circulation relies on motive force from heart qi.

Blood deficiency involves all possible dysfunctions of the above-mentioned organs, predominantly the spleen and kidney. Blood deficiency caused by deficient spleen pertains to a mild case, while that caused by deficiency of both the spleen and kidney is severe and critical.

B. Subcutaneous and mucosal hemorrhage:

Hemorhage can be caused by excess or deficiency etiology.

- Excessive bleeding with acute onset, fresh red blood, large purpura, and high fever are caused by excess heat in the blood, forcing the blood to move recklessly. When depletion of the marrow and blood are complicated by exterior warm-febrile pathogenic invasion, signs and symptoms of infection are apparent.
- Gradual blood loss in an intermittent fashion, aggravated by exertion, pertains to qi deficiency. The pathogenesis is deficient spleen failing to control the blood; the pattern is spleen deficiency with blood depletion. Manifestations of infection are not common.

C. Fever:

Fever can be induced by exterior factors or internal disequilibrium.

- Fever due to exterior influences can be mild or severe. Mild cases involve the protective and qi levels. During the invasion of exterior influence from the superficial layers into the interior, manifestations of high fever, headache, and sores on the tongue and in the mouth are detectable. The severe cases involve the nutritive and blood levels. High fever is accompanied by alteration of consciousness, hemorrhages and purpura. Infection is common in both mild and severe cases.
- Fever caused by internal disequilibrium consists of two major subtypes, yin deficient fever and qi deficient fever. The former is marked by longstanding, unremitting and persistent low grade fever, five-centers heat, and night sweating; the common pattern is kidney yin depletion. The latter is manifested by low grade fever, shortness of breath, spontaneous sweating and aggravation of the condition by exertion; the common pattern is spleen deficiency with blood depletion. Fever of internal disequilibrium is usually not related to infection.

Basic Patterns

- Depleted blood with contraction of warm-febrile toxins
- Spleen deficiency with blood depletion
- Kidney yin depletion
- Spleen and kidney yang deficiency
- Kidney deficiency with blood stasis

Progression of Pattern

In the initial stage of acute exacerbation, deficient righteous qi with contraction of warm-febrile toxins constitutes the primary pathogenesis, pertaining to a pattern of deficient root with excess branch. Prompt treatment can make a difference; by expelling the toxic heat, bleeding will stop. The remaining concern is deficient righteous qi. However, various deficiencies determine the individualized patterns. If a patient has a constitutional yin deficiency or severe yin injury during an acute exacerbation, progression into kidney yin depletion is most likely. Constitutional yang deficiency or insignificant yin injury during exacerbation is followed by spleen deficiency with blood depletion, and spleen and kidney yang deficiency.

These deficiencies signify major deprivation of righteous qi; therefore, recurrent contractions to exterior pathogenic factors are inevitable, leading to frequent exacerbations. In addition, chronic illness leads to qi deficiency and blood stasis or kidney deficiency with blood stasis.

Excessive toxic heat cause bleeding. During severe condition, qi collapse will follow excessive blood loss; crisis of intracranial hemorrhage is possible.

Treatment Principle

Aplastic anemia roots from depletion of both the essence and blood, and the contraction of warm-febrile toxicity forms the branch of the illness. Favorable treatment should satisfy both needs of the root and branch. During the acute phase, the primary strategy is to expel the pathogens by relieving the toxicity and cooling the blood, and the auxiliary strategy is to support righteous qi. During remission, the main focus is to tonify righteous qi based on the differentiations; various approaches include warming the yang and benefiting the qi, nourishing the yin and blood, and tonifying both the yin and yang.

Pattern and Suggested Measure

Depleted blood with contraction of warm-febrile toxins

High fever, epistaxis, bleeding gums, large purpura, possible hematemesis, hematuria, hematochezia and tarry stool, thirst, sore throat, oral erosion, palpitations and shortness of breath. Dry red tongue with grayish-yellow greasy coating, and rapid flooding pulse.

- Cool the blood and stop bleeding; nourish the yin and clear heat.
- Modified *Xi Jiao Di Huang Tang*

Shui Niu Jiao 30g. (substitute *Xi Jiao*)		*Sheng Di Huang* 15g.
Chi Shao 10g.	*Mu Dan Pi* 10g.	*Xuan Shen* 10g.
Dan Shen 15g.	*Jin Yin Hua* 10g.	*Lian Qiao* 10g.
Zhu Ye 6g.	*Bai Mao Gen* 10g.	*Xi Yang Shen* 6g.

- Intractable high fever and listlessness. + *An Gong Niu Huang Wan*
  Extreme heat triggering internal wind with convulsions or contractions of the extremities. + *Zi Xue Dan*
  Excessive bleeding with large purpura. + *Da Qing Ye* 10g., *Zi Cao* 10g.
  Constrained heat complicated by dampness with focal distention and fullness in the chest and epigastrium, red tongue with yellow greasy coating. + *Qing Hao* 10g., *He Ye* 10g., *Dan Dou Chi* 6g.

Spleen deficiency with blood depletion

Gradual onset, sallow complexion, malaise and weakness, shortness of breath, palpitations, dizziness, insomnia, dream-disturbed sleep, possibly bleeding gums, unremitting uterine bleeding, and advanced menstruation. White tongue coating and weak pulse.

- Strengthen the spleen, augment the qi and nourish the blood.
- Modified *Gui Pi Tang*

  Dang Shen 15g. *Huang Qi* 10g. *Bai Zhu* 10g.
  Dang Gui 10g. *Suan Zao Ren* 15g. *Long Yan Rou* 10g.
  He Shou Wu 10g. *Mu Xiang* 10g. *Fu Shen* 15g.
  Gan Cao 6g.
- Significant bleeding. + *E Jiao* 10g., *Xian He Cao* 10g.

Kidney yin depletion

Dizziness, blurred vision, irritability, palpitations, fatigue, lack of strength, and purpura. Dry red tongue, and rapid thready pulse.

- Nourish and tonify kidney yin.
- Modified *Liu Wei Di Huang Wan*

  Shu Di Huang 10g. *Shan Yao* 10g. *Shan Zhu Yu* 10g.
  Fu Ling 15g. *Mu Dan Pi* 10g. *Ze Xie* 15g.
  Zhi Mu 10g. *Han Lian Cao* 10g. *Nu Zhen Zi* 15g.
  Tu Si Zi 10g. *Gou Qi Zi* 10g.
- Significant yin deficiency. + *Gui Ban* 20g., *Bie Jia* 20g., *Mai Men Dong* 10g., *Tian Men Dong* 10g.

  Significant qi deficiency with shortness of breath and fatigue, take the decoction of *Xi Yang Shen* 15g. in addition to the primary formula.

  Significant bleeding. + *Qian Cao Gen* 10g., *Xuan Shen* 10g., *Chi Shao* 10g.

  If complicated by kidney yang deficiency or chronic condition turning into deficiency of both the yin and yang, add herbs that warm and tonify the kidney. Herbs of choice may be selected from the next pattern.

Spleen and kidney yang deficiency

Pale complexion, cold intolerance and cold limbs, shortness of breath, fatigue, lassitude, poor appetite, loose stool, edematous lower extremities, impotence, and possibly bleeding gums or scattered purpura. Flabby pale tongue with white coating, and deep thready and forceless pulse.

- Warm the kidney and spleen, augment the qi and generate the fluid.
- Modified *Shi Si Wei Jian Zhong Tang*

Huang Qi 15g.	*Dang Shen* 10g.	*Bai Zhu* 10g.
Fu Ling 15g.	*Ban Xia* 6g.	*Shu Di Huang* 10g.
Dang Gui 10g.	*Bai Shao* 10g.	*Chuan Xiong* 6g.
Mai Men Dong 10g.	*Rou Cong Rong* 10g.	*Zhi Fu Zi* 6g.
Rou Gui 10g.	*Da Zao* 10g.	*Xian He Cao* 10g.

- Significant bleeding. + *E Jiao* 10g.
  Preponderance by spleen yang deficiency with poor appetite and loose stool. + *Pao Jiang* 10g.
  Preponderance by kidney yang deficiency with significant edematous lower extremities. + *Yin Yang Huo* 10g., *Hu Lu Ba* 10g.

Kidney deficiency with blood stasis

Dusky complexion, soreness and weakness of the lower back and knees, lack of strength, shortness of breath, cold intolerance, cold limbs, flaky skin, possibly dark purpura and bleeding gums, recurrent conditions. Pale-purple tongue with petechiae, and thready choppy pulse.

- Warm the kidney and assist the yang, invigorate the blood and expel stasis.
- Modified *You Gui Wan* and *Tao Hong Si Wu Tang*

Zhi Fu Zi 6g.	*Rou Gui* 10g.	*Shu Di Huang* 10g.
Shan Yao 10g.	*Shan Zhu Yu* 10g.	*Gou Qi Zi* 10g.
Tu Si Zi 10g.	*Lu Jiao Jiao* 6g.	*Du Zhong* 10g.
Dang Gui 10g.	*Chuan Xiong* 6g.	*Tao Ren* 10g.
Hong Hua 10g.	*Niu Xi* 10g.	

Other Modality

A. Acupuncture: is appropriate for remission and stable conditions.

- **Manipulation:** Reinforcing method:
- **Prescription:** BL43 Gaohuangshu, CV6 Qihai, SP10 Xuehai, BL15 Xinshu, BL23 Shenshu, ST36 Zusanli, CV17 Tanzhong
- **Supplementary points:**
  - Liver and kidney yin deficiency. + SP6 Sanyinjiao; LR2 Xingjian; LR8 Ququan
  - Spleen and kidney yang deficiency. + GV4 Mingmen; HT6 Yinxi

B. Experiential remedies:

❶ Single effective herbs for anemia:

Huang Qi, Dang Gui, Bai Shao, Dang Shen, Ren Shen, Long Yan Rou, Lu Jiao Jiao, E Jiao.

❷ Single effective herbs for leukocytopenia:

Ji Xue Teng, Bu Gu Zhi, Zi He Che, Lu Jiao Jiao, Huang Qi, Ren Shen, Shi Wei.

❸ Single effective herbs for thrombocytopenia:

Zi Cao, Tu Da Huang, Juan Bai, Shi Shu Ye, Shui Niu Jiao, San Qi, Zi He Che, Long Yan Rou.

CHAPTER 64

Thrombotic Thrombocytopenia Purpura

With unknown etiology, thrombotic thrombocytopenia purpura (TTP) is an infrequent syndrome that encompasses microangiopathic hemolytic anemia, thrombocytopenia and a significant elevation of serum lactic dehydrogenase (LDH); it primarily affects young adults between the ages of 20 and 50.

Current proposed pathogenesis is an autoimmune response that antibodies directly attack the Von Willebrand factor-cleaving protease leading to deficit of coagulation. Blood smear shows fragmental red blood cells and laboratory tests may indicate variable degrees of decreasing platelets. Bleeding time may be extended; abnormal prothrombin time (PT) and partial thromboplastin time (PTT) indicate progression into disseminated intravascular coagulation (DIC). Pathological finding may also include presence of thrombi in the capillaries and small arteries. Precipitated factors include estrogen usage, pregnancy, pharmaceutical factors or infectious diseases. It is found that higher incidence of TTP is associated with HIV infection.

Purpura and fever are the principal symptoms of TTP. Nevertheless, the primary reason for majority of patients seek medical attention are anemia, bleeding or neurological symptoms, including headache and dizziness. In severe cases, symptoms, such as hemiplegia, aphasia, seizure or alteration in consciousness from lethargy to coma, signify occurrence of complication.

Fresh frozen plasma (FFP) replacement is the most common treatment during a crisis. Prednisone and antiplatelet agents, such as aspirin or dipyridamole, are also administered in addition to FFP replacement. Prompt medical measures favors optimistic prognosis; however, twenty percent of patients suffer from chronic and relapsing TTP.

Reference:

Linker, C. A. (2003). Blood- Anemia: Trombotic thrombocytopenia purpura. In L. M. Tierney, Jr., et. al. (Eds.), *Current Medical Diagnosis & Treatment* (42nd ed. chap 13). New York, NY: McGraw-Hill Companies, Inc.

Based on the primary clinical presentations, TTP can be categorized into TCM differentiation and treatment of hemorrhage.

Pathogeneses of TTP include excessive heat toxicity and deficient qi and blood of the organs. Excessive heat toxicity induces acute episode while deficiency of qi and blood is associated with chronic progression of the disease. The incidence of TTP is closely related to the following contributing factors:

Wind-heat and heat toxicity invade from the exterior environment. By either damaging the blood vessels or entering the blood level to force the blood moving recklessly, emission of blood from its normal reservoirs occurs. Bleeding from orifices follows and manifests as epistaxis and subcutaneous and mucosal bleeding.

Emotional stress: Frustration and anger affect the normal function of the liver. Liver qi stagnation further turns into fire to injure the blood vessels. Pensiveness injuring the spleen impairs the function of the spleen's function to control the blood.

General deficiency due to chronic illness or overexertion: Deficient spleen qi is unable to control the blood, while kidney yin deficiency will generate empty fire, which may disturb the blood and force it to move recklessly.

Blood stasis obstructing in the collaterals: Blood stasis is an etiology as well as a pathological derivative. The contributing factors mentioned previously may induce formation of blood stasis. Poor blood circulation due to obstruction of stasis leads to the detour of the blood flow, manifesting as purpura or epistaxis.

Analysis of Primary Symptom

A. Purpura and bleeding:

Purpura and bleeding signify the ongoing or recurrence of TTP. They can be differentiated into either excess or deficiency pattern.

- Multiple large red, purple, even black purpura with acute onset or fresh red bleeding at particularly the upper parts of the body may signify excess heat in the blood, leading to reckless movement of the blood.
- Intermittent onset of purplish-red purpura in the lower limbs, insignificant epistaxis and bleeding gums, tidal fever and night sweating are caused by deficient fire flaring and forcing the blood to move recklessly.
- Intermittent onset of light red purpura, aggravated by slight exertion, shortness of breath and fatigue indicate a deficient qi pattern. When TTP becomes chronic and manifests with dusky purpura, cold intolerance and cold limbs,

spleen and kidney yang deficiency is apparent. As the deficiency is rooted in the deeper part of the body, the course is prolonged and intractable.

- Large bluish-purple purpura or bleeding in dark red color, excessive clots in menstrual flow, and palpable hypochondriac masses characterize the pattern of blood stasis obstructing in the collaterals.

B. Fever:

Fever is the primary symptom signifying acute phase of TTP.

- High fever and past medical history of exterior-contracted illnesses indicate the presence of wind-heat or heat toxicity, which invades into the qi level, leading to excess heat accumulated in the qi level or flaring fire in both qi and blood levels.
- Tidal fever or five-centers heat accompanied by night sweating results from yin deficiency with empty heat.
- Low grade fever or subjective hot sensation that is aggravated by slight exertion is related to deficiency of qi, also known as qi deficiency fever.
- An afebrile patient with cold intolerance, cold limbs, lassitude, and shortness of breath may experience spleen and kidney yang deficiency.

Basic Patterns

- Heat in the blood
- Yin deficiency with empty fire
- Deficient qi failing to restrain the blood
- Spleen and kidney yang deficiency
- Blood stasis obstructing in the collaterals

Progression of Pattern

Acute episodes of TTP are closely related to heat toxicity attacking and reckless movement of the blood, pertaining to excess pattern. As the illness progresses, heat toxicity consumes nutritive qi and yin fluid, leading to yin deficiency with empty fire. Heat toxicity may also consume the qi, leading to qi deficiency, which fails to restrain the blood. As qi deficiency continue to progress, spleen and kidney yang deficiency is inevitable. Obviously, deficient patterns develop. Some patients might experience excessive heat triggering internal wind, and intracranial bleeding is possible. Neurological symptoms including seizures, hemiplegia, aphasia or altered consciousness may be evident. The presence of neurological symptoms signifies the development of a crisis situation.

Chronic and intermittent onsets are mostly caused by yin deficiency with empty fire or deficient qi failing to restrain the blood. When these chronic courses are complicated by invasion of exterior wind-heat, disturbance of the blood will lead to bleeding. This is a complicated condition of excess pathogens with deficient righteous qi. Blood stasis may occur in all patterns mentioned.

Treatment Principle

The core presentations of acute episodes include excessive heat toxicity and bleeding; therefore, the treatment principle focuses on clearing heat, relieving toxicity, cooling the blood and stopping bleeding. The chronic and intermittent phases are characterized by internal deficiency and recurrent bleeding; therefore, modify the strategy of tonification based on relevant organs in order to stop bleeding. If blood stasis manifests, incorporate method of invigorating the blood and expelling stasis.

Pattern and Suggested Measure

Heat in the blood

Acute onset, aversion to cold and fever initially, large red, purple or dark purpura, possible epistaxis, bleeding gum or hematuria with fresh red color, red face, irritability and thirst. Dark red tongue with dry yellow coating, and rapid slippery pulse.

- Clear heat, relieve toxicity, cool the blood and stop bleeding.
- Modified *Xi Jiao Di Haung Tang*
  Shui Niu Jiao 30g. (substitute *Xi Jiao*) *Sheng Di Huang* 15g.
  Chi Shao 10g. *Mu Dan Pi* 10g. *Xuan Shen* 10g.
  Zi Cao 10g. *Da Qing Ye* 15g.
- Heavy bleeding. + *Ou Jie* 10g., *Di Yu* 10g., *Qian Cao Gen* 10g.
  Profuse bleeding followed by pale complexion, frigid extremities and minute pulse, administer *Du Shen Tang*.

Yin deficiency with empty fire

Scattered purpura, purplish-red in color, mainly affects the lower extremities with intermittent onset, possible mild epistaxis, bleeding gum, dizziness, tidal fever and night sweating. Dry red tongue, and rapid thready pulse.

- Nourish the yin, clear heat and stop bleeding.
- Modified *Qian Gen San*

Qian Cao Gen 10g. *Ce Bai Ye* 10g. *E Jiao* 6g.
Huang Qin 6g. *Sheng Di Huang* 10g. *Xuan Shen* 10g.
Gui Ban 20g. *Nu Zhen Zi* 15g. *Han Lian Cao* 10g.

- Tidal fever and night sweating. + *Di Gu Pi* 10g., *Yin Chai Hu* 10g.

Deficient qi failing to restrain the blood

Scanty and scattered purpura that is slightly red in color and not easy to detect, intermittent onset, aggravated by slight exertion, palpitations, shortness of breath, weakness, poor appetite, and heavy pale menstrual flow. Pale tongue, and decelerating soft pulse.

- Augment the qi to strengthen the spleen, restrain and nourish the blood.
- Modified *Gui Pi Tang*

Dang Shen 10g. *Huang Qi* 15 g. *Bai Zhu* 10g.
Fu Ling 10g. *Dang Gui* 10g. *E Jiao* 6g.
Bai Shao 10g. *Mu Xiang* 10g. *Zhi Gan Cao* 6g.
Xian He Cao 10g. *Pu Huang* 6g.

Spleen and kidney yang deficiency

Insignificant dusky purpura, prolonged course of the disease, pale complexion, lassitude, weak, cold intolerance and cold limbs, and soreness and weakness of the lower back and knees. Pale tongue with white coating, and deep thready and forceless pulse.

- Warm and tonify the spleen and kidney, nourish the blood and stop bleeding.
- Modified *Jin Gui Shen Qi Wan*

Zhi Fu Zi 6g. *Rou Gui* 10g. *Shu Di Huang* 10g.
Shan Yao 10g. *Shan Zhu Yu* 10g. *Fu Ling* 15g.
E Jiao 10g. *Bai Zhu* 10g. *Pao Jiang Tan* 6g.

- Significant cold intolerance, cold limbs, and soreness and weakness of the lower back and knees. + *Xian Ling Pi* 10g., *Ba Ji Tian* 10g.

Blood stasis obstructing in the collaterals

Dermal or muscular hematoma, large bluish-purple purpura, possible epistaxis, hematemesis or hematochezia with blood that is dark purple in color, and the menstrual flow with excessive blood clots, and dusky complexion. Dark purple tongue with petechiae, and thready or choppy pulse.

- Invigorate the blood, expel stasis and stop bleeding.
- Modified *Tao Hong Si Wu Tang*

Tao Ren 10g.	*Hong Hua* 10g.	*Chuan Xiong* 6g.
Chi Shao 10g.	*Dang Gui* 10g.	*Shu Di Huang* 10g.
Xian He Cao 10g.	*Qian Cao Gen* 10g.	*Gan Cao* 3g.

- Large dark purple purpura. + *San Qi* 3g. (powder)
  Distending or stabbing pain in the hypochondriac regions. + *Yan Hu Suo* 10g., *Xiang Fu* 10g.

Other Modality

A. Acupuncture:

Refer to "Hemorrhage" in Chapter 37 for differentiation and treatment (see page 263).

B. Experiential remedies:

❶ *Hong Zao* 100g. (taking in decoction or the entire fruit daily to reduce the formation of purpura).

❷ Single hemostatic herbs:

San Qi 3g. (powder, four times per day).

E Jiao Zhu 15g. (melted in boiling water, once or twice per day).

Zi Zhu Cao 5g. (powder, four times per day).

C. Single herbs with therapeutic effects on TTP:

Ling Zhi, *Zhong Jie Feng*.

CHAPTER 65

Hyperthyroidism

Hyperthyroidism is an endocrine disorder characterized by increased serum levels of thyroid hormones (T_4 and T_3). Hyperthyroidism can result from increased synthesis and secretion of thyroid hormones due to autonomous thyroid hyperfunction or due to circulation of thyroid stimulating substances in the blood; hyperthyroidism can also result from increased secretion of thyroid hormone in the cases of destruction of the thyroid gland as a result of thyroiditis. Deliberate or accidental overdose of thyroid hormone is another cause of hyperthyroidism and is known as thyrotoxicosis factitia.

Of all the causes of hyperthyroidism, Grave's disease is the most common. It is characterized by goiter, exophthalmos and pretibial myxedema. Grave's disease is an autoimmune disease, in which antibodies target the thyroid-stimulating hormone (TSH) receptors of the thyroid, resulting in constant synthesis and release of thyroid hormones. Its chronic course is remitting and relapsing. Autoimmune insulin-dependent diabetes mellitus, vitiligo, premature graying of the hair, pernicious anemia, collagen diseases and polyglandular deficiency syndrome are frequently associated with Grave's disease. Although the pathogenesis is not clear, infiltrative ophthalmopathy is closely related to active hyperthyroidism. In addition to Grave's disease, other etiologies of hyperthyroidism include toxic solitary or multinodular goiter (common in elderly patients), non-autoimmune autosomal dominant hyperthyroidism (familial and occurring during infancy), inflammatory disease (various types of thyroiditis), thyrotoxicosis factitia (overdose of thyroid hormone), iodine ingestion, metastatic thyroid cancer, and struma ovarii (teratomatous ovarian tumor).

Symptoms of hyperthyroidism may be dramatic or subtle. Since the thyroid is in charge of basal metabolism, symptoms of hyperthyroidism are related to an increased metabolic rate affecting the body systems. Common signs related to hyperthyroidism include goiter, palpitations, tachycardia, atrial fibrillation, widened pulse pressure, warm, fine and moist skin, tremors, abnormalities of the eyes (stare, lid lag, lid retraction, and mild conjunctival injection), nervousness, increased activity, perspiration, heat sensitivity, fatigue, increased appetite, weight loss, insomnia, weakness, and frequent bowel movements. In the case of Grave's disease, there may be infiltrative dermopathy (pretibial myxedema) with pruritus and erythema at the early stage, turning brawny during later stages. Atypical signs that occur with an abrupt onset may indicate a crisis of hyperthyroidism, also known as thyroid storm; it manifests as acute onset of fever, marked weakness and muscle wasting, extreme restlessness, severe mood swings, confusion, psychosis, or even coma. Hepatomegaly with mild jaundice as well as cardiovascular collapse and shock are possible.

Diagnosing hyperthyroidism is not complicated. A clinical history and physical examination together with laboratory findings (thyroid hormone function tests) are very useful in formulating the diagnosis. TSH is suppressed except in those cases with a TSH-secreting pituitary tumor or pituitary resistance to thyroid hormone. Serum elevations of free T_4 and free T_3 are diagnostic in a majority of the cases; the presence of antibodies confirms a diagnosis of Grave's disease. Depending on the etiology, treatment for hyperthyroidism varies. Pharmaceutical agents, radiation therapy and surgery are applicable.

Reference:

Beers, M. H. & Berkow, R. et. al., (Eds.). (1999). Thyroid disorders: Hyperthyroidism. *The Merck Manual of Diagnosis and Therapy* (17th ed. chap 8). West Point, PA: Merck Co., Inc.

Qi stagnation and phlegm accumulation surrounding the thyroid cartilage at the neck characterize hyperthyroidism and goiter; when they are chronic, these factors precipitate blood stasis. In some cases, the stagnant qi and accumulated phlegm can turn into fire to injure the yin. Manifestations of heart and liver yin deficiency with empty fire may be present. Emotional stress, such as longstanding anger, frustration and depression, causes liver qi stagnation, which can interfere with proper metabolism of the body fluid and lead to phlegm accumulation. As qi stagnation combines with phlegm accumulation in the neck region, goiter forms. Unremitting, chronic qi stagnation and phlegm accumulation will cause blood stasis, manifesting as hard nodular goiters. Females generally have a higher morbidity rate of goiter compared to their male counterparts, because many developmental stages of the female body are related to the qi and blood of the liver and women are more susceptible to emotional stress.

Goiter is the major and most common symptom of hyperthyroidism, thus TCM differentiation and treatment is presented in Chapter 34, "Goiter" (see pages 231-236).

CHAPTER 66

Hypothyroidism

Hypothyroidism is an endocrine disorder with a systemic effect on the body. The extent of this disease ranges from mild and asymptomatic to severe myxedema, which is an accumulation of hydrophilic mucopolysaccharides in the interstitial layer. Mild hypothyroidism can be detected by screening, while myxedema and cretinism are clinically recognizable. A higher prevalence is found in females. Hypothyroidism can result from a primary deficit of the thyroid gland or be secondary to deficient pituitary thyroid-stimulating hormone (TSH). Goiter may or may not be present in hypothyroidism, depending on the pathogenesis. Goiter is associated with lack of iodine in the diet, genetic thyroid enzyme defects, and goitrogenic drugs such as lithium and amiodarone. Hashimoto's thyroiditis may present with goiter; however, goiter is absent when hypothyroidism is associated with deficient pituitary TSH or destruction of the gland secondary to surgery and radiation.

A diagnosis of hypothyroidism is usually based on laboratory findings. Elevated serum TSH indicates primary hypothyroidism, while a low or normal TSH level is found in hypothyroidism secondary to deficient pituitary TSH secretion. Other abnormal laboratory evidence includes hypercholesterolemia, increased serum liver enzymes, hyponatremia, hypoglycemia and anemia. Serum triiodothyronine (T_3) is not a good indicator of hypothyroidism.

Clinical presentation varies depending on progression of the disease. Common complaints during the initial stage of hypothyroidism include pallor, fatigue, weakness, lethargy, arthralgia and myalgia, headache, cold intolerance, dry skin, thin and brittle nails, thinning of hair, and constipation. When left untreated, hypothyroidism progresses; the previous symptoms worsen and there will also be slow speech with hoarseness, absence of sweating, decreased sense of taste, smell and hearing, dyspnea, and weight changes. Some women have amenorrhea while others have menorrhagia. Some patients present with carotenoid skin tone, hard pitting edema, and puffy face and eyelids. When myxedema affects the cardiopulmonary system and joints, effusion into pleural, pericardial and joint spaces will manifest. A decreased heart rate is detectable, and hypothermia will be apparent. The severe complications of hypothyroidism are mostly cardiac, including advanced coronary artery disease and congestive heart failure. Susceptibility to infection is increased. The medication of choice is levothyroxine, which should be taken in the early morning with an empty stomach. Hypothyroidism is clinically manageable, but once myxedema coma occurs, death from this medical emergency is very likely.

References:

Fitzgerald, P. A. (2003). Endocrinology-Diseases of the thyroid gland: Hypothyroidism and myxedema. In L. M. Tierney, Jr., et al. (Eds.), *Current Medical Diagnosis & Treatment* (42nd ed. chap. 26). New York, NY: McGraw-Hill Companies, Inc.

Larson, P. R. & Davies, T. E. (2003). Hypothyroidism and thyroiditis: Hypopthyroidism. In P. R. Larson, et. al. (Eds.), *Williams Textbook of Endocrinology* (10th ed. chap. 12). St. Louis, MO: W. B. Saunders.

The clinical manifestations of hypothyroidism can be referred to TCM differentiation and treatment for consumptive deficiency, edema and goiter.

The characteristics of hypothyroidism arise from a slow and declining metabolism. From the perspective of TCM, the core pathogenesis is yang qi deficiency, and the clinical manifestations develop subsequently to yang qi's failure to warm, motivate and transform. The primary organs involved include the spleen and kidney; heart involvement becomes apparent in the advanced stage. The contributing factors to hypothyroidism are:

Constitutional factors may be the result of congenital deficiency or acquired malnourishment, depriving essence and dietary nutrients; the kidney and spleen are primarily affected.

Improper diet, including irregular dietary habits and excessive consumption of raw and cold food, injures the spleen yang. Long-term deficiency of specific nutrients, such as iodine, also contributes to the occurrence of hypothyroidism.

Iatrogenic factors, including high doses of bitter and cold herbs, emetics and purgatives, have a direct impact on the spleen, stomach, and yang qi.

Overexertion during physical, sexual or mental activity exhausts the kidney.

Hypothyroidism is a gradually progressive disorder characterized by chronic deficiency of spleen and kidney yang and declining organ functions. When spleen qi is deficient, the generating source of qi and blood is insufficient, followed by decline of kidney essence, particularly kidney yang. Deficient kidney yang fails to warm the spleen yang, leading to yang deficiency of both organs. When deficient yang can no longer metabolize fluids, water overflows towards the heart, manifesting as heart dysfunction. Heart involvement can also occur when the fire in the gate of vitality declines, failing to warm heart yang and leading to secondary heart yang deficiency.

As indicated, hypothyroidism derives from both qi and blood deficiency, and develops into both yin and yang deficiency.

Analysis of Primary Symptom

Symptoms of hypothyroidism are multifaceted according to its progression; nevertheless, all symptoms originate from the core pathogenesis of deficient yang qi failing to warm, defend, consolidate and transform.

A. Cold intolerance:

This is the earliest and most common symptom. "Qi warms." Qi maintains the body temperature by its warming effect. When yang qi is deficient, inadequate warming of the body causes cold intolerance. Cold intolerance is a subjective sensation of cold that can be alleviated by adding clothing and coverings or by increasing room temperature. This phenomenon is also known as yang deficiency generating internal cold. Cold intolerance is accompanied by absence of sweating. As an end product of fluid metabolism, generation of sweat relies on the transforming effectsof yang qi. Failure of fluid metabolism secondary to deficient spleen and kidney yang leads to internal fluid accumulation and lack of sweat. A differential diagnosis is important to rule out exterior wind-cold excess, in which absence of sweating is accompanied by aversion to cold.

B. Constipation:

Constipation is usually accompanied by poor appetite, epigastric and abdominal cold pain relieved by warmth and pressure, and a deep slow pulse. Constipation due to hypothyroidism is closely related to yang deficiency with internal cold obstructing the large intestine.

C. Edema:

The kidney stores basal yang which metabolizes fluids. When kidney yang is deficient, this metabolic function will be disturbed, leading to accumulation of pathogenic derivatives that are cold and yin in nature, namely various types of water retention. When fluids diffuse into the interstitial layer, superficial edema is apparent. When fluids accumulate in the joints, swollen joints are evident. In an advanced condition, when water overflows towards the heart or lung, pericardial and pleural effusion will manifest with palpitations, bradypnea, chest congestion and coma. In TCM, myxedema coma is perceived as accumulation of turbid, cold, yin pathogens in the pericardium.

D. Dry and flaky skin, thinning of hair or hair loss:

Not only is deficient spleen yang incapable of generating qi, blood and essence, it also fails to distribute nutrients to the body. The state of the kidney manifests in the condition of the hair. When the hair is deprived of nutrients due to kidney deficiency, there will be thinning of hair or loss of hair. Dry and flaky skin, thinning of the hair or hair loss originates from a complicated condition of spleen and kidney yang deficiency with essence and blood depletion.

E. Irregular menstruation:

Irregular menses, including amenorrhea and menorrhagia, are evidence of qi dysfunction. Qi serves dual functions for the blood; it promotes blood circulation as well as keeps the blood circulating in the vessels. When dysfunction is more pronounced in activating blood circulation and is complicated by blood and essence deficiency, patients suffer from amenorrhea; if dysfunction is predominantly failure to control the blood in the vessels, pale menorrhagia is apparent. In male patients, kidney yang deficiency leads to impotence.

Basic Patterns

- Spleen yang deficiency
- Spleen and kidney yang deficiency
- Heart and kidney yang deficiency
- Depletion and devastation of yang qi

Progression of Pattern

Organ involvement in the initial stage of hypothyroidism can be limited to the spleen only or include both spleen and kidney, particularly yang deficiency. The progressing condition involves the heart, manifesting as heart and kidney yang deficiency, analogous to pericardial and pleural effusion in modern medicine. The end stage of hypothyroidism, or myxedema coma, is a condition of cold-yin pathogen accumulation and depletion of yang qi with an unfavorable prognosis.

Treatment Principle

Since the essential pathogenesis of hypothyroidism is spleen and kidney yang deficiency, the treatment should focus on warming and tonifying the spleen and kidney. Replenish the deficiencies of qi, blood, yin and essence accordingly. When the heart is involved, warm and unblock the flow of heart yang for mild cases; transform turbidity, open the orifices, reverse peripheral frigidity and rescue the yang from collapse in critical and severe cases.

Pattern and Suggested Measure

Spleen yang deficiency

Cold intolerance, cold limbs, poor appetite, pallor, fatigue, epigastric and abdominal cold pain relieved by warm compresses, possibly abdominal distention and constipation, and excessive thin white leukorrhea. Flabby pale tongue with teeth marks and white slippery coating, and deep slow and forceless pulse.

- Warm the yang, disperse cold, and strengthen the spleen.
- Modified *Fu Zi Li Zhong Wan*

Fu Zi 10g.	*Ren Shen* 6g.	*Gan Jiang* 10g.
Bai Zhu 10g.	*Fu Ling* 15g.	*Zhi Gan Cao* 10g.
Huang Qi 10g.	*Chen Pi* 10g.	

- Significant cold intolerance and cold limbs. + *Rou Gui* 6g., *Wu Zhu Yu* 10g.
  Severe abdominal distention and constipation. + *Rou Cong Rong* 10g., *Dang Gui* 10g., *Mu Xiang* 10g.
  Thick white greasy tongue coating. + *Cang Zhu* 10g., *Hou Po* 10g.

Spleen and kidney yang deficiency

Lassitude, lethargy, cold intolerance, cold limbs, absence of sweating, systemic edema, dizziness, soreness and weakness of the lower back and knees, dry and flaky skin, dry and thinning hair or hair loss, poor appetite, constipation, and possibly impotence in male patients or irregular menses in female patients. Flabby pale tongue with white moist coating, and deep slow and forceless pulse.

- Warm the kidney and strengthen the spleen.
- Modified *You Gui Wan*

Fu Zi 6g.	*Rou Gui* 10g.	*Lu Jiao Jiao* 6g.
Tu Si Zi 10g.	*Shu Di Huang* 10g.	*Shan Yao* 15g.
Shan Zhu Yu 10g.	*Gou Qi Zi* 10g.	*Dang Gui* 10g.
Du Zhong 15g.		

- Lassitude, lack of strength, lethargy and fatigue. + *Ren Shen* 6g., *Huang Qi* 10g.
  Significant edema. + *Fu Ling* 30g., *Ze Xie* 15g., *Bai Zhu* 10g.
  Poor appetite and constipation. + *Sha Ren* 6g., *Mu Xiang* 10g., *Rou Cong Rong* 10g.

Heart and kidney yang deficiency

Palpitations, chest congestion or pain, lassitude, lethargy, cold intolerance, cold limbs, absence of sweating, soreness and weakness of the lower back and knees, hoarse voice, slow response to stimuli, dry hair and severe systemic edema. Tender, flabby and pale tongue, and deep, slow, intermittent or knotted pulse.

- Warm and unblock the flow of heart yang, warm the kidney to promote urination.
- Modified *Zhi Gan Cao Tang* and *Zhen Wu Tang*

Gui Zhi 10g.	*Zhi Gan Cao* 15g.	*Ren Shen* 6g.
Fu Zi 10g.	*Bai Zhu* 10g.	*Fu Ling* 15g.
Bai Shao 10g.	*Mai Men Dong* 10g.	*E Jiao* 10g.
Shu Di Huang 10g.	*Da Zao* 10g.	*Sheng Jiang* 6g.

- Significant palpitations. + *Long Gu* 30g., *Mu Li* 30g.
  Chest congestion and pain. + *Gua Lou* 20g., *Xie Bai* 10g., *Chuan Xiong* 6g.
  Lassitude and lethargy. + *Huang Qi* 15g.

Depletion and devastation of yang qi

Pale and dusky complexion, dizziness and blurred vision, icy-cold extremities, shallow and weak respiration, flaccid and weak muscles, somnolence, or even coma. Dusky pale tongue and minute pulse.

- Warm the yang, transform turbidity, reverse peripheral frigidity and rescue yang from collapse.
- Modified *Si Ni Jia Ren Shen Tang*

Ren Shen 15g.	*Fu Zi* 10g.	*Gan Jiang* 10g.
Zhi Gan Cao 15g.		

- For coma, take *Su He Xiang Wan* with *Si Ni Jia Ren Shen Tang*.

Other Modality

Acupuncture:

- **Manipulation:** Reinforcing method; moxibustion is applicable.
- **Prescription:**

GV4 Mingmen	CV4 Guanyuan	CV6 Qihai
BL17 Geshu	ST36 Zusanli	PC6 Neiguan
SP6 Sanyinjiao	LI4 Hegu	

- **Supplementary points:**
  - Constipation. + CV8 Shenque; BL20 Pishu; BL21 Weishu
  - Edema. + BL20 Pishu; BL23 Shenshu; CV9 Shuifen; KI7 Fuliu
  - Hair loss. + BL18 Ganshu; BL23 Shenshu; KI3 Taixi
  - Palpitations. + BL15 Xinshu; CV14 Juque; HT7 Shenmen; SP9 Yinlingquan
  - Irregular menses. + CV3 Zhongji; SP10 Xuehai

CHAPTER 67

Diabetes Mellitus

Causing about 13,000 new cases every year and affecting more than 125,000 children in the Unites States, diabetes mellitus has a major impact on our society. Diabetes mellitus is characterized by impaired carbohydrate metabolism due to inadequate insulin action or secretion; it can be acute and fatal, as in diabetic ketoacidosis, and it can be chronic, leading to complications in other organ systems as a result of hyperglycemia. The traditional oral glucose tolerance test (OGTT) has been replaced by testing for fasting plasma glucose, which is cheaper and more convenient. Research indicates that the risk for later vascular disease from chronic hyperglycemia increases when the fasting glucose level is greater than 125 mg/dL. Current classification of diabetes mellitus is etiology-based rather than treatment-based, because treatment-based classification does not cover other uncommon disorders.

Type I diabetes mellitus is caused by defective β cells, which are responsible for synthesis and secretion of insulin. Resulting from a cell-mediated autoimmune response, type I diabetes mellitus causes catabolism, weight loss, and a tendency toward diabetic ketoacidosis. Patients suffering from this type of diabetes mellitus usually are not obese. It was once thought that this type of diabetes mellitus had a juvenile onset; however, it can occur at any age. During an acute event, insulin injection is required; when stabilized, oral agents may be sufficient and the need for insulin is reduced.

Type II diabetes mellitus is ten times more common than type I. Even though it is the most common type of diabetes mellitus, an estimated 50 percent of those affected are unaware of their condition. It was once thought to have an adult onset; however, type II is becoming increasingly prevalent in children and adolescents. A predisposition to type II diabetes has genetic antecedents, in which several genes have defects, and it is represented by a heterogeneous group of conditions. It has a complicated pathogenesis of insulin resistance and insufficient insulin secretion. Type II diabetes mellitus is closely related to obesity. Diabetic ketoacidosis is not commonly associated with this type. Unless a crisis of diabetic ketoacidosis occurs, it is treated with oral agents.

Other etiologies of diabetes mellitus include disease of the exocrine pancreas, endocrinopathy, drug or chemical agents, infection and pregnancy.

Effects of diabetes mellitus can be acute or chronic. Disturbances in protein and lipid metabolism will follow the defective carbohydrate metabolism. Acute diabetic ketoacidosis is a fatal crisis. It has a mortality rate of three percent due to cerebral edema. Chronic hyperglycemia affects nervous, vascular and renal systems, sensory organs such as eyes and ears, and promotes infections.

Long-term management, including blood sugar monitoring, compliance with dietary and nutritional guidelines, infection prevention and control, foot care, and medication, should be incorporated in patient education.

References:

Centers of Disease Control and Prevention (2002). National diabetes fact sheet: General information and national estimates on diabetes in the United States, 2000. Retrieved July 20, 2003 from http://www.cdc.gov/diabetes/pubs/pdf/ndfs.pdf

Gitelman, S. E. (2002). Diabetes mellitus. In A. H. Ruldolph & C. D. Ruldolph et. al. (Eds), *Rudolph's Pediatrics* (21st ed. chap. 24). New York, NY: McGraw-Hill Companies, Inc.

From the perspective of TCM, diabetes mellitus has a principal pathogenesis of yin deficiency as the root and heat-dryness as the branch; these two patterns mutually influence and aggravate each other. The major organs responsible for occurrence of diabetes mellitus include the lung, stomach and kidney. Because the lung is the upper source of the body fluid, lung yin deficiency with heat-dryness will result in failure of the lung to disseminate the body fluid. When body fluid is not distributed by the lung, the stomach and kidney will suffer from secondary yin deficiency. In a similar manner, excess stomach heat can injure stomach yin as well as consume lung and kidney yin. Kidney yin is the foundation that supplies the fluid for the entire body. Once kidney yin is deficient, lung and stomach yin will not have their source and eventually become deficient, too.

TCM classifies diabetes mellitus, which is known as *xiao ke*, into three categories according to the primary organ involved. The lung is the major organ in upper *xiao*, manifesting as polydipsia and increased fluid intake. The stomach is responsible for middle *xiao*, presenting as excessive hunger and polyphagia. The kidney is the root of lower *xiao* with increased fluid intake and polyuria. In chronic diabetes mellitus, insufficient yin fails to support the functions of yang. As a result, the yang becomes deficient, and deficiency of both the yin and yang ensues; complications involve multiple organ systems.

The description of diabetes mellitus and details of its management are well-documented in TCM literature. For comprehensive TCM differentiation and treatment of diabetes mellitus, refer to Chapter 41, "Wasting and Thirsting Disorder" (see pages 287-294).

CHAPTER 68

Hyperlipidemia

Hyperlipidemia, or hyperlipoproteinemia, refers to a primary or secondary condition of elevated plasma lipoprotein levels. Plasma lipids, mainly cholesterol and triglycerides, rely on certain proteins for free transport in the plasma. The bound lipid and protein complexes are known as lipoproteins; four major lipoproteins are chylomicrons, very low-density lipoproteins (VLDL), low-density lipoproteins (LDL), and high-density lipoproteins (HDL). Chylomicrons, the largest lipoproteins, are in charge of transportation of the major plasma lipids, triglycerides; chylomicrons transport exogenous triglycerides from the intestinal tract via the thoracic duct into the venous system; VLDL transports the endogenous triglycerides from the liver. When triglycerides arrive at their peripheral destination, the adipocytes and muscle cells, they will be hydrolyzed by lipase into fatty acids and glycerol, which then enter the two types of cells for usage or storage. The liver plays an important role in the metabolism of LDL by removing approximately 70 percent of LDL from the blood and by providing active receptor sites on the surfaces of the hepatocytes. The level of plasma cholesterol is related to VLDL and LDL. Overproduction and defective clearance of VLDL or increased conversion of VLDL to LDL contributes to hypercholesterolemia. Conditions predisposing to hypercholesterolemia and hypertriglyceridemia are obesity, diabetes mellitus, nephritic syndromes or genetic disorders, and excessive consumption of alcohol.

Clinically, hyperlipoproteinemia is classified into five major categories. The majority of patients with hyperlipidemia are treated accordingly to primary type II hyperlipoproteinemia.

Type I is characterized by deficits in clearance of chylomicrons and VLDL, and has a higher prevalence in children or young adults, with manifestations of pancreatitis-like abdominal pain, eruptive xanthomas over pressure points and extensor surfaces, lipemia retinalis and hepatosplenomegaly; these symptoms are aggravated by increased dietary fat. Primary treatment is a low-fat diet to prevent pancreatitis, as severe and fatal hemorrhagic pancreatitis is a possible development. There is no evidence of correlation with atherosclerosis.

Type II is characterized by primary

or secondary elevated LDL, which follows a familial pattern. Clinical manifestations may range from asymptomatic to xanthomas, especially in the achilles, patellar and digital extensors. Family history of premature coronary artery disease (CAD before age 55) is possible. When left untreated, complications of corneal arcus juvenilis, atherosclerosis, and early death from myocardial infarction (MI) may develop. The treatment for type II integrates diet and medications to reduce the LDL and cholesterol levels via various mechanisms.

Type III is less often a familial disease; it is characterized by elevations of VLDL and both tryglycerides and total cholesterol (TC). The first symptoms may be tuberoeruptive xanthomas on the elbow and knees. A higher rate of prevalence is found during early adulthood in men, with occurrences 10 to 15 years later in women. Weight reduction and dietary restriction compose the principal treatment.

Type IV hyperlipidemia is often a familial pattern, and it is frequently related to insulin resistance and obesity. A fat-restricted and carbohydrate-rich diet can aggravate the condition. The prognosis is uncertain and premature CAD may be possible. Weight reduction and restricted alcohol consumption are the most effective treatment measures.

Type V is rare; it is characterized by a deficit in clearance of triglycerides and a risk of fatal pancreatitis. Symptoms, including sudden onset of severe eruptive xanthomas, lipemia retinalis, hepatosplenomegaly and abdominal pain, can be aggravated by increased dietary fat or alcohol. The prognosis is unpredictable and unfavorable.

References:

Beers, M. H. & Berkow, R., et. al. (Eds.). (1999). Hyperlipidemia. *The Merck Manual of Diagnosis and Therapy* (17th ed. chap. 15). West Point, PA: Merck & Co., Inc.

Witztum, J. L. & Steinberg, D. (2000). The hyperlipoproteinemias. In L. Goldman, J. C., Benett, et. al. (Eds.), *Cecil Textbook of Medicine* (21st ed. chap 206). Philadelphia, PA: W. B. Saunders.

Depending on the clinical manifestations, TCM differentiation and treatment of hyperlipidemia can be referred to congested fluids.

The clinical manifestations of hyperlipidemia are typical of its branch, phlegm-dampness accumulation, and its root, spleen qi deficiency. Phlegm is an excessive turbid and viscous metabolic byproduct that can be deposited in any area of the body, including the blood. This perception of hyperlipidemia is similar to that of modern medicine. The following etiological factors contribute to hyperlipidemia:

Improper diet injures the spleen and stomach, leading to phlegm-dampness accumulation. The digestive function is deficient and cannot extract the essence from diet, causing aggregation of lipids in the blood stream.

Emotional stress: Pensiveness injures the heart and spleen; anger and frustration injure the liver, which then overacts on the spleen. When the spleen is injured, it will fail to transform and transport, leading to phlegm-dampness accumulation.

Constitution: Constitutional obesity is related to a higher incidence of phlegm accumulation. For those with constitutional liver and kidney yin deficiency, empty heat consumes the fluid and generates phlegm, aggravating the pre-existing phlegm-dampness accumulation.

Among all the etiological factors, improper diet is the major predisposing factor to phlegm-dampness accumulation, or hyperlipidemia; this concept is analogous to that of modern medicine. Therefore, among all treatment measures, reasonable diet management plays the key role to prevent and limit the disease.

Analysis of Primary Symptom

Hyperlipidemia is diagnosed by elevated levels of lipoproteins and lipids in the blood. Some patients may be asymptomatic whereas others may have xanthomas at any part of the body. Xanthomas are a typical sign of hyperlipidemia; in TCM, xanthomas are phlegm-cores resulting from phlegm-dampness accumulation or from phlegm formation due to heat consuming the fluid.

- Light yellow xanthomas of various sizes, located predominantly in the extremities and trunk, and accompanied by fatigue, and heaviness of the head and body, indicate phlegm-dampness accumulation that may be primary, or secondary to spleen deficiency. The deposition of xanthomas, or phlegm-cores, is allocated to the surface and subcutaneous layers.
- Bright yellow, oval or tubercular xanthomas located on eyelids and extensor surfaces, with symptoms of a sticky sensation and bitter taste in the mouth, and dry stool or a sensation of incomplete defecation, indicate heat secondary to phlegm-dampness accumulation and damp-heat steaming upwards.
- Erupted rashes of brownish-yellow xanthomas, accompanied by dizziness, blurred vision, malar flush and night sweating, signifies phlegm secondary to liver and kidney yin deficiency with empty heat consuming the fluid.

Basic Patterns

- Phlegm-dampness accumulation
- Damp-heat accumulation
- Constrained liver with spleen qi deficiency
- Liver and kidney yin deficiency
- Phlegm-blood stasis complex

Progression of Pattern

Phlegm-dampness accumulation or spleen deficiency with phlegm formation composes the initial stage of hyperlipidemia. Chronic accumulated dampness transforms into heat, developing into damp-heat accumulation. In those where damp-heat has consumed the yin or in the elderly with weak constitution, liver and kidney yin deficiency is apparent. When blood circulation is disturbed due to liver qi stagnation or to phlegm obstruction secondary to spleen qi deficiency, blood stasis forms, followed by a phlegm-blood stasis complex.

Treatment Principle

The characteristic pathogenesis is spleen deficiency with phlegm-dampness accumulation. Treatment for hyperlipidemia focuses on strengthening the spleen, drying dampness, and transforming phlegm. Modify the treatment by clearing heat when there are heat signs, facilitating the qi flow and invigorating the blood for blood stasis, and nourishing the liver and kidney when there is yin deficiency.

Pattern and Suggested Measure

Phlegm-dampness accumulation

Elevated plasma lipids or lipoproteins, obesity, fatigue, lassitude, focal distention and fullness in the epigastrium and abdomen, heaviness of the head and extremities, nausea, acid regurgitation, thirst without desire to drink, and possibly eruptive light or dark yellow xanthomas. Flabby pale tongue with teeth marks and greasy coating, and soft pulse.

- Dry dampness, transform phlegm and strengthen the spleen.
- Modified *Xiang Sha Liu Jun Zi Tang*

Ban Xia 10g.	*Chen Pi* 10 g.	*Fu Ling* 15g.
Bai Zhu 10g.	*Dang Shen* 10g.	*Sha Ren* 10g.
Mu Xiang 10g.	*Gua Lou* 20g.	*Sheng Jiang* 6g.

- Accompanied by food retention. + *Lai Fu Zi* 10g., *Shen Qu* 10g., *Jiao Shan Zha* 10g., *Bing Lang* 10g.

  Headache and dizziness. + *Tian Ma* 10g., *Zhi Shi* 10g.

  Chest congestion, dyspnea and palpitations. + *Yuan Zhi* 10g., *Gua Lou* 20g., *Shi Chang Pu* 10g.

  Focal distention and fullness in the epigastrium and abdomen, thick and greasy tongue coating. + *Cang Zhu* 10g., *Hou Po* 10g.

Damp-heat accumulation

Elevated plasma lipids or lipoproteins, focal distention and fullness in the epigastrium and abdomen, sticky dry mouth or bitter taste in the mouth, thirst without desire to drink, cough with yellow sputum, dry stool or loose stool with a foul odor and sensation of incomplete defecation, and possibly bright yellow xanthomas. Red tongue with yellow greasy coating, and rapid slippery pulse.

- Clear heat and dry dampness.
- Modified *Lian Po Yin*

Huang Lian 10g.	*Hou Po* 10g.	*Ban Xia* 10g.
Zhi Zi 10g.	*Shi Chang Pu* 10g.	*Ze Xie* 15g.
Yi Yi Ren 15g.	*Bian Dou* 15g.	

- Distending hypochondriac pain, irritability, and bitter taste in the mouth. + *Long Dan Cao* 6g., *Huang Qin* 10g.
  Cough with yellow sputum. + *Zhu Ru* 10g., *Dan Nan Xing* 6g.
  Constipation and distention in the epigastrium and abdomen. + *Zhi Shi* 10g., *Gua Lou Ren* 20g., *Sheng Da Huang* 3g.

Constrained liver with spleen qi deficiency

Elevated plasma lipids or lipoproteins, depression or irritability, dizziness, blurred vision, distending chest and hypochondriac pain, poor appetite, abdominal distention, or irregular menstruation. Pale tongue with white or greasy coating, and wiry thready pulse.

- Soothe the liver and strengthen the spleen.
- Modified *Xiao Yao San*

Chai Hu 10g.	*Dang Gui* 10g.	*Bai Shao* 10g.
Fu Ling 15g.	*Bai Zhu* 10g.	*Sheng Jiang* 10g.
Ze Xie 15g.	*Shan Zha* 10g.	*Yu Jin* 10g.

- Severe distending hypochondriac pain. + *Qing Pi* 10g., *Zhi Qiao* 10g.
  Severe dizziness and blurred vision. + *Zhi Zi* 6g., *Ju Hua* 10g.

Liver and kidney yin deficiency

Elevated plasma lipids or lipoproteins, dizziness, blurred vision, tinnitus, insomnia, poor memory, soreness and weakness of the lower back and knees, malar flush, night sweating, and possibly eruptive rashes of brownish-yellow xanthomas. Red tongue with scanty coating, and rapid thready pulse.

- Tonify and nourish the liver and kidney, and eliminate deficient heat.
- Modified *Qi Ju Di Huang Wan*

Shu Di Huang 10g.	*Shan Yao* 10g.	*Shan Zhu Yu* 10g.
Gou Qi Zi 10g.	*Ju Hua* 10g.	*Ze Xie* 15g.
Mu Dan Pi 10g.	*Fu Ling* 15g.	*Han Lian Cao* 10g.

- Severe internal heat due to yin deficiency. + *Zhi Mu* 10g., *Huang Bai* 6g.
  Blurred vision. + *Qing Xiang Zi* 10g., *Chong Wei Zi* 10g.
  Severe dizziness. + *Tian Ma* 10g., *Gou Teng* 10g.

Phlegm-blood stasis complex

Elevated plasma lipids or lipoproteins, chest congestion or chest pain, shortness of breath, palpitations, possibly palpable hypochondriac masses with stabbing pain that is aggravated by pressure, and possibly light yellow or brownish-yellow xanthomas. Dark purple tongue with petechiae, and choppy pulse.

- Transform phlegm and dispel blood stasis.
- Modified *Gua Lou Xie Bai Ban Xia Tang* and *Xue Fu Zhu Yu Tang*

Gua Lou 30g.	*Xie Bai* 10g.	*Ban Xia* 10g.
Tao Ren 6g.	*Hong Hua* 10g.	*Chuan Xiong* 6g.
Chi Shao 15g.	*Sheng Di Huang* 10g.	*Dang Gui* 10g.
Chai Hu 10g.	*Zhi Qiao* 10g.	*Jie Geng* 6g.
Niu Xi 10g.		

- Severe chest pain. + *Dan Shen* 20g., *Yu Jin* 10g.
  Palpable hard masses. + *Bie Jia* 15g., *San Leng* 10g.

Other Modality

A. Acupuncture:

- **Manipulation:** Even method.
- **Prescription:** PC6 Neiguan LR3 Taichong ST36 Zusanli SP6 Sanyinjiao

The four points listed above are the principal points for hyperlipidemia, especially PC6 Neiguan, which effectively reduces plasma lipid levels according to recent research. Modify the point selection according to the relevant pattern.

B. Experiential remedies:

Herbs that reduce the plasma lipoproteins and lipids are:

Dan Shen, *Da Huang*, *Dang Gui*, *He Shou Wu*, *Ze Xie*, *Shan Zha*, *Pu Huang*, *San Qi*, *Yin Chen Hao*, *Hu Zhang*, *Ling Zhi*, *Nu Zhen Zi*.

CHAPTER 69

Obesity

Obesity is one of the most frustrating and difficult to managed disorder in healthcare industry; it has significant physical and psychosocial influences. Diagnosis of obesity involves an accurate measurement on the body mass index (BMI). The National Institute of Health defines a desire body weight as BMI of 18.5-24.9. Overweight individual has an increased body weight in relation to height, in comparison to acceptable or desirable weight, or BMI of 25-29.9. Class I obesity has a BMI of 30-34.9, class II obesity has a BMI of 35-39.9, and Class III obesity has a BMI > 40. BMI is calculated by dividing measured body weight in kilograms by the height in meters squared. Specific antecedents to obesity proposed include environmental, behavioral and biological factors. Environmental and behavioral factors play significant roles in both causing and managing overweight and obesity disorder. Biological factors, such as genetics, metabolism rate, some endocrinal diseases or drug usage, are other contributing factors of overweight or obesity. In general, overweight or obesity is a result of energy imbalance, in which the amount of calories consumed exceeds the amount of calories used.

Obesity is related to considerable rise in both morbidity and mortality. The primary complaint by the patients is an uneven distribution of body fat resulting in appearance of "big at certain areas of the body" or general "big" appearance in relation to height. Its complicated symptoms include palpitations, lower back pain, edema, sweating and fatigue. The most common physiological complications related to obesity include hypertension, type II diabetes mellitus, coronary artery disease, and degenerative joint disease; in addition, higher incidence of certain cancers, thromboembolic disorders, and gastrointestinal dysfunction are also found in obesity. The psychosocial disabilities are low self-esteem, poor coping mechanism and depression. Conservative managements in weight control include diet, exercises, behavioral modifications, social support and medications. Multidisciplinary approach to weight loss is found to be beneficial. Surgical approaches, such as vertical banded gastroplasty (VBP), roux-en-Y gastric bypass (GBP) via laparotomy or laparoscopy, are available for treatment of morbid obesity and its associated complications. Herbal supplement and acupuncture modality are also popular for mostly weight control and complication management.

References:

Baron, R. B. (2003). Nutrition: Obesity. In L. M. Tierney, Jr., et. al. (Eds.), *Current Medical Diagnosis & Treatment* (42nd ed. chap 29). New York, NY: McGraw-Hill Companies, Inc.

Centers of Disease Control and Prevention (2003). Overweight and obesity: Defining overweight and obesity. Retrieved on June 8, 2003 from http://www.cdc.gov/nccdphp/dnpa/obesity/defining.htm

Centers of Disease Control and Prevention (2003). Overweight and obesity: Factors contributing to obesity. Retrieved on June 8, 2003 from http://www.cdc.gov/nccdphp/dnpa/obesity/contributing_factors.htm

Centers of Disease Control and Prevention (2003). Overweight and obesity: Health consequences. Retrieved on June 8, 2003 from http://www.cdc.gov/nccdphp/dnpa/obesity/consequences.htm

Centers of Disease Control and Prevention (2003). Overweight and obesity: Overview. Retrieved on June 8, 2003 from http://www.cdc.gov/nccdphp/dnpa/obesity/index.htm

Based on the theories, "Obesity is related to phlegm", and "Obesity is related to dampness", obesity can be referred to TCM differentiation and treatment of congested fluids.

The first documentation of TCM regarding overweight and obesity was found in <u>Nei Jing</u>. The incidence of obesity is closely related to the following contributing factors:

Insufficient righteous qi are caused by chronic illness, constitutional deficiency, and aging. Gradual deprivation of kidney essence leads to insufficient fire failing to generate earth. When dysfunction of the spleen is not able to transform and transport, dampness, turbidity, phlegm and stasis will accumulate.

Lack of physical exercise causes poor circulation of the qi and blood. As a result, fluids, food and digestive essence will not be evenly distributed. These metabolic derivatives turn into turbidity, dampness and fat; they accumulate and stagnate in the organs, channels, muscles and skin.

Improper diet: Overindulgence in rich, greasy and sweet diet injures the spleen and stomach, leading to generation of damp-heat and phlegm. Metabolism of fluids and food is interrupted and these digestive derivatives accumulate. Dysfunction of the spleen and stomach aggravates the formation and accumulation of dampness, heat and phlegm.

Constitutional factors: <u>Nei Jing</u> clearly stated that occurrence of obesity is related to constitutional status and traits inherited from parental generations. In addition, it also described and categorized the physical appearances into five elements. For instance, physical appearance pertaining to earth has a round face, large head, wide and expanded shoulders, big abdomen, relatively small and muscular extremities, resembling general overweight or obesity.

Analysis of Primary Symptom

A. Overweight and obesity:

Overweight and obesity are mostly a complicated pattern of deficient root with excess branch. Different perspectives from historical practitioners indicated that "Obesity is mostly qi deficiency" and "Obesity is related to phlegm-dampness". In addition, a new concept of "Obesity is highly related to stasis" is presented by contemporary scholars. With "body weight exceeding normal" as the primary symptom, secondary symptoms may help with differentiations:

- Overweight accompanied by edema, heaviness and weakness of the extremities is mostly related to dysfunction of the spleen and stomach. Poor metabolism leads to formation of dampness and stagnation of nutritive essences. As these digestive derivatives accumulate in the muscles and skin, obesity manifests.
- Overweight together with excessive hunger and increased consumption of food indicates constrained heat in the stomach, which may also injure the spleen. This is a state of hyperactivity of the stomach with hypoactivity of the spleen. Even though consumption of food is increased to meet the desire of a hyperactive stomach, dysfunction of the hypoactive spleen failing to metabolize will lead to accumulation of whatever was consumed.
- Constitutional overweight with indulgence in rich, sweet and greasy diet, focal distention and fullness in the epigastrium and abdomen signifies phlegm-dampness accumulation in the middle burner. Phlegm-dampness accumulation hinders the spleen's function, leading to turbidity and fat accumulation.
- Overweight, distending pain in the chest and hypochondria, and irregular menstruation are symptoms of qi stagnation and blood stasis. Turbidity accumulation follows the malfunction of ascending and descending function of organs.
- Overweight with edematous lower extremities, cold intolerance and cold limbs is associated with longstanding illness, in which spleen and kidney yang deficiency is not able to transform fluids.

B. Symptoms of the complications:

- Palpitations, shortness of breath or breathlessness may be the results of phlegm-dampness obstructed in the chest leading to inactive heart yang, or may be the results of yang deficiency with water overflowing towards the heart.
- Sweating and heat intolerance are caused by stomach heat, or hyperactive stomach with hypoactive spleen. It can also result from phlegm-turbidity turning into heat and a contest between heat and dampness.
- Lower back pain and painful swollen joints in the lower limbs are symptoms of phlegm-dampness, which are heavy and adhesive, and they descend and affect the lower part of the body. Pain may also result from malnourishment and lacking warmth of the sinews and bones due to spleen and kidney yang deficiency.

Basic Patterns

- Spleen deficiency with dampness accumulation
- Hyperactive stomach with hypoactive spleen
- Phlegm-dampness obstruction in the middle burner
- Qi stagnation and blood stasis
- Spleen and kidney yang deficiency

Progression of Pattern

Initially, obesity can be an excess pattern, including stomach heat with hypoactive spleen or phlegm-dampness accumulated in the middle burner; as the function of the spleen and stomach is hindered over time, deficient patterns can be expected. Spleen yang deficiency further consumes kidney yang, leading to spleen and kidney yang deficiency. Deficient patterns of obesity may also progress to a relatively excess pattern. When dysfunction of spleen fails to transform and transport, excessive dampness accumulation manifests. Spleen deficiency may also lead to secondary liver qi stagnation, which further causes blood stasis.

Treatment Principle

Supporting the righteous qi to expel the pathogens is the primary principle. Augment the qi, strengthen the spleen and warm the spleen and kidney to address the root. Promote the movement of qi, transform dampness, resolve phlegm, invigorate the blood, promote urination and unblock the bowel to address the branch.

Pattern and Suggested Measure

Spleen deficiency and dampness accumulation

Overweight or obesity with edema, heaviness and weakness of the extremities, fatigue, abdominal distention, poor appetite and loose stool. Pale and flabby tongue with white coating and soft thready pulse.

- Strengthen the spleen and transform dampness.
- Modified *Shen Ling Bai Zhu San*

Dang Shen 10g.	*Fu Ling* 15g.	*Cang Zhu* 10g.
Bai Zhu 10g.	*Ze Xie* 20g.	*Zhu Ling* 10g.

Che Qian Zi 10g. *Sha Ren* 6g. *Chen Pi* 10g.

- Severe pitting edema in the extremities. + *Da Fu Pi* 10g., *Sheng Jiang Pi* 6g.
  Severe abdominal distention. + *Hou Po* 10g., *Zhi Qiao* 10g.

Hyperactive stomach with hypoactive spleen

Overweight or obesity, hunger with excessive indulgence, intense thirst and desire to drink, fever, abdominal distention and constipation. Red tongue with yellow coating, and rapid slippery pulse.

- Clear heat, purge fire, and unblock the bowel.
- Modified *Zhi Shi Dao Zhi Wan*
  Huang Lian 6g. *Huang Qin* 10g. *Zhi Shi* 10g.
  Da Huang 3g. *Shen Qu* 15g. *Bai Zhu* 10g.
  Fu Ling 15g. *Ze Xie* 15g.

Phlegm-dampness obstruction in the middle burner

Constitutional overweight or obesity, craving for greasy or sweet food, dizziness with distending sensation in the head, thick and sticky sputum, heaviness and numbness of the extremities. Greasy or yellow greasy tongue coating, and wiry slippery pulse.

- Harmonize the stomach and transform phlegm.
- Modified *Er Chen Tang* and *Ze Xie Tang*
  Ban Xia 10g. *Chen Pi* 10g. *Fu Ling* 15g.
  Shi Chang Pu 10g. *Yuan Zhi* 10g. *Ze Xie* 15g.
  Dong Gua Pi 10g. *Gua Lou Pi* 6g.
- When congested phlegm-dampness turns into heat with yellow greasy tongue coating, use *Wen Dan Tang*.

Qi stagnation and blood stasis

Overweight or obesity, distending or stabbing pain in the chest, hypochondria, epigastium and abdomen, irregular menstruation or amenorrhea. Dark or purple tongue with petechiae, and wiry thready or choppy pulse.

- Facilitate the qi flow and invigorate the blood.
- Modified *Chai Hu Shu Gan San*
  Chai Hu 10g. *Zhi Qiao* 10g. *Chi Shao* 15g.
  Bai Shao 15g. *Chuan Xiong* 6g. *Xiang Fu* 10g.
  Chen Pi 6g. *Gan Cao* 3g.
- Significant qi stagnation. + *Qing Pi* 10g., *Chuan Lian Zi* 10g., *Fo Shou* 6g.
  Significant blood stasis. + *Tao Ren* 10g., *Hong Hua* 6g., *Dan Shen* 30g.

Spleen and kidney yang deficiency

Overweight or obesity with edema, especially in the lower extremities, cold intolerance, cold limbs, soreness and weakness in the lower back and knees, lassitude and fatigue aggravated by exertion, palpitations, breathlessness, scanty urination and loose stool. Pale tongue with white slippery coating, and deep thready and weak pulse.

- Warm the yang and transform dampness.
- Modified *Zhen Wu Tang*

Zhi Fu Zi 6g.	*Huang Qi* 10g.	*Bai Zhu* 10g.
Fu Ling 15g.	*Bai Shao* 10g.	*Che Qian Zi* 10g.
Sheng Jiang 6g.		

- Severe pitting edema. + *Zhu Ling* 10g., *Ze Xie* 15g., *Da Fu Pi* 10g.
  Severe deficient cold. + *Rou Gui* 6g.

Other Modality

A. Acupuncture:

- **Manipulation:** Combination of reinforcing and reducing methods.
- **Prescription:** ST34 Liangqiu SP4 Gongsun ST40 Fenglong ST36 Zusanli
- **Supplementary points:**
  - Spleen and kidney yang deficiency. + CV4 Guanyuan; KI3 Taixi
  - Qi stagnation and blood stasis. + TE4 Yangchi; SP10 Xuehai
  - Phlegm-heat. + TE6 Zhigou; LI11 Quchi
- **Auricular points:**

  Spleen; Stomach; Endocrine; Ear-Shenmen

B. Experiential remedies:

❶ *He Ye, Shan Zha, Ze Xie.*

These herbs can be made into tea and be taken daily with non-specific dosage.

❷ *Fang Feng Tong Sheng Wan* 6-10g. (patent medicine, three times a day).

C. Single herbs for weight loss or weight control:

He Ye, Zhi Shou Wu, Jue Ming Zi, Shan Zha, Yu Zhu, Xia Ku Cao, Ze Xie, Cang Zhu, Kun Bu, Hai Zao, Huo Ma Ren, Ma Huang.

CHAPTER 70

Gout

Gout is a metabolic disorder that is characterized by recurrent acute arthritis, usually monarticular and later by chronic deforming arthritis. Although some people with hyperuricemia never develop gout, hyperuricemia is still believed to be highly associated with formation of gout. Heredity is another major hypothesized contributing factor to gout, especially in secondary gout. Even though pathogenesis of early stage of acute gout is not well comprehended, lately, chronic stage of gout is better understood. Tophaceous deposition in the articular and periarticular tissues with structural derangement characterizes the pathology. Ninety percent of primary gout patients are male. Elevated serum uric acid is found in ninety-five percent of patients who have serial measurements during the course of an attack. During acute phase, erythrocyte sedimentation rate (ESR) and leukocyte count are elevated. Imaging diagnosis is more meaningful during chronic stage. Biopsy can be useful for differentiating tophi from rheumatoid nodules.

Sudden onset of intense pain, and usually nocturnal, and swollen joints characterize acute gouty arthritis. Tense, warm, and dusky red skin, as well as fever manifest during an acute attack. Desquamation and pruritus may appear during recovery stage from acute arthritis. Tophi on the external ears, hands, feet, olecranon and prepatellar bursa are common. Gouty arthritis predominantly affects the metatarsophalangeal joint of the great toe, usually monarticular and asymmetrical. Joints of the lower extremities are also commonly affected. Approximately 5-10 percent of gout patients developed uric acid renal calculi. Pharmaceutical agents lowering uric acids are not recommended for asymptomatic hyperuricemia until appearance of arthritis, renal calculi and tophi. Nonsteroidal anti-inflammatory drugs, colchicine, corticosteroids and analgesics are used to manage acute arthritis; sudden reduction of serum uric acid usually precipitates recurrent attacks. Management between the acute attacks emphasizes on avoiding causes that may induce hyperuricemia.

Reference:

Hellmann, D. B. & Stone, J. H. (2003). Arthritis & musculoskeletal disorders: gouty arthritis. In L. M. Tierney, Jr., et. al. (Eds.), *Current Medical Diagnosis & Treatment* (42nd ed. chap. 20). New York, NY: McGraw-Hill Companies, Inc.

Based on the clinical manifestations, TCM differentiation and treatment of gout can be categorized into painful obstruction; it may also be referred to lin syndrome.

From the perspective of TCM, both exterior and interior pathogenic factors contribute to the occurrence of gout, especially dampness. Due to the diffusing downwards characteristic of dampness, joints in the lower extremities are commonly affected; respectively, the nature of dampness is to adhere and linger, gout tends to be recurrent and persistent.

Exterior pathogenic influences: Invasion of wind, cold and dampness or combine thereof may first affect the joints and channels at the early stage, causing qi and blood stagnation. Later, chronic unremitting condition involves the internal organs, such as the liver, bladder, spleen and kidney. The tendency of progression is from superficial to interior.

Interior pathogenic influences: Righteous qi deficiency due to chronic illness or congenital insufficiency increases the susceptibility to exterior pathogenic invasion via an unconsolidated interstitial layer between the muscle and skin. Failure of the spleen to metabolize water will lead to the generation of dampness or damp-heat.

Analysis of Primary Symptom

A. Swollen painful joints:

From the characteristics of this primary symptom, pathogenic influences of wind, cold, dampness or heat are identifiable.

- Joints that are swollen, red, warm to the touch and painful, alleviated by cold and aggravated by heat, indicates a pathogen of heat.
- For swollen joints with migrating pain from joint to joint, especially the upper limbs, the major precipitating factor is wind.
- Swollen painful joints, with fixed location of pain that is alleviated by warmth, is caused by cold, which is congealing and constricting.
- In addition to swelling and pain, if the heavy sensation is also felt over the joints or limbs, especially the lower extremities, excessive dampness is expected. Dampness is heavy and adhesive in nature and it diffuses downwards.

B. Tophaceous deposition (known as phlegm-core in TCM):

During the course, tophi can be detected around the affected joints, external ears, hands and feet. Accumulation of damp-heat is the major contributor to the formation of tohpi. As heat consumes the fluid, which becomes concentrated and sticky, phlegm-core accompanied by blood stasis is inevitable. When these pathological by-products accumulate on the tissue or around the joints, tophi manifests.

C. Renal calculi:

Small and insignificant renal calculi can be asymptomatic; however, if calculi are large and lodged in the urinary tract, severe lower back or flank pain, and urgent, frequent, difficult and painful urination will present. Renal calculi are caused by damp-heat accumulating in the bladder. Even though this symptom is categorized into stone *lin* syndrome, elevation of serum uric acid confirms the diagnosis of gout.

Basic Patterns

- Cold-dampness in the collaterals
- Damp-heat obstruction
- Damp-heat in the bladder
- Phlegm-blood stasis complex
- Qi and blood deficiency

Progression of Pattern

At initial stage, an excess pattern is identified via sudden onset of red, swollen and painful joints that are warm to the touch. As the disease progresses, subcutaneous phlegm-core, or tophi, phlegm-blood stasis complex will result; renal calculi indicate damp-heat in the bladder. Recurrent persistent gout will gradually consume righteous qi, leading to chronic qi and blood deficiency.

Treatment Principle

Dampness, phlegm and blood stasis are the major pathologies of excess patterns of gout; therefore, to expel dampness, transform phlegm and eliminate stasis generate the principle of treating acute episode. When condition is stabilized, modify the treatment to a combination of expelling the pathogens and supporting the righteous qi.

Pattern and Suggested Measure

Cold-dampness in the collaterals

Stiff and deformed joints, limited range of motion, dark-red color on the periarticular skin, cold intolerance and cold limbs. Dark tongue with thin white coating, and deep thready pulse.

- Eliminate dampness, warm the channels and unblock the collaterals.
- Modified *Yi Yi Ren Tang*

  Cang Zhu 10g. *Yi Yi Ren* 20g. *Qiang Huo* 10g.
  Du Huo 10g. *Fang Feng* 10g. *Zhi Chuan Wu* 3g.
  Ma Huang 6g. *Gui Zhi* 10g. *Chuan Xiong* 6g.
  Dang Gui 10g. *Shen Jin Cao* 10g.

- Migrating pain or gout of the upper extremities, increase the dose of *Qiang Huo* to 20g. + *Sang Zhi* 10g., *Jiang Huang* 10g.

  Fixed pain alleviated by warmth. + *Xi Xin* 3g.

  Swollen joints with heavy sensation, mainly affecting the lower extremities. + *Mu Gua* 10g., *Fang Ji* 10g.

Damp-heat obstruction

Red swollen joints that are warm to the touch, severe pain aggravated by pressure and alleviated by cold, possibly fever, dark scanty urination and constipation. Red tongue with yellow greasy coating, and rapid slippery pulse.

- Clear heat and eliminate dampness, unblock obstruction and invigorate the collaterals.
- Modified *Si Miao Wan*

  Cang Zhu 10g. *Huang Bai* 10g. *Yi Yi Ren* 15g.
  Chuan Niu Xi 15g. *Ren Dong Teng* 10g. *Sang Zhi* 10g.
  Mu Gua 10g. *Can Sha* 6g.

- Excessive heat. + *Shi Gao* 30g., *Zhi Mu* 10g.

  Periarticular erythema. + *Mu Dan Pi* 10g., *Chi Shao* 15g.

  Excessive dampness. + *Han Fang Ji* 10g., *Wei Ling Xian* 10g.

Phlegm-blood stasis complex

Subcutaneous nodules, or tophi, painless and normal skin color on palpation, possibly erosion and forming fistula. Dark tongue with petechiae, and deep slippery pulse.

- Eliminate phlegm, dissipate nodules, and transform blood stasis.
- Modified *Xiao Tan Tang* and *Tao Hong Yin*

  Kun Bu 10g. *Hai Zao* 10g. *Bai Jie Zi* 10g.
  Zhe Bei Mu 10g. *Xuan Shen* 10g. *Tao Ren* 10g.
  Hong Hua 10g. *Chuan Xiong* 6g. *Dang Gui* 10g.
  Wei Ling Xian 10g. *Tian Nan Xing* 6g.

- Erosion of tophi. + *Huang Qi* 15g.

Damp-heat in the bladder

Dysuria with urgency, increased frequency and pain, urination with sands or stones, colic pain in the lower back, flank and abdomen, and swollen painful joints. Red tongue with yellow coating, and rapid slippery pulse.

- Clear heat, drain dampness, unblock obstruction in the urinary tract and eliminate stones.
- Modified *Shi Wei San*

Shi Wei 10g.	*Qu Mai* 10g.	*Hua Shi* 15g.
Che Qian Zi 10g.	*Bian Xu* 10g.	*Huang Bai* 6g.
Jin Qian Cao 15g.	*Hai Jin Sha* 15g.	*Wu Yao* 10g.

- Hematuria. + *Bai Mao Gen* 10g., *Xiao Ji* 10g.

Qi and blood deficiency

Recurrent swollen and painful joints, migrating pain from joint to joint or soreness and heaviness in the joints, limited range of motion of the affected joints, possibly joint deformity, pale complexion, lassitude and general weakness. Pale flabby tongue with thin white coating, and deep thready and weak pulse.

- Tonify the qi and blood, nourish the liver and kidney, unblock obstruction and invigorate the collaterals.
- Modified *Du Huo Ji Sheng Tang*

Du Huo 15g.	*Qin Jiao* 10g.	*Fang Feng* 10g.
Xi Xin 3g.	*Du Zhong* 10g.	*Niu Xi* 10g.
Sang Ji Sheng 15g.	*Dang Gui* 10g.	*Chuan Xiong* 6g.
Bai Shao 15g.	*Rou Gui* 6g.	*Xu Duan* 10g.
Shen Jin Cao 10g.		

- Significant cold pain in the joint. + *Fu Zi* 3g.
  Numbness of the limbs. + *Ji Xue Teng* 30g., *Luo Shi Teng* 15g.

Other Modality

A. Acupuncture:

Refer to Chapter 31, "Painful Obstruction Syndrome", for differentiation and treatment (see page 217).

- **Supplementery points:** based on affected joints.
  - Shoulder. + LI15 Jianyu; SI9 Jianzhen; Ashi points
  - Wrist. + TE5 Waiguan; LI4 Hegu

- Elbow. + LI4 Hegu; LI10 Shousanli; LI11 Quchi
- Knee. + Extra36 Xiyan; GB34 Yanglingquan
- Ankle. + LR4 Zhongfeng; UB60 Kunlun; ST41 Jiexi; GB40 Qiuxu

B. Experiential remedies:

❶ Single herbs promoting uric acid elimination:
Che Qian Zi, Di Long, Shan Ci Gu.

❷ Single herbs with anti-inflammatory effect:
Mu Gua, Qing Feng Teng, Qin Jiao, Chuan Wu, Ci Wu Jia, Du Zhong, Huai Niu Xi.

❸ Single herbs promoting microcirculation:
Wu Tou, Han Fang Ji, Gui Zhi, Xi Xin, Luo Shi Teng, Sang Ji Sheng, Niu Xi.

❹ Herbal analgesics:
Du Huo, Yan Hu Suo, Han Fang Ji, Chuan Wu, Xi Xin.

CHAPTER 71

Systemic Lupus Erythematosus

Systemic lupus erythematosus (SLE) is a chronic systemic inflammatory disorder that follows a course of alternating exacerbations and remissions. It is caused by autoimmune responses. SLE involves multiple systems, and its symptoms are the results of antigen-antibody complex trapped in the capillaries on the visceral structures or those of autoantibody-mediated destruction of host cells. Multiple factors contribute to the occurrence of SLE. SLE seems to be gender and racial specific; female accounts approximately 85% of the total patients; morbidity rate for an African American woman is about four times of her Caucasian counterpart. Sexual hormone appears to be significant since most patients develop SLE after menarche and before menopause. Some drug might induce lupus-like syndrome. Therefore, ruling out causes from pharmaceutical agents is important prior to diagnosing SLE. Laboratory evidence of autoantibodies is currently available for confirmation of diagnosis.

Nonspecific as well as systematic symptoms vary from individuals to individuals. Nonspecific symptoms are fever, anorexia, malaise and weight loss. However, most patients have skin lesions at some time; less than half of the patients will exhibit typical "butterfly rash" on their face. The erythematous rash may also be present at any area of the body where exposed to ultraviolet ray. Complicated symptoms depend on the systems affected. Cutaneous symptoms include discoid lupus, typical fingertip lesions, nail fold infarcts, periungual erythma, splinter hemorrhages or alopecia. Joint symptoms can be the first and persistent manifestation in some patients. Pulmonary symptoms including pleurisy, plural effusion and pneumonia are common. Neurological involvement is apparent with psychosis, seizure or stroke. Glomerulonephritis may manifest in various forms. Hemodynamic instability may be present. Available treatments include corticosteroids and immunosuppressants. Patients who suffer from joint symptoms or lupus rashes and poor response to nonsteroidal anti-inflammatory drugs (NSAIDs) may find antimalarials to be helpful.

References:

Hellmann, D. B. & Stone, J. H. (2003). Arthritis & musculoskeletal disorders: Systemic lupus erythematosus. In L. M. Tierney, Jr., et. al. (Eds.), *Current Medical Diagnosis & Treatment* (42nd ed. chap. 20). New York, NY: McGraw-Hill Companies, Inc.

Sack, K. E. & Fye, K. H. (2001). Rheumatic diseases: Systemic lupus erythematosus. In T. G. Parslow, D. P. Stites, A. I. Terr, & J. B. Imboden (Eds.), *Medical Immunology* (10th ed. chap. 31). New York, NY: McGraw-Hill Companies, Inc.

Based on the manifestations, SLE can be referred to TCM differentiation and treatment of fever of internal disequilibrium, hemorrhage, painful obstruction and edema.

Pathogeneses for SLE are thought to be closely related to excessive heat toxicity and insufficient yin and fluid. The contributing factors are as follows:

Insufficient yin and fluid, resulting from constitutional yin deficiency or yin injury by various pathogens, lead to disharmony between nutritive and protective qi. Therefore, increases the susceptibility to exterior attacks. As stated in Ling Shu, Chapter 78, "Blood occlusion forms when the pathogens enter the yin level."

Exterior pathogenic factors, including wind, cold, summer heat, dampness, dryness and heat, may invade the body all year round. Invasion of the exterior pathogens, especially heat toxicity, may elicit the occurrence of SLE.

Exposure to sunlight elicits and exacerbates SLE. As indicated, insufficient yin and fluid account for the underlying pathologies, whereas exterior invasion of heat toxicity plays a triggering role in the disease course. When heat toxicity injures the blood vessels, emission of blood into the interstitial layers between the skin and muscles manifests as rashes (erythema); emission of the blood into the joints leads to swollen painful joints. Heat toxicity may also attack the internal organs and induce corresponding dysfunctions and symptoms.

Analysis of Primary Symptom

A. Erythematous rash:

- Gradual emerging of erythematous rash signifies a classic progression of the course. However, if the erythematous rash disappears and other symptoms exacerbate, a condition of retrogression is very likely.
- Bright red rash indicates a heat sign. Excess and deficient heat should be differentiated. Rapid revealing and rapid disappearing of the rash pertain to excess heat, or excess heat toxicity. Slow revealing and slow disappearing of the rash pertain to deficient heat, or yin deficiency with empty heat.
- Dark red rash signifies blood stasis. It also slowly reveals and slowly disappears.

B. Fever:

- Persistent high fever is a sign of excessive heat toxicity.
- Low-grade fever, tidal fever or five-centers heat indicates deficient heat. When these heat signs are accompanied by night sweating and dry throat, a complication of yin deficiency with empty fire is evident. With additional symptoms of shortness of breath and malaise, consider the condition to be deficiency of both the qi and yin.

C. Joint pain:

- Red, swollen, painful joint that is warm to the touch is caused by excessive heat.
- Migrating joint pain indicates preponderance of wind.
- Painful joints with heavy sensation are results from excessive dampness.
- Severe joint pain at a fixed location signifies blood stasis.
- Joint pain accompanied by limited range of motion, cold intolerance, and cold limbs are mostly related to spleen and kidney yang deficiency with excessive internal cold.

D. Edema:

Minimal proteinuria and hematuria are possible during early stage of SLE. However, when the pathogenesis progresses from spleen pathology to kidney involvement, failure of water metabolism leads to edema. Severe pitting edema at the lower extremities and tympanic abdominal distention are symptoms of advanced stage of deficiency of both the spleen and kidney.

Basic Patterns

- Excessive heat toxicity
- Yin deficiency with empty heat
- Constrained heat with congested fluids
- Blood stasis with heat
- Spleen and kidney deficiency

Progression of Pattern

From excess to deficiency: Excess branch is seen in early stage of SLE, mainly presented as excessive heat injuring the yin. Yin deficiency with empty fire consuming the yin and body fluid dominates the chronic active phase. Later stage of SLE pertains to deficiency of both the qi and yin, or to deficiency of both the yin and yang.

From exterior to interior: The disease course develops from superficial layers, such as the skin, mucosa, muscles, blood vessels and joints, to the involvement of the internal organs. Palpitations and chest pain indicate heart involvement. Dyspnea, cough and breathlessness signify lung involvement. When the liver is affected, hypochondriac pain, impaired vision, and nail pathology are evident. If the spleen is affected, poor appetite, nausea, vomiting and abdominal pain are common. Following kidney complication are symptoms of lower back pain, oliguria or edema.

If high fever appears at the initial onset of SLE, signs and symptoms pertaining to excessive heat flaring in both qi and nutritive levels will immediately follow. This progression is very different from warm-febrile disease. High fever, intense thirst and profuse sweating are accompanied by erythematous rash, and subcutaneous and mucosal bleeding. The symptoms may last as long as three months or longer. During this period, high fever may alternate with low-grade fever; however, the major complaint is joint pain.

Treatment Principle

Insufficiency of the yin and fluid accompanied by excessive heat is the primary pathogenesis. The key is to address the insufficient yin for treating deficient pattern or during chronic remission phases. Focus the treatment on excessive heat for excess pattern or during acute active phases. Incorporating methods of invigorating stasis, diuresis and unblocking the collaterals are recommended.

Pattern and Suggested Measure

Excessive heat toxicity

High fever that is temporarily reduced after perspiration followed by immediate elevation of temperature, red face with erythematous rash, soreness and pain of the muscles and joints, irritability, and thirst with desire for cold beverages. Dark red tongue, and rapid slippery or rapid flooding pulse.

- Clear heat and purge fire.
- Modified *San Shi Tang* and *Qing Wen Bai Du Yin*

Sheng Shi Gao 30g.	*Han Shui Shi* 30g.	*Hua Shi* 20g.
Sheng Di Huang 10g.	*Xuan Shen* 10g.	*Jin Yin Hua* 10g.
Huang Qin 10g.	*Mu Dan Pi* 10g.	*Chi Shao* 15g.
Yi Yi Ren 15g.	*Bai Mao Gen* 10g.	

- Unremitting high fever. + *Ling Yang Jiao* 0.5g. (powder); or + *Zi Xue Dan*
  Chills, headache, vomiting and thick yellow tongue coating. + *Da Huang* 6g., *Guan Zhong* 10g., *Ban Lan Gen* 10g.
  Soreness and painful joints. + *Ren Dong Teng* 10g., *Sang Zhi* 10g., *Fang Ji* 10g.

Yin deficiency with empty heat

Typical facial butterfly rash aggravated after exposure to sunlight. The rash may turn bright red and the redness spreads all over the face with low-grade fever, dry mouth, red eyes, epistaxis, irritability, insomnia, painful swollen joints that are warm to the touch. Red tongue with no coating, and rapid thready pulse.

- Nourish the yin and clear heat.
- Modified *Yu Nu Jian* and *Zeng Ye Tang*

Sheng Di Huang 15g.	*Shi Gao* 30g.	*Mai Men Dong* 10g.
Xuan Shen 10g.	*Zhi Mu* 10g.	*Ren Dong Teng* 10g.
Hu Zhang 6g.	*Chuan Niu Xi* 15g.	*Sheng Gan Cao* 6g.

- Persistent low-grade fever. + *Di Gu Pi* 10g., *Qing Hao* 10g.
  Joint pain. + *Hai Feng Teng* 10g., *Sang Zhi* 10g.

Constrained heat with congested fluids

Facial erythematous rash, stifling sensation and pain in the chest, palpitations, dyspnea, irritability, dry throat and thirst. Red tongue with thick greasy coating, rapid and slippery pulse, knotted and intermittent pulse occasionally.

- Clear heat, transform congested fluids and force out fluids.
- Modified *Ting Li Da Zao Xie Fei Tang* and *Xie Bai San*

Ting Li Zi 10g.	*San Bai Pi* 10g.	*Sheng Di Huang* 10g.
Zhi Mu 10g.	*Sha Shen* 10g.	*Huang Qin* 10g.
Yi Yi Ren 15g.	*Zhu Ling* 15g.	*Fu Ling* 15g.
Zhi Qiao 10g.	*Xing Ren* 10g.	*Sheng Gan Cao* 6g.

- Excessive congested fluids in robust constitution. + *Gan Sui* 0.5g. (powder), discontinue when the therapeutic effect is achieved.
  Palpitations and knotted or intermittent pulse. + *Long Chi* 30g., *Dan Shen* 10g., *Wu Wei Zi* 10 g.
  Dyspnea and congested chest. + *Su Zi* 10g., *Gua Lou Pi* 10g., *Hou Po* 10g.

Blood stasis with heat

Erythematous rash in dark red color, varicose veins in the lower extremities, petechiae spreading all over the limbs, possible epistaxis, hematuria or delayed menstruation, hair loss, sore in the mouth and on the tongue, joints pain, hot flashes, irritability, short temper, dark and scanty urination. Red tongue with patechiae, and thready choppy pulse.

- Cool and invigorate the blood to stop bleeding.
- Modified *Sheng Di Huang San*

Sheng Di Huang 15g.	*Dan Shen* 10g.	*Mu Dan Pi* 10g.
Chi Shao 15g.	*Chuan Xiong* 6g.	*Xuan Shen* 10g.
Zhi Mu 10g.	*Yi Mu Cao* 10g.	*Chuan Niu Xi* 15g.
Qian Cao Gen 10g.	*Ou Jie* 6g.	*Hu Zhang* 6g.

Spleen and kidney deficiency

Dusky complexion, malar flush, typical fingertip lesions, splinter hemorrhage, malaise, tidal fever in the afternoon, dry mouth, scanty urine and constipation, severe pitting edema in the lower limbs. Pale or red and flabby tongue with thin greasy coating, and thready weak pulse.

- Nourish the kidney and replenish the essence, strengthen the spleen and promote urination.
- Modified *Ji Sheng Shen Qi Wan*

Shu Di Huang 10g.	*Gui Ban* 10g.	*Shan Zhu Yu* 10g.
Gou Qi Zi 10g.	*Bai Zhu* 10g.	*Zhu Ling* 10g.
Fu Ling 15g.	*Ze Xie* 15g.	*Che Qian Zi* 10g.
Da Fu Pi 10g.	*Chuan Niu Xi* 15g.	*Fu Zi* 6g.

- Significant qi deficiency with shortness of breath and fatigue. + *Huang Qi* 10g.
  Malar flush. + *Zhi Mu* 10g.
  Severe joint pain. + *Xu Chang Qing* 10g., *Ji Xue Teng* 10g., *Xu Duan* 10g.

Other Modality

A. Acupuncture:

Refer to Chapter 37 on "Hemorrhage" for differentiation and treatment (see page 263).

B. Experiential remedies:

❶ Single effective herbs:

Lei Gong Teng, *Kun Ming Shan Hai Tang*.

❷ Experiential formula:

Ren Shen	*Bai Mu Er*	*Huang Qi*	*Gou Qi Zi*
Mei Gui Hua	*Ze Xie*	*Ling Xiao Hua*	*Qin Jiao*
Wu Shao She	*Yu Xing Cao*	*Bai Mao Gen*	*Yu Mi Xu*

Use routine dosage for each herb.

Taking the decoction for 4-5 months to control the symptoms of SLE and to stabilize the condition.

CHAPTER 72

Cerebrovascular Accident

Cerebrovascular accident (CVA), also known as stroke, is an acute neurological disorder secondary to vascular pathology that causes ischemic damage to the brain cells. It is the third leading cause of death in the United States. Annual incidence is estimated at 200 cases per 100,000 population. The magnitude of its implications goes beyond death; severe disability due to the residual effects of a stroke can be devastating to patients and their families. 20% of patients have their first stroke between the ages of 45 and 65. Risk factors include hypertension, hyperlipidemia, diabetes mellitus, obesity, ischemic heart disease, and peripheral vascular disease. Young adults are at higher risk if they take oral contraceptives, or if they have migraine headache, cardiac lesions and aneurysms. Many studies now point out that ischemic heart disease and CVA are closely related; in fact, myocardial infarction (MI) is the most common causal factor for death in stroke patients. Hyperlipidemia and cigarette smoking also are important contributing factors to both ischemic heart disease and CVA.

Currently, classification of CVA is based on pathogenesis: ischemic infarction and hemorrhagic CVA. The most common type of ischemic infarction is transient ischemic attack (TIA). A TIA occurs when there is a brief deprivation of blood supply to the brain cells; it resolves within 24 hours without significant residual deficits. Emboli are the most common cause of TIAs. Symptoms usually originate from the carotid or vertebrobasilar system with a typical complaint of amaurosis fugax, or transient monocular blindness, which is described as an abrupt, painless loss of vision like a "curtain being drawn" over part of the visual field. Other symptoms are monoparesis, hemiparesis, a clumsy limb, paresthesia, dysphasia, and ipsilateral blurred vision. 20% of TIAs occur within 5 years after a MI.

Embolic or thrombotic infarctions, together known as atherothrombotic brain infarcts, are closely related to MI. It is now believed that TIAs are better risk indicators for MI than angina pectoris. Acute infarction has a sudden onset and an rapid progression to drowsiness, confusion, and stupor. Patients will not necessarily lose consciousness unless the brainstem is affected. Embolic and thrombotic infarctions usually occur at night and patients wake up with the sequelae. Symptoms vary depending on the areas of the brain affected and include dysphasia, sensory deficits, facial weakness, and contralateral spastic hemiparesis involving the arms more than the legs. Weak and flaccid muscle tone is followed by spasticity during the ensuing days or weeks.

Hemorrhagic CVA results from intracerebral hemorrhage, often related to hypertension. Sudden onset with a higher incidence during the daytime characterizes hemorrhagic stroke. Bleeding can occur in any part of the brain, producing various symptoms. Patients often lose consciousness after complaining of a headache accompanied by nausea and vomiting. Sudden death is possible. Grand mal seizures may occur. When patients regain consciousness, they experience various residual deficits, such as slurred speech or dysarthria, aphasia, clumsy hands, decerebrate rigidity, conjugate deviation of the eyes, and hemiparesis and hemiplegia.

Usually the symptoms speak for themselves; however, CT and MRI of the brain confirm the pathogenesis and diagnosis. Cerebrospinal fluid (CSF) analysis can be helpful but there is potential harm associated with lumbar puncture. Differential diagnosis of CVA from brain tumor is necessary prior to intervention. Management in the acute stage depends on the patient's presentation. Reassurance accompanied by explanations is very important to patients and their families; supportive measures are required for comatose patients. Long-term management focuses on rehabilitation, prevention of additional strokes, and treatment of depression. For end-of-life care, quality of life becomes an important issue.

Reference:

Pryse-Phillips, W. & Murray, T. L. (2001). Stroke. In J. Nobel, et. al. (Eds.), *Noble: Textbook of Primary Care Medicine* (3rd ed. chap. 164). St. Lois, MO: Mosby, Inc.

From the perspective of TCM, CVA has multiple pathogeneses, including deficiencies of the qi and blood, and disharmony of the heart, liver and kidney. When the root deficiency is complicated by emotional stimulation, overindulgence in alcohol, excessive sexual activity, and exterior pathogenic factors, the resulting pathology is one of deficiency below with excess above. Liver and kidney yin deficiency and hyperactive liver yang combining with phlegm or fire mist the clear orifices, and obstruct the channels and collaterals, inducing stroke. In critical cases, the yin and yang disconnect from each other, and death is the likely outcome.

TCM recognizes an identical syndrome with all the clinical presentations of CVA and names it wind stroke; differentiation and treatment of CVA is categorized in Chapter 27, "Wind Stroke" (see pages 181-190).

CHAPTER 73

Parkinson's Disease

Affecting 500,000 people in the U.S. and with new incidence of 50,000 cases reported annually, Parkinson's disease is a chronic, progressive irreversible disorder. It is a degenerative disease in which the neurons responsible for releasing motor regulating neurotransmitters, or dopamine, are deteriorated. The prevalence of Parkinson's disease increases with advancing age. Parkinson's disease is not a new challenge to medical science; the first Chinese medical text, <u>*Nei Jing*</u>, had documented this disease as "*feng fei*". For more than a century the scientists believe that Parkinson's disease is an inherited condition. Current theory holds that one or more environmental implications contribute to this disease, especially exposure to chemical 1-methyl-4-phenyl-1,2,3,6-tetrahydropyridine (MPTP) associated with heroin addiction, and to herbicides and pesticides. Genetic factors are now believed to increase the susceptibility to the environmental factors. In addition, some medications, including haloperidol, chlorpromazine, metoclopromide and valproate, may induce some Parkinson-like symptoms, particularly severe tremors. The major pathogenesis of Parkinson's disease is the degeneration and damage of the neurons in the substantia nigra, which releases the neurotransmitter, dopamine. Dopamine is essential in motor coordination and balance by transmitting signals between the substantia nigra and corpus striatum. When there is a lack of dopamine, muscular movements become rigid and uncontrollable.

Diagnosis of Parkinson's disease is usually based on common symptoms evaluated by a neurologist. Advanced non-invasive diagnostic imaging, such as positron emission tomography (PET scan), can provide supportive evidence to the diagnosis. There are four criteria to diagnosis: 1) the presence of two of the three typical symptoms, tremors, muscle rigidity and bradykinesia, 2) absence of other possible neurological signs, such as overactivity of reflexes or sensory loss, 3) ruling out medication mediated Parkinson-like symptoms, and other possible medical diagnoses, and 4) responsiveness to medications for Parkinson's disease, such as Levodopa.

The first symptom is tremor of a limb, usually initiated unilaterally in one hand. Gradually, other symptoms develop, including slow movement (bradykinesia), inability to move (akinesia), rigid limbs, a shuffling gait, and a stooped posture. Gradual loss of facial expressions and speaking in a soft tone are common. Occasionally, there will be depression, personality change, dementia, sleep disturbances, speech impairments, and sexual difficulties. The course will inevitably worsen. Parkin-son's disease is treatable yet not curable. The classic medication treatment aims to increase the concentration of neurotransmitters, by which the motor coordination and balance can be improved; common medication is Levodopa. There is also adjunctive medication used together with Levodopa to enhance the therapeutic effects; a combination of Levodopa and Carbidopa (Sinemet) is a typical example. The advanced treatments include various surgeries, such as thalamotomy, pallidotomy and deep brain stimulation.

References:

National Institute of Neurological Disorders and Stroke (2001). Parkinson's disease backgrounder. Retrieved on June 21, 2003 from http://www.ninds.nih.gov/health_and_medical/pubs/parkinson's_disease_backgrounder.htm

Mayo Foundation for Medical Education & Research (2003). Parkinson's disease. Retrieved on June 21, 2003 from http://www.mayoclinic.com/invoke.cfm?id=DS00295

American Association of Neurological Surgeons- Congress of Neurological Surgeons. (2000). Parkinson's disease. Retrieved on June 21, 2003 from http://www.neurosurgery.org/health/patient/detail.asp?DisorderID=46

Based on the clinical manifestations, Parkinson's disease can be categorized into TCM differentiation and treatment of wind stroke; it may also be referred to hypertonicity.

Discussed in the imperial TCM classic, Su Wen, Chapter 74, " all signs of wind, tremors and dizziness pertains to disorder of the liver; all signs of cold, constriction and contracture are categorized into dysfunction of the kidney; all signs of acute onset, rigidity and stiffness are closely related to wind..." Based on its major presentations, such as tremors, muscle rigidity, and inability to move the joints, Parkinson's disease should fall into the extent of wind disorder. The basic pathogenesis results from a malnourishment of the sinews secondary to depleted liver and kidney, and insufficient qi and blood.

Liver and kidney depletion: Insufficient essence and blood results from advanced age or weak constitution. Failure of water to nourish the wood leads to deficient wind swirling internally, and malnourishment of the sinews, manifesting in tremors, rigidity and stiffness.

Qi and blood deficiency results from deficient heart and spleen secondary to overexertion or improper diet. Emptiness in the vessels and channels leads to lack of strength to bear weight. Transient tremors manifest in mild cases, and muscular contraction, rigidity and inability to move will present in severe cases.

Based on the pathologies stated above, extent of qi deficiency may lead to yang failure. Insufficient yang and qi will not be able to distribute the fluid evenly and circulate the blood properly, leading to secondary phlegm-dampness and blood stasis. Therefore, it is thought that Parkinson's disease might also be related to phlegm-dampness accumulation and blood stasis in the collaterals. Another theory of phlegm-heat activating internal wind was proposed based on the pathogenesis of congested phlegm turning into heat.

Analysis of Primary Symptom

The three typical symptoms are tremors, muscle rigidity and bradykinesia. A combination and gradual progression of these three symptoms are common. Differentiations of deficient and excess pathogeneses are as follows:

- Constant tremors accompanied by numbness of the limbs or contracture are most likely a result of liver and kidney yin deficiency failing to nourish the sinews and vessels.
- Constant tremors and muscle rigidity accompanied by significant lack of strength, cold limbs, bradykinesia, shortness of breath, and spontaneous sweating usually result from qi and blood deficiency with emptiness in the vessels and channels.
- Condition of intermittent tremors accompanied by heaviness of the body, excessive sputum and salivation is caused by wind-phlegm complex. Swirling wind manifests tremors and obstructed phlegm presents as heaviness and stiffness. Deficient qi failing to metabolize water is the pathogenesis of phlegm accumulation.
- As the disease progress to its severe stage, tremors worsen; there is possible dysphagia, dark purplish skin, and/or dark quivering tongue. This is due to qi deficiency with blood stasis obstructed in the channels.

Basic Patterns

- Liver and kidney yin deficiency
- Qi and blood deficiency
- Wind-phlegm obstruction in the collaterals
- Qi deficiency with blood stasis

Progression of Pattern

At the early stage of Parkinson's disease, the primary pathogeneses are liver and kidney yin deficiency, and qi and blood deficiency, which activate internal wind; however, it is predominately a deficiency condition. As deficient qi fails to metabolize fluids and circulate the blood, the result is secondary phlegm-dampness accumulation and blood stasis obstruction; this stage is a complicated condition of deficient root with excess branch. Finally, the inexorable progress continues, and extreme depletion of essence with unstoppable wind occurs, which cause constant tremors to the extent of total loss of musculoskeletal functions, including inability to ambulate, aphasia and aphagia.

Treatment Principle

Basic pathogenesis of Parkinson's disease is deficiency, including liver and kidney deficiency, qi and blood deficiency, and deficient wind swirling internally. The treatment principle aims on nourishing the liver and kidney, tonifying the qi and blood, and subduing the yang and extinguishing wind. Adjuvant approaches are needed to treat secondary pathogenesis, such as drying dampness and transforming phlegm, and invigorating the blood and expelling stasis. As the disease progress to its end stage, strongly tonify the basal qi and replenish the essence to refill the marrow are necessary.

Pattern and Suggested Measure

Liver and kidney yin deficiency

Unremitting, progressive tremors, possible numbness or contraction of the limbs, soreness and weakness of the lower back and knees, bradykinesia, stooped posture, dizziness, vertigo, tinnitus, and five-centers heat. Red tongue with scanty coating, and rapid thready pulse.

- Nourish and tonify the liver and kidney, extinguish wind and stop tremors.
- Modified *Da Ding Feng Zhu*

  Bai Shao 15g. *E Jiao* 10g. *Sheng Di Huang* 10g.
  Mai Men Dong 10g. *Sheng Gui Ban* 20g. *Sheng Bie Jia* 20g.
  Sheng Mu Li 30g. *Ma Zi Ren* 10g. *Wu Wei Zi* 10g.
  Gan Cao 6g.

- Significant tremors. + *Tian Ma* 10g., *Gou Teng* 10g.
  Contractions of the limbs. + *Mu Gua* 10g., *Shen Jin Cao* 10g.

Five-centers heat. + *Zhi Mu* 10g., *Mu Dan Pi* 10g.
When the condition stabilizes, use *Qi Ju Di Huang Wan*.

Qi and blood deficiency

Tremors, weak extremities or cold limbs, pale complexion, shortness of breath, reluctance to speak, dizziness, vertigo, spontaneous sweating and poor appetite. Flabby pale tongue with teeth marks, and weak thready pulse.

- Augment the qi and nourish the blood, extinguish wind, and nourish and unblock the collaterals.
- Modified *Ba Zhen Tang*

Dang Shen 15g.	*Bai Zhu* 10g.	*Fu Ling* 15g.
Zhi Gan Cao 6g.	*Shu Di Huang* 10g.	*Dang Gui* 10g.
Bai Shao 15g.	*Chuan Xiong* 6g.	*Tian Ma* 6g.
Gou Teng 10g.	*Shi Jue Ming* 25g.	*Ju Hua* 10g.

- Severe qi and blood deficiency. + *Huang Qi* 10g., *Ren Shen* 10g., *E Jiao* 10g.
  Significant tremors. + *Quan Xie* 6g., *Mu Gua* 10g.

Wind-phlegm obstruction in the collaterals

Intermittent tremors, general heaviness, lack of strength, focal distention and fullness in the chest and epigastrium, dizziness, retching, excessive sputum and salivation, abdominal distention, poor appetite, and loose stool. White greasy tongue coating and slippery pulse.

- Dry dampness, strengthen the spleen, resolve phlegm and extinguish wind.
- Modified *Dao Tan Tang*

Zhi Nan Xing 10g.	*Ban Xia* 10g.	*Chen Pi* 10g.
Fu Ling 15g.	*Zhi Shi* 10g.	*Tian Ma* 10g.
Gou Teng 10g.	*Quan Xie* 6g.	*Bai Zhu* 10g.

- Excessive sputum and salivation. + *Zhu Ru* 10g., *Shi Chang Pu* 10g.
  Significant dizziness. + *Shi Jue Ming* 30g., *Zhen Zhu Mu* 30g.
  Bitter taste in the mouth with yellow greasy tongue coating. + *Huang Lian* 6g., *Huang Qin* 10g.

Qi deficiency with blood stasis

Progressive tremors, lack of facial expression, dysphagia, contracture of the joints with pain and limited range of motion, dark purplish skin tone, and possible varicose veins. Dark quivering tongue, and thready choppy pulse.

- Augment the qi, invigorate the blood and extinguish wind.
- Modified *Bu Yang Huan Wu Tang* and *Da Ding Feng Zhu*

Huang Qi 30g.	*Tao Ren* 10g.	*Hong Hua* 10g.
Chuan Xiong 6g.	*Chi Shao* 15g.	*Dang Gui* 20g.
Di Long 6g.	*Bai Shao* 10g.	*Mai Men Dong* 10g.
Sheng Gui Ban 30g.	*Sheng Bie Jia* 30g.	*Sheng Mu Li* 30g.

- Dysphagia. + *Qi Ge San*

Other Modality

Acupuncture:

- **Manipulation:** Even method.
- **Prescription:** GV14 Dazhui; LI4 Hegu; LR3 Taichong; KI3 Taixi; SP6 Sanyinjiao; BL18 Ganshu
- **Supplementary points:**

- Tremors of the upper extremities. + LI15 Jianyu; LI11 Quchi; TE5 Waiguan

- Tremors of the lower extremities. + ST31 Biguan; GB34 Yanglingquan; ST44 Neiting; BL60 Kunlun

- Tremor of the head. + GB20 Fengchi; Extra16 Bailao

- Dysphagia. + CV23 Lianquan

- Difficulty of mobilizing the temporomandibular joint. + GB3 Shangguan; ST7 Xiaguan

CHAPTER 74

Myasthenia Gravis

Myasthenia gravis is an idiopathic motor disorder resulting from an autoimmune response, in which antibodies target the postsynaptic acetylcholine receptors. Characterized by episodic muscle weakness and fatigue, symptoms of myasthenia gravis worsen with repetitive muscle use and improve with rest. Myasthenia gravis is not a common disease, affecting 60 out of 1 million people. The incidence is higher in women and young adults between 20 and 40 years of age, yet it may occur at any age. Ocular muscles are often the first affected; approximately 85 percent of patients eventually develop ocular-related symptoms. Ptosis (droop of the upper eyelid), diplopia (double vision) and muscle fatigue on exertion are the most common symptoms. Dysarthria, dysphagia and proximal limb weakness may also occur. Severe generalized quadriparesis is possible during a relapse. In about 10 percent of patients, myasthenia gravis affects the respiratory muscles and leads to myasthenic crisis with difficulty breathing.

When symptoms and signs point to myasthenia gravis, the disease can be confirmed by an edrophonium test. Short-term improvement of symptoms after intravenous injection of edrophonium, an anticholinesterase drug, establishes a diagnosis of myasthenia gravis; on the other hand, if the condition worsens, the patient is experiencing a cholinergic crisis. Ninety percent of myasthenia gravis patients will have acetylcholine-receptor antibodies present in their blood. In some patients, a thymoma can be detected with CT and MRI.

Myasthenia gravis can be very difficult to manage. Pharmaceutical agents, especially anticholinesterase medicine, account for the major treatment for myasthenia gravis by preventing the breakdown of acetylcholine at the neuromuscular junctions. Immunosuppresive agents, plasmapheresis and immunoglobulin therapy are also commonly prescribed. Thymectomy is indicated for most patients with a generalized condition. Corticosteroids are indicated for long-term treatment. Patients should be informed about the nature and course of the disease, and about treatment options. Emotional support and positive coping mechanisms are encouraged.

References:

Beers, M. H. & Berkow, R. et. al. (Eds.) (1999). Disorders of the peripheral nervous system. *The Merck Manual of Diagnosis and Therapy* (17th ed. chap. 183). West Point, PA: Merck & Co., Inc.

Venes, D. et. al. (2001). *Taber's Cyclopedic Medical Dictionary* (19th ed.). Philadelphia, PA: F. A. Davis Company.

Myasthenia gravis, according to TCM theory, is caused by injury to the internal organs and deficiencies of the essence, blood, and yin accompanied by excessive fire. Its symptoms pertain to vital essence deficiency and malnourishment of the muscles and extremities. The affected organs are the lung, spleen, stomach, liver and kidney.

Lung heat injures the body fluid and the lung cannot disperse and descend. Because the lung is unable to disseminate and distribute moisture and nourishment to the internal organs, the extremities become malnourished and motor function is impaired. The extremities become weak and flaccid with decreased mobility. The deficient spleen and stomach contribute to myasthenia by failing to transform and transport or receive and ripen; consequently, there is inadequate production of the qi, blood, body fluid and essence. Deficient qi fails to circulate the blood and body fluid; deficient blood and body fluid fail to nourish and moisten the sinews, bones and muscles; pathology of the sinews, bones, joints and muscles ensues. The liver governs the sinews and stores blood to nourish them, while the kidney governs the bones and stores essence that produces marrow to nourish the bones. When both the liver and kidney are deficient, they are unable to support their related tissues and the sinews and bones become flaccid and weak.

Although many organs are affected in myasthenia gravis, the spleen and stomach are the focus of treatment. The spleen and stomach are the source of the qi, blood, essence and body fluid. Located in the middle burner, they raise vital substances to the lung for dissemination to the entire body. They also supply the liver and kidney with the blood and essence to nourish the sinews and bones. The spleen governs the muscles and provides them with nourishment. Strengthening the spleen and stomach will ensure an adequate supply of vital substances to all the other organs and tissues. Sufficient nourishment and moisture contribute to remission from myasthenia gravis.

TCM differentiation and treatment for myasthenia gravis is presented in Chapter 32, "Atrophy Syndrome" (see page 219-224).

CHAPTER 75

Multiple Sclerosis

Multiple sclerosis (MS) is named after its pathology of scarification at multiple sites on the neurons, leading to impairment or blockage of the neural transmission. The leading theory of etiology causing MS is autoimmune disease. During the autoimmune process, antibodies are drawn to white matter and induce an inflammatory response. Results of inflammation include demyelination, in which the myelin was stripped off the axons, and causing destruction of the underlying axonal membrane. Also, the maintenance cells, or the oligodendrocytes, are killed during inflammation. Oligodendrocytes are accountable for creating and repairing myelin, as well as supplying essential factors to the axon. These damages will further decelerate or block neural transmission, affecting the functions of the target tissues that the damaged nerves serve. Diagnosing MS is actually a process of eliminating all other possibilities. Currently, the most effective diagnostic examination is magnetic resonance imaging (MRI), under which the MS lesions show up as paler areas. The diagnostic role of MRI is two facets. Not only does it indicate the actual demyelination events, but also explain the presence and potential clinical manifestations.

Symptoms of MS involve multiple systems. When affecting the sensory systems, blurred vision, double vision, color blindness or blindness, nystagmus, paresthesia or anesthesia, and neuralgia are possible. If the musculoskeletal system is involved, paresis, plegia, spasticity, spasm, muscle atrophy, slurred speech or foot drop can occur. Ataxia, intention tremor, vertigo, speech ataxia and dystonia are also common symptoms due to impaired coordination and balance. It is not uncommon for MS patient to develop depression, dementia, mood swing, fatigue, and sleeping disorder. Other symptoms involving the elimination or reproductive systems are also reported. There is no cure for MS. Medications are used to treat both MS and its symptoms. In addition to cortisone, ABC treatment may be the most effective. A stands for Avonex, B stands for Betaseron/Betaferon, and C stands for Copaxone. Some evidence indicates that acupuncture may cause releasing peptides in the central nervous system (CNS) and promote modulation of sensory input from the body to the brain.

References:

All About Multiple Sclerosis (2003). What is multiple sclerosis. Retrieved on June 21, 2003 from http://www.mult-sclerosis.org/whatisms.html

All About Multiple Sclerosis (2003). How does multiple sclerosis do its damage? Retrieved on June 21, 2003 from http://www.mult-sclerosis.org/howms.html

All About Multiple Sclerosis (2003). Diagnosing multiple sclerosis. Retrieved on June 21, 2003 from http://www.mult-sclerosis.org/diagnosingms.html

All About Multiple Sclerosis (2003). Multiple sclerosis symptoms. Retrieved on June 21, 2003 from http://www.mult-sclerosis.org/mssymptoms.html

All About Multiple Sclerosis (2003). MS treatments: ABC drugs. Retrieved on June 21, 2003 from http://www.mult-sclerosis.org/abctreatments.html

All About Multiple Sclerosis (2003). Acupuncture. Retrieved on June 21, 2003 from http://www.mult-sclerosis.org/acupuncture.html

Based on the primary clinical manifestations, MS can be categorized into TCM differentiation and treatment of atrophy syndrome, dizziness and wind stroke.

Based on the TCM fundamental theories, pathogeneses of MS include the deficiency of the liver, spleen and kidney, as well as malnourishment to their extended tissues.

Kidney stores the essence and governs the bones, and generates the marrow to fill the brain; it is the congenital source of pre-heaven qi. Liver stores the blood, governs the sinews, and connects to the external environment via its orifice, the eyes. Essence and blood share the same source; therefore, the liver and kidney have a common origin. The spleen is the origin of the qi and blood generation, becoming an acquired root of post-heaven energy; it also governs the muscles. Chronic illness or consumptive conditions, secondary to exterior, interior factors and aging, results in dysfunctions of these three organs, leading to inadequate production and distribution of the qi and blood, and malnourishment from the insufficient essence. This multiple systems disorder, which exhibits in numerous manifestations and various degrees of debilities, reflects the disequilibrium of the three organs of the liver, spleen and kidney, and the dysfunctions of relevant tissues.

Analysis of Primary Symptom

A. Blurred or double vision:

Eyes are the orifices, or the extended tissue, of the liver, and they rely on liver blood for nourishment. Blurred and double visions manifest malnourishment of the eyes from the insufficient liver yin and blood. Other signs and symptoms related to liver deficiency include dizziness, vertigo, tinnitus or depression. If the condition worsens and there are additional symptoms of distention and pain of the eyes, irritability and agitation, consider that the yin is deficient and unable to restrain the yang, known as yin deficiency with yang rising.

B. Paresthesia and tremors:

These are signs of liver wind swirling internally. Both excess and deficiency patterns are possible. Internal wind can be elicited by either liver and kidney yin deficiency or yin deficiency with yang rising.

C. Ataxia and slurred speech:

Ataxia and slurred speech were first documented in *Nei Jing* as symptoms of "*feng fei*", a subtype of wind stroke. When kidney essence is deficient, production of marrow and nourishment to the brain will be inadequate, leading to disturbance of the brain to control mobility of the limbs. In addition, the collateral of kidney channel travels around the root of the tongue. Difficult in speech or slurred speech occurs due to poor circulation in the collateral secondary to kidney deficiency.

D. Paresis and atrophy:

The spleen governs the muscles, the liver governs the sinews, and the kidney governs the bone and generates the marrow. Spleen and stomach deficiency failing to generate the qi and blood may further progress to insufficient essence and blood of the liver and kidney. Paresis and atrophy indicate the critical phase of exhaustion of the essence and depletion of the blood.

E. Urinary symptoms:

Including increased frequency, urgency and incontinence, urinary symptoms may be caused by kidney yang deficiency and bladder's dysfunction in transforming qi. These symptoms occur during the advanced stage of MS, and they are usually accompanied by many other symptoms of yang deficiency with internal cold.

Basic Patterns

- Liver and kidney yin deficiency
- Yin deficiency with yang rising
- Essence exhaustion and blood depletion
- Kidney yang deficiency

Progression of Pattern

The deficiency of these three organs, liver, kidney and spleen, and their inter-influencing relationships are the center of the progression and the transformation of the patterns. Deficiency dominates the majority of the patterns.

Liver yin deficiency and kidney yin deficiency have a mutual causal-effect relationship; they may coexist simultaneously. Yin deficiency failing to restrain the yang will lead to the pattern of yin deficiency with yang rising. Essence exhaustion and blood depletion may result from failure of deficient spleen to generate the blood, and essence insufficiency due to kidney deficiency. A progress from longstanding illness is yang deficiency due to chronic yin consumption, finally kidney yang deficiency.

Treatment Principle

Deficiencies of the liver, kidney and spleen are the primary conflicts in MS. Replenishing the essence and securing the foundation should be the primary principle. Integrate the following methods, including benefiting the qi, nourishing the blood, augmenting the yin and warming the yang, according to different clinical presentations. Also incorporate the strategies on nourishing the liver, tonifying the kidney and strengthening the spleen based on the organs involved.

Pattern and Suggested Measure

Liver and kidney yin deficiency

Blurred vision, double vision, dizziness, tinnitus, numbness in the extremities, depression and thirst. Red tongue with scanty coating, and wiry thready pulse.

- Nourish the liver and kidney.
- Modified *Qi Ju Di Huang Wan*
  Gou Qi Zi 10g. *Ju Hua* 10g. *Shu Di Huang* 10g.
  Shan Yao 10g. *Shan Zhu Yu* 10g. *Mu Dan Pi* 10g.
  Ze Xie 10g. *Fu Ling* 15g.
- Dry eyes and blurred vision. + *Shi Hu* 10g., *Nu Zhen Zi* 10g.
  Numbness in the limbs. + *Bai Shao* 10g., *Dang Gui* 10g., *Mu Gua* 10g.
  Depression. + *Xiang Fu* 10g., *Bai Shao* 10g., *Chuan Lian Zi* 6g.

Yin deficiency with yang rising

Dizziness, tinnitus or deafness, agitation, blurred vision, distending pain of the eyes, spasms or tremors in the extremities, slurred speech, ataxia, or lack of coordination. Red tongue with thin yellow coating, and wiry rapid and thready pulse.

- Nourish the yin and subdue the yang.
- Modified *Tian Ma Gou Teng Yin*

Tian Ma 10g.
Gou Teng 15g.
Shi Jue Ming 30g.
Zhi Zi 6g.
Huang Qin 10g.
Chuan Niu Xi 15g.
Du Zhong 10g.
Yi Mu Cao 10g.
Sang Ji Sheng 15g.
Fu Shen 15g.
Gui Ban 30g.

- Blurred vision and distention of the eyes. + *Ju Hua* 10g., *Gou Qi Zi* 10g.
  Muscle and sinew spasms. + *Bai Shao* 10g., *Sang Zhi* 10g., *Jiang Can* 10g.
  Abnormal gaits and lack of coordination. + *Mu Gua* 12g., *Xu Duan* 10g.

Essence exhaustion and blood depletion

Numbness in the limbs, soreness and weakness in the lower back and knees, muscular atrophy, pain or weakness, even loss of mobility; also dizziness, tinnitus or slurred speech, shortness of breath and fatigue. Pale tongue and rapid thready pulse.

- Replenish the essence and nourish the blood.
- Modified *Zuo Gui Wan*

Shu Di Huang 10g.
Shan Yao 15g.
Gou Qi Zi 10g.
Shan Zhu Yu 10g.
Tu Si Zi 10g.
Lu Jiao Jiao 10g.
Gui Ban Jiao 10g.
Niu Xi 15 g.
Du Zhong 10g.
Xu Duan 10g.
Dang Gui 10g.
Bai Shao 10g.

- Shortness of breath and fatigue. + *Ren Shen* 6g.
  Severe essence depletion and blood exhaustion with slurred speech or aphasia, use *Di Huang Yin Zi*.

Kidney yang deficiency

Including all manifestations from pattern of essence exhaustion and blood depletion, there are also cold intolerance, cold limbs, lassitude, frequent urination, possible urinary incontinence. Flabby and pale tongue, and thready and weak pulse, especially in the both rear positions.

- Warm and tonify kidney yang.
- Modified *You Gui Wan*

Zhi Fu Zi 6g.
Rou Gui 10g.
Shu Di Huang 10g.
Shan Yao 10g.
Shan Zhu Yu 10g.
Gou Qi Zi 10g.
Tu Si Zi 10g.
Lu Jiao Jiao 10g.
Du Zhong 10g.
Dang Gui 10g.
Ba Ji Tian 10g.
Rou Cong Rong 10g.

- Urinary incontinence. + *Yi Zhi Ren* 10g., *Fu Pen Zi* 15g., *Sang Piao Xiao* 10g.
  Lassitude. + *Ren Shen* 6g., *Huang Qi* 15g.
  Ataxia or loss mobility with muscular atrophy. + *Xu Duan* 10g., *Gou Ji* 10g.

Other Modality

Acupuncture:

- **Manipulation:** Reinforcing method.
- **Prescription:** HT7 Shenmen GB20 Fengchi BL23 Shenshu BL18 Ganshu SP6 Sanyinjiao LR3 Taichong BL2 Zanzhu
- **Supplementary points:**

  - Paralysis of the upper limbs. + LI15 Jianyu; LI11 Quchi; TE5 Waiguan; LI4 Hegu

  - Paralysis of the lower limbs. + ST31 Biguan; GB30 Huantiao; SP10 Xuehai; ST34 Liangqiu; ST36 Zusanli; GB34 Yanglingquan; GB39 Xuanzhong; ST41 Jiexi

  - Slurred speech. + GV15 Yamen; CV23 Lianquan

  - Urinary incontinence. + CV3 Zhongji; CV4 Guanyuan; CV6 Qihai

CHAPTER 76

Seizure Disorders

A seizure is an episode of spontaneous, transient, and abnormal electrical discharge in the brain, manifesting with sudden loss of consciousness, involuntary motor activities and altered sensory phenomena. Seizures are transient and usually self-limiting; however, when they become recurrent, a diagnosis of epilepsy is established. Approximately 2.3 million Americans are affected by seizure and epilepsy, costing estimated $12.5 billion in medical charges and loss of production. About 10 percent of Americans experience a seizure once in their lifetimes; of those, 3 percent develop epilepsy before 80 years of age. The highest incidence is in children aged 0 to 9 years. Factors contributing to seizure disorders include pathology of the central nervous system (anoxic degeneration, focal neuronal loss, neoplasia and sclerosis), stressors (fever and pulsating light), and specific genetic inheritance (autosomal-dominant pattern of tuberous sclerosis). Acquired etiologies for secondary seizure disorders are usually detectable, including intracranial hematoma (30 percent), depressed skull fracture (15 percent), and brain tumor (40 percent).

Seizure disorders are classified into two major types, generalized seizures and partial seizures. The former arise from both cerebral hemispheres and are characterized by sudden onset of altered consciousness with tonic muscular contraction, apnea, cyanosis, and rolled-back eyes; the tonic phase is short and followed by clonus. An episode often initiates with a short, high-pitched cry. The convulsions last approximately 1 to 3 minutes, in some cases as long as 15 minutes. Partial seizures, on the other hand, derive from a single cerebral hemisphere and manifest with motor, sensory or psychic symptoms. Depending on whether consciousness remains clear during the episode, partial seizures can be further classified as simple, in which the patient remains aware, or complex, in which the patient experiences alterations in consciousness. Detailed history intake is a critical element in establishing diagnosis. When patients are unable to report events due to amnesia, obtain information from witnesses and consider the patient's age, present complaints, birth history, childhood illnesses, family history and psychological stresses. Certain medications and substances, especially alcohol, can provoke seizure activity; therefore, a history regarding substance and alcohol consumption is important. MRI and CT scan provide accurate detection of lesions in the brain; laboratory studies usually are of limited help in diagnosis, although basic investigations, including serum electrolytes, glucose, calcium, magnesium, and a complete blood count, are mandatory. Elevated serum prolactin and creatinine phosphokinase levels are possible within 30 minutes after a seizure; therefore, these two findings can help establish the diagnosis. An EEG is diagnostic for 30 to 50 percent of first-time seizures and repetitive testing can effectively categorize up to 90 percent of patients. If meningitis, encephalitis or central nervous system trauma is suspected, lumbar puncture is valuable.

The goals of treatment for seizure disorders are different during episode and remission. During the seizure, the first priority is to protect the patient and prevent injuries; the airway is to be kept clear. Biting the tongue is the most common injury. Turn the patient onto one side and loosen clothing and jewelry around the neck. Do not attempt to place anything into the mouth. Medical assistance may be needed if the seizure lasts longer than 3 to 5 minutes. During remission, several pharmaceutical agents are available for preventing seizures. Valproate treats primary generalized seizures in 80 percent of patients. Lamotrigine, carbamazepine and phenytoin are often prescribed for tonic-clonic seizures. Patients taking valproate or phenytoin must have their serum drug levels monitored.

References:

Centers of Disease Control and Prevention (2003). Epilepsy: One of the nation's most common disabling neurological disorders. Retrieved July 20, 2003 from http://www.cdc.gov/nccdphp/epilepsy/index.htm

Middleton, D. B. (2003). Seizure disorders. In A. K. David et. al. (Eds), *Family Medicine: Principles and Practice* (6th ed. chap. 64). New York, NY: Springer-Verlag New York, Inc.

Emotional stimulation, congenital factors, head injuries, improper diet and overexertion are contributing factors to seizures. From the TCM viewpoint, phlegm and internal wind are the primary pathogens, and the liver, spleen and kidney are the primary organs responsible for seizures. Existing phlegm, when stirred by liver wind or hyperactive liver yang, travels to cover the clear orifices and obstruct the channels, resulting in seizures. Recurrent and unremitting seizures aggravate organ deficiency and make phlegm accumulation worse, developing into intractable epilepsy.

The description and name of seizure disorder in TCM is identical to that in modern medicine. Differentiation and treatment of seizure disorders are categorized in Chapter 24, "Epilepsy" (see page 163-168).

CHAPTER 77

Bipolar Disorder

Bipolar disorder is an affective disorder distinguished by episodes of mania and depression. The *Diagnostic and Statistical Manual of Mental Disorders, Fourth Edition (DSM-IV)* provides criteria for diagnosing bipolar disorder and its subtypes. The depressive phase is identified by loss of interest or pleasure in life; it is sometimes described as being in a "blue mood." Depression is characterized by alterations in sleep, activities, energy level, cognition and judgment. The manic phase is identified by an abnormally elevated, expansive or irritable mood accompanied by impaired judgment that interferes with social and occupational functioning. It is characterized by delusional grandiosity, increased energy level, and goal-directed activities that are often potentially hazardous to self or others. Bipolar disorder is equally prevalent in both genders, although a higher incidence is associated with higher socioeconomic status. There is also high comorbidity of alcohol and substance dependence; however, the mechanisms of this cooccurrence are not clear.

The etiology of bipolar disorder is multifaceted, consisting of genetic and environmental factors. Current studies indicate that familial factors are the most important predictors for occurrence. Familial factors include shared genetic material, congenital factors, and physiological and psychological environmental factors. Some researchers hypothesize that neurotransmitter, neuroendocrine, neuroanatomical and physiological factors play important roles in pathogenesis.

The medical model of symptom assessment, disorder diagnosis and outcome-oriented treatment directs the treatment and choice of modalities for bipolar disorder. Common approaches include mood-stabilizing agents, antidepressants, anticonvulsants and electroconvulsive therapy (ECT), as well as psychotherapy and psychoeducation. Psychoeducation should be adjusted to the patient's culture and motivational factors; effective therapy should include both general knowledge of the disorder as well as exploration of individual specific needs.

Reference:

Bauer, M. S. (1997). Bipolar disorders. In S. M. Goldfinder, et. al. (Eds), *Tasman: Psychiatry* (1st ed. chap. 53). St. Louis, MO: W. B. Saunders Company.

From the perspective of TCM, bipolar disorder is a result of disequilibrium between the yin and yang. Preponderance of either the yin or yang determines the clinical presentations of mental disorders. Both an absolute and relative excess of the yang can lead to manic episodes, or *kuang*; whereas an absolute or relative excess of the yin can lead to depressive episodes, or *dian*. The etiopathology of yin-yang imbalance includes emotional stress, turbid phlegm, qi stagnation and blood stasis, heredity and a weak constitution.

Excessive anger, joy, pensiveness, sadness, worry, fear or shock can injure the internal organs. These emotions induce manic episodes when they transform into fire and disturb the mind; they lead to depressive episodes when they injure the spleen and cause secondary qi and blood deficiency, which fails to nourish the mind. When turbid phlegm covers the heart's orifice, mental clarity is impaired and awareness of reality and the ability to form judgments are lost, leading to abnormal behavior and depressed demeanor. While turbid phlegm is the major pathogenic factor causing depressive psychosis, turbid phlegm complicated by fire is the cause of manic behaviors. Qi stagnation and blood stasis in the brain due to head injury obstruct the flow of qi and cause disassociation between the internal organs and the brain. The brain is one of the organs controlling thinking and mental activities; when it is inadequately supplied with qi, it cannot properly manage the mind and manic-depressive psychosis can arise. The influence of miscellaneous causative factors, including heredity and constitution, should not be underestimated. Individuals with weaker constitutions are vulnerable to and unable to cope with emotional stress. Imbalance of the yin and yang is more likely to occur in these individuals and equilibrium is more difficult to restore; therefore, a weak constitution is associated with a higher risk of bipolar disorder. Family history is also relevant to the occurrence of mental disorders.

TCM recognizes and treats a disorder identical to bipolar disorder; refer to Chapter 23, "Manic-Depressive Psychosis", for comprehensive TCM differentiation and treatment of bipolar disorder (see page 157-162).

CHAPTER 78

Alzheimer's Disease

Dementia is a chronically debilitating disorder involving severe deterioration of intellectual function and cognitive skills, resulting in debility to perform ordinary activities of daily life. Traditionally, dementia has been classified as Alzheimer's or non-Alzheimer's type. More than 65% of dementias in the elderly are Alzheimer's disease. Alzheimer's disease is a chronic, progressive and inexorable loss of cognitive function. It is associated with excessive number of senile plaques in the cerebral cortex and subcortical gray matter. Four million Americans are diagnosed with Alzheimer's disease. The annual cost for medical and nursing care, social services, lost productivity and early death is approximately $90 billion. Alzheimer's disease also accounts for more than 50% of admissions into long-term care facility. The actual cause of Alzheimer's disease remains unclear. However, genetic influences seem to be possible. Approximately 15-20% of the cases are familial-related. Four distinct genes, located on chromosomes 1, 14, 19 and 21, are identified and they seem capable of influencing the initiation and progression of the disease. Environmental factors are still under research.

There are four clinical stages of Alzheimer's disease. Various progressive patterns may not be in any specific order. Early stage is characterized by loss of recent memory, inability to learn and retain new information, language problems, mood swings and personality changes. Complaints of difficulty in performing daily tasks are possible. In the intermediate stage, the above symptoms become worse, and remote memory is affected. Assistances in the activities of daily living (ADL) such as bathing, eating, dressing or toileting become a necessity. Behavioral disorganization, such as wandering, agitation and hostility, also manifests. Disorientation and confusion increase the risk of falls or accidents. When Alzheimer's disease progresses into the severe stage, patients may not be able to ambulate. Recent and remote memory is totally lost. Failing to perform ADL puts the patients under high risk of pressure sore, malnutrition and pneumonia. Mute is inevitable. At the end stage of Alzheimer's disease, motor impairment is severe. Coma and death resulting from infection may terminate the progression of this disease.

Diagnosis of Alzheimer's disease relies on history intake and physical examination (H&P), laboratory tests and exclusion of other causes of dementia. There is no known cure for Alzheimer's disease although temporarily memory improvement might be achieved with the use of cholinergic agonists at an early stage. Antioxidants, estrogen therapy, nonsteroidal anti-inflammatory drugs (NSAIDs) and Gingko biloba are still under study. Family education on disease progress is also important.

Reference:

Beers, M. H. & Berkow, R., et. al. (Eds.). (1999). Delirium and dementia: dementia. *The Merck Manual of Diagnosis and Therapy* (17th ed. chap. 171). West Point, PA: Merck & Co, Inc.

Based on the clinical manifestations, Alzheimer's disease can be categorized into TCM differentiation and treatment of dementia, or chi dai.

The presentations of Alzheimer's disease are very similar to that of dementia, *chi dai*, in TCM. *Chi dai*, dementia or retarded mental activities and disorientation, has been clearly described and documented in numerous ancient texts.

As early as in *Nei Jin*, partial manifestations and pathogeneses were elaborated. For instance, in *Ling Shu* Chapter 33, "Brain is sea of the marrow… sufficient sea of the marrow ensures rigorous strength, and intact voluntary movement and coordination of the body parts… deficient sea of the marrow causes dizziness, tinnitus, vertigo, soreness of the lower back, impaired visual acuity, weakness and loss of control to the body parts." In Ming dynasty, scholar Zhang, Jingyue first formally named this disorder *chi dai*. In Qing dynasty, the scholar, Chen, Shiduo, dedicated a single chapter to discuss *chi dai* as a distinctive disorder in his book, *Bian Zheng Lu*. According to this publication, *chi dai* is "Initiated by liver qi stagnation and ended as stomach qi failure; constrained liver leads to wood overacting on the earth; phlegm is accumulated in the chest and lodged around the heart; spirit is misted and the mind's function is deteriorated, manifested as *chi dai*." However, it was the other scholar, Wang, Qingren, during the Qing Dynasty, categorized *chi dai* into pathology of the brain, "Poor memory in children is caused by unfilled sea of the marrow since the development and growth has not been fully matured; however, poor memory in advanced age signifies a deficiency in sea of the marrow."

Conclude from the previous discussion, *chi dai*, or dementia, pertains to pathology of the heart and kidney; the spleen and liver also play significant roles to the pathogenesis. Deficiency of sea of the marrow results from multiple pathologies, including congenital deficiency, depletion due to chronic illness, and deterioration of the essence related to advanced age. Spleen and stomach deficiency with phlegm generation and emotional stress, induced liver constraint with qi stagnation and blood stasis, may contribute to the occurrence of *chi dai* by causing malnourishment of the mind or phlegm misting the clear orifices.

Analysis of Primary Symptom

Following the progression of the course, Alzheimer's disease is characterized by gradual diminishment to complete loss of the following basic physiological functions and activities:

A. Alteration in cognition:

Such as loss of memory, inability to learn and retain new information, disorientation and confusion, language problem and coma, these cognitive symptoms are closely related to dysfunction of the heart and kidney, phlegm misting the clear orifices and blood stasis obstruction.

- The statement, "Heart dominates the mind," clearly illustrates that the cognitive activities and consciousness are primarily governed by the heart. Heart blood deficiency will cause malnourishment of the mind; phlegm-turbidity misting the heart's orifice or blood stasis obstructing the heart's vessels will manifest with alteration of memory and cognition; the heart opens at the tongue; factors contributing to the heart's dysfunction may be observable as curled tongue, difficulty in speech, slurred speech or aphasia.
- "The kidney stores the essence, generates the marrow and fills up the brain." According to the publication, <u>Ben Cao Cong Xin</u>, by the scholar, Wang, Ang in Qing dynasty, "All memories are stored in the brain". He categorized the sensory function, such as memory, visual, auditory, olfactory and speech activities, into the responsibilities of the brain. Therefore, this disease may be elicited by empty sea of the marrow when the liver and kidney is insufficient or when kidney essence is deficient.

B. Behavioral disorganization:

Mood swing, depression, wandering, agitation and hostility can result from an excess or deficiency pattern. Excess pattern is constrained liver with qi stagnation or phlegm-qi complex due to emotional stress; deficient pattern is deficiency of both the spleen and heart due to injury of the mind by worry and grief.

- "The liver is in charge of the smooth flow of qi." Therefore, the liver assures proper coping mechanism. When liver qi is stagnant or phlegm-qi complex is formed, manifestations of congestion or suffocating sensation in the chest, distention and fullness in the chest and hypochondria, propensity to sighing, irritability and agitation are apparent.
- The physiological function of the spleen is closely related to activities of think-

ing. Overthinking and pensiveness may injure the spleen and heart. When both the spleen and heart are deficient or when the mind is injured by worry and grief, presentations of mood swing, depression and wandering will follow.

C. Motor dysfunction:

Motor dysfunctions consist of difficulty and inability in performing ADL, ambulating, and increased risk of falling. The spleen dominates the muscles; the liver dominates the sinews and the kidney dominates the bones. Qi and blood deficiency secondary to spleen insufficiency will lead to malnourishment of the muscles. Yin and essence insufficiency secondary to liver and kidney deficiency will cause failure of moistening the sinews and filling the bones. Motor dysfunctions follow the pathologies of the muscles, sinews and bones. These deficits will also exacerbate the condition caused by obstruction from phlegm-dampness or blood stasis. Implications from both deficiency and excess contribute to the progression of the course to a total loss of the motor ability.

Basic Patterns

- Liver and kidney depletion
- Deficiency of both the heart and spleen
- Liver contraint with blood deficiency
- Phlegm-turbidity obstructing the orifices
- Stasis obstruction in the collaterals of the brain

Progression of Pattern

Deficient pathogenesis is related to liver and kidney insufficiency with essence and blood deficiency. Excess pathogenesis is associated with phlegm-turbidity obstructing the orifices and blood stasis obstructing in the collaterals of the brain. Inter-transformation among these patterns is possible. Chronic liver qi stagnation leads to blood stasis, and follows the pattern of blood stasis obstructing in the collaterals in the brain; liver qi stagnation often overacts on the spleen; failure to transform and transport the dampness due to spleen deficiency will cause secondary phlegm accumulation, and the pattern of phlegm-turbidity obstructing the orifices then follows. Phlegm and stasis can further fuse together and elicit Alzheimer's disease. Although this disease has complicated pathogeneses, the root arises from depletion of the essence and blood.

Treatment Principle

The basic principle is to replenish the essence and fill the marrow. Adjunct tonifying approaches, based on various vital substance deficiencies in the heart, kidney, liver and spleen, are equally important. Treat the branch as the priority when excess symptom is obvious; treatments include facilitating the qi flow, transforming phlegm and invigorating the blood. Avoiding any unnecessary tonification prevents qi stagnation.

Pattern and Suggested Measure

Liver and kidney depletion

Apathy, dull eyes, dizziness, tinnitus, bradykinesia or akinesia, soreness and weakness of the lower back and knees, isolated aphasia, possible occasionally mute, inability to manage ADL, possible smiling or crying to self. Dusky tongue, and weak thready pulse.

- Nourish the kidney, replenish the essence, augment the marrow and strengthen the brain.
- Modified *Huan Shao Dan*

Shu Di Huang 10g.	*Shan Zhu Yu* 15g.	*Shan Yao* 10g.
Gou Qi Zi 15g.	*Chu Shi Zi* 10g.	*Du Zhong* 10g.
Niu Xi 10g.	*Rou Cong Rong* 6g.	*Ba Ji Tian* 6g.
Xiao Hui Xiang 6g.	*Wu Wei Zi* 10g.	*Yuan Zhi* 10g.
Shi Chang Pu 10g.	*Fu Ling* 10g.	

- Predominately yin deficiency. + *Gui Ban Jiao* 10g., *Nu Zhen Zi* 15g.
  Predominately yang deficiency. + *Lu Jiao Jiao* 10g., *Rou Gui* 6g.
  Unremitting exhaustion and depletion of the essence, and irresponsive to treatment. + *Ren Shen* 10g., *E Jiao* 10g., *Lu Rong* 3g.

Deficiency of both the heart and spleen

Wandering mind, apathy, bradykinesia, palpitations, shortness of breath, insomnia, forgetfulness, poor appetite and loose stool. Pale tongue, and thready pulse.

- Augment the qi, nourish the blood, tonify the heart and strengthen the spleen.
- Modified *Gui Pi Tang*

Huang Qi 15g.	*Dang Shen* 10g.	*Bai Zhu* 10g.
Dang Gui 10g.	*Suan Zao Ren* 10g.	*Long Yan Rou* 10g.
Fu Shen 15g.	*Yuan Zhi* 10g.	*Mu Xiang* 10g.

- Preponderance by blood deficiency. + *E Jiao* 10g., *He Shou Wu* 10g.
  Preponderance by qi deficiency. + *Ren Shen* 6g.

Liver constraint with blood deficiency

Apathy, wandering mind, propensity to sighing, melancholy, possible distention and fullness in the chest, irritability, impatience, short temper and insomnia. Pale tongue, and wiry thready pulse.

- Spread the constrained liver qi, nourish the heart and tonify the blood.
- Modified *Xiao Yao San* and *Gan Mai Da Zao Tang*

Chai Hu 10g.	*Dang Gui* 15g.	*Bai Shao* 15g.
Bai Zhu 10g.	*Fu Ling* 10g.	*Huai Xiao Mai* 15g.
Zhi Gan Cao 10g.	*Da Zao* 10g.	*Xiang Fu* 10g.
Fo Shou 6g.	*He Huan Pi* 10g.	*Bo He* 6g.

- Distention and pain in the chest and hypochondriac regions. + *Qing Pi* 10g., *Yu Jin* 10g.
  Irritability and insomnia. + *Ye Jiao Teng* 10g., *Suan Zao Ren* 10g.

Phlegm-turbidity obstructing the orifices

Depression, non-verbal or talking to self, self-isolation, disorientation to time, place and person, distention and fullness of the epigastrium and abdomen, poor appetite and vomiting clear fluids. White greasy tongue coating, and deep slippery pulse.

- Transform phlegm, open the orifices, strengthen the spleen and drain dampness.
- Modified *Wen Dan Tang*

Ban Xia 10g.	*Chen Pi* 10g.	*Fu Ling* 15g.
Bai Zhu 10g.	*Zhi Shi* 10g.	*Zhu Ru* 10g.
Shi Chang Pu 10g.	*Yuan Zhi* 10g.	*Long Chi* 30g.

- Distention and fullness in the epigastrium and abdomen with thick greasy tongue coating. + *Cang Zhu* 10g., *Hou Po* 10g.
  Accumulated phlegm turning into fire with yellow greasy tongue coating. + *Huang Lian* 10g., *Huang Qin* 10g.

Stasis obstruction in the collaterals of the brain

Longstanding condition, retarded mental activities, non-verbal or delusion, headache or distending headache, congested chest, impatience, slurred speech or aphasia, impairment or total loss of motor activities. Dark purple tongue with petechiae, and thready choppy pulse.

- Invigorate the blood, expel stasis, unblock the obstruction in the collaterals and open the orifices.
- Modified *Tong Qiao Huo Xue Tang*

Tao Ren 10g.	*Hong Hua* 10g.	*Chuan Xiong* 6g.
Chi Shao 15g.	*Cong Bai* 10g.	*Shi Chang Pu* 15g.
Yu Jin 10g.	*Di Long* 10g.	

- Chronic condition with qi and blood insufficiency. + *Huang Qi* 15g., *Dang Shen* 10g., *Dang Gui* 10g.

  Longstanding stasis transforming into heat with irritability and impatience. + *Gou Teng* 10g., *Ju Hua* 10g., *Xia Ku Cao* 6g.

Other Modality

A. Acupuncture:

- **Manipulation:** Even method, select one of the following three groups of points and alternate to different group daily for a therapeutic cycle of 15 days.
- **Prescription:**

❶ GV15 Yamen	PC8 Laogong	ST36 Zusanli	BL23 Shenshu
❷ GV14 Dazhui	CV15 Jiuwei	SP6 Sanyinjiao	KI1 Yongquan
❸ GV15 Yamen	Extra24 Shixuan	LI10 Shousanli	LR3 Taichong

B. Experiential remedies:

❶ Single effective herbs for improving memory:

Ci Wu Jia, *Chuan Xiong*, *Tu Si Zi*, *Huang Qi*, *He Shou Wu*, *Yuan Zhi*, *Gou Qi Zi*, *Du Zhong*.

❷ Common single herbs to decelerate aging:

Yin Yang Huo, *He Shou Wu*, *Yi Zhi Ren*, *Suo Yang*, *Bai Zhu*, *Huang Qi*, *Nu Zhen Zi*, *Tu Si Zi*, *Fu Ling*.

CHAPTER 79

Chronic Fatigue Syndrome

Chronic fatigue syndrome (CFS) is a debilitating and complex disorder with an unknown etiology. It is characterized by extreme fatigue that is not improved by bed rest and it may be aggravated by physical or mental activity. The diagnosis of CFS has to meet two criteria: 1) Having severe chronic fatigue for a minimum of six month's duration with all other possible diagnoses ruled out; and 2) concurrently experiencing at least four of the following symptoms: significant impairment of short-term memory or concentration, sore throat, tender lymph nodes, muscle pain, multi-joint pain without swelling or redness, headache, unrefreshing sleep, and post-exertional malaise lasting for more than 24 hours. Other commonly reported symptoms in CFS involve nonspecific gastrointestinal discomforts, various pains, respiratory or cardiologic symptoms, psychological complaints, paresthesias, and night sweating or weight loss.

Diagnosis of CFS requires excluding other possible medical conditions. Differential diagnoses, including fibromyalgia syndrome, myalgic encephalomyelitis, neurasthenia, multiple chemical sensitivities, and chronic mononucleosis, should be ruled out.

Current available evidence indicates that CFS can affect both genders and all ethnic groups. The causes of CFS are not identified yet. Some proposed theories suggest that viral infections, transient traumatic conditions, stress and toxins may be contributing factors. Researchers presume that immunology, the endocrine and nervous systems, and nutritional deficits may play important roles in the occurrence of CFS.

There is little known about CFS and there is much more needing to be explored. The course of CFS varies and the actual recovery rate is not estimated. Indeed, the definition of recovery is not yet determined and remains controversial. Due to its unexplained etiology, treatment for CFS consists of symptomatic management. The goal aims to re-establish energy, alleviate discomfort and regain pre-illness condition. Patients need to be informed that rapid recovery is not realistic.

References:

Centers of Disease Control and Prevention (2003). Chronic fatigue syndrome: CFS information. Retrieved on June 8, 2003 from http://www.cdc.gov/ncidod/diseases/cfs/info.htm

Centers of Disease Control and Prevention (2003). Chronic fatigue syndrome: Diagnosis of CFS. Retrieved on June 8, 2003 from http://www.cdc.gov/ncidod/diseases/cfs/diagnosis.htm

Centers of Disease Control and Prevention (2003). Chronic fatigue syndrome: Treatment. Retrieved on June 8, 2003 from http://www.cdc.gov/ncidod/diseases/cfs/treat.htm

National Institute of Allergy and Infectious Diseases (2001). Chronic fatigue syndrome. Retrieved on June 8, 2003 from http://niaid.nih.gov/factsheets/cfs.htm

CFS can be referred to TCM differentiation and treatment for consumptive deficiency, painful obstruction syndrome, headache and insomnia, according to the clinical manifestations.

As indicated by its name, CFS is characterized by longstanding tiredness or fatigue that is not alleviated by rest. TCM documentation of fatigue can be found in the disorders of consumptive deficiency. The first discussion of consumptive deficiency can be traced to Chapter 28 in Su Wen, which clearly stated that deprivation and consumption of essence and qi elicit deficiency; this statement is a concise description of consumptive deficiency. According to Chapter 13 in Su Wen, "Overuse of the eyes consumes the blood; prolonged reclining consumes the qi; longstanding sitting consumes the muscles; excessive standing consumes the bones; intensive ambulation consumes the sinews." Therefore, overexertion is the primary cause of consumptive deficiency.

The multifaceted clinical manifestations of CFS reflect the physiological dysfunctions of multiple organs and systems; quantitative insufficiency of vital substances may not be evident. The liver is the primary organ affected. Chapter 9 of Su Wen stated that "The liver is the root of extreme fatigue". The liver dominates the sinews, which connect the muscles to the bones, and motor functions. When the liver fails to nourish the sinews, patients will experience difficulty in or intolerance to activity, resulting in fatigue. In addition, from the holistic viewpoint of TCM, the internal organs are interdependent; deficiency of the liver can easily affect other organs. The liver stores the blood, which nourishes the internal and external organs. Malfunction of the liver leads to secondary dysfunction of the spleen, kidney, heart and lung. Etiologically, emotional stress, overexertion or exterior pathogenic factors contribute to the prevalence of CFS.

Although they share common clinical manifestations, i.e. chronic fatigue, CFS and consumptive deficiency have distinguishing qualities. Insufficiency of vital substances, including the qi, blood, yin and yang of various organs, comprises the primary pathogenesis of consumptive deficiency. It follows a chronic, consumptive and progressive course; thus, consumptive deficiency is a relatively severe condition with a poor prognosis. On the other hand, malfunction of multiple organs and systems comprises the primary pathogenesis of CFS. It is characterized by chronic persistent fatigue. When exertion exceeds physiological compensation, deficiency follows; thus, CFS may develop into consumptive deficiency.

Analysis of Primary Symptom

A. Unremitting chronic fatigue that is not relieved by rest:

Motor function relies on the following organs.

- The liver dominates the sinews; it is the root of extreme fatigue. The liver plays an important role in normal motor functions. Liver blood deficiency deprives the sinews of nourishment, leading to lack of strength and intolerance for exertion.
- The spleen dominates the muscles; it generates the qi and blood to nourish the extremities. Spleen deficiency with secondary insufficiency of the qi and blood manifests as soreness and weakness of the muscles; this is a deficient pattern. Excessive dampness hindering the spleen is considered an excess pattern; spleen qi stagnation secondary to heavy and sticky dampness manifests as heaviness and weakness of the extremities.
- The kidney dominates the bones; it resides in the lower back. In the case of kidney essence deficiency, there will be symptoms of soreness and weakness of the lower back and lack of strength to walk or stand. Sore and painful joints without redness or swelling are possible, a symptom of lack of marrow nourishing the bone.

B. Significant impairment of memory or concentration, and headache:

Impairment of memory, or forgetfulness, is related to debility of the brain.

- The kidney stores the essence that generates the marrow, which fills the brain. Depletion of kidney essence leads to secondary deprivation of the marrow, resulting in malnourishment of the brain. This pathology is reflected in the symptoms of forgetfulness and dull or empty headache. The functions of thinking and memorization also pertain to the spleen. Pensiveness, therefore, has a direct effect on the spleen and the heart, manifesting as insomnia or unrefreshing sleep, forgetfulness and trance. Patterns related to the kidney and spleen are obviously deficient in nature.
- Both liver qi stagnation secondary to emotional stress and spleen deficiency with excessive phlegm-dampness are excess patterns. Depression, irritability, insomnia, distending headache, and inability to concentrate result from liver qi stagnation; fatigue, lethargy and impairment of memory result from phlegm-dampness misting the clear orifice.

C. Tender lymph nodes:

Swollen or tender lymph nodes are known as phlegm-core or scrofula in TCM. Phlegm-core is a palpable, nodular accumulation of phlegm, distinct from a diffused accumulation of phlegm. They are precipitated by disturbance in water metabolism secondary to liver qi stagnation or spleen qi deficiency. When the accumulations of pathological derivatives, or tender lymph nodes, are located in the subcutaneous layer, they are called phlegm-cores; when phlegm-cores are located in the neck, they are more specifically called scrofula.

Basic Patterns

- Exterior pathogenic invasion in existing deficiency
- Spleen deficiency with liver qi stagnation
- Heart and spleen deficiency
- Spleen qi deficiency
- Liver and kidney essence deficiency

Progression of Pattern

Based on the theory of interdependence among the internal organs, patterns of CFS can inter-transform. Liver qi stagnation may overact on the spleen; spleen deficiency failing to generate the blood may result in heart and spleen deficiency. Liver yin insufficiency will affect the kidney essence and deficient kidney essence can lead to secondary liver yin deprivation, resulting in liver and kidney essence deficiency. Spleen qi deficiency causes unconsolidated protective qi, increasing the risk of contracting exterior pathogens due to deficiency. CFS involves multiple organ systems and multifaceted dysfunctions; consequently, complicated cases that reflect disharmony among multiple organs, the liver, the kidney, the spleen, the heart and the lung, are common in clinical practice.

Treatment Principle

Being a disorder with a deficient root and an excess branch, CFS derives from disharmony of the righteous qi, including the qi, blood, yin and yang, and manifests as secondary qi stagnation due to liver failing to ensure smooth qi flow and as secondary dampness obstruction due to accumulation of pathological derivatives. The treatment plan should support the righteous qi to expel pathogens, as well as restore the physiological functions of the organs.

Pattern and Suggested Measure

Exterior pathogenic invasion in existing deficiency

Fatigue, lassitude, fever, slight aversion to wind-cold, perspiration, itchy or sore throat, headache and body ache or muscle and joint pain, tender and swollen lymph nodes, and recurrent symptoms of common cold. Thin tongue coating and soft rootless pulse.

- Support the righteous qi and consolidate the surface; disperse wind and expel the pathogens.
- Modified *Shen Su Yin*

Dang Shen 10g.	*Fu Ling* 10g.	*Su Ye* 6g.
Ge Gen 15g.	*Qian Hu* 10g.	*Jie Geng* 6g.
Zhi Qiao 10g.	*Chen Pi* 10g.	*Gan Cao* 3g.

- Severe fever and aversion to cold. + *Fang Feng* 10g., *Jing Jie Sui* 6g.
  Muscle and joint pain. + *Qiang Huo* 10g., *Du Huo* 10g., *Chuan Xiong* 6g.
  Sore throat. + *Xing Ren* 10g., *Chan Tui* 6g.
  Qi deficiency with spontaneous sweating, aversion to wind, and recurrent common cold, use *Yu Ping Feng San*.
  Yin deficiency with exterior pathogens attacking, use *Jia Jian Wei Rui Tang*.

Spleen deficiency with liver qi stagnation

Fatigue and malaise, migrating hypochondriac pain or general body ache, depression, mood swings, sadness, crying spells or restlessness, irritability, short temper, insomnia, impairment of memory or concentration, poor appetite and abdominal distention. Pale tongue with thin coating, and wiry and thready pulse.

- Soothe the liver, regulate the qi flow and strengthen the spleen.
- Modified *Xiao Yao San*

Chai Hu 10g.	*Dang Gui* 10g.	*Bai Shao* 10g.
Bai Zhu 10g.	*Fu Ling* 15g.	*Huang Qi* 10g.
Chen Pi 10g.	*Dan Shen* 20g.	*Zhi Gan Cao* 6g.

- Severe distending hypochondriac pain. + *Yu Jin* 10g., *Xiang Fu* 10g.
  Severe muscle and joint pain. + *Mu Gua* 10g., *Sang Zhi* 10g., *Gui Zhi* 6g.
  Depression, frequent attacks of melancholy, and crying spells. + *Gan Mai Da Zao Tang*
  Restlessness, agitation and short temper with red tongue and rapid wiry pulse. + *Mu Dan Pi* 10g., *Zhi Zi* 10g.

Heart and spleen deficiency

Pale or sallow complexion, fatigue, malaise, lack of strength in the extremities, symptoms aggravated by exertion, palpitations, shortness of breath, insomnia or dream-disturbed sleep, unrefreshing sleep, impairment of memory or concentration, poor appetite, abdominal distention and loose stool. Pale tongue, and thready weak pulse.

- Benefit the qi and nourish the blood; strengthen the spleen and augment the heart.
- Modified *Gui Pi Tang*

Dang Shen 10g.	*Bai Zhu* 10g.	*Huang Qi* 10g.
Dang Gui 10g.	*Suan Zao Ren* 15g.	*Long Yan Rou* 10g.
Yuan Zhi 10g.	*Fu Shen* 15g.	*Mu Xiang* 10g.
Zhi Gan Cao 6g.		

- Heart blood deficiency with pale complexion and palpitations. + *Shu Di Huang* 10g., *E Jiao* 6g., *Wu Wei Zi* 10g.
  Severe insomnia or dream-disturbed sleep. + *Bai Zi Ren* 10g., *Ye Jiao Teng* 10g., *Long Gu* 30g., *Mu Li* 30g.

Spleen qi deficiency

Fatigue and malaise, muscle soreness and pain, shortness of breath, reluctance to speak, perspiration, subjective fever, symptoms worsening in the afternoon or post-exertion, lethargy or somnolence after meals, headache, dizziness, and loose stool. Pale tongue with thin white coating, and weak thready pulse.

- Tonify and lift the qi.
- Modified *Bu Zhong Yi Qi Tang*

Huang Qi 15g.	*Chai Hu* 10g.	*Sheng Ma* 10g.
Bai Zhu 10g.	*Dang Shen* 10g.	*Dang Gui* 10g.
Chen Pi 10g.	*Gan Cao* 6g.	

- Muscle soreness and pain. + *Mu Gua* 10g., *Bai Shao* 10g., *Sang Zhi* 10g.
  Heavy sensation in the extremities or head, and greasy tongue coating. + *Ban Xia* 10g., *Sha Ren* 6g., *Yi Yi Ren* 15g., *Fu Ling* 15g.

Liver and kidney essence deficiency

Weakness, fatigue, malaise, soreness and weakness in the lower back, knees and heels; dull and empty headache, malar flush, night sweating, dry mouth, sore throat and tender lymph nodes. Red tongue with scanty coating, and thready or rapid pulse.

- Tonify the liver and kidney, replenish the yin and essence.
- Modified *Da Bu Yuan Jian*

Ren Shen 10g.	*Shan Yao* 10g.	*Shu Di Huang* 10g.
Du Zhong 10g.	*Gou Qi Zi* 10g.	*Dang Gui* 10g.
Shan Zhu Yu 10g.	*Bai Shao* 10g.	*Huang Jing* 10g.
Zhi Gan Cao 6g.		

- Night sweating and malar flush. + *Mu Dan Pi* 10g., *Zhi Mu* 10g.
  Tender lymph nodes. + *Xuan Shen* 10g., *Mu Li* 30g.
  Soreness and weakness in the lower back, knees and heels or joints. + *Ba Ji Tian* 10g., *Niu Xi* 10g., *Ji Xue Teng* 10g.

Other Modality

Acupuncture:

- **Manipulation:** Reinforcing method and moxibustion for deficient patterns; reducing method for excess patterns.
- **Prescription:** GV20 Baihui; Extra6 Sishencong; LR3 Taichong; ST36 Zusanli; LI4 Hegu
- **Supplementary points based on patterns:**
  - Qi deficiency. + BL20 Pishu; LR13 Zhangmen; CV12 Zhongwan; CV6 Qihai
  - Blood deficiency. + CV4 Guanyuan; BL18 Ganshu; BL20 Pishu
  - Essence deficiency. + BL23 Shenshu; KI6 Zhaohai; BL18 Ganshu
  - Qi stagnation. + GB40 Qiuxu; LR14 Qimen
- **Supplementary points based on symptoms:**
  - Sore throat. + CV23 Lianquan; LI18 Futu; KI6 Zhaohai; LU7 Lieque
  - Tender lymph nodes. + TE10 Tianjing; LR13 Zhangmen
  - Forgetfulness. + BL15 Xinshu; BL20 Pishu; KI6 Zhaohai; BL23 Shenshu
  - Insomnia. + HT7 Shenmen; SP6 Sanyinjiao; Extra13 Anmian
  - Muscle and joint pain, refer to Chapter 31, "*Bi* Syndrome" (see page 217).

Index of Western Medical Diseases

D

E

F

G

H

I

R

S

T

U

V

X

Pinyin-Latin Cross Reference of Herb Names

A

A Wei . . . *Resina Ferulae*
Ai Ye . . . *Folium Artemisiae Argyi*
An Xi Xiang . . . *Benzoinum*

B

Ba Dou . . . *Fructus Crotonis*
Ba Ji Tian . . . *Radix Morindae Officinalis*
Bai Bian Dou . . . *Semen Lablab Album*
Bai Bu . . . *Radix Stemonae*
Bai Dou Kou . . . *Fructus Amomi Rotundus*
Bai Fan . . . *Alumen*
Bai Fu Zi . . . *Rhizoma Typhonii*
Bai Guo . . . *Semen Ginkgo*
Bai He . . . *Bulbus Lilii*
Bai Hua She . . . *Agkistrodon*
Bai Hua She She Cao . . . *Herba Hedyotidis Diffusae*
Bai Ji . . . *Rhizoma Bletillae*
Bai Ji Li . . . *Fructus Tribuli*
Bai Jiang Can . . . *Bombyx Batryticatus*
Bai Jiang Cao . . . *Herba cum Radice Patriniae*
Bai Jie Zi . . . *Semen Sinapis*
Bai Lian . . . *Radix Ampelopsis*
Bai Mao Gen . . . *Rhizoma Imperatae*
Bai Mu Er . . . *Fructificatio Tremellae Fuctformis*
Bai Qian . . . *Rhizoma Cynanchi Stauntonii*
Bai Shao . . . *Radix Paeoniae Alba*
Bai Tou Weng . . . *Radix Pulsatillae*
Bai Wei . . . *Radix Cynanchi Atrati*
Bai Xian Pi . . . *Cortex Dictamni*
Bai Zhi . . . *Radix Angelicae Dahuricae*
Bai Zhu . . . *Rhizoma Atractylodis Macrocephalae*
Bai Zi Ren . . . *Semen Platycladi*
Ban Bian Lian . . . *Herba Lobeliae Chinensis*
Ban Lan Gen . . . *Radix Isatidis*
Ban Xia . . . *Rhizoma Pinelliae*
Ban Zhi Lian . . . *Herba Scutellariae Barbatae*
Bei Sha Shen . . . *Radix Glehniae*
Bi Ba . . . *Fructus Piperis Longi*
Bi Xie . . . *Rhizoma Dioscoreae Septemlobae*
Bian Xu . . . *Herba Polygoni Avicularis*
Bie Jia . . . *Carapax Trionycis*
Bing Lang . . . *Semen Arecae*
Bing Pian . . . *Borneolum Syntheticum*
Bo He . . . *Herba Menthae*
Bu Gu Zhi . . . *Fructus Psoraleae*

C

Cang Er Zi . . . *Fructus Xanthii*
Cang Zhu . . . *Rhizoma Atractylodis*
Cao Dou Kou . . . *Semen Alpiniae Katsumadai*
Cao Guo . . . *Fructus Tsaoko*
Ce Bai Ye . . . *Cacumen Platycladi*
Chai Hu . . . *Radix Bupleuri*
Chan Tui . . . *Periostracum Cicadae*
Che Qian Zi . . . *Semen Plantaginis*

Chen Pi . . . . *Pericarpium Citri Reticulatae*
Chen Xiang . . *Lignum Aquilariae Resinatum*
Chi Shao . . . . *Radix Paeoniae Rubra*
Chi Shi Zhi . . . . *Halloysitum Rubrum*
Chi Xiao Dou . . . . *Semen Phaseoli*
Chong Wei Zi . . . . *Fructus Leonuri*
Chou Wu Tong . . . . *Folium et Ramulus Clerodendri Trichotomi*
Chu Shi Zi . . . . *Fructus Broussonetiae*
Chuan Bei Mu . *Bulbus Fritillariae Cirrhosae*
Chuan Lian Zi . . . . *Fructus Toosendan*
Chuan Niu Xi . . . . *Radix Cyathulae*
Chuan Shan Jia . . . . *Squama Manis*
Chuan Xin Lian . . . . . *Herba Andrographis*
Chuan Xiong . . . . *Rhizoma Chuanxiong*
Chui Pen Cao . . . . *Herba Sedi*
Chun Pi . . . . *Cortex Ailanthi*
Ci Shi . . . . *Magnetitum*
Ci Wu Jia . . . . *Radix et Caulis Acanthopanacis Senticosi*
Cong Bai . . . . *Bulbus Allii Fistulosi*

D

Da Fu Pi . . . . *Pericarpium Arecae*
Da Huang . . . . *Radix et Rhizoma Rhei*
Da Jiˇ . . . . *Radix Euphorbiae Pekinensis*
Da Ji` . . . . . *Herba seu Radix Cirsii Japonici*
Da Qing Ye . . . . *Folium Isatidis*
Da Zao . . . . *Fructus Jujubae*
Dai Mao . *Carapax Eretmochelydis Imbricatae*
Dai Zhe Shi . . . . *Haematitum*
Dan Dou Chi . . . . *Semen Sojae Preparatum*
Dan Nan Xing . . . . *Arisaema cum Bile*
Dan Shen . . . . . . *Radix Salviae Miltiorrhizae*
Dang Gui . . . . *Radix Angelicae Sinensis*
Dang Shen . . . . *Radix Codonopsis*
Deng Xin Cao . . . . *Medulla Junci*
Di Fu Zi . . . . *Fructus Kochiae*
Di Gu Pi . . . . *Cortex Lycii*
Di Long . . . . *Pheretima*
Di Yu . . . . *Radix Sanguisorbae*
Ding Xiang . . . . *Flos Caryophylli*
Dong Chong Xia Cao . . . . *Cordyceps*
Dong Guo Ren . . . . *Semen Benincasae*
Dong Kui Zi . . . . *Semen Abutili seu Malvae*
Du Huo . . . . . . *Radix Angelicae Pubescentis*
Du Zhong . . . . *Cortex Eucommiae*

E

E Jiao . . . . *Gelatinum Corii Asini*
E Zhu . . . . *Rhizoma Curcumae*
Er Cha . . . . *Catechu*

F

Fan Xie Ye . . . . *Folium Sennae*
Fang Feng . . . . *Radix Saposhnikoviae*
Fang Ji . . . . *Radix Stephaniae Tetrandrae*
Feng Mi . . . . *Mel*
Fo Shou . . . . . . *Fructus Citri Sarcodactylis*
Fu Hai Shi . . . . *Pumice*
Fu Ling . . . . *Poria*
Fu Ling Pi . . . . *Cortex Poria*
Fu Pen Zi . . . . *Fructus Rubi*
Fu Xiao Mai . . *Fructus Tritici Levis Immaturus*
Fu Zi . . . . *Radix Aconiti Lateralis Preparata*

G

Gan Cao . . . . *Radix Glycyrrhizae*
Gan Jiang . . . . *Rhizoma Zingiberis*
Gan Sui . . . . *Radix Kansui*
Gao Ben . . . . *Rhizoma Ligustici*
Gao Liang Jiang . . . . *Rhizoma Alpiniae Officinarum*
Ge Gen . . . . *Radix Puerariae*
Ge Jie . . . . *Gecko*
Gou Ji . . . . *Rhizoma Cibotii*
Gou Qi Zi . . . . *Fructus Lycii*
Gou Teng . . . . *Ramulus Uncariae cum Uncis*
Gu Jing Cao . . . . *Flos Eriocauli*
Gu Sui Bu . . . . *Rhizoma Drynariae*
Gu Ya . . . . . . *Fructus Setariae Germinatus*
Gua Lou . . . . *Fructus Trichosanthis*

Gua Lou Pi .....*Pericarpium Trichosanthis*
Gua Lou Ren ....*Semen Trichosanthis*
Guan Zhong ....
Rhizoma Dryopteris Crassirhizomatis
Gui Ban ....*Carapax et Plastrum Testudinis*
Gui Ban Jiao ....
Gelatinum Carapax et Plastrum Testudinis
Gui Zhi ....*Ramulus Cinnamomi*

H

Hai Feng Teng ....*Caulis Piperis Kadsurae*
Hai Ge Ke ..*Concha Meretricis seu Cyclinae*
Hai Jin Sha ....*Spora Lygodii*
Hai Piao Xiao ....*Endoconcha Sepiae*
Hai Tong Pi ....*Cortex Erythrinae*
Hai Zao ....*Sargassum*
Han Lian Cao ....*Herba Ecliptae*
Han Shui Shi ....*Calcitum*
He Huan Hua ....*Flos Albiziae*
He Huan Pi ....*Cortex Albiziae*
He Shou Wu ....*Radix Polygoni Multiflori*
He Ye ....*Folium Nelumbinis*
He Zi ....*Fructus Chebulae*
Hei Zhi Ma ....*Semen Sesami Nigrum*
Hong Hua ....*Flos Carthami*
Hou Po ......*Cortex Magnoliae Officinalis*
Hu Huang Lian ......*Rhizoma Picrorhizae*
Hu Lu Ba ....*Semen Trigonellae*
Hu Po ....*Succinum*
Hu Tao Rou ....*Semen Juglandis*
Hu Zhang ....*Rhizoma Polygoni Cuspidati*
Hua Jiao ....*Pericarpium Zanthoxyli*
Hua Ju Hong ....*Exocarpium Citri Grandis*
Hua Shi ....*Talcum*
Huai Hua ....*Flos Sophorae*
Huang Bai ....*Cortex Phellodendri*
Huang Jing ....*Rhizoma Polygonati*
Huang Lian ....*Rhizoma Coptidis*
Huang Qi ....*Radix Astragali*
Huang Qin ....*Radix Scutellariae*
Huo Ma Ren ....*Fructus Cannabis*
Huo Xiang ....*Herba Pogostemonis*

J

Ji Gu Cao ....*Herba Abri*
Ji Nei Jin ....
Endothelium Corneum Gigeriae Galli
Ji Xue Teng ....*Caulis Spatholobi*
Jiang Huang ...*Rhizoma Curcumae Longae*
Jiang Xiang .*Lignum Dalbergiae Odoriferae*
Jiao Mu ....*Semen Zanthoxyli*
Jie Geng ....*Radix Platycodonis*
Jin Fei Cao ....*Herba Inulae*
Jin Qian Cao ....*Herba Lysimachiae*
Jin Yin Hua ....*Flos Lonicerae*
Jin Ying Zi ......*Fructus Rosae Laevigatae*
Jing Jie ....*Herba Schizonepetae*
Jiu Zi ....*Semen Allii Tuberosi*
Ju He ....*Semen Citri Reticulatae*
Ju Hua ....*Flos Chrysanthemi*
Juan Bai ....*Herba Selaginellae*
Jue Ming Zi ....*Semen Cassiae*

K

Ku Ding Cha ....*Folium Ilicis Cornutae*
Ku Lian Pi ....*Cortex Meliae*
Ku Shen ......*Radix Sophorae Flavescentis*
Kuan Dong Hua ....*Flos Farfarae*
Kun Bu ....*Thallus Eckloniae*
Kun Bu ....*Thallus Laminariae*
Kun Ming Shan Hai Tang ....
Herba Begonia Yunnanensis

L

Lai Fu Zi ....*Semen Raphani*
Lei Gong Teng ..*Herba Tripterygium Wilfordii*
Li Zhi He ....*Semen Litchi*
Lian Fang ......*Receptaculum Nelumbinis*
Lian Qiao ....*Fructus Forsythiae*
Lian Xu ....*Stamen Nelumbinis*
Lian Zi ....*Semen Nelumbinis*
Lian Zi Xin ....*Plumula Nelumbinis*

Ling Xiao Hua . . . . *Flos Campsis*
Ling Yang Jiao . . . . *Cornu Saigae Tataricae*
Ling Zhi . . . . *Ganoderma*
Liu Huang . . . . *Sulfur*
Long Chi . . . . *Dens Draconis Fossilia*
Long Dan Cao . . . . *Radix Gentianae*
Long Gu . . . . *Os Draconis Fossilia*
Long Yan Rou . . . . *Arillus Longan*
Lu Feng Fang . . . . *Nidus Vespae*
Lu Gan Shi . . . . *Galamina*
Lu Gen . . . . *Rhizoma Phragmitis*
Lu Hui . . . . *Aloe*
Lu Jiao . . . . *Cornu Cervi*
Lu Jiao Jiao . . . . *Gelatinum Cornu Cervi*
Lu Jiao Shuang . *Cornu Cervi Degelatinatum*
Lu Rong . . . . . . *Cornu Cervi Pantotrichum*
Luo Bu Ma Ye . . . . . . *Folium Apocyni Veneti*
Luo Shi Teng . . . . . . *Caulis Trachelospermi*

M

Ma Bo . . . . *Lasiosphaera seu Calvatia*
Ma Chi Xian . . . . *Herba Portulacae*
Ma Dou Ling . . . . *Fructus Aristolochiae*
Ma Huang . . . . *Herba Ephedrae*
Ma Huang Gen . . . . *Radix Ephedrae*
Mai Men Dong . . . . . . *Radix Ophiopogonis*
Mai Ya . . . . *Fructus Hordei Germinatus*
Man Jing Zi . . . . *Fructus Viticis*
Mang Xiao . . . . *Natrii Sulfas*
Mei Gui Hua . . . . *Flos Rosae Rugosae*
Mi Meng Hua . . . . *Flos Buddlejae*
Mo Yao . . . . *Myrrha*
Mu Dan Pi . . . . *Cortex Moutan*
Mu Gua . . . . *Fructus Chaenomelis*
Mu Hu Die . . . . *Semen Oroxyli*
Mu Li . . . . *Concha Ostreae*
Mu Tong . *Caulis Aristolochiae Manshuriensis*
Mu Xiang . . . . *Radix Aucklandiae*

N

Nan Sha Shen . . . . *Radix Adenophorae*
Niu Bang Zi . . . . *Fructus Arctii*
Niu Huang . . . . *Calculus Bovis*
Niu Xi . . . . . . *Radix Achyranthis Bidentatae*
Nu Zhen Zi . . . . *Fructus Ligustri Lucidi*

O

Ou Jie . . . . . . *Nodus Nelumbinis Rhizomatis*

P

Pang Da Hai . *Semen Sterculiae Lychnohorae*
Pao Jiang . . *Rhizoma Zingiberis Preparatum*
Pei Lan . . . . *Herba Eupatorii*
Pi Pa Ye . . . . *Folium Eriobotryae*
Pu Gong Ying . . . . *Herba Taraxaci*
Pu Huang . . . . *Pollen Typhae*

Q

Qian Cao . . . . *Radix Rubiae*
Qian Hu . . . . *Radix Peucedani*
Qian Nian Jian . . . . *Rhizoma Homalomenae*
Qian Niu Zi . . . . *Semen Pharbitidis*
Qian Shi . . . . *Semen Euryales*
Qiang Huo . . . *Rhizoma et Radix Notopterygii*
Qin Jiao . . . *Radix Gentianae Macrophyllae*
Qin Pi . . . . *Cortex Fraxini*
Qing Dai . . . . *Indigo Naturalis*
Qing Fen . . . . *Calomelas*
Qing Feng Teng . . . . *Caulis Sinomenii*
Qing Hao . . . . *Herba Artemisiae Annuae*
Qing Meng Shi . . . . *Lapis Chloriti*
Qing Mu Xiang . . . . *Radix Aristolochiae*
Qing Pi . *Pericarpium Citri Reticulatae Viride*
Qing Xiang Zi . . . . *Semen Celosiae*
Qu Mai . . . . *Herba Dianthi*
Quan Xie . . . . *Scorpio*

R

Ren Dong Teng . . . . *Caulis Lonicerae*
Ren Shen . . . . *Radix Ginseng*
Rou Cong Rong . . . . *Herba Cistanches*
Rou Dou Kou . . . . *Semen Myristicae*
Rou Gui . . . . *Cortex Cinnamomi*
Ru Xiang . . . . *Resina Olibani*

S

San Leng ... *Rhizoma Sparganii*
San Qi ... *Radix Notoginseng*
Sang Bai Pi ... *Cortex Mori*
Sang Ji Sheng ... *Herba Taxilli*
Sang Piao Xiao ... *Ootheca Mantidis*
Sang Shen ... *Fructus Mori*
Sang Ye ... *Folium Mori*
Sang Zhi ... *Ramulus Mori*
Sha Ren ... *Fructus Amomi*
Sha Yuan Zi ... *Semen Astragali Complanati*
Shan Ci Gu ... *Pseudobulbus Cremastrae seu Pleiones*
Shan Dou Gen ... *Radix Sophorae Tonkinensis*
Shan Yang Jiao ... *Cornu Naemorhedus Goral*
Shan Yao ... *Rhizoma Dioscoreae*
Shan Zha ... *Fructus Crataegi*
Shan Zhu Yu ... *Fructus Corni*
Shang Lu ... *Radix Phytolaccae*
She Chuang Zi ... *Fructus Cnidii*
She Gan ... *Rhizoma Belamcandae*
She Xiang ... *Moschus*
Shen Jin Cao ... *Herba Lycopodii*
Shen Qu ... *Massa Fermentata*
Sheng Di Huang ... *Radix Rehmanniae*
Sheng Jiang ... *Rhizoma Zingiberis Recens*
Sheng Jiang Pi ... *Cortex Zingiberis Recens*
Sheng Ma ... *Rhizoma Cimicifugae*
Shi Chang Pu ... *Rhizoma Acori Tatarinowii*
Shi Di ... *Calyx Kaki*
Shi Gao ... *Gypsum Fibrosum*
Shi Hu ... *Herba Dendrobii*
Shi Jue Ming ... *Concha Haliotidis*
Shi Jun Zi ... *Fructus Quisqualis*
Shi Liu Pi ... *Pericarpium Granati*
Shi Shu Ye ... *Folium Kaki*
Shi Wei ... *Folium Pyrrosiae*
Shu Di Huang ... *Radix Rehmanniae Preparata*
Shui Niu Jiao ... *Cornu Bubali*
Si Gua Luo ... *Retinervus Luffae Fructus*
Song Zi Ren ... *Semen Pini*
Su He Xiang ... *Styrax*
Su Mu ... *Lignum sappan*
Su Zi ... *Fructus Perillae*
Suan Zao Ren ... *Semen Ziziphi Spinosae*
Suo Yang ... *Herba Cynomorii*

T

Tai Zi Shen ... *Radix Pseudostellariae*
Tan Xiang ... *Lignum Santali Albi*
Tao Ren ... *Semen Persicae*
Tian Hua Fen ... *Radix Trichosanthis*
Tian Ji Huang ... *Herba Hyperici Japonici*
Tian Ma ... *Rhizoma Gastrodiae*
Tian Men Dong ... *Radix Asparagi*
Tian Nan Xing ... *Rhizoma Arisaematis*
Tian Zhu Huang ... *Concretio Silicea Bambusae*
Ting Li Zi ... *Semen Descurainiae*
Ting Li Zi ... *Semen Lepidii*
Tong Cao ... *Medulla Tetrapanacis*
Tu Da Huang ... *Radix Rumex Madaio*
Tu Fu Ling ... *Rhizoma Smilacis Glabrae*
Tu Si Zi ... *Semen Cuscutae*

W

Wa Leng Zi ... *Concha Arcae*
Wang Bu Liu Xing ... *Semen Vaccariae*
Wei ling Xian ... *Radix Clematidis*
Wu Bei Zi ... *Galla Chinensis*
Wu Gong ... *Scolopendra*
Wu Jia Pi ... *Cortex Acanthopanacis*
Wu Ling Zhi ... *Excrementum Trogopteri seu Pteromi*
Wu Mei ... *Fructus Mume*
Wu Shao She ... *Zaocys*
Wu Tou ... *Radix Aconiti*
Wu Wei Zi ... *Fructus Schisandrae Chinensis*
Wu Yao ... *Radix Linderae*
Wu Zhu Yu ... *Fructus Evodiae*

X

Xi Hong Hua . . . . *Stigma Croci*
Xi Jiao . . . . *Cornu Rhinoceri*
Xi Xian Cao . . . . *Herba Siegesbeckiae*
Xi Xin . . . . *Herba Asari*
Xi Yang Shen . . *Radix Panacis Quinquefolii*
Xia Ku Cao . . . . *Spica Prunellae*
Xia Tian Wu *Rhizoma Corydalis Decumbentis*
Xian He Cao . . . . *Herba Agrimoniae*
Xian Mao . . . . *Rhizoma Curculiginis*
Xiang Fu . . . . *Rhizoma Cyperi*
Xiang Ru . . . . *Herba Moslae*
Xiang Yuan . . . . *Fructus Citri*
Xiao Hui Xiang . . . . *Fructus Foeniculi*
Xiao Ji . . . . *Herba Cirsii*
Xiao Mai . . . . *Fructus Tritici Levis*
Xie Bai . . . . . . *Bulbus Allii Macrostemonis*
Xin Yi Hua . . . . *Flos Magnoliae*
Xing Ren . . . . *Semen Armeniacae Amarum*
Xiong Huang . . . . *Realgar*
Xu Chang Qing . . . *Radix Cynanchi Paniculati*
Xu Duan . . . . *Radix Dipsaci*
Xuan Fu Hua . . . . *Flos Inulae*
Xuan Shen . . . . *Radix Scrophulariae*
Xue Jie . . . . *Sanguis Draxonis*

Y

Yan Hu Suo . . . . *Rhizoma Corydalis*
Ye Jiao Teng . . . *Caulis Polygoni Multiflori*
Ye Ju Hua . . . . . . *Flos Chrysanthemi Indici*
Yi Mu Cao . . . . *Herba Leonuri*
Yi Tang . . . . *Saccharum Granorum*
Yi Yi Ren . . . . *Semen Coicis*
Yi Zhi Ren . . . *Fructus Alpiniae Oxyphyllae*
Yin Chai Hu . . . . *Radix Stellariae*
Yin Chen Hao . *Herba Artemisiae Scopariae*
Yin Xing Ye . . . . *Folium Ginkgo*
Yin Yang Huo . . . . *Herba Epimedii*
Yu Jin . . . . *Radix Curcumae*
Yu Li Ren . . . . *Semen Pruni*
Yu Xing Cao . . . . *Herba Houttuyniae*
Yu Zhu . . . . . . *Rhizoma Polygonati Odorati*
Yuan Hua . . . . *Flos Genkwa*
Yuan Zhi . . . . *Radix Polygalae*

Z

Zao Jiao Ci . . . . *Spina Gleditsiae*
Zao Xin Tu . . . . *Terra Flava Usta*
Ze Lan . . . . *Herba Lycopi*
Ze Xie . . . . *Rhizoma Alismatis*
Zhe Bei Mu . . *Bulbus Fritillariae Thunbergii*
Zhe Chong . . . *Eupolyphaga seu Steleophaga*
Zhen Zhu . . . . *Margarita*
Zhen Zhu Mu . . . . . . *Concha Margaritifera*
Zhi Cao Wu . . . .
Radix Aconiti Kusnezoffii Preparata
Zhi Chuan Wu . . . *Radix Aconiti Preparapa*
Zhi Gan Cao . . *Radix Glycyrrhizae Preparata*
Zhi Mu . . . . *Rhizoma Anemarrhenae*
Zhi Qiao . . . . *Fructus Aurantii*
Zhi Shi . . . . *Fructus Aurantii Immaturus*
Zhi Zi . . . . *Fructus Gardeniae*
Zhong Jie Feng . . . . *Herba Sarcandrae*
Zhu Ling . . . . *Polyporus*
Zhu Ru . . . . *Caulis Bambusae in Taenia*
Zhu Sha . . . . *Cinnabaris*
Zhu Ye . . . . *Herba Lophatheri*
Zi Bei Tian Kui . . . .
Herba Begonie Fimbristipulatae
Zi Cao . . . . *Radix Arnebiae*
Zi Cao . . . . *Radix Lithospermi*
Zi He Che . . . . *Placenta Hominis*
Zi Hua Di Ding . . . . *Herba Violae*
Zi Shi Ying . . . . *Fluoritum*
Zi Su Geng . . . . *Caulis Perillae*
Zi Su Ye . . . . *Folium Perillae*
Zi Wan . . . . *Radix Asteris*
Zi Wei . . . . *Flos Lagerstroemia Indica*
Zi Zhu Cao . *Herba Callicarpae Formosanae*
Zong Lu . . . . *Petiolus Trachycarpi*

List of Formulas by Pinyin

(Herbs in the following formulas are presented by Pinyin name, followed by the abbreviated Latin pharmaceutical name. Refer to page 547 for a list of common abbreviations.)

A

An Gong Niu Huang Wan:

Niu Huang *Calculus Bovis*
Yu Jin *Rx. Curcumae*
Xi Jiao *Cornu Rhinoceri*
Huang Lian *Rz. Coptidis*
Zhu Sha *Cinnabaris*
Bing Pian *Borneolum Syntheticum*
Zhen Zhu *Margarita*
Zhi Zi *Fr. Gardenia*
Xiong Huang *Realgar*
Huang Qin *Rx. Scutellariae*
She Xiang *Moschus*

An Shen Ding Zhi Wan:

Fu Ling *Poria*
Fu Shen *Sclerotium Poriae Pararadicis*
Yuan Zhi *Rx. Polygalae*
Ren Shen *Rx. Ginseng*
Shi Chang Pu *Rz. Acori Tatarinowii*
Long Chi *Dens Draconis Fossilia*

B

Ba Zhen Tang:

Ren Shen *Rx. Ginseng*
Bai Zhu *Rz. Atractylodis Macrocephala*
Fu Ling *Poria*
Gan Cao *Rx. Glycyrrhizae*
Dang Gui *Rx. Angelicae Sinensis*
Bai Shao *Rx. Paeoniae Alba*
Chuan Xiong *Rz. Chuanxiong*
Shu Di Huang *Rx. Rehmanniae Preparata*
Sheng Jiang *Rz. Zingiberis Recens*
Da Zao *Fr. Jujubae*

Ba Zheng San:

Mu Tong *Caulis Aristolochiae Manshuriensis*
Che Qian Zi *Sm. Plantaginis*
Bian Xu *Hb. Polygoni Avicularis*
Qu Mai *Hb. Dianthi*
Hua Shi *Talcum*
Gan Cao Shao *Rx. Glycyrrhizae*
Da Huang *Rx. et Rz. Rhei*
Zhi Zi *Fr. Gardenia*
Deng Xin Cao *Medulla Junci*

Bai He Gu Jin Wan:

Sheng Di Huang *Rx. Rehmanniae*
Shu Di Huang *Rx. Rehmanniae Preparata*
Mai Men Dong *Rx. Ophiopogonis*
Bei Mu *Blb. Fritillariae Thunbergii*
Bai He *Blb. Lilii*
Dang Gui *Rx. Angelicae Sinensis*
Bai Shao *Rx. Paeoniae Alba*
Gan Cao *Rx. Glycyrrhizae*
Xuan Shen *Rx. Scrophulariae*
Jie Geng *Rx. Platycodonis*

Bai Hu Jia Gui Zhi Tang:

Shi Gao *Gypsum Fibrosum*
Zhi Mu *Rz. Anemarrhenae*

Gan Cao *Rx. Glycyrrhizae*
Jing Mi *Nonglutinous Rice*
Gui Zhi *Rml. Cinnamomi*

Bai Hu Jia Ren Shen Tang:
Shi Gao *Gypsum Fibrosum*
Zhi Mu *Rz. Anemarrhenae*
Gan Cao *Rx. Glycyrrhizae*
Jing Mi *Nonglutinous Rice*
Ren Shen *Rx. Ginseng*

Bai Hu Tang:
Shi Gao *Gypsum Fibrosum*
Zhi Mu *Rz. Anemarrhenae*
Gan Cao *Rx. Glycyrrhizae*
Jing Mi *Nonglutinous Rice*

Bai Tou Weng Tang:
Bai Tou Weng *Rx. Pulsatillae*
Qin Pi *Cx. Fraxini*
Huang Lian *Rz. Coptidis*
Huang Bai *Cx. Phellodendri*

Ban Xia Bai Zhu Tian Ma Tang:
Ban Xia *Rz. Pinelliae*
Bai Zhu *Rz. Atractylodis Macrocephala*
Tian Ma *Rz. Gastrodiae*
Chen Pi *Pc. Citri Reticulatae*
Fu Ling *Poria*
Gan Cao *Rx. Glycyrrhizae*
Sheng Jiang *Rz. Zingiberis Recens*
Da Zao *Fr. Jujubae*

Ban Xia Hou Po Tang:
Ban Xia *Rz. Pinelliae*
Hou Po *Cx. Magnoliae Officinalis*
Zi Su Ye *Fm. Perillae*
Fu Ling *Poria*
Sheng Jiang *Rz. Zingiberis Recens*

Bao He Wan:
Shen Qu *Massa Fermentata*
Shan Zha *Fr. Crataegi*
Fu Ling *Poria*
Ban Xia *Rz. Pinelliae*
Chen Pi *Pc. Citri Reticulatae*
Lai Fu Zi *Sm. Raphani*
Lian Qiao *Fr. Forsythiae*

Bie Jia Jian Wan:
Bie Jia *Carapax Trionycis*
She Gan *Rz. Belamcandae*
Huang Qin *Rx. Scutellariae*
Gan Jiang *Rz. Zingiberis*
Da Huang *Rx. et Rz. Rhei*
Gui Zhi *Rml. Cinnamomi*
Shi Wei *Fm. Pyrrosiae*
Hou Po *Cx. Magnoliae Officinalis*
Qu Mai *Hb. Dianthi*
Zi Wei *Fl. Lagerstroemia Indica*
E Jiao *Gelatinum Corii Asini*
Chai Hu *Rx. Bupleuri*
Shao Yao *Rx. Paeoniae Alba*
Mu Dan Pi *Cx. Moutan*
Zhe Chong *Eupolyphaga seu Steleophaga*
Lu Feng Fang *Nidus Vespae*
Mang Xiao *Natrii Sulfas*
Tao Ren *Sm. Persicae*
Ren Shen *Rx. Ginseng*
Ban Xia *Rz. Pinelliae*
Ting Li Zi *Sm. Descurainiae*

Bu Fei Tang:
Ren Shen *Rx. Ginseng*
Huang Qi *Rx. Astragali*
Shu Di Huang *Rx. Rehmanniae Preparata*
Wu Wei Zi *Fr. Schisandrae Chinensis*
Zi Wan *Rx. Asteris*
Sang Bai Pi *Cx. Mori*

Bu Yang Huan Wu Tang:
Huang Qi *Rx. Astragali*
Dang Gui Wei *Rx. Angelicae Sinensis*
Chuan Xiong *Rz. Chuanxiong*
Tao Ren *Sm. Persicae*
Hong Hua *Fl. Carthami*
Chi Shao *Rx. Paeoniae Rubra*
Di Long *Pheretima*

Bu Zhong Yi Qi Tang:

Ren Shen *Rx. Ginseng*
Huang Qi *Rx. Astragali*
Bai Zhu *Rz. Atractylodis Macrocephala*
Gan Cao *Rx. Glycyrrhizae*
Dang Gui *Rx. Angelicae Sinensis*
Chen Pi *Pc. Citri Reticulatae*
Sheng Ma *Rz. Cimicifugae*
Chai Hu *Rx. Bupleuri*

C

Chai Ge Jie Ji Tang:

Chai Hu *Rx. Bupleuri*
Ge Gen *Rx. Puerariae*
Gan Cao *Rx. Glycyrrhizae*
Huang Qin *Rx. Scutellariae*
Qing Hao *Hb. Artemisiae Annuae*
Bai Zhi *Rx. Angelicae Dahuricae*
Shao Yao *Rx. Paeoniae Alba*
Jie Geng *Rx. Platycodonis*

Chai Hu Shu Gan San:

Chai Hu *Rx. Bupleuri*
Zhi Qiao *Fr. Aurantii*
Xiang Fu *Rz. Cyperi*
Shao Yao *Rx. Paeoniae Alba*
Chuan Xiong *Rz. Chuanxiong*
Gan Cao *Rx. Glycyrrhizae*

Chen Xiang San:

Chen Xiang *Lignum Aquilariae Resinatum*
Shi Wei *Fm. Pyrrosiae*
Hua Shi *Talcum*
Dang Gui *Rx. Angelicae Sinensis*
Chen Pi *Pc. Citri Reticulatae*
Bai Shao *Rx. Paeoniae Alba*
Dong Kui Zi *Sm. Abutili seu Malvae*
Wang Bu Liu Xing *Sm. Vaccariae*

Cheng Shi Bi Xie Fen Qing Yin:

Bi Xie *Rz. Dioscoreae Septemlobae*
Che Qian Zi *Sm. Plantaginis*
Fu Ling *Poria*
Lian Zi Xin *Plumula Nelumbinis*
Shi Chang Pu *Rz. Acori Tatarinowii*
Huang Bai *Cx. Phellodendri*
Dan Shen *Rx. Salviae Miltiorrhizae*
Bai Zhu *Rz. Atractylodis Macrocephala*

Chuan Xiong Cha Tiao San:

Chuan Xiong *Rz. Chuanxiong*
Jing Jie *Hb. Schizonepetae*
Bo He *Hb. Menthae*
Qiang Huo *Rz. et Rx. Notopterygii*
Xi Xin *Hb. Asari*
Bai Zhi *Rx. Angelicae Dahuricae*
Gan Cao *Rx. Glycyrrhizae*
Fang Feng *Rx. Saposhnikoviae*

D

Da Bu Yin Wan:

Zhi Mu *Rz. Anemarrhenae*
Huang Bai *Cx. Phellodendri*
Shu Di Huang *Rx. Rehmanniae Preparata*
Gui Ban *Carapax et Plastrum Testudinis*
Zhu Ji Sui *Pork Spinal Cord*

Da Bu Yuan Jian:

Ren Shen *Rx. Ginseng*
Shan Yao *Rz. Dioscoreae*
Shu Di Huang *Rx. Rehmanniae Preparata*
Du Zhong *Cx. Eucommiae*
Gou Qi Zi *Fr. Lycii*
Dang Gui *Rx. Angelicae Sinensis*
Shan Zhu Yu *Fr. Corni*
Zhi Gan Cao *Rx. Glycyrrhizae Preparata*

Da Chai Hu Tang:

Chai Hu *Rx. Bupleuri*
Huang Qin *Rx. Scutellariae*
Ban Xia *Rz. Pinelliae*
Zhi Shi *Fr. Aurantii Immaturus*
Bai Shao *Rx. Paeoniae Alba*
Da Huang *Rx. et Rz. Rhei*
Sheng Jiang *Rz. Zingiberis Recens*
Da Zao *Fr. Jujubae*

Da Cheng Qi Tang:

Da Huang *Rx. et Rz. Rhei*
Mang Xiao *Natrii Sulfas*
Hou Po *Cx. Magnoliae Officinalis*
Zhi Shi *Fr. Aurantii Immaturus*

Da Ding Feng Zhu:

Bai Shao *Rx. Paeoniae Alba*
E Jiao *Gelatinum Corii Asini*
Sheng Gui Ban *Carapax et Plastrum Testudinis*
Sheng Bie Jia *Carapax Trionycis*
Sheng Di Huang *Rx. Rehmanniae*
Huo Ma Ren *Fr. Cannabis*
Wu Wei Zi *Fr. Schisandrae Chinensis*
Sheng Mu Li *Concha Ostreae*
Mai Men Dong *Rx. Ophiopogonis*
Zhi Gan Cao *Rx. Glycyrrhizae Preparata*
Ji Zi Huang *Egg Yolk*

Da Jian Zhong Tang:

Chuan Jiao *Pc. Zanthoxyli*
Gan Jiang *Rz. Zingiberis*
Ren Shen *Rx. Ginseng*
Yi Tang *Saccharum Granorum*

Da Qin Jiao Tang:

Qin Jiao *Rx. Gentianae Macrophyllae*
Dang Gui *Rx. Angelicae Sinensis*
Gan Cao *Rx. Glycyrrhizae*
Qiang Huo *Rz. et Rx. Notopterygii*
Fang Feng *Rx. Saposhnikoviae*
Bai Zhi *Rx. Angelicae Dahuricae*
Shu Di Huang *Rx. Rehmanniae Preparata*
Fu Ling *Poria*
Shi Gao *Gypsum Fibrosum*
Chuan Xiong *Rz. Chuanxiong*
Bai Shao *Rx. Paeoniae Alba*
Du Huo *Rx. Angelicae Pubescentis*
Huang Qin *Rx. Scutellariae*
Sheng Di Huang *Rx. Rehmanniae*
Bai Zhu *Rz. Atractylodis Macrocephala*
Xi Xin *Hb. Asari*

Dai Di Dang Wan:

Da Huang *Rx. et Rz. Rhei*
Dang Gui Wei *Rx. Angelicae Sinensis*
Sheng Di Huang *Rx. Rehmanniae*
Chuan Shan Jia *Squama Manis*
Mang Xiao *Natrii Sulfas*
Tao Ren *Sm. Persicae*
Rou Gui *Cx. Cinnamomi*

Dai Ge San:

Qing Dai *Indigo Naturalis*
Hai Ge Ke *Concha Meretricis seu Cyclinae*

Dan Shen Yin:

Dan Shen *Rx. Salviae Miltiorrhizae*
Tan Xiang *Lignum Santali Albi*
Sha Ren *Fr. Amomi*

Dan Zhi Xiao Yao San:

Dang Gui *Rx. Angelicae Sinensis*
Bai Shao *Rx. Paeoniae Alba*
Bai Zhu *Rz. Atractylodis Macrocephala*
Chai Hu *Rx. Bupleuri*
Fu Ling *Poria*
Gan Cao *Rx. Glycyrrhizae*
Sheng Jiang *Rz. Zingiberis Recens*
Bo He *Hb. Menthae*
Mu Dan Pi *Cx. Moutan*
Zhi Zi *Fr. Gardenia*

Dang Gui Bu Xue Tang:

Huang Qi *Rx. Astragali*
Dang Gui *Rx. Angelicae Sinensis*

Dang Gui Liu Huang Tang:

Dang Gui *Rx. Angelicae Sinensis*
Sheng Di Huang *Rx. Rehmanniae*
Shu Di Huang *Rx. Rehmanniae Preparata*
Huang Lian *Rz. Coptidis*
Huang Qin *Rx. Scutellariae*
Huang Bai *Cx. Phellodendri*
Huang Qi *Rx. Astragali*

Dang Gui Long Hui Wan:

Dang Gui *Rx. Angelicae Sinensis*
Long Dan Cao *Rx. Gentianae*
Zhi Zi *Fr. Gardenia*
Huang Lian *Rz. Coptidis*
Huang Qin *Rx. Scutellariae*
Huang Bai *Cx. Phellodendri*
Da Huang *Rx. et Rz. Rhei*
Qing Dai *Indigo Naturalis*
Lu Hui *Aloe*
Mu Xiang *Rx. Aucklandia*
She Xiang *Moschus*

Dao Chi San:

Sheng Di Huang *Rx. Rehmanniae*
Mu Tong *Caulis Aristolochiae Manshuriensis*
Zhu Ru *Caulis Bambusae in Taenia*
Gan Cao *Rx. Glycyrrhizae*

Dao Tan Tang:

Ban Xia *Rz. Pinelliae*
Chen Pi *Pc. Citri Reticulatae*
Zhi Shi *Fr. Aurantii Immaturus*
Fu Ling *Poria*
Gan Cao *Rx. Glycyrrhizae*
Tian Nan Xing *Rz. Arisaematis*

Di Huang Yin Zi:

Sheng Di Huang *Rx. Rehmanniae*
Ba Ji Tian *Rx. Morindae Officinalis*
Shan Zhu Yu *Fr. Corni*
Shi Hu *Hb. Dendrobii*
Rou Cong Rong *Hb. Cistanches*
Wu Wei Zi *Fr. Schisandrae Chinensis*
Rou Gui *Cx. Cinnamomi*
Fu Ling *Poria*
Mai Men Dong *Rx. Ophiopogonis*
Pao Fu Zi *Rx. Aconiti Lateralis Preparata*
Shi Chang Pu *Rz. Acori Tatarinowii*
Yuan Zhi *Rx. Polygalae*
Sheng Jiang *Rz. Zingiberis Recens*
Da Zao *Fr. Jujubae*
Bo He *Hb. Menthae*

Di Tan Tang:

Ban Xia *Rz. Pinelliae*
Tian Nan Xing *Rz. Arisaematis*
Chen Pi *Pc. Citri Reticulatae*
Zhi Shi *Fr. Aurantii Immaturus*
Fu Ling *Poria*
Ren Shen *Rx. Ginseng*
Shi Chang Pu *Rz. Acori Tatarinowii*
Zhu Ru *Caulis Bambusae in Taenia*
Gan Cao *Rx. Glycyrrhizae*
Sheng Jiang *Rz. Zingiberis Recens*

Di Yu San:

Di Yu *Rx. Sanguisorbae*
Qian Cao *Rx. Rubiae*
Huang Qin *Rx. Scutellariae*
Huang Lian *Rz. Coptidis*
Zhi Zi *Fr. Gardenia*
Fu Ling *Poria*

Ding Chen Tou Ge San:

Bai Zhu *Rz. Atractylodis Macrocephala*
Xiang Fu *Rz. Cyperi*
Ren Shen *Rx. Ginseng*
Sha Ren *Fr. Amomi*
Ding Xiang *Fl. Caryophylli*
Mai Ya *Fr. Hordei Germinatus*
Mu Xiang *Rx. Aucklandia*
Rou Dou Kou *Sm. Myristicae*
Shen Qu *Massa Fermentata*
Zhi Gan Cao *Rx. Glycyrrhizae Preparata*
Chen Xiang *Lignum Aquilariae Resinatum*
Qing Pi *Pc. Citri Reticulatae Viride*
Hou Po *Cx. Magnoliae Officinalis*
Huo Xiang *Hb. Pogostemonis*
Chen Pi *Pc. Citri Reticulatae*
Ban Xia *Rz. Pinelliae*
Cao Guo *Fr. Tsaoko*

Ding Chuan Tang:

Bai Guo *Sm. Ginkgo*
Ma Huang *Hb. Ephedrae*
Sang Bai Pi *Cx. Mori*

Kuan Dong Hua *Fl. Farfarae*
Ban Xia *Rz. Pinelliae*
Xing Ren *Sm. Armeniacae Amarum*
Su Zi *Fr. Perillae*
Huang Qin *Rx. Scutellariae*
Gan Cao *Rx. Glycyrrhizae*

Ding Xian Wan:
Tian Ma *Rz. Gastrodiae*
Chuan Bei Mu *Blb. Fritillariae Cirrhosae*
Dan Nan Xing *Arisaema cum Bile*
Ban Xia *Rz. Pinelliae*

Ding Xiang San:
Ding Xiang *Fl. Caryophylli*
Shi Di *Calyx Kaki*
Gao Liang Jiang *Rz. Alpiniae Officinarum*
Zhi Gan Cao *Rx. Glycyrrhizae Preparata*

Ding Zhi Wan:
Dang Shen *Rx. Codonopsis*
Fu Shen *Sclerotium Poriae Pararadicis*
Shi Chang Pu *Rz. Acori Tatarinowii*
Yuan Zhi *Rx. Polygalae*
Gan Cao *Rx. Glycyrrhizae*
Fu Ling *Poria*
Bai Zhu *Rz. Atractylodis Macrocephala*
Mai Men Dong *Rx. Ophiopogonis*

Du Huo Ji Sheng Tang:
Du Huo *Rx. Angelicae Pubescentis*
Sang Ji Sheng *Hb. Taxilli*
Qin Jiao *Rx. Gentianae Macrophyllae*
Fang Feng *Rx. Saposhnikoviae*
Xi Xin *Hb. Asari*
Dang Gui *Rx. Angelicae Sinensis*
Shao Yao *Rx. Paeoniae Alba*
Chuan Xiong *Rz. Chuanxiong*
Di Huang *Rx. Rehmanniae*
Du Zhong *Cx. Eucommiae*
Niu Xi *Rx. Achyranthis Bidentatae*
Ren Shen *Rx. Ginseng*
Fu Ling *Poria*
Gan Cao *Rx. Glycyrrhizae*
Rou Gui *Cx. Cinnamomi*

Du Shen Tang:
Ren Shen *Rx. Ginseng*

E

Er Chen Tang:
Ban Xia *Rz. Pinelliae*
Chen Pi *Pc. Citri Reticulatae*
Fu Ling *Poria*
Zhi Gan Cao *Rx. Glycyrrhizae Preparata*

Er Long Zuo Ci Wan:
Shu Di Huang *Rx. Rehmanniae Preparata*
Shan Zhu Yu *Fr. Corni*
Shan Yao *Rz. Dioscoreae*
Mu Dan Pi *Cx. Moutan*
Fu Ling *Poria*
Ze Xie *Rz. Alismatis*
Chai Hu *Rx. Bupleuri*
Ci Shi *Magnetitum*

Er Xian Tang:
Xian Mao *Rz. Curculiginis*
Yin Yang Huo *Hb. Epimedii*
Ba Ji Tian *Rx. Morindae Officinalis*
Huang Bai *Cx. Phellodendri*
Zhi Mu *Rz. Anemarrhenae*
Dang Gui *Rx. Angelicae Sinensis*

Er Yin Jian:
Sheng Di Huang *Rx. Rehmanniae*
Mai Men Dong *Rx. Ophiopogonis*
Suan Zao Ren *Sm. Ziziphi Spinosae*
Gan Cao *Rx. Glycyrrhizae*
Xuan Shen *Rx. Scrophulariae*
Fu Ling *Poria*
Huang Lian *Rz. Coptidis*
Mu Tong *Caulis Aristolochiae Manshuriensis*
· Deng Xin Cao *Medulla Junci*
Zhu Ye *Hb. Lophatheri*

Er Zhi Wan:

Nu Zhen Zi *Fr. Ligustri Lucidi*
Han Lian Cao *Hb. Ecliptae*

F

Fang Feng Tang:

Fang Feng *Rx. Saposhnikoviae*
Dang Gui *Rx. Angelicae Sinensis*
Fu Ling *Poria*
Xing Ren *Sm. Armeniacae Amarum*
Huang Qin *Rx. Scutellariae*
Qin Jiao *Rx. Gentianae Macrophyllae*
Ge Gen *Rx. Puerariae*
Ma Huang *Hb. Ephedrae*
Rou Gui *Cx. Cinnamomi*
Sheng Jiang *Rz. Zingiberis Recens*
Gan Cao *Rx. Glycyrrhizae*
Da Zao *Fr. Jujubae*

Fang Feng Tong Sheng San:

Fang Feng *Rx. Saposhnikoviae*
Jing Jie *Hb. Schizonepetae*
Lian Qiao *Fr. Forsythiae*
Ma Huang *Hb. Ephedrae*
Bo He *Hb. Menthae*
Chuan Xiong *Rz. Chuanxiong*
Dang Gui *Rx. Angelicae Sinensis*
Bai Shao *Rx. Paeoniae Alba*
Bai Zhu *Rz. Atractylodis Macrocephala*
Zhi Zi *Fr. Gardenia*
Da Huang *Rx. et Rz. Rhei*
Mang Xiao *Natrii Sulfas*
Shi Gao *Gypsum Fibrosum*
Huang Qin *Rx. Scutellariae*
Jie Geng *Rx. Platycodonis*
Gan Cao *Rx. Glycyrrhizae*
Hua Shi *Talcum*
Sheng Jiang *Rz. Zingiberis Recens*

Fu Yuan Huo Xue Tang:

Chai Hu *Rx. Bupleuri*
Tian Hua Fen *Rx. Trichosanthis*
Dang Gui *Rx. Angelicae Sinensis*
Hong Hua *Fl. Carthami*
Gan Cao *Rx. Glycyrrhizae*
Chuan Shan Jia *Squama Manis*
Da Huang *Rx. et Rz. Rhei*
Tao Ren *Sm. Persicae*

Fu Zi Li Zhong Wan:

Pao Fu Zi *Rx. Aconiti Lateralis Preparata*
Ren Shen *Rx. Ginseng*
Bai Zhu *Rz. Atractylodis Macrocephala*
Pao Jiang *Rz. Zingiberis Preparatum*
Zhi Gan Cao *Rx. Glycyrrhizae Preparata*

G

Gan Jiang Ling Zhu Tang:

Gan Cao *Rx. Glycyrrhizae*
Gan Jiang *Rz. Zingiberis*
Fu Ling *Poria*
Bai Zhu *Rz. Atractylodis Macrocephala*

Gan Lu Xiao Du Dan:

Hua Shi *Talcum*
Yin Chen Hao *Hb. Artemisiae Scopariae*
Huang Qin *Rx. Scutellariae*
Shi Chang Pu *Rz. Acori Tatarinowii*
Chuan Bei Mu *Blb. Fritillariae Cirrhosae*
Mu Tong *Caulis Aristolochiae Manshuriensis*
Huo Xiang *Hb. Pogostemonis*
She Gan *Rz. Belamcandae*
Lian Qiao *Fr. Forsythiae*
Bo He *Hb. Menthae*
Bai Dou Kou *Fr. Amomi Rotundus*

Gan Mai Da Zao Tang:

Gan Cao *Rx. Glycyrrhizae*
Xiao Mai *Fr. Tritici Levis*
Da Zao *Fr. Jujubae*

Gao Lin Tang:

Shan Yao *Rz. Dioscoreae*
Qian Shi *Sm. Euryale*
Long Gu *Os Draconis Fossilia*

Mu Li *Concha Ostreae*
Sheng Di Huang *Rx. Rehmanniae*
Dang Shen *Rx. Codonopsis*
Bai Shao *Rx. Paeoniae Alba*

Ge Gen Qin Lian Tang:
Ge Gen *Rx. Puerariae*
Huang Qin *Rx. Scutellariae*
Huang Lian *Rz. Coptidis*
Zhi Gan Cao *Rx. Glycyrrhizae Preparata*

Ge Gen Tang:
Ge Gen *Rx. Puerariae*
Ma Huang *Hb. Ephedrae*
Gui Zhi *Rml. Cinnamomi*
Sheng Jiang *Rz. Zingiberis Recens*
Gan Cao *Rx. Glycyrrhizae*
Shao Yao *Rx. Paeoniae Alba*
Da Zao *Fr. Jujubae*

Ge Xia Zhu Yu Tang:
Wu Ling Zhi *Excrementum Trogopteri seu Pteromi*
Dang Gui *Rx. Angelicae Sinensis*
Chuan Xiong *Rz. Chuanxiong*
Tao Ren *Sm. Persicae*
Mu Dan Pi *Cx. Moutan*
Chi Shao *Rx. Paeoniae Rubra*
Wu Yao *Rx. Linderae*
Yan Hu Suo *Rz. Corydalis*
Gan Cao *Rx. Glycyrrhizae*
Xiang Fu *Rz. Cyperi*
Hong Hua *Fl. Carthami*
Zhi Qiao *Fr. Aurantii*

Gua Lou Xie Bai Bai Jiu Tang:
Gua Lou *Fr. Trichosanthis*
Xie Bai *Blb. Allii Macrostemonis*
Bai Jiu *White Wine*

Gua Lou Xie Bai Ban Xia Tang:
Gua Lou *Fr. Trichosanthis*
Xie Bai *Blb. Allii Macrostemonis*
Bai Jiu *White Wine*
Ban Xia *Rz. Pinelliae*

Gui Pi Tang:
Dang Shen *Rx. Codonopsis*
Huang Qi *Rx. Astragali*
Bai Zhu *Rz. Atractylodis Macrocephala*
Fu Shen *Sclerotium Poriae Pararadicis*
Suan Zao Ren *Sm. Ziziphi Spinosae*
Long Yan Rou *Arillus Longan*
Mu Xiang *Rx. Aucklandia*
Zhi Gan Cao *Rx. Glycyrrhizae Preparata*
Dang Gui *Rx. Angelicae Sinensis*
Yuan Zhi *Rx. Polygalae*
Sheng Jiang *Rz. Zingiberis Recens*
Da Zao *Fr. Jujubae*

Gui Zhi Gan Cao Long Gu Mu Li Tang:
Gui Zhi *Rml. Cinnamomi*
Gan Cao *Rx. Glycyrrhizae*
Long Gu *Os Draconis Fossilia*
Mu Li *Concha Ostreae*

Gui Zhi Jia Hou Po Xing Zi Tang:
Gui Zhi *Rml. Cinnamomi*
Shao Yao *Rx. Paeoniae Alba*
Zhi Gan Cao *Rx. Glycyrrhizae Preparata*
Sheng Jiang *Rz. Zingiberis Recens*
Da Zao *Fr. Jujubae*
Hou Po *Cx. Magnoliae Officinalis*
Xing Ren *Sm. Armeniacae Amarum*

Gui Zhi Tang:
Gui Zhi *Rml. Cinnamomi*
Shao Yao *Rx. Paeoniae Alba*
Sheng Jiang *Rz. Zingiberis Recens*
Zhi Gan Cao *Rx. Glycyrrhizae Preparata*
Da Zao *Fr. Jujubae*

H

Hai Zao Yu Hu Tang:
Hai Zao *Sargassum*
Kun Bu *Thallus Ecklonae seu Thallus Laminariae*
Ban Xia *Rz. Pinelliae*

Chen Pi *Pc. Citri Reticulatae*
Qing Pi *Pc. Citri Reticulatae Viride*
Lian Qiao *Fr. Forsythiae*
Bei Mu *Blb. Fritillariae Thunbergii*
Dang Gui *Rx. Angelicae Sinensis*
Chuan Xiong *Rz. Chuanxiong*
Du Huo *Rx. Angelicae Pubescentis*
Gan Cao *Rx. Glycyrrhizae*

Hu Qian Wan:
Gui Ban *Carapax et Plastrum Testudinis*
Huang Bai *Cx. Phellodendri*
Zhi Mu *Rz. Anemarrhenae*
Shu Di Huang *Rx. Rehmanniae Preparata*
Bai Shao *Rx. Paeoniae Alba*
Suo Yang *Hb. Cynomorii*
Chen Pi *Pc. Citri Reticulatae*
Gan Jiang *Rz. Zingiberis*

Hua Gan Jian:
Qing Pi *Pc. Citri Reticulatae Viride*
Chen Pi *Pc. Citri Reticulatae*
Shao Yao *Rx. Paeoniae Alba*
Mu Dan Pi *Cx. Moutan*
Zhi Zi *Fr. Gardenia*
Ze Xie *Rz. Alismatis*
Bei Mu *Blb. Fritillariae Thunbergii*

Hua Ji Wan:
San Leng *Rz. Sparganii*
E Zhu *Rz. Curcumae*
A Wei *Resina Ferulae*
Fu Hai Shi *Pumice*
Xiang Fu *Rz. Cyperi*
Xiong Huang *Realgar*
Bing Lang *Sm. Arecae*
Su Mu *Lignum Sappan*
Wa Leng Zi *Concha Arcae*
Wu Ling Zhi *Excrementum Trogopteri seu Pteromi*

Huan Shao Dan:
Shu Di Huang *Rx. Rehmanniae Preparata*
Niu Xi *Rx. Achyranthis Bidentatae*
Ba Ji Tian *Rx. Morindae Officinalis*
Rou Cong Rong *Hb. Cistanches*
Shan Yao *Rz. Dioscoreae*
Gou Qi Zi *Fr. Lycii*
Shan Zhu Yu *Fr. Corni*
Fu Ling *Poria*
Du Zhong *Cx. Eucommiae*
Yuan Zhi *Rx. Polygalae*
Wu Wei Zi *Fr. Schisandrae Chinensis*
Chu Shi Zi *Fr. Broussonetine*
Xiao Hui Xiang *Fr. Foeniculi*
Shi Chang Pu *Rz. Acori Tatarinowii*

Huang Lian E Jiao Tang:
Huang Lian *Rz. Coptidis*
E Jiao *Gelatinum Corii Asini*
Huang Qin *Rx. Scutellariae*
Ji Zi Huang *Egg Yolk*
Shao Yao *Rx. Paeoniae Alba*

Huang Lian Jie Du Tang:
Huang Lian *Rz. Coptidis*
Huang Qin *Rx. Scutellariae*
Huang Bai *Cx. Phellodendri*
Zhi Zi *Fr. Gardenia*

Huang Lian Wen Dan Tang:
Ban Xia *Rz. Pinelliae*
Chen Pi *Pc. Citri Reticulatae*
Fu Ling *Poria*
Gan Cao *Rx. Glycyrrhizae*
Zhi Shi *Fr. Aurantii Immaturus*
Zhu Ru *Caulis Bambusae in Taenia*
Huang Lian *Rz. Coptidis*
Da Zao *Fr. Jujubae*

Huang Qi Jian Zhong Tang:
Huang Qi *Rx. Astragali*
Bai Shao *Rx. Paeoniae Alba*
Gui Zhi *Rml. Cinnamomi*
Zhi Gan Cao *Rx. Glycyrrhizae Preparata*
Sheng Jiang *Rz. Zingiberis Recens*
Da Zao *Fr. Jujubae*
Yi Tang *Saccharum Granorum*

Huang Qi Tang:

Huang Qi *Rx. Astragali*
Chen Pi *Pc. Citri Reticulatae*
Huo Ma Ren *Fr. Cannabis*
Feng Mi *Mel*

Huang Tu Tang:

Fu Long Gan *Terra Flava Usta*
Gan Cao *Rx. Glycyrrhizae*
Di Huang *Rx. Rehmanniae*
Bai Zhu *Rz. Atractylodis Macrocephala*
Fu Zi *Rx. Aconiti Lateralis Preparata*
E Jiao *Gelatinum Corii Asini*
Huang Qin *Rx. Scutellariae*

Huo Xiang Zheng Qi San:

Huo Xiang *Hb. Pogostemonis*
Zi Su Ye *Fm. Perillae*
Bai Zhi *Rx. Angelicae Dahuricae*
Jie Geng *Rx. Platycodonis*
Bai Zhu *Rz. Atractylodis Macrocephala*
Hou Po *Cx. Magnoliae Officinalis*
Ban Xia *Rz. Pinelliae*
Da Fu Pi *Pc. Arecae*
Fu Ling *Poria*
Chen Pi *Pc. Citri Reticulatae*
Gan Cao *Rx. Glycyrrhizae*
Da Zao *Fr. Jujubae*

J

Ji Chuan Jian:

Dang Gui *Rx. Angelicae Sinensis*
Niu Xi *Rx. Achyranthis Bidentatae*
Rou Cong Rong *Hb. Cistanches*
Ze Xie *Rz. Alismatis*
Sheng Ma *Rz. Cimicifugae*
Zhi Qiao *Fr. Aurantii*

Ji Jiao Li Huang Wan:

Fang Ji *Rx. Stephaniae Tetrandrae*
Jiao Mu *Sm. Zanthoxyli*
Ting Li Zi *Sm. Descurainiae*
Da Huang *Rx. et Rz. Rhei*

Ji Sheng Shen Qi Wan:

Sheng Di Huang *Rx. Rehmanniae*
Shan Yao *Rz. Dioscoreae*
Shan Zu Yu *Fr. Corni*
Mu Dan Pi *Cx. Moutan*
Fu Ling *Poria*
Ze Xie *Rz. Alismatis*
Fu Zi *Rx. Aconiti Lateralis Preparata*
Gui Zhi *Rml. Cinnamomi*
Niu Xi *Rx. Achyranthis Bidentatae*
Che Qian Zi *Sm. Plantaginis*

Jia Jian Wei Rui Tang:

Yu Zhu *Rz. Polygonati Odorati*
Cong Bai *Blb. Allii Fistulosi*
Jie Geng *Rx. Platycodonis*
Bai Wei *Rx. Cynanchi Atrati*
Dan Dou Chi *Sm. Sojae Preparatum*
Bo He *Hb. Menthae*
Gan Cao *Rx. Glycyrrhizae*
Da Zao *Fr. Jujubae*

Jia Wei Jie Geng Tang:

Jie Geng *Rx. Platycodonis*
Gan Cao *Rx. Glycyrrhizae*
Bei Mu *Blb. Fritillariae Thunbergii*
Ju Hong *Exocarpium Citri Grandis*
Jin Yin Hua *Fl. Lonicerae*
Yi Yi Ren *Sm. Coicis*
Ting Li Zi *Sm. Descurainiae*
Bai Ji *Rz. Bletillae*

Jiao Tai Wan:

Huang Lian *Rz. Coptidis*
Rou Gui *Cx. Cinnamomi*

Jie Yu Dan:

Bai Fu Zi *Rz. Typhonii*
Shi Chang Pu *Rz. Acori Tatarinowii*
Yuan Zhi *Rx. Polygalae*
Tian Ma *Rz. Gastrodiae*
Quan Xie *Scorpio*
Qiang Huo *Rz. et Rx. Notopterygii*
Tian Nan Xing *Rz. Arisaematis*
Mu Xiang *Rx. Aucklandia*
Gan Cao *Rx. Glycyrrhizae*

Jin Gui Shen Qi Wan:

Gui Zhi *Rml. Cinnamomi*
Fu Zi *Rx. Aconiti Lateralis Preparata*
Shu Di Huang *Rx. Rehmanniae Preparata*
Shan Zhu Yu *Fr. Corni*
Shan Yao *Rz. Dioscoreae*
Fu Ling *Poria*
Mu Dan Pi *Cx. Moutan*
Ze Xie *Rz. Alismatis*

Jin Ling Zi San

Chuan Lian Zi *Fr. Toosendan*
Yan Hu Suo *Rz. Corydalis*

Jin Suo Gu Jing Wan:

Sha Yuan Ji Li *Sm. Astragali Complanati*
Qian Shi *Sm. Euryale*
Lian Xu *Stamen Nelumbinis*
Long Gu *Os Draconis Fossilia*
Mu Li *Concha Ostreae*
Lian Zi *Sm. Nelumbinis*

Jing Fang Bai Du San:

Jing Jie *Hb. Schizonepetae*
Fang Feng *Rx. Saposhnikoviae*
Qiang Huo *Rz. et Rx. Notopterygii*
Du Huo *Rx. Angelicae Pubescentis*
Chai Hu *Rx. Bupleuri*
Qian Hu *Rx. Peucedani*
Chuan Xiong *Rz. Chuanxiong*
Zhi Qiao *Fr. Aurantii*
Fu Ling *Poria*
Jie Geng *Rx. Platycodonis*
Gan Cao *Rx. Glycyrrhizae*

Ju Pi Zhu Ru Tang:

Ren Shen *Rx. Ginseng*
Chen Pi *Pc. Citri Reticulatae*
Zhu Ru *Caulis Bambusae in Taenia*
Gan Cao *Rx. Glycyrrhizae*
Sheng Jiang *Rz. Zingiberis Recens*
Da Zao *Fr. Jujubae*

L

Li Zhong Wan:

Ren Shen *Rx. Ginseng*
Bai Zhu *Rz. Atractylodis Macrocephala*
Gan Jiang *Rz. Zingiberis*
Zhi Gan Cao *Rx. Glycyrrhizae Preparata*

Lian Li Tang:

Ren Shen *Rx. Ginseng*
Bai Zhu *Rz. Atractylodis Macrocephala*
Gan Jiang *Rz. Zingiberis*
Huang Lian *Rz. Coptidis*
Zhi Gan Cao *Rx. Glycyrrhizae Preparata*
Fu Ling *Poria*

Lian Po Yin:

Huang Lian *Rz. Coptidis*
Hou Po *Cx. Magnoliae Officinalis*
Dan Dou Chi *Sm. Sojae Preparatum*
Zhi Zi *Fr. Gardenia*
Ban Xia *Rz. Pinelliae*
Shi Chang Pu *Rz. Acori Tatarinowii*
Lu Gen *Rz. Phragmitis*

Liang Fu Wan:

Gao Liang Jiang *Rz. Alpiniae Officinarum*
Xiang Fu *Rz. Cyperi*

Ling Gan Wu Wei Jiang Xin Tang:

Fu Ling *Poria*
Gan Cao *Rx. Glycyrrhizae*
Wu Wei Zi *Fr. Schisandrae Chinensis*
Gan Jiang *Rz. Zingiberis*
Xi Xin *Hb. Asari*

Ling Gui Zhu Gan Tang:

Fu Ling *Poria*
Gui Zhi *Rml. Cinnamomi*
Bai Zhu *Rz. Atractylodis Macrocephala*
Gan Cao *Rx. Glycyrrhizae*

Ling Jiao Gou Teng Tang:

Ling Yang Jiao *Cornu Saigae Tataricae*
Sang Ye *Fm. Mori*
Chuan Bei Mu *Blb. Fritillariae Cirrhosae*
Sheng Di Huang *Rx. Rehmanniae*
Gou Teng *Rml. Uncariae cum Uncis*
Ju Hua *Fl. Chrysanthemi*
Bai Shao *Rx. Paeoniae Alba*
Gan Cao *Rx. Glycyrrhizae*
Zhu Ru *Caulis Bambusae in Taenia*
Fu Shen *Sclerotium Poriae Pararadicis*

Liu Jun Zi Tang:

Ren Shen *Rx. Ginseng*
Zhi Gan Cao *Rx. Glycyrrhizae Preparata*
Fu Ling *Poria*
Bai Zhu *Rz. Atractylodis Macrocephala*
Chen Pi *Pc. Citri Reticulatae*
Ban Xia *Rz. Pinelliae*

Liu Mo Tang:

Chen Xiang *Lignum Aquilariae Resinatum*
Mu Xiang *Rx. Aucklandia*
Bing Lang *Sm. Arecae*
Wu Yao *Rx. Linderae*
Zhi Shi *Fr. Aurantii Immaturus*
Da Huang *Rx. et Rz. Rhei*

Liu Wei Di Huang Wan:

Shu Di Huang *Rx. Rehmanniae Preparata*
Shan Yao *Rz. Dioscoreae*
Shan Zhu Yu *Fr. Corni*
Fu Ling *Poria*
Mu Dan Pi *Cx. Moutan*
Ze Xie *Rz. Alismatis*

Long Dan Xie Gan Tang:

Long Dan Cao *Rx. Gentianae*
Ze Xie *Rz. Alismatis*
Mu Tong *Caulis Aristolochiae Manshuriensis*
Che Qian Zi *Sm. Plantaginis*
Dang Gui *Rx. Angelicae Sinensis*
Chai Hu *Rx. Bupleuri*
Sheng Di Huang *Rx. Rehmanniae*
Huang Qin *Rx. Scutellariae*
Zhi Zi *Fr. Gardenia*

M

Ma Huang Fu Zi Xi Xin Tang:

Ma Huang *Hb. Ephedrae*
Fu Zi *Rx. Aconiti Lateralis Preparata*
Xi Xin *Hb. Asari*

Ma Huang Lian Qiao Chi Xiao Dou Tang:

Ma Huang *Hb. Ephedrae*
Xing Ren *Sm. Armeniacae Amarum*
Sang Bai Pi *Cx. Mori*
Lian Qiao *Fr. Forsythiae*
Chi Xiao Dou *Sm. Phaseoli*
Gan Cao *Rx. Glycyrrhizae*
Sheng Jiang *Rz. Zingiberis Recens*
Da Zao *Fr. Jujubae*

Ma Huang Tang:

Ma Huang *Hb. Ephedrae*
Gui Zhi *Rml. Cinnamomi*
Xing Ren *Sm. Armeniacae Amarum*
Zhi Gan Cao *Rx. Glycyrrhizae Preparata*

Ma Xing Shi Gan Tang:

Ma Huang *Hb. Ephedrae*
Xing Ren *Sm. Armeniacae Amarum*
Shi Gao *Gypsum Fibrosum*
Gan Cao *Rx. Glycyrrhizae*

Ma Zi Ren Wan:

Ma Zi Ren *Fr. Cannabis*
Shao Yao *Rx. Paeoniae Alba*
Zhi Shi *Fr. Aurantii Immaturus*
Hou Po *Cx. Magnoliae Officinalis*
Xing Ren *Sm. Armeniacae Amarum*
Da Huang *Rx. et Rz. Rhei*

Mai Men Dong Tang:

Mai Men Dong *Rx. Ophiopogonis*
Ren Shen *Rx. Ginseng*
Ban Xia *Rz. Pinelliae*
Gan Cao *Rx. Glycyrrhizae*
Jing Mi *Nonglutinous Rice*
Da Zao *Fr. Jujubae*

Mai Wei Di Huang Wan:

Shu Di Huang *Rx. Rehmanniae Preparata*
Shan Zhu Yu *Fr. Corni*
Shan Yao *Rz. Dioscoreae*
Mu Dan Pi *Cx. Moutan*
Ze Xie *Rz. Alismatis*
Fu Ling *Poria*
Mai Men Dong *Rx. Ophiopogonis*
Wu Wei Zi *Fr. Schisandrae Chinensis*

Meng Shi Gun Tan Wan:

Qing Meng Shi *Lapis Chloriti*
Chen Xiang *Lignum Aquilariae Resinatum*
Da Huang *Rx. et Rz. Rhei*
Huang Qin *Rx. Scutellariae*
Pu Xiao *Natrii Sulfas*

Mu Xiang Bing Lang Wan:

Mu Xiang *Rx. Aucklandia*
Xiang Fu *Rz. Cyperi*
Qing Pi *Pc. Citri Reticulatae Viride*
Chen Pi *Pc. Citri Reticulatae*
Zhi Qiao *Fr. Aurantii*
Hei Chou *Sm. Pharbitidis*
Bing Lang *Sm. Arecae*
Huang Lian *Rz. Coptidis*
Huang Bai *Cx. Phellodendri*
San Leng *Rz. Sparganii*
E Zhu *Rz. Curcumae*
Da Huang *Rx. et Rz. Rhei*
Mang Xiao *Natrii Sulfas*

N

Niu Huang Zhi Bao Dan:

Zhu Sha *Cinnabaris*
Xiong Huang *Realgar*
Dai Mao *Carapax Eretmochelydis*
Hu Po *Succinum*
She Xiang *Moschus*
Niu Huang *Calculus Bovis*
An Xi Xiang *Benzoinum*

P

Ping Wei San:

Cang Zhu *Rz. Atractylodis*
Hou Po *Cx. Magnoliae Officinalis*
Chen Pi *Pc. Citri Reticulatae*
Gan Cao *Rx. Glycyrrhizae*
Sheng Jiang *Rz. Zingiberis Recens*
Da Zao *Fr. Jujubae*

Q

Qi Ge San:

Sha Shen *Rx. Glehniae*
Fu Ling *Poria*
Dan Shen *Rx. Salviae Miltiorrhizae*
Chuan Bei Mu *Blb. Fritillariae Cirrhosae*
Yu Jin *Rx. Curcumae*
Sha Ren *Fr. Amomi*
He Ye *Fm. Nelumbinis*

Qi Ju Di Huang Wan:

Gou Qi Zi *Fr. Lycii*
Ju Hua *Fl. Chrysanthemi*
Shu Di Huang *Rx. Rehmanniae Preparata*
Shan Zhu Yu *Fr. Corni*
Shan Yao *Rz. Dioscoreae*
Ze Xie *Rz. Alismatis*
Mu Dan Pi *Cx. Moutan*
Fu Ling *Poria*

Qi Wei Du Qi Wan:

Shu Di Huang *Rx. Rehmanniae Preparata*
Shan Zhu Yu *Fr. Corni*
Shan Yao *Rz. Dioscoreae*
Fu Ling *Poria*
Mu Dan Pi *Cx. Moutan*
Ze Xie *Rz. Alismatis*
Wu Wei Zi *Fr. Schisandrae Chinensis*

Qian Gen San:

Qian Cao *Rx. Rubiae*
Huang Qin *Rx. Scutellariae*
E Jiao *Gelatinum Corii Asini*
Ce Bai Ye *Cacumen Platycladi*
Sheng Di Huang *Rx. Rehmanniae*

Qian Jin Wei Jing Tang:

Xian Lu Gen *Rz. Phragmitis*
Yi Yi Ren *Sm. Coicis*
Dong Guo Ren *Sm. Benincasae*
Tao Ren *Sm. Persicae*

Qian Zheng San:

Bai Fu Zi *Rz. Typhonii*
Bai Jiang Can *Bombyx Batryticatus*
Quan Xie *Scorpio*

Qiang Huo Sheng Shi Tang:

Qiang Huo *Rz. et Rx. Notopterygii*
Du Huo *Rx. Angelicae Pubescentis*
Chuan Xiong *Rz. Chuanxiong*
Man Jing Zi *Fr. Viticis*
Gan Cao *Rx. Glycyrrhizae*
Fang Feng *Rx. Saposhnikoviae*
Gao Ben *Rz. Ligustici*

Qing Fei Yin:

Fu Ling *Poria*
Huang Qin *Rx. Scutellariae*
Sang Bai Pi *Cx. Mori*
Mai Men Dong *Rx. Ophiopogonis*
Che Qian Zi *Sm. Plantaginis*
Zhi Zi *Fr. Gardenia*
Mu Tong *Caulis Aristolochiae Manshuriensis*

Qing Jin Hua Tan Tang:

Huang Qin *Rx. Scutellariae*
Zhi Zi *Fr. Gardenia*
Jie Geng *Rx. Platycodonis*
Mai Men Dong *Rx. Ophiopogonis*
Sang Bai Pi *Cx. Mori*
Bei Mu *Blb. Fritillariae Thunbergii*
Zhi Mu *Rz. Anemarrhenae*
Gua Lou Ren *Sm. Trichosanthis*
Ju Hong *Exocarpium Citri Grandis*
Fu Ling *Poria*

Qing Wei San:

Dang Gui *Rx. Angelicae Sinensis*
Sheng Di Huang *Rx. Rehmanniae*
Mu Dan Pi *Cx. Moutan*
Huang Lian *Rz. Coptidis*
Sheng Ma *Rz. Cimicifugae*

Qing Wen Bai Du Yin:

Sheng Shi Gao *Gypsum Fibrosum*
Sheng Di Huang *Rx. Rehmanniae*
Xi Jiao *Cornu Rhinoceri*
Huang Lian *Rz. Coptidis*
Zhi Zi *Fr. Gardenia*
Jie Geng *Rx. Platycodonis*
Huang Qin *Rx. Scutellariae*
Zhi Mu *Rz. Anemarrhenae*
Chi Shao *Rx. Paeoniae Rubra*
Xuan Shen *Rx. Scrophulariae*
Lian Qiao *Fr. Forsythiae*
Mu Dan Pi *Cx. Moutan*
Zhu Ye *Hb. Lophatheri*

Qing Ying Tang:

Xi Jiao *Cornu Rhinoceri*
Huang Lian *Rz. Coptidis*
Sheng Di Huang *Rx. Rehmanniae*
Xuan Shen *Rx. Scrophulariae*
Zhu Ye *Hb. Lophatheri*
Jin Yin Hua *Fl. Lonicerae*
Lian Qiao *Fr. Forsythiae*
Dan Shen *Rx. Salviae Miltiorrhizae*
Mai Men Dong *Rx. Ophiopogonis*

Qing Zao Jiu Fei Tang:

Sang Ye *Fm. Mori*
Shi Gao *Gypsum Fibrosum*
Xing Ren *Sm. Armeniacae Amarum*
Gan Cao *Rx. Glycyrrhizae*
Mai Men Dong *Rx. Ophiopogonis*
Ren Shen *Rx. Ginseng*
E Jiao *Gelatinum Corii Asini*
Hu Ma Ren *Sm. Sesami Nigrum*
Pi Pa Ye *Fm. Eriobotryae*

R

Ren Shen Yang Ying Tang:

Ren Shen *Rx. Ginseng*
Gan Cao *Rx. Glycyrrhizae*
Dang Gui *Rx. Angelicae Sinensis*
Bai Shao *Rx. Paeoniae Alba*
Shu Di Huang *Rx. Rehmanniae Preparata*
Rou Gui *Cx. Cinnamomi*
Da Zao *Fr. Jujubae*
Huang Qi *Rx. Astragali*
Bai Zhu *Rz. Atractylodis Macrocephala*
Fu Ling *Poria*
Wu Wei Zi *Fr. Schisandrae Chinensis*
Yuan Zhi *Rx. Polygalae*
Chen Pi *Pc. Citri Reticulatae*
Sheng Jiang *Rz. Zingiberis Recens*

Run Chang Wan:

Dang Gui *Rx. Angelicae Sinensis*
Sheng Di Huang *Rx. Rehmanniae*
Ma Zi Ren *Fr. Cannabis*
Tao Ren *Sm. Persicae*
Zhi Qiao *Fr. Aurantii*

S

San Ao Tang:

Ma Huang *Hb. Ephedrae*
Xing Ren *Sm. Armeniacae Amarum*
Gan Cao *Rx. Glycyrrhizae*

San Ren Tang:

Xing Ren *Sm. Armeniacae Amarum*
Bai Dou Kou *Fr. Amomi Rotundus*
Yi Yi Ren *Sm. Coicis*
Hou Po *Cx. Magnoliae Officinalis*
Ban Xia *Rz. Pinelliae*
Tong Cao *Medulla Tetrapanacis*
Hua Shi *Talcum*
Zhu Ye *Hb. Lophatheri*

San Shi Tang:

Hua Shi *Talcum*
Han Shui Shi *Calcitum*
Shi Gao *Gypsum Fibrosum*
Xing Ren *Sm. Armeniacae Amarum*
Jin Yin Hua *Fl. Lonicerae*
Zhu Ru *Caulis Bambusae in Taenia*
Tong Cao *Medulla Tetrapanacis*

San Zi Yang Qin Tang:

Su Zi *Fr. Perillae*
Bai Jie Zi *Sm. Sinapis*
Lai Fu Zi *Sm. Raphani*

Sang Bai Pi Tang:

Sang Bai Pi *Cx. Mori*
Ban Xia *Rz. Pinelliae*
Su Zi *Fr. Perillae*
Xing Ren *Sm. Armeniacae Amarum*
Bei Mu *Blb. Fritillariae Thunbergii*
Huang Qin *Rx. Scutellariae*
Huang Lian *Rz. Coptidis*
Zhi Zi *Fr. Gardenia*

Sang Ju Yin:

Sang Ye *Fm. Mori*
Ju Hua *Fl. Chrysanthemi*
Lian Qiao *Fr. Forsythiae*
Bo He *Hb. Menthae*
Jie Geng *Rx. Platycodonis*
Xing Ren *Sm. Armeniacae Amarum*
Lu Gen *Rz. Phragmitis*
Gan Cao *Rx. Glycyrrhizae*

Sang Xing Tang:

Sang Ye *Fm. Mori*
Xing Ren *Sm. Armeniacae Amarum*
Sha Shen *Rx. Glehniae*
Zhe Bei Mu *Blb. Fritillariae Thunbergii*
Dan Dou Chi *Sm. Sojae Preparatum*
Zhi Zi *Fr. Gardenia*

Sha Shen Mai Dong Tang:

Sha Shen *Rx. Glehniae*
Mai Men Dong *Rx. Ophiopogonis*
Yu Zhu *Rz. Polygonati Odorati*
Gan Cao *Rx. Glycyrrhizae*
Sang Ye *Fm. Mori*
Tian Hua Fen *Rx. Trichosanthis*
Bai Bian Dou *Sm. Lablab Album*

Sha Shen Qing Fei Tang:

Sha Shen *Rx. Glehniae*
Huang Qi *Rx. Astragali*
Tai Zi Shen *Rx. Pseudostellariae*
He Huan Pi *Cx. Albiziae*
Bai Ji *Rz. Bletillae*
Gan Cao *Rx. Glycyrrhizae*
Jie Geng *Rx. Platycodonis*
Yi Yi Ren *Sm. Coicis*
Dong Guo Ren *Sm. Benincasae*

Shao Fu Zhu Yu Tang:

Xiao Hui Xiang *Fr. Foeniculi*
Gan Jiang *Rz. Zingiberis*
Yan Hu Suo *Rz. Corydalis*
Mo Yao *Myrrha*
Dang Gui *Rx. Angelicae Sinensis*
Chuan Xiong *Rz. Chuanxiong*
Rou Gui *Cx. Cinnamomi*
Chi Shao *Rx. Paeoniae Rubra*
Pu Huang *Pollen Typhae*
Wu Ling Zhi *Excrementum Trogopteri seu Pteromi*

Shao Yao Gan Cao Tang:

Bai Shao *Rx. Paeoniae Alba*
Zhi Gan Cao *Rx. Glycyrrhizae Preparata*

Shao Yao Tang:

Huang Qin *Rx. Scutellariae*
Shao Yao *Rx. Paeoniae Alba*
Zhi Gan Cao *Rx. Glycyrrhizae Preparata*
Huang Lian *Rz. Coptidis*
Da Huang *Rx. et Rz. Rhei*
Bing Lang *Sm. Arecae*
Dang Gui *Rx. Angelicae Sinensis*
Mu Xiang *Rx. Aucklandia*
Rou Gui *Cx. Cinnamomi*

She Gan Ma Huang Tang:

She Gan *Rz. Belamcandae*
Ma Huang *Hb. Ephedrae*
Xi Xin *Hb. Asari*
Zi Wan *Rx. Asteris*
Kuan Dong Hua *Fl. Farfarae*
Ban Xia *Rz. Pinelliae*
Wu Wei Zi *Fr. Schisandrae Chinensis*
Sheng Jiang *Rz. Zingiberis Recens*
Da Zao *Fr. Jujubae*

Shen Fu Tang:

Ren Shen *Rx. Ginseng*
Fu Zi *Rx. Aconiti Lateralis Preparata*
Sheng Jiang *Rz. Zingiberis Recens*
Da Zao *Fr. Jujubae*

Shen Ge San:

Ren Shen *Rx. Ginseng*
Ge Jie *Gecko*

Shen Ling Bai Zhu San:

Ren Shen *Rx. Ginseng*
Fu Ling *Poria*
Bai Zhu *Rz. Atractylodis Macrocephala*
Jie Geng *Rx. Platycodonis*
Shan Yao *Rz. Dioscoreae*
Gan Cao *Rx. Glycyrrhizae*
Bai Bian Dou *Sm. Lablab Album*
Lian Zi *Sm. Nelumbinis*
Sha Ren *Fr. Amomi*
Yi Yi Ren *Sm. Coicis*

Shen Su Yin:

Ren Shen *Rx. Ginseng*
Zi Su Ye *Fm. Perillae*
Ge Gen *Rx. Puerariae*
Qian Hu *Rx. Peucedani*
Ban Xia *Rz. Pinelliae*
Fu Ling *Poria*
Hua Ju Hong *Exocarpium Citri Grandis*
Gan Cao *Rx. Glycyrrhizae*
Jie Geng *Rx. Platycodonis*
Zhi Qiao *Fr. Aurantii*
Mu Xiang *Rx. Aucklandia*
Chen Pi *Pc. Citri Reticulatae*
Sheng Jiang *Rz. Zingiberis Recens*
Da Zao *Fr. Jujubae*

Shen Tong Zhu Yu Tang:

Qin Jiao *Rx. Gentianae Macrophyllae*
Chuan Xiong *Rz. Chuanxiong*
Tao Ren *Sm. Persicae*
Hong Hua *Fl. Carthami*
Gan Cao *Rx. Glycyrrhizae*
Qiang Huo *Rz. et Rx. Notopterygii*
Mo Yao *Myrrha*
Xiang Fu *Rz. Cyperi*
Wu Ling Zhi *Excrementum Trogopteri seu Pteromi*
Niu Xi *Rx. Achyranthis Bidentatae*
Di Long *Pheretima*
Dang Gui *Rx. Angelicae Sinensis*

Sheng Di Huang San:

Sheng Di Huang *Rx. Rehmanniae*
Chuan Xiong *Rz. Chuanxiong*
Chi Shao *Rx. Paeoniae Rubra*
Ling Yang Jiao *Cornu Saigae Tataricae*
Mu Xiang *Rx. Aucklandia*
Zhi Qiao *Fr. Aurantii*
Da Huang *Rx. et Rz. Rhei*

Sheng Mai San:

Ren Shen *Rx. Ginseng*
Mai Men Dong *Rx. Ophiopogonis*
Wu Wei Zi *Fr. Schisandrae Chinensis*

Shi Hui San:

Da Ji *Hb. seu Rx. Cirsii Japonici*
Xiao Ji *Hb. Cirsii*
Ce Bai Ye *Cacumen Platycladi*
He Ye *Fm. Nelumbinis*
Qian Cao *Rx. Rubiae*
Zhi Zi *Fr. Gardenia*
Bai Mao Gen *Rz. Imperatae*
Da Huang *Rx. et Rz. Rhei*
Mu Dan Pi *Cx. Moutan*
Zong Lu Pi *Petiolus Trachycarpi*

Shi Pi Yin:

Fu Zi *Rx. Aconiti Lateralis Preparata*
Gan Jiang *Rz. Zingiberis*
Bai Zhu *Rz. Atractylodis Macrocephala*
Gan Cao *Rx. Glycyrrhizae*
Hou Po *Cx. Magnoliae Officinalis*
Mu Xiang *Rx. Aucklandia*
Cao Guo *Fr. Tsaoko*
Bing Lang *Sm. Arecae*
Mu Gua *Fr. Chaenomelis*
Sheng Jiang *Rz. Zingiberis Recens*
Da Zao *Fr. Jujubae*
Fu Ling *Poria*

Shi Quan Da Bu Tang:

Shu Di Huang *Rx. Rehmanniae Preparata*
Bai Shao *Rx. Paeoniae Alba*
Dang Gui *Rx. Angelicae Sinensis*
Chuan Xiong *Rz. Chuanxiong*
Ren Shen *Rx. Ginseng*
Bai Zhu *Rz. Atractylodis Macrocephala*
Fu Ling *Poria*
Gan Cao *Rx. Glycyrrhizae*
Huang Qi *Rx. Astragali*
Rou Gui *Cx. Cinnamomi*

Shi Si Wei Jian Zhong Tang:

Ren Shen *Rx. Ginseng*
Huang Qi *Rx. Astragali*
Dang Gui *Rx. Angelicae Sinensis*
Bai Zhu *Rz. Atractylodis Macrocephala*
Gan Cao *Rx. Glycyrrhizae*
Bai Shao *Rx. Paeoniae Alba*
Fu Ling *Poria*
Sheng Di Huang *Rx. Rehmanniae*
Chuan Xiong *Rz. Chuanxiong*
Mai Men Dong *Rx. Ophiopogonis*
Fu Zi *Rx. Aconiti Lateralis Preparata*
Rou Gui *Cx. Cinnamomi*
Rou Cong Rong *Hb. Cistanches*
Ban Xia *Rz. Pinelliae*
Sheng Jiang *Rz. Zingiberis Recens*
Da Zao *Fr. Jujubae*

Shi Wei San:

Shi Wei *Fm. Pyrrosiae*
Dong Kui Zi *Sm. Abutili seu Malvae*
Qu Mai *Hb. Dianthi*
Hua Shi *Talcum*
Che Qian Zi *Sm. Plantaginis*

Shi Xiao San:

Pu Huang *Pollen Typhae*
Wu Ling Zhi *Excrementum Trogopteri seu Pteromi*

Shi Zao Tang:

Da Ji *Rx. Euphorbiae Pekinensis*
Yuan Hua *Fl. Genkwa*
Gan Sui *Rx. Kansui*
Da Zao *Fr. Jujubae*

Shu Zao Yin Zi:

Shang Lu *Rx. Phytolaccae*
Ze Xie *Rz. Alismatis*
Chi Xiao Dou *Sm. Phaseoli*
Jiao Mu *Sm. Zanthoxyli*
Mu Tong *Caulis Aristolochiae Manshuriensis*
Fu Ling Pi *Cx. Poria*
Da Fu Pi *Pc. Arecae*
Bing Lang *Sm. Arecae*
Sheng Jiang *Rz. Zingiberis Recens*
Qiang Huo *Rz. et Rx. Notopterygii*
Qin Jiao *Rx. Gentianae Macrophyllae*

Si Hai Shu Yu Wan:

Hai Ge Ke *Concha Meretricis seu Cyclinae*
Hai Zao *Sargassum*
Hai Piao Xiao *Endoconcha Sepiae*
Kun Bu *Thallus Eckloniae seu Thallus Laminariae*
Chen Pi *Pc. Citri Reticulatae*
Qing Mu Xiang *Rx. Aristolochiae*

Si Jun Zi Tang:

Ren Shen *Rx. Ginseng*
Bai Zhu *Rz. Atractylodis Macrocephala*
Fu Ling *Poria*
Zhi Gan Cao *Rx. Glycyrrhizae Preparata*

Si Miao Wan:

Cang Zhu *Rz. Atractylodis*
Huang Bai *Cx. Phellodendri*
Niu Xi *Rx. Achyranthis Bidentatae*
Yi Yi Ren *Sm. Coicis*

Si Ni Jia Ren Shen Tang:

Fu Zi *Rx. Aconiti Lateralis Preparata*
Gan Jiang *Rz. Zingiberis*
Gan Cao *Rx. Glycyrrhizae*
Ren Shen *Rx. Ginseng*

Si Ni San:

Chai Hu *Rx. Bupleuri*
Gan Cao *Rx. Glycyrrhizae*
Zhi Shi *Fr. Aurantii Immaturus*
Shao Yao *Rx. Paeoniae Alba*

Si Ni Tang:

Fu Zi *Rx. Aconiti Lateralis Preparata*
Gan Jiang *Rz. Zingiberis*
Gan Cao *Rx. Glycyrrhizae*

Si Shen Wan:

Bu Gu Zhi *Fr. Psoraleae*
Rou Dou Kou *Sm. Myristicae*
Wu Zhu Yu *Fr. Evodiae*
Wu Wei Zi *Fr. Schisandrae Chinensis*
Sheng Jiang *Rz. Zingiberis Recens*
Da Zao *Fr. Jujubae*

Si Wu Tang:

Dang Gui *Rx. Angelicae Sinensis*
Bai Shao *Rx. Paeoniae Alba*
Chuan Xiong *Rz. Chuanxiong*
Shu Di Huang *Rx. Rehmanniae Preparata*

Su He Xiang Wan:

Bai Zhu *Rz. Atractylodis Macrocephala*
Qing Mu Xiang *Rx. Aristolochiae*
Xi Jiao *Cornu Rhinoceri*
Xiang Fu *Rz. Cyperi*

Zhu Sha *Cinnabaris*
He Zi *Fr. Chebulae*
Tan Xiang *Lignum Santali Albi*
An Xi Xiang *Benzoinum*
Chen Xiang *Lignum Aquilariae Resinatum*
She Xiang *Moschus*
Ding Xiang *Fl. Caryophylli*
Bi Ba *Fr. Piperis Longi*
Su He Xiang *Styrax*
Bing Pian *Borneolum Syntheticum*

Su Zi Jiang Qi Tang:
Su Zi *Fr. Perillae*
Chen Pi *Pc. Citri Reticulatae*
Ban Xia *Rz. Pinelliae*
Dang Gui *Rx. Angelicae Sinensis*
Qian Hu *Rx. Peucedani*
Hou Po *Cx. Magnoliae Officinalis*
Rou Gui *Cx. Cinnamomi*
Gan Cao *Rx. Glycyrrhizae*
Sheng Jiang *Rz. Zingiberis Recens*

Suan Zao Ren Tang:
Suan Zao Ren *Sm. Ziziphi Spinosae*
Zhi Mu *Rz. Anemarrhenae*
Chuan Xiong *Rz. Chuanxiong*
Fu Ling *Poria*
Gan Cao *Rx. Glycyrrhizae*

T

Tao Hong Si Wu Tang:
Tao Ren *Sm. Persicae*
Hong Hua *Fl. Carthami*
Dang Gui *Rx. Angelicae Sinensis*
Bai Shao *Rx. Paeoniae Alba*
Chuan Xiong *Rz. Chuanxiong*
Sheng Di Huang *Rx. Rehmanniae*

Tao Hong Yin:
Tao Ren *Sm. Persicae*
Hong Hua *Fl. Carthami*
Chuan Xiong *Rz. Chuanxiong*
Dang Gui Wei *Rx. Angelicae Sinensis*
Wei ling Xian *Rx. Clematidis*

Tao Hua Tang:
Chi Shi Zhi *Halloysitum Rubrum*
Gan Jiang *Rz. Zingiberis*
Jing Mi *Nonglutinous Rice*

Tian Ma Gou Teng Yin:
Tian Ma *Rz. Gastrodiae*
Gou Teng *Rml. Uncariae cum Uncis*
Shi Jue Ming *Concha Haliotidis*
Chuan Niu Xi *Rx. Cyathulae*
Sang Ji Sheng *Hb. Taxilli*
Du Zhong *Cx. Eucommiae*
Zhi Zi *Fr. Gardenia*
Huang Qin *Rx. Scutellariae*
Yi Mu Cao *Hb. Leonuri*
Fu Shen *Sclerotium Poriae Pararadicis*
Ye Jiao Teng *Caulis Polygoni Multiflori*

Tian Wang Bu Xin Dan:
Ren Shen *Rx. Ginseng*
Xuan Shen *Rx. Scrophulariae*
Dan Shen *Rx. Salviae Miltiorrhizae*
Fu Ling *Poria*
Wu Wei Zi *Fr. Schisandrae Chinensis*
Yuan Zhi *Rx. Polygalae*
Jie Geng *Rx. Platycodonis*
Dang Gui *Rx. Angelicae Sinensis*
Tian Men Dong *Rx. Asparagi*
Mai Men Dong *Rx. Ophiopogonis*
Bai Zi Ren *Sm. Platycladi*
Suan Zao Ren *Sm. Ziziphi Spinosae*
Sheng Di Huang *Rx. Rehmanniae*
Zhu Sha *Cinnabaris*

Tiao Wei Cheng Qi Tang:
Da Huang *Rx. et Rz. Rhei*
Gan Cao *Rx. Glycyrrhizae*
Mang Xiao *Natrii Sulfas*

Tiao Ying Yin:
E Zhu *Rz. Curcumae*
Chuan Xiong *Rz. Chuanxiong*
Dang Gui *Rx. Angelicae Sinensis*

Yan Hu Suo *Rz. Corydalis*
Chi Shao *Rx. Paeoniae Rubra*
Qu Mai *Hb. Dianthi*
Da Huang *Rx. et Rz. Rhei*
Bing Lang *Sm. Arecae*
Chen Pi *Pc. Citri Reticulatae*
Da Fu Pi *Pc. Arecae*
Ting Li Zi *Sm. Descurainiae*
Fu Ling *Poria*
Sang Bai Pi *Cx. Mori*
Xi Xin *Hb. Asari*
Rou Gui *Cx. Cinnamomi*
Zhi Gan Cao *Rx. Glycyrrhizae Preparata*
Bai Zhi *Rx. Angelicae Dahuricae*
Sheng Jiang *Rz. Zingiberis Recens*
Da Zao *Fr. Jujubae*

Ting Li Da Zao Xie Fei Tang:
Ting Li Zi *Sm. Descurainiae*
Da Zao *Fr. Jujubae*

Tong Qiao Huo Xue Tang:
Chi Shao *Rx. Paeoniae Rubra*
Chuan Xiong *Rz. Chuanxiong*
Tao Ren *Sm. Persicae*
Hong Hua *Fl. Carthami*
She Xiang *Moschus*
Cong Bai *Blb. Allii Fistulosi*
Sheng Jiang *Rz. Zingiberis Recens*
Da Zao *Fr. Jujubae*
Bai Jiu *White Wine*

Tong Xie Yao Fang:
Bai Zhu *Rz. Atractylodis Macrocephala*
Bai Shao *Rx. Paeoniae Alba*
Fang Feng *Rx. Saposhnikoviae*
Chen Pi *Pc. Citri Reticulatae*

Tong You Tang:
Sheng Di Huang *Rx. Rehmanniae*
Shu Di Huang *Rx. Rehmanniae Preparata*
Tao Ren *Sm. Persicae*
Hong Hua *Fl. Carthami*
Dang Gui *Rx. Angelicae Sinensis*
Zhi Gan Cao *Rx. Glycyrrhizae Preparata*
Sheng Ma *Rz. Cimicifugae*

Tong Yu Jian:
Dang Gui Wei *Rx. Angelicae Sinensis*
Shan Zha *Fr. Crataegi*
Xiang Fu *Rz. Cyperi*
Hong Hua *Fl. Carthami*
Wu Yao *Rx. Linderae*
Qing Pi *Pc. Citri Reticulatae Viride*
Mu Xiang *Rx. Aucklandia*
Ze Xie *Rz. Alismatis*

W

Wei Ling Tang:
Cang Zhu *Rz. Atractylodis*
Hou Po *Cx. Magnoliae Officinalis*
Chen Pi *Pc. Citri Reticulatae*
Gan Cao *Rx. Glycyrrhizae*
Sheng Jiang *Rz. Zingiberis Recens*
Da Zao *Fr. Jujubae*
Gui Zhi *Rml. Cinnamomi*
Bai Zhu *Rz. Atractylodis Macrocephala*
Ze Xie *Rz. Alismatis*
Fu Ling *Poria*
Zhu Ling *Polyporus*

Wen Dan Tang:
Ban Xia *Rz. Pinelliae*
Chen Pi *Pc. Citri Reticulatae*
Gan Cao *Rx. Glycyrrhizae*
Zhi Shi *Fr. Aurantii Immaturus*
Zhu Ru *Caulis Bambusae in Taenia*
Sheng Jiang *Rz. Zingiberis Recens*
Fu Ling *Poria*

Wen Pi Tang:
Fu Zi *Rx. Aconiti Lateralis Preparata*
Ren Shen *Rx. Ginseng*
Da Huang *Rx. et Rz. Rhei*
Gan Cao *Rx. Glycyrrhizae*
Gan Jiang *Rz. Zingiberis*

Wu Bi Shan Yao Wan:

Shan Yao *Rz. Dioscoreae*
Rou Cong Rong *Hb. Cistanches*
Shu Di Huang *Rx. Rehmanniae Preparata*
Shan Zhu Yu *Fr. Corni*
Fu Shen *Sclerotium Poriae Pararadicis*
Tu Si Zi *Sm. Cuscutae*
Wu Wei Zi *Fr. Schisandrae Chinensis*
Chi Shi Zhi *Halloysitum Rubrum*
Ba Ji Tian *Rx. Morindae Officinalis*
Ze Xie *Rz. Alismatis*
Du Zhong *Cx. Eucommiae*
Niu Xi *Rx. Achyranthis Bidentatae*

Wu Ling San:

Gui Zhi *Rml. Cinnamomi*
Bai Zhu *Rz. Atractylodis Macrocephala*
Fu Ling *Poria*
Zhu Ling *Polyporus*
Ze Xie *Rz. Alismatis*

Wu Mei Wan:

Wu Mei *Fr. Mume*
Huang Lian *Rz. Coptidis*
Huang Bai *Cx. Phellodendri*
Ren Shen *Rx. Ginseng*
Dang Gui *Rx. Angelicae Sinensis*
Fu Zi *Rx. Aconiti Lateralis Preparata*
Gui Zhi *Rml. Cinnamomi*
Chuan Jiao *Pc. Zanthoxyli*
Gan Jiang *Rz. Zingiberis*
Xi Xin *Hb. Asari*

Wu Mo Yin Zi:

Wu Yao *Rx. Linderae*
Chen Xiang *Lignum Aquilariae Resinatum*
Bing Lang *Sm. Arecae*
Zhi Shi *Fr. Aurantii Immaturus*
Mu Xiang *Rx. Aucklandia*

Wu Pi San:

Sang Bai Pi *Cx. Mori*
Chen Pi *Pc. Citri Reticulatae*
Sheng Jiang Pi *Cx. Zingiberis Recens*
Da Fu Pi *Pc. Arecae*
Fu Ling Pi *Cx. Poria*

Wu Ren Wan:

Tao Ren *Sm. Persicae*
Xing Ren *Sm. Armeniacae Amarum*
Bai Zi Ren *Sm. Platycladi*
Song Zi Ren *Sm. Pini*
Yu Li Ren *Sm. Pruni*
Chen Pi *Pc. Citri Reticulatae*

Wu Tou Tang:

Zhi Chuang Wu *Rx. Aconiti Preparapa*
Ma Huang *Hb. Ephedrae*
Shao Yao *Rx. Paeoniae Alba*
Huang Qi *Rx. Astragali*
Gan Cao *Rx. Glycyrrhizae*

Wu Wei Xiao Du Yin:

Jin Yin Hua *Fl. Lonicerae*
Ye Ju Hua *Fl. Chrysanthemi Indici*
Pu Gong Ying *Hb. Taraxaci*
Zi Hua Di Ding *Hb. Violae*
Zi Bei Tian Kui *Hb. Begonie Fimbristipulatae*

Wu Zhi An Zhong Yin:

Jiu Zhi *Fm. AlliiTtuberosi*
Niu Ru *Cow Milk*
Sheng Jiang Zhi *Rz. Zingiberis Recens*
Li Zhi *Pear Juice*
Ou Zhi *Lotus Juice*

Wu Zhu Yu Tang:

Wu Zhu Yu *Fr. Evodiae*
Ren Shen *Rx. Ginseng*
Sheng Jiang *Rz. Zingiberis Recens*
Da Zao *Fr. Jujubae*

Wu Zi Yan Zong Wan:

Gou Qi Zi *Fr. Lycii*
Fu Peng Zi *Fr. Rubi*

Tu Si Zi *Sm. Cuscutae*
Wu Wei Zi *Fr. Schisandrae Chinensis*
Che Qian Zi *Sm. Plantaginis*

X

Xi Jiao Di Huang Tang:
Xi Jiao *Cornu Rhinoceri*
Sheng Di Huang *Rx. Rehmanniae*
Mu Dan Pi *Cx. Moutan*
Shao Yao *Rx. Paeoniae Alba*

Xi Jiao San:
Xi Jiao *Cornu Rhinoceri*
Huang Lian *Rz. Coptidis*
Sheng Ma *Rz. Cimicifugae*
Zhi Zi *Fr. Gardenia*
Yin Chen Hao *Hb. Artemisiae Scopariae*

Xiang Lian Wan:
Huang Lian *Rz. Coptidis*
Mu Xiang *Rx. Aucklandia*

Xiang Sha Liu Jun Zi Tang:
Mu Xiang *Rx. Aucklandia*
Sha Ren *Fr. Amomi*
Chen Pi *Pc. Citri Reticulatae*
Ban Xia *Rz. Pinelliae*
Dang Shen *Rx. Codonopsis*
Bai Zhu *Rz. Atractylodis Macrocephala*
Fu Ling *Poria*
Gan Cao *Rx. Glycyrrhizae*

Xiao Ban Xia Tang:
Ban Xia *Rz. Pinelliae*
Sheng Jiang *Rz. Zingiberis Recens*

Xiao Chai Hu Tang:
Chai Hu *Rx. Bupleuri*
Huang Qin *Rx. Scutellariae*
Ban Xia *Rz. Pinelliae*
Ren Shen *Rx. Ginseng*
Gan Cao *Rx. Glycyrrhizae*
Sheng Jiang *Rz. Zingiberis Recens*
Da Zao *Fr. Jujubae*

Xiao Cheng Qi Tang:
Da Huang *Rx. et Rz. Rhei*
Hou Po *Cx. Magnoliae Officinalis*
Zhi Shi *Fr. Aurantii Immaturus*

Xiao Ji Yin Zi:
Sheng Di Huang *Rx. Rehmanniae*
Xiao Ji *Hb. Cirsii*
Hua Shi *Talcum*
Tong Cao *Medulla Tetrapanacis*
Pu Huang *Pollen Typhae*
Zhu Ye *Hb. Lophatheri*
Ou Jie *Nodus Nelumbinis Rz.tis*
Dang Gui *Rx. Angelicae Sinensis*
Zhi Zi *Fr. Gardenia*
Gan Cao *Rx. Glycyrrhizae*

Xiao Jian Zhong Tang:
Gui Zhi *Rml. Cinnamomi*
Bai Shao *Rx. Paeoniae Alba*
Gan Cao *Rx. Glycyrrhizae*
Sheng Jiang *Rz. Zingiberis Recens*
Da Zao *Fr. Jujubae*
Yi Tang *Saccharum Granorum*

Xiao Ke Fang:
Huang Lian *Rz. Coptidis*
Tian Hua Fen *Rx. Trichosanthis*
Sheng Di Huang *Rx. Rehmanniae*
Ou Zhi *Lotus Root Juice*
Ren Ru *Human Milk*
Sheng Jiang Zhi *Rz. Zingiberis Recens*
Feng Mi *Mel*

Xiao Qing Long Tang:
Ma Huang *Hb. Ephedrae*
Gui Zhi *Rml. Cinnamomi*
Shao Yao *Rx. Paeoniae Alba*
Gan Cao *Rx. Glycyrrhizae*
Gan Jiang *Rz. Zingiberis*
Xi Xin *Hb. Asari*
Ban Xia *Rz. Pinelliae*
Wu Wei Zi *Fr. Schisandrae Chinensis*

Xiao Tan Tang:
Kun Bu *Thallus Eckloniae seu Thallus Laminariae*

Hai Zao *Sargassum*
Bai Jie Zi *Sm. Sinapis*
Zhe Bei Mu *Blb. Fritillariae Thunbergii*
Tian Nan Xing *Rz. Arisaematis*
Fu Ling *Poria*
Ban Xia *Rz. Pinelliae*
Ren Shen *Rx. Ginseng*
Gan Cao *Rx. Glycyrrhizae*
Jie Geng *Rx. Platycodonis*
Fu Zi *Rx. Aconiti Lateralis Preparata*

Xiao Yao San:
Chai Hu *Rx. Bupleuri*
Bai Shao *Rx. Paeoniae Alba*
Bai Zhu *Rz. Atractylodis Macrocephala*
Dang Gui *Rx. Angelicae Sinensis*
Fu Ling *Poria*
Zhi Gan Cao *Rx. Glycyrrhizae Preparata*
Bo He *Hb. Menthae*
Wei Jiang *Rz. Zingiberis Preparatum*

Xie Bai San:
Sang Bai Pi *Cx. Mori*
Di Gu Pi *Cx. Lycii*
Gan Cao *Rx. Glycyrrhizae*
Jing Mi *Nonglutinous Rice*

Xie Xin Tang:
Da Huang *Rx. et Rz. Rhei*
Huang Qin *Rx. Scutellariae*
Huang Lian *Rz. Coptidis*

Xin Jia Xiang Ru Yin:
Xiang Ru *Hb. Moslae*
Bai Bian Dou *Sm. Lablab Album*
Hou Po *Cx. Magnoliae Officinalis*
Jin Yin Hua *Fl. Lonicerae*
Lian Qiao *Fr. Forsythiae*

Xin Zhi Ju Pi Zhu Ru Tang:
Chen Pi *Pc. Citri Reticulatae*
Zhu Ru *Caulis Bambusae in Taenia*
Shi Di *Calyx Kaki*
Sheng Jiang *Rz. Zingiberis Recens*

Xing Su San:
Xing Ren *Sm. Armeniacae Amarum*
Zi Su Ye *Fm. Perillae*
Chen Pi *Pc. Citri Reticulatae*
Ban Xia *Rz. Pinelliae*
Sheng Jiang *Rz. Zingiberis Recens*
Zhi Qiao *Fr. Aurantii*
Jie Geng *Rx. Platycodonis*
Qian Hu *Rx. Peucedani*
Fu Ling *Poria*
Gan Cao *Rx. Glycyrrhizae*
Da Zao *Fr. Jujubae*

Xiong Zhi Shi Gao Tang:
Chuan Xiong *Rz. Chuanxiong*
Bai Zhi *Rx. Angelicae Dahuricae*
Shi Gao *Gypsum Fibrosum*
Ju Hua *Fl. Chrysanthemi*
Gao Ben *Rz. Ligustici*
Qiang Huo *Rz. et Rx. Notopterygii*

Xuan Fu Hua Tang:
Xuan Fu Hua *Fl. Inulae*
Xin Jiang *Silk*
Cong *Green Onion*

Xue Fu Zhu Yu Tang:
Dang Gui *Rx. Angelicae Sinensis*
Sheng Di Huang *Rx. Rehmanniae*
Tao Ren *Sm. Persicae*
Hong Hua *Fl. Carthami*
Zhi Qiao *Fr. Aurantii*
Chi Shao *Rx. Paeoniae Rubra*
Chai Hu *Rx. Bupleuri*
Gan Cao *Rx. Glycyrrhizae*
Jie Geng *Rx. Platycodonis*
Chuan Xiong *Rz. Chuanxiong*
Niu Xi *Rx. Achyranthis Bidentatae*

Y

Yang Xin Tang:
Huang Qi *Rx. Astragali*
Fu Ling *Poria*
Fu Shen *Sclerotium Poriae Pararadicis*
Dang Gui *Rx. Angelicae Sinensis*

Chuan Xiong *Rz. Chuanxiong*
Gan Cao *Rx. Glycyrrhizae*
Ban Xia *Rz. Pinelliae*
Bai Zi Ren *Sm. Platycladi*
Suan Zao Ren *Sm. Ziziphi Spinosae*
Yuan Zhi *Rx. Polygalae*
Wu Wei Zi *Fr. Schisandrae Chinensis*
Ren Shen *Rx. Ginseng*
Rou Gui *Cx. Cinnamomi*

Yi Guan Jian:
Sha Shen *Rx. Glehniae*
Mai Men Dong *Rx. Ophiopogonis*
Dang Gui *Rx. Angelicae Sinensis*
Sheng Di Huang *Rx. Rehmanniae*
Gou Qi Zi *Fr. Lycii*
Chuan Lian Zi *Fr. Toosendan*

Yi Qi Cong Ming Tang:
Huang Qi *Rx. Astragali*
Ren Shen *Rx. Ginseng*
Sheng Ma *Rz. Cimicifugae*
Ge Gen *Rx. Puerariae*
Man Jing Zi *Fr. Viticis*
Shao Yao *Rx. Paeoniae Alba*
Huang Bai *Cx. Phellodendri*
Zhi Gan Cao *Rx. Glycyrrhizae Preparata*

Yi Wei Tang:
Sha Shen *Rx. Glehniae*
Mai Men Dong *Rx. Ophiopogonis*
Sheng Di Huang *Rx. Rehmanniae*
Yu Zhu *Rz. Polygonati Odorati*

Yi Yi Ren Tang:
Yi Yi Ren *Sm. Coicis*
Chuan Xiong *Rz. Chuanxiong*
Dang Gui *Rx. Angelicae Sinensis*
Ma Huang *Hb. Ephedrae*
Gui Zhi *Rml. Cinnamomi*
Qiang Huo *Rz. et Rx. Notopterygii*
Du Huo *Rx. Angelicae Pubescentis*
Fang Feng *Rx. Saposhnikoviae*
Zhi Chuang Wu *Rx. Aconiti Preparapa*
Cang Zhu *Rz. Atractylodis*
Gan Cao *Rx. Glycyrrhizae*
Sheng Jiang *Rz. Zingiberis Recens*

Yin Chen Hao Tang:
Yin Chen Hao *Hb. Artemisiae Scopariae*
Zhi Zi *Fr. Gardenia*
Da Huang *Rx. et Rz. Rhei*

Yin Chen Wu Ling San:
Yin Chen Hao *Hb. Artemisiae Scopariae*
Gui Zhi *Rml. Cinnamomi*
Fu Ling *Poria*
Bai Zhu *Rz. Atractylodis Macrocephala*
Ze Xie *Rz. Alismatis*
Zhu Ling *Polyporus*

Yin Chen Zhu Fu Tang:
Yin Chen Hao *Hb. Artemisiae Scopariae*
Bai Zhu *Rz. Atractylodis Macrocephala*
Fu Zi *Rx. Aconiti Lateralis Preparata*
Gan Jiang *Rz. Zingiberis*
Zhi Gan Cao *Rx. Glycyrrhizae Preparata*
Rou Gui *Cx. Cinnamomi*

Yin Qiao San:
Jin Yin Hua *Fl. Lonicerae*
Lian Qiao *Fr. Forsythiae*
Dan Dou Chi *Sm. Sojae Preparatum*
Niu Bang Zi *Fr. Arctii*
Bo He *Hb. Menthae*
Jing Jie *Hb. Schizonepetae*
Jie Geng *Rx. Platycodonis*
Gan Cao *Rx. Glycyrrhizae*
Zhu Ye *Hb. Lophatheri*
Lu Gen *Rz. Phragmitis*

You Gui Wan:
Shu Di Huang *Rx. Rehmanniae Preparata*
Shan Yao *Rz. Dioscoreae*
Shan Zhu Yu *Fr. Corni*

Gou Qi Zi *Fr. Lycii*
Du Zhong *Cx. Eucommiae*
Tu Si Zi *Sm. Cuscutae*
Fu Zi *Rx. Aconiti Lateralis Preparata*
Rou Gui *Cx. Cinnamomi*
Dang Gui *Rx. Angelicae Sinensis*
Lu Jiao Jiao *Gelatinum Cornu Cervi*

You Gui Yin:
Shu Di Huang *Rx. Rehmanniae Preparata*
Shan Yao *Rz. Dioscoreae*
Shan Zhu Yu *Fr. Corni*
Gou Qi Zi *Fr. Lycii*
Fu Ling *Poria*
Gan Cao *Rx. Glycyrrhizae*

Yu Nu Jian:
Shi Gao *Gypsum Fibrosum*
Shu Di Huang *Rx. Rehmanniae Preparata*
Mai Men Dong *Rx. Ophiopogonis*
Zhi Mu *Rz. Anemarrhenae*
Niu Xi *Rx. Achyranthis Bidentatae*

Yu Ping Feng San:
Huang Qi *Rx. Astragali*
Bai Zhu *Rz. Atractylodis Macrocephala*
Fang Feng *Rx. Saposhnikoviae*

Yue Bi Jia Zhu Tang:
Ma Huang *Hb. Ephedrae*
Shi Gao *Gypsum Fibrosum*
Gan Cao *Rx. Glycyrrhizae*
Da Zao *Fr. Jujubae*
Bai Zhu *Rz. Atractylodis Macrocephala*
Sheng Jiang *Rz. Zingiberis Recens*

Yue Ju Wan:
Chuan Xiong *Rz. Chuanxiong*
Cang Zhu *Rz. Atractylodis*
Xiang Fu *Rz. Cyperi*
Zhi Zi *Fr. Gardenia*
Shen Qu *Massa Fermentata*

Z

Ze Xie Tang:
Ze Xie *Rz. Alismatis*
Bai Zhu *Rz. Atractylodis Macrocephala*

Zeng Ye Cheng Qi Tang:
Da Huang *Rx. et Rz. Rhei*
Mang Xiao *Natrii Sulfas*
Xuan Shen *Rx. Scrophulariae*
Mai Men Dong *Rx. Ophiopogonis*
Sheng Di Huang *Rx. Rehmanniae*

Zeng Ye Tang:
Xuan Shen *Rx. Scrophulariae*
Mai Men Dong *Rx. Ophiopogonis*
Sheng Di Huang *Rx. Rehmanniae*

Zhen Gan Xi Feng Tang:
Huai Niu Xi *Rx. Achyranthis Bidentatae*
Long Gu *Os Draconis Fossilia*
Bai Shao *Rx. Paeoniae Alba*
Tian Men Dong *Rx. Asparagi*
Mai Ya *Fr. Hordei Germinatus*
Dai Zhe Shi *Haematitum*
Mu Li *Concha Ostreae*
Xuan Shen *Rx. Scrophulariae*
Chuan Lian Zi *Fr. Toosendan*
Yin Chen Hao *Hb. Artemisiae Scopariae*
Gan Cao *Rx. Glycyrrhizae*
Gui Ban *Carapax et Plastrum Testudinis*

Zhen Wu Tang:
Fu Zi *Rx. Aconiti Lateralis Preparata*
Bai Zhu *Rz. Atractylodis Macrocephala*
Fu Ling *Poria*
Shao Yao *Rx. Paeoniae Alba*
Sheng Jiang *Rz. Zingiberis Recens*

Zhi Bai Di Huang Wan:
Zhi Mu *Rz. Anemarrhenae*
Huang Bai *Cx. Phellodendri*

Shu Di Huang *Rx. Rehmanniae Preparata*
Shan Zhu Yu *Fr. Corni*
Shan Yao *Rz. Dioscoreae*
Fu Ling *Poria*
Mu Dan Pi *Cx. Moutan*
Ze Xie *Rz. Alismatis*

Zhi Bao Dan:

Zhu Sha *Cinnabaris*
She Xiang *Moschus*
An Xi Xiang *Benzoinum*
Xi Jiao *Cornu Rhinoceri*
Hu Po *Succinum*
Xiong Huang *Realgar*
Dai Mao Carapax *Eretmochelydis Imbricatae*
Niu Huang *Calculus Bovis*

Zhi Gan Cao Tang:

Zhi Gan Cao *Rx. Glycyrrhizae Preparata*
Ren Shen *Rx. Ginseng*
Gui Zhi *Rml. Cinnamomi*
Sheng Jiang *Rz. Zingiberis Recens*
E Jiao *Gelatinum Corii Asini*
Sheng Di Huang *Rx. Rehmanniae*
Mai Men Dong *Rx. Ophiopogonis*
Huo Ma Ren *Fr. Cannabis*
Da Zao *Fr. Jujubae*

Zhi Shi Dao Zhi Wan:

Da Huang *Rx. et Rz. Rhei*
Zhi Shi *Fr. Aurantii Immaturus*
Huang Qin *Rx. Scutellariae*
Huang Lian *Rz. Coptidis*
Shen Qu *Massa Fermentata*
Bai Zhu *Rz. Atractylodis Macrocephala*
Fu Ling *Poria*
Ze Xie *Rz. Alismatis*

Zhi Sou San:

Jing Jie *Hb. Schizonepetae*
Jie Geng *Rx. Platycodonis*
Gan Cao *Rx. Glycyrrhizae*
Bai Qian *Rz. Cynanchi Stauntonii*
Chen Pi *Pc. Citri Reticulatae*
Bai Bu *Rx. Stemonae*
Zi Wan *Rx. Asteris*

Zhong Man Fen Xiao Wan:

Hou Po *Cx. Magnoliae Officinalis*
Zhi Shi *Fr. Aurantii Immaturus*
Huang Qin *Rx. Scutellariae*
Huang Lian *Rz. Coptidis*
Zhi Mu *Rz. Anemarrhenae*
Ban Xia *Rz. Pinelliae*
Ren Shen *Rx. Ginseng*
Gan Cao *Rx. Glycyrrhizae*
Chen Pi *Pc. Citri Reticulatae*
Fu Ling *Poria*
Zhu Ling *Polyporus*
Ze Xie *Rz. Alismatis*
Sha Ren *Fr. Amomi*
Gan Jiang *Rz. Zingiberis*
Jiang Huang *Rz. Curcumae Longae*
Bai Zhu *Rz. Atractylodis Macrocephala*

Zhou Che Wan:

Gan Sui *Rx. Kansui*
Yuan Hua *Fl. Genkwa*
Da Ji *Rx. Euphorbiae Pekinensis*
Da Huang *Rx. et Rz. Rhei*
Qian Niu Zi *Sm. Pharbitidis*
Mu Xiang *Rx. Aucklandia*
Qing Pi *Pc. Citri Reticulatae Viride*
Chen Pi *Pc. Citri Reticulatae*
Bing Lang *Sm. Arecae*

Zhu Che Wan:

Huang Lian *Rz. Coptidis*
E Jiao *Gelatinum Corii Asini*
Dang Gui *Rx. Angelicae Sinensis*
Gan Jiang *Rz. Zingiberis*

Zhu Ling Tang:

Zhu Ling *Polyporus*
Fu Ling *Poria*
Ze Xie *Rz. Alismatis*
Hua Shi *Talcum*

E Jiao *Gelatinum Corii Asini*

Zhu Sha An Shen Wan:

Huang Lian *Rz. Coptidis*
Zhu Sha *Cinnabaris*
Sheng Di Huang *Rx. Rehmanniae*
Dang Gui *Rx. Angelicae Sinensis*
Zhi Gan Cao *Rx. Glycyrrhizae Preparata*

Zi Shui Qing Gan Yin:

Sheng Di Huang *Rx. Rehmanniae*
Shan Zhu Yu *Fr. Corni*
Fu Ling *Poria*
Dang Gui *Rx. Angelicae Sinensis*
Shan Yao *Rz. Dioscoreae*
Mu Dan Pi *Cx. Moutan*
Ze Xie *Rz. Alismatis*
Bai Shao *Rx. Paeoniae Alba*
Chai Hu *Rx. Bupleuri*
Zhi Zi *Fr. Gardenia*
Suan Zao Ren *Sm. Ziziphi Spinosae*

Zi Xue Dan:

Hua Shi *Talcum*
Shi Gao *Gypsum Fibrosum*
Han Shui Shi *Calcitum*
Ci Shi *Magnetitum*
Ling Yang Jiao *Cornu Saigae Tataricae*
Qing Mu Xiang *Rx. Aristolochiae*
Xi Jiao *Cornu Rhinoceri*
Chen Xiang *Lignum Aquilariae Resinatum*
Ding Xiang *Fl. Caryophylli*
Sheng Ma *Rz. Cimicifugae*
Xuan Shen *Rx. Scrophulariae*
Gan Cao *Rx. Glycyrrhizae*
Mang Xiao *Natrii Sulfas*
Zhu Sha *Cinnabaris*
She Xiang *Moschus*

Zuo Gui Wan:

Shu Di Huang *Rx. Rehmanniae Preparata*
Shan Yao *Rz. Dioscoreae*
Shan Zhu Yu *Fr. Corni*
Tu Si Zi *Sm. Cuscutae*
Gou Qi Zi *Fr. Lycii*
Chuan Niu Xi *Rx. Cyathulae*
Lu Jiao Jiao *Gelatinum Cornu Cervi*
Gui Ban Jiao *Gelatinum Carapax et Plastrum Testudinis*

Zuo Gui Yin:

Shu Di Huang *Rx. Rehmanniae Preparata*
Shan Yao *Rz. Dioscoreae*
Shan Zhu Yu *Fr. Corni*
Gou Qi Zi *Fr. Lycii*
Du Zhong *Cx. Eucommiae*
Gan Cao *Rx. Glycyrrhizae*
Fu Zi *Rx. Aconiti Lateralis Preparata*
Rou Gui *Cx. Cinnamomi*

Zuo Jin Wan:

Huang Lian *Rz. Coptidis*
Rou Gui *Cx. Cinnamomi*

Cross Reference for Latin Abbreviations:

Blb.	*Bulbus*	*Pc.*	*Pericarpium*
Cx	*Cortex*	*Rml.*	*Ramulus*
Fl.	*Flos*	*Rx.*	*Radix*
Fm.	*Folium*	*Rz.*	*Rhizoma*
Fr.	*Fructus*	*Sm.*	*Semen*
Hb.	*Herba*		

Bibliography

Pharmacopoeia (2000). (vol. 1). Beijing: Chemical Industry Press.

Chang, B., et. al. (Eds.). (1999). *Zhongyi neikexue* [Science of TCM internal medicine] (21st print). Shanghai: Shanghai Science and Technology Press.

Chen, G., & Yang, S., et. al. (Eds.). (1995). *Shiyong zhongxiyijiehe zhenduanzhiliaoxue: Practical diagnostics and therapeutics of integrated traditional Chinese and Western medicine*. Beijing: China Medical Science and Technology Press.

Chen, K., et. al. (Eds.). (1998). *Shiyong zhongxiyijiehe neikexue* [Practical science of internal medicine of integrated Chinese and Western medicine]. Beijing: Beijing Medical University and China Xiehe Medical University United Press.

Cheng, X. et. al. (Eds.). (1999). *Chinese acupuncture and moxibustion*. Beijing: Foreign Languages Press.

Huangdi neijing suwen jiaoshi [Interpretation of the Yellow Emperor's inner classic- simple question] (1995). (vols. 1-2). Beijing: The People's Medical Publishing House.

Jiangsu New Medical School. (1975). *Zhongyao dacidian* [Chinese herbal dictionary]. Shanhai: Shanghai People's Publishing House.

Li, E., et. al. (Eds.). (1996). *Integrated clinical encyclopedia of traditional and western medicine*. Beijing: TCM Classic Press

Lingshujing jiaoshi [Interpretation of the spiritual axis] (1995). (vols. 1-2). Beijing: The People's Medical Publishing House.

MacLean, W. & Lyttleton, J. (1998-2002). *Clinical handbook of internal medicine* (vols. 1-2). Campbeltown, NSW: University of Western Sydney.

Peng, H., et. al. (Eds.). (1995). *Zhongyi fangji dacidian* [Dictionary of Chinese herbal formulas] (2nd print). Beijing: The People's Medical Publishing House.

The American heritage college dictionary (4th ed.) (2002). Boston, MA: Houghton Mifflin Company.

Thomas, C. L., et. al. (Eds.) (1989). *Taber's cyclopedic medical dictionary*. (16th ed.). Philadelphia, PA: F. A. Davis.

Wang, Y., et. al. (Eds.). (1994). *Linchuang zhongyi neikexue* [Clinical science of TCM internal medicine]. Beijing: Beijing Publishing House.

Xu, J, et. al. (Eds.). (2003). *Fangjixue* [Formulas] (30th print). Shanghai: Shanghai Science and Technology Press.

Yuan, Y. et. al. (Eds.). (1997). *Chinese-English dictionary of traditional Chinese medicine*. Beijing: The People's Medical Publishing House.

Zeng, D., et. al. (1987). Zhongguoyiyaoxue [Chinese medicine]. In *Zhongguo baike dacidian*. Beijing: Huaxia Publishing House.

Zeng, D. (2003). *Essentials of Chinese medicine: Materia medica*. Walnut, CA: Bridge Publishing Group.

$ 64.95 U.S.D.